1991

The Maintenance of Arterial Reconstruction

The Maintenance of Arterial Reconstruction

Edited by

R. M. Greenhalgh, MA, MD, MChir, FRCS
Professor of Surgery and Chairman,
Department of Surgery,
Charing Cross & Westminster Medical School
London, England

and

L. H. Hollier, MD
Chairman, Department of Surgery,
Ochsner Clinic and Alton Ochsner Medical Foundation
Clinical Professor of Surgery, Tulane Medical Center and
Louisiana State University Medical Center,
New Orleans, USA

W. B. SAUNDERS COMPANY LTD
London · Philadelphia · Toronto · Sydney · Tokyo

W. B. Saunders 24–28 Oval Road
London NW1 7DX

The Curtis Center
Independence Square West
Philadelphia, PA 19106–3399

55 Horner Avenue
Toronto, Ontario M8Z 4X6, Canada

Harcourt Brace Jovanovich (Australia) Pty Ltd,
30–52 Smidmore St
Marrickville, NSW 2204, Australia

Harcourt Brace Jovanovich Japan Inc.
Ichibancho Central Building, 22–1 Ichibancho
Chiyoda-ku, Tokyo, 102, Japan

British Library Cataloguing in Publication Data
A catalogue record for this book is available from the British Library.

ISBN 0-7020-1564-4

This book is printed on acid-free paper ∞

Editorial and Production Services by Fisher Duncan
10 Barley Mow Passage, London W4 4PH

Typeset by Dobbie Typesetting Limited, Tavistock, Devon
and printed and bound in Great Britain by The University Press, Cambridge

Contents

ASSOCIATED PROCEDURES AFFECTING LONG-TERM RESULTS

List of Contributors

S. S. AHN, MD
Assistant Professor of Surgery
Vascular Surgery Section
UCLA School of Medicine
10833 Le Conte Avenue, Los Angeles
California 90024–1749, USA

C. H. DE ALMEIRA, MD
Specialist in Vascular Surgery
Hospital de Santa Maria
(also Professor of Surgery, Faculty of Medicine, Lisbon Medical School)
Av Rainha D Amelia,
1600 Lisbon, Portugal

M. B. BAARS
Department of Surgery
St Antonius Hospital
Koekoekslaan 1, 3430 EM Nieuwegein
The Netherlands

P. R. F. BELL
Department of Surgery
Clinical Sciences Building
The Leicester Royal Infirmary
Leicester LE2 7LX, UK

G. A. BERLAKOVICH, MD
GK 1st Department of Surgery
University of Vienna
A-1090 Vienna, Alserstrasse 4
Austria

J. BRENNAN
Department of Surgery
Clinical Sciences Building
The Leicester Royal Infirmary
Leicester LE2 7LX, UK

B. BRENER, MD
Department of Surgery
Newark-Beth-Israel Medical Center
201 Lyons Avenue
Newark, New Jersey
NJ 07112, USA

S.-E. BERGENTZ, MD
Department of Surgery
Lund University
Malmö General Hospital
S-214 01 Malmö
Sweden

D. BERGQVIST, MD PhD
Associate Professor
Department of Surgery
University of Lund
General Hospital
S-214 01 Malmö
Sweden

J. BLUTH
Department of Surgery
Catharina Hospital
Eindhoven, The Netherlands

D. CALCAGNO, MD
Assistant Professor of Surgery
Department of Surgery
Georgetown University School of Medicine
Washington DC 20007–2197, USA

H. M. H. CARR
Department of Vascular Surgery
Manchester Royal Infirmary and Medical School
Oxford Road
Manchester, UK

A. D. B. CHANT, MS FRCS
Consultant Vascular Surgeon
Southampton General Hospital
Tremonan Road
Shirley
Southampton SO9 4XY, UK

A. W. CLOWES, MD
University of Washington
Department of Surgery RF-25
Seattle, Washington 98195, USA

M. P. COLGAN, MD
Director of the Vascular Laboratories
St James Hospital
James Street
PO Box 580
Dublin 6
Ireland

F. L. CROSS, MD
Department of Surgery
Newark-Beth-Israel Medical Center
201 Lyons Avenue
Newark, New Jersey
NJ 07112, USA

R. CUMING, BSc
Vascular Technician
King Edward VII Hospital
St Leonard's Road
Windsor
Berkshire SL4 3DP, UK

A. DAMIÃO, MD
Specialist in Vascular Surgery
Hospital de Santa Maria
(also Professor of Surgery, Faculty of Medicine, Lisbon Medical School)
Av Rainha D Amelia
1600 Lisbon
Portugal

S. G. DARKE, MS FRCS
Consultant Surgeon
Oaks
6 Leicester Road
Branksome Park
Poole, Dorset, UK

B. DISSELHOFF
Department of Surgery
Catharina Hospital
Eindhoven, The Netherlands

R. J. C. M. DONDERS
Department of Surgery
St Antonius Hospital
Koekoekslaan 1
3430 EM Nieuwegein
The Netherlands

A. EDWARDS, FRCS
Vascular Research Fellow
Department of Surgery
University Hospital of South Manchester
Research & Teaching Building
Nell Lane, West Didsbury
Manchester M20 8LR, UK

B. C. EIKELBOOM
Professor of Vascular Surgery
University of Utrecht
St Antonius Hospital
Koekoekslaan 1
3430 EM Nieuwegein
The Netherlands

E. EINARSSON, MD PhD
Associate Professor
Department of Surgery
University of Lund
General Hospital
S-214 01 Malmö
Sweden

D. E. EISENBUD
Department of Surgery
Newark-Beth-Israel Medical Center
201 Lyons Avenue
Newark, New Jersey
NJ 07112, USA

J. FERNANDES e FERNANDES, MD
Chief of Service
Department of Vascular Surgery
Hospital de Santa Maria
(also Professor of Surgery, Faculty of Medicine, Lisbon Medical School)
Av Rainha D Amelia,
1600 Lisbon, Portugal

M. FERRARA-RYAN, BS
Department of Surgery
Newark-Beth-Israel Medical Center
201 Lyons Avenue
Newark, New Jersey
NJ 07112, USA

P. FIORANI
Cattedra di Chirurgia Vascolare
dell'Universita di Roma
'La Sapienza'
Policlinico Umberto 1
00161 Roma, Italy

C. N. FISHER, BSc(Med) FRACS
Irvine Laboratory for Cardiovascular
Investigation and Research
Vascular Section
Academic Surgical Unit
St Mary's Hospital Medical School
Praed Street, London W2, UK

F. FLÜCKIGER, MD
Karl-Franzens University and Medical
School
Auenbrugger Platz 9
A-8036 Graz
Austria

P. J. FRANKS, PhD
Lecturer in Epidemiology
Department of Surgery
Charing Cross and Westminster
Medical School
London W6 8RF, UK

R. G. GAYLE, MD
Norfolk Surgical Group, Ltd
250 West Brambleton Avenue,
Suite 101
Norfolk, Virginia 23510, USA

R. T. GREGORY, MD
Norfolk Surgical Group, Ltd
250 West Brambleton Avenue,
Suite 101
Norfolk, Virginia 23510, USA

M. C. GROUDEN
Vascular Technologist
Department of Surgery
St James Hospital
James Street
PO Box 580
Dublin 6, Ireland

E. J. GUSSENHOVEN, MD PhD
Department of Vascular Surgery
Room HM 1049
University Hospital Rotterdam
Dr Molewaterplein 40,
3015 GD Rotterdam
The Netherlands

J. W. HALLETT, Jr, MD
Associate Professor of Surgery
Section of Vascular Surgery
Mayo Medical School and Mayo
Foundation
Rochester, Minnesota 55905, USA

G. HAMILTON, MB ChB FRCS
Consultant General and Vascular
Surgeon
Royal Free Hospital
Pond Street, London NW3 2QG, UK

P. L. HARRIS
Broadgreen Hospital
Vascular Surgery Unit
Thomas Drive
Liverpool L14 3LB, UK

K. HAUSEGGER, MD
Karl-Franzens University and Medical
School
Auenbrugger Platz 9
A-8036 Graz, Austria

F. HERBST, MD
GK 1st Department of Surgery
University of Vienna
A-1090 Vienna
Alserstrasse 4
Austria

L. H. HOLLIER, MD
Ochsner Clinic
Department of Surgery
1514 Jefferson Highway
New Orleans
LA 70121, USA

B. R. HOPKINSON, MB ChM FRCS
Consultant General and Vascular Surgeon
University Hospital
Queens Medical Centre
Nottingham NG7 2UH, UK

M. HORROCKS, MS FRCS
Vascular Studies Unit
Department of Surgery
Bristol Royal Infirmary
Marlborough Street
Bristol BS2 8HW, UK

R. JAKOB
Surgical Resident
Surgical Clinic, 8900 Augsburg
Germany

G. JOHNSON, MD
Roscoe B. G. Cowper Distinguished Professor of Surgery
University of North Carolina
Campus Box no 7210
Chapel Hill
NC 27599–7210
USA

G. E. KLEIN, MD
Karl-Franzens University and Medical School
Auenbrugger Platz 9
A-8036 Graz
Austria

TED R. KOHLER, MD
University of Washington
Department of Surgery RF-25
Seattle,
Washington 98195, USA

G. KRETSCHMER, MD
Assistant Professor
GK 1st Department of Surgery
University of Vienna
A-1090 Vienna
Alserstrasse 4
Austria

U. KUGELMANN
Surgical Resident
Surgical Clinic, 8900 Augsburg
Germany

J. LAMMER, MD
Karl-Franzens University and Medical School
Auenbrugger Platz 9
A-8036 Graz
Austria

H. LOEPRECHT
Professor of Surgery
Surgical Clinic, 8900 Augsburg
Germany

K. LOPYAN, MD
Department of Surgery
Newark-Beth-Israel Medical Center
201 Lyons Avenue
Newark
New Jersey
NJ 07112, USA

R. L. McCANN, MD
Associate Professor of Surgery
Duke University Medical Center
PO Box 2190
Durham NC 27710, USA

C. N. McCOLLUM, MD FRCS
Professor of Surgery
Department of Surgery
University Hospital of South Manchester
Research & Teaching Building
Nell Lane, West Didsbury
Manchester M20 8LR, UK

A. MEEK, FRCS MD
Senior Registrar
King Edward VII Hospital
St Leonard's Road
Windsor
Berkshire SL4 3DP
UK

D. C. MITCHELL, FRCS
Research Fellow
Professorial Surgical Unit
St Bartholomew's Hospital
West Smithfield
London EC1A 7BE
UK

M. P. MOLLOY, FRCR
Consultant Radiologist
Department of Radiology
St James Hospital
James Street
PO Box 580
Dublin 6
Ireland

A. P. MOODY
Broadgreen Hospital
Vascular Surgery Unit
Thomas Drive
Liverpool L14 3LB
UK

D. J. MOORE, MD
Consultant Vascular Surgeon
Department of Surgery
St James Hospital
James Street
PO Box 580
Dublin 6
Ireland

W. M. MOORE Jr, MD
Ochsner Clinic
Department of Surgery
1514 Jefferson Highway
New Orleans
LA 70121, USA

H. MULLER-WIEFEL, MD
Professor of Surgery
Chief, Vascular Surgical Clinic
Academic Teaching Hospital
St Johannes
D-4100 Duisburg-11
Germany

A. MURRAY, MS FRCS
Lecturer in Surgery
Professorial Surgical Unit
St Bartholomew's Hospital
West Smithfield
London EC1A 7BE
UK

H. O. MYHRE, MD
Department of Surgery
Trondheim University
7006 Trondheim
Norway

G. E. NEWMAN, MD
Associate Professor of Radiology
Duke University Medical Center
PO Box 2990
Durham NC 27710
USA

A. N. NICOLAIDES
Professor of Vascular Surgery
Irvine Laboratory for Cardiovascular Investigation and Research
Vascular Section
Academic Surgical Unit
St Mary's Hospital Medical School
Praed Street
London W2
UK

L. NORGREN, MD PhD
Associate Professor
Department of Surgery
University of Lund
General Hospital
S-214 01 Malmö
Sweden

M. K. O'MALLEY, MCh FRCSI
Department of Surgery
Charing Cross and Westminster Medical School
London W6 8RF, UK

J. C. PALMAZ, MD
Department of Radiology
University of Texas Health Center at San Antonio
7703 Sloyd Curl Drive
San Antonio
Texas 78284–7800
USA

F. N. PARENT III, MD
Norfolk Surgical Group, Ltd
250 West Brambleton Avenue
Suite 101
Norfolk, Virginia 23510, USA

V. PARSONNET, MD
Department of Surgery
Newark-Beth-Israel Medical Center
201 Lyons Avenue
Newark, New Jersey
NJ 07112, USA

E. PILGER, MD
Karl-Franzens University and Medical School
Auenbrugger Platz 9
A-8036 Graz
Austria

J. T. POWELL, PhD MD
Department of Surgery
Charing Cross and Westminster Medical School
London W6 8RF, UK

M. PRAGER, MD
GK 1st Department of Surgery
University of Vienna
A-1090 Vienna
Alserstrasse 4
Austria

E. J. PRENDIVILLE FRCSI
Acting Senior Registrar in General Surgery
Department of Surgery
St James Hospital
James Street
PO Box 580
Dublin 6
Ireland

C. DANIEL PROCTOR Sr, MD
Ochsner Clinic
Department of Surgery
1514 Jefferson Highway
New Orleans
LA 70121
USA

T. S. RILES, MD
Professor of Surgery
Director, Division of Vascular Surgery
New York University Medical Center
550 First Avenue
New York
NY 10016
USA

O. D. SAETHER, MD
Department of Surgery
Trondheim University
7006 Trondheim
Norway

T. H. SAUTNER, MD
GK 1st Department of Surgery
University of Vienna
A-1090 Vienna
Alserstrasse 4
Austria

M. SCHEMPER, PhD
GK 1st Department of Surgery
University of Vienna
A-1090 Vienna
Alserstrasse 4
Austria

T. SCHMITZ-RIXEN, MD
Department of Surgery
University of Cologne
Josef-Stelzmann-Str 9
D-5000 Koln 41
Germany

G. D. SHANIK, MD
Professor of Surgery
Department of Surgery
St James Hospital
James Street
PO Box 580
Dublin 6
Ireland

M. H. SKETCH Jr, MD
Fellow, Cardiology
Duke University Medical Center
Durham NC 27710, USA

S. O. SNYDER Jr, MD
Norfolk Surgical Group, Ltd
250 West Brambleton Avenue
Suite 101
Norfolk
Virginia 23510, USA

L. STAM
Department of Surgery
Catharina Hospital
Eindhoven
The Netherlands

C. M. TALKINGTON, MD FACS
Suite 505
3600 Gaston Avenue
Dallas
Texas 75246
USA

J. E. THOMPSON, MD
Suite 505
3600 Gaston Avenue
Dallas
Texas 75246
USA

M. TRENT, MD
Department of Surgery
Newark-Beth-Israel Medical Center
201 Lyons Avenue
Newark, New Jersey
NJ 07112, USA

T. TROENG, MD
Department of Surgery
University of Lund
General Hospital
S-214 01 Malmö
Sweden

E. TRUYEN
Department of Surgery
Catharina Hospital
Eindhoven
The Netherlands

M. R. TYRRELL, FRCS FRCSEd
St Mary's Hospital
Praed Street
London W2 1NY, UK

H. C. de VALOIS
Consultant Radiologist
St Antonius Hospital
Koekoekslaan 1
3430 EM Nieuwegein
The Netherlands

H. VAN URK, MD PhD
Department of Vascular Surgery
Room HM 1049
University Hospital Rotterdam
Dr Molewaterplein 40,
3015 GD Rotterdam
The Netherlands

F. VEITH, MD
Divisions of Vascular Surgery and
Radiology
Montefiore Medical Center
Albert Einstein College of Medicine
111 East 210 Street
New York, NY 10467, USA

M. G. VELLER, MMED(Surg) FCS(SA)
Irvine Laboratory for Cardiovascular Investigation and Research
Vascular Section
Academic Surgical Unit
St Mary's Hospital Medical School
Praed Street
London W2, UK

A. VILLANUEVA, BA
Department of Surgery
Newark-Beth-Israel Medical Center
201 Lyons Avenue
Newark
New Jersey
NJ 07112, USA

R. VOHRA
Department of Vascular Surgery
Manchester Royal Infirmary and Medical School
Oxford Road
Manchester, UK

MICHAEL G. WALKER
Department of Vascular Surgery
Manchester Royal Infirmary and Medical School
Oxford Road
Manchester, UK

H. WEIBULL
Department of Surgery
Lund University
Malmö General Hospital
S-214 01 Malmö
Sweden

M. WELCH
Department of Vascular Surgery
Manchester Royal Infirmary and Medical School
Oxford Road
Manchester, UK

J. R. WHEELER, MD
Norfolk Surgical Group, Ltd
250 West Brambleton Avenue
Suite 101
Norfolk, Virginia 23510, USA

K. D. WOELFLE
Oberarzt in Vascular Surgery
Surgical Clinic, 8900 Augsburg
Germany

J. H. N. WOLFE, MS FRCS
Department of Surgery
St Mary's Hospital
Praed Street
London W2 1NY, UK

R. F. M. WOOD, MD FRCS
Professor of Surgery
Professorial Surgical Unit
St Bartholomew's Hospital
West Smithfield
London EC1A 7BE, UK

M. G. WYATT, MSc FRCS
Vascular Studies Unit
Department of Surgery
Bristol Royal Infirmary
Marlborough Street
Bristol BS2 8HW, UK

Preface

The techniques of arterial reconstruction are now well established. This book is concerned with the long-term durability of these procedures. It is no longer enough for the vascular surgeon to recommend and perform a technique without knowing what the inherent recurrence rate of the procedure is. It has long been known that the development of intimal hyperplasia wrecks some technically excellent reconstructive procedures. The thickening which can occur can be so extensive on some occasions that the outflow of blood can be reduced so severely that a reconstruction completely fails. How this intimal hyperplasia develops and what regulates it is discussed at the beginning of the book. Some factors which encourage excessive intimal hyperplasia are known. If, for example, a somewhat inelastic prosthetic graft is anastomosed to a more elastic host artery, the mismatch of compliance can encourage excessive intimal hyperplasia and surgeons are already developing ways to reduce this problem. Grafts are being lined with endothelial cells and this is being done largely in the hope that the graft will stay patent longer with less inappropriate thickening along its length and at the anastomosis site.

A number of factors which affect the durability of arterial patency are known. Many of these have been highlighted recently in the Femoropopliteal Bypass Trial which has been undertaken in Britain. This Femoropopliteal Bypass Trial involved 46 centres and recruited 801 patients. The clinical trial was funded by the Medical Research Council and the British Heart Foundation funded the additional portion concerned with factors associated with maintained patency. A major purpose of this trial was to examine the efficacy of platelet inhibitory therapy on femoropopliteal vein bypass procedures. These results are reviewed in the chapter by Edwards and McCollum. The second arm of the trial concerned a comparison of different prosthetic procedures, each receiving platelet inhibitory therapy and this is reviewed in the chapter by Franks. Avoidance of smoking and a low fibrinogen were the factors which were associated with best maintenance of arterial reconstruction and these results are reviewed in Dr Powell's chapter. The Viennese group had firm data on the role of anticoagulants and this is reviewed in the chapter by Kretschmer.

The days when a patient was no longer followed-up after an arterial procedure should be over. Even now, surgeons are apt to prescibe and dispense bypass procedures and then hand out a visiting card inviting the patient to get in touch should symptoms redevelop. This is simply not good enough at this state of our knowledge. It is known that many bypasses show signs of failure quite soon after the procedure and that there can be an asymptomatic phase of such failure. This has given rise to a spate of communications on the need for surveillance of grafts. That surveillance is desirable is broadly agreed but the method of this surveillance is still debated. Duplex scan, intravenous digital subtraction angiography and pressure measurements with and without a treadmill head the list and many draw attention to the need for proper intra-operative techniques to guarantee long-term satisfactory patency results. The use of the angioscope, for example, is recommended for complete valve ablation in a femoropopliteal *in situ* vein bypass procedure but the management of vein bypass stricture, either by observation, transluminal angioplasty or repeat surgery remains somewhat controversial.

Newer endovascular techniques have been introduced recently and there are a number of centres which have adopted these with some enthusiasm. Other established vascular surgeons have been somewhat reluctant to even consider discarding established techniques for the newer methods but it emerges that these procedures may be performed requiring a very short stay in hospital. For economic reasons, therefore, it is essential to evaluate these techniques fairly and with an open mind. The precise position of percutaneous transluminal angioplasty is not yet established without controversy let alone the debate on who should do it, the radiologist, the vascular surgeon, or a physician or angiologist. Whether a laser should be used to assist the angioplasty is also controversial. Adequate trials justifying this laser assistance are few and far between. Then there are different types of laser which are available to assist the angioplasty and claims for one against the other type are difficult to evaluate. The three chapters on these subjects represent reviews of the present knowledge in this field and contain such information as there is on these comparisons.

Atherectomy devices are appealing in principle and can be introduced either at open operation or in some cases percutaneously. The value of the procedure is clear, that the atheroma is pulverized and the artery lumen widened. There is much we need to know about these devices and whether a single device can do the whole job, or whether a combination of devices is required. It is also important to know the cost of these procedures and the durability of atherectomy and angioplasty must be compared with established surgical procedures and conservative measures. The stent has been introduced recently to hold open a stenosing lesion. It would seem to have the theoretical disadvantage that part of the artery wall is inelastic and this once again introduces a compliance change at either end of the stent and surveillance of these procedures is vital but some initial results are encouraging. These newer procedures also have their down side. Complications can occur with these procedures like any surgical procedure and these must be carefully documented. In economic and patient satisfaction terms, it would be easy to see how some of the newer techniques are appealing from the point of view of the potential short period of time in hospital but the durability of these procedures and freedom from intimal hyperplasia must be evaluated over a reasonable period of time. Established surgical procedures must also be looked at again from the same point of view. They may be more expensive, more painful and more undesirable at the beginning but if the results are durable, it may be that in terms of patient suffering and even cost, they can beat the newer methods.

For these reasons, we have reviewed many of the established arterial reconstructive procedures from the point of view of the maintenance of the procedure and its durability. The authors have been asked to concentrate essentially upon the long-term outcome of the procedures. Finally, towards the end of the book, other factors which may affect long-term results are considered. Clearly, if the operation is not properly designed and the wrong procedure performed on a patient through poor preoperative assessment, the result will not be satisfactory at all, let alone durable. It necessarily follows that, as always, careful preoperative assessments are essential and will influence the outcome of the operation, instantly perceived in the immediate postoperative period but also appreciated over the years that follow. The place of sympathectomy affecting long-term patency is discussed. Many believe that this procedure has long ago had its obituary but surgeons still perform it in combination with arterial reconstruction. What is the evidence that sympathectomy influences any arterial reconstruction? Arteriovenous fistulas with femorodistal bypass give one example of an adjunctive technique which can be performed to increase patency results and maintenance of arterial reconstruction, but at the price of reducing distal perfusion. Tests are now being introduced which assess impedance in grafts in the postoperative period. These are being used to ascribe a prognosis for some arterial reconstructions. It could be argued that the information is derived too late to be of value but it is not too late to influence a surgeon who may perform a similar technique on another patient the next day. The book concludes on the need for careful audit of results and none has been performed more conclusively than the vascular registry in Sweden which is described by Bergqvist. We are not intending to address in any depth what should be done when grafts fail but the use of tissue plasminogen activator and other thrombolytic agents has mushroomed in recent months, is topical and is, therefore, included as a final chapter.

It is hoped that the reader will derive benefit from these reviews of established and new methods of performing arterial reconstruction as well as an analysis of surveillance methods and factors associated with optimal maintenance of arterial reconstruction.

R.M.G.
L.H.H.

Acknowledgements

We are pleased to acknowledge the contribution of the Femoropopliteal Bypass Trial in the section: Factors Prolonging Patency. This Trial was supported by the Medical Research Council and represented a collaboration between 46 vascular surgeons who are co-ordinated from the Department of Surgery at Charing Cross Hospital and the Department of Surgery at the Queen Elizabeth Hospital, Birmingham. Charles McCollum who co-writes the chapter on Platelet Inhibitory Therapy was then Reader in Surgery at Charing Cross and directed the Trial. He, Ken MacRae, Reader in Statistics at Charing Cross and Westminster Medical School and Roger Greenhalgh designed the Trial, the data from which were collected and analysed by Peter Franks, who also writes a chapter in this section. Dr Janet Powell, Senior Lecturer in Surgery and Biochemistry at Charing Cross and Westminster Medical School received funding from the British Heart Foundation for additional studies on this Trial and reports much of the data in her chapter also in this section. The Trial was co-ordinated in London successively by Nicola Flannery, Rachel Dain and Christine Alexander and for the whole time in Birmingham by Glenda Kenchington. The Trial participant surgeons are listed below. They recruited 801 patients in these centres for femoropopliteal bypass.

London: M. Adisheshiah, M. Birnstingl, J. W. P. Bradley, J. Collin, J. M. Edwards, J. R. C. Gardham, A. E. B. Giddings, R. M. Greenhalgh, I. G. Kidson, A. O. Mansfield, J. A. P. Marston, A. R. L. May, C. N. McCollum, W. M. Mee, P. J. Morris, J. A. Murie, D. Negus, A. N. Nicholaides, B. D. Pardy, P. H. Pattisson, B. D. Pentlow, M. C. Pietroni, J. H. Scurr, R. S. Taylor, J. C. Williams, J. H. N. Wolfe.

Birmingham: P. R. Armistead, F. Ashton, E. T. Bainbridge, W. W. Barrie, P. R. F. Bell, J. M. Dolphin, R. Downing, J. W. L. Fielding, D. B. Hamer, J. D. Hamer, L. J. Lawson, J. B. Marczak, D. S. Macpherson, D. M. Matheson, M. L. Obeid, S. J. A. Powis, P. N. Roberts, G. Slaney and D. A. K. Woodward.

We also acknowledge the skill, understanding and support of Sean Duggan, the Publishing Director, who commissioned this book, as well as his very able production team.

R.M.G.
L.H.H.

INTIMAL HYPERPLASIA AND ENDOTHELIAL CELLS

The Development of Intimal Hyperplasia and its Possible Prevention

M. K. O'Malley

As with so much else in vascular surgery Alexis Carrell was responsible for the first description of intimal hyperplasia. Having described a successful technique for arterial anastomosis he investigated the outcome of vein transplanted into the arterial circulation and accurately described the subsequent intimal thickening.[1,2] Intimal hyperplasia is the vessel wall's response to endothelial denudation and is characterized by smooth muscle cell (SMC) proliferation (Fig. 1). Endothelial denudation occurs during many common clinical procedures such as balloon

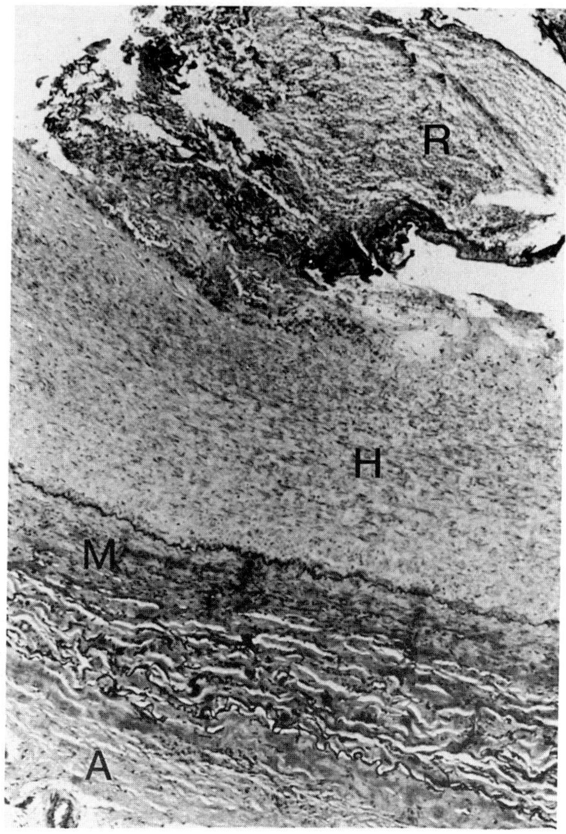

Fig. 1. Photomicrograph of a cross-section through a human infrainguinal vein bypass graft showing extensive intimal hyperplasia. A: adventitia; M: media; H: intimal hyperplasia; R: red blood cells. (H + E stain × 50)

thromboembolectomy, balloon dilatation angioplasty, endarterectomy, organ transplantation, vein bypass grafting, vascular access and angiography. Whether the trauma is due to surgical excision, compliance mismatch, shear forces, hypoxia or hypothermia the vessel wall responds with SMC proliferation. However, while the actual response is quite predictable the extent of it is not. Thus, what in some circumstances may be a normal and beneficial process of repairing the vessel wall, may be clearly harmful if it continues unchecked.

The major disadvantage of coronary artery balloon angioplasty is the 30% restenosis rate at 6 months[3] and, in vascular surgery, upwards of 25% of all vein graft failures after the initial few weeks are due to intimal hyperplasia.[4–6] Similar results have been reported in cardiac surgery[7] and following carotid endarterectomy a restenosis rate of 15% is representative.[8] Moreover, it is not just established techniques in vascular surgery which are complicated by intimal hyperplasia as it appears that the rate limiting step for the more recent endovascular techniques, such as atherectomy and laser angioplasty, will also be the restenosis rate. The continued development of less invasive devices in the treatment of cardiovascular disease is only going to be of lasting benefit when we can control the cellular response of the vessel wall.

THE MORPHOLOGY OF INTIMAL HYPERPLASIA

Baumgartner first used the embolectomy balloon catheter to denude endothelium experimentally[9] and this model has since been used extensively to follow the

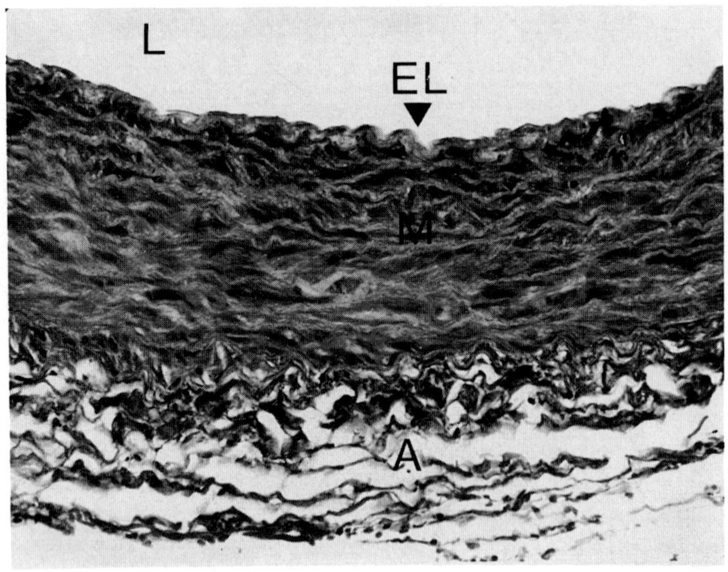

Fig. 2. Photomicrograph of rabbit aorta immediately after endothelial denudation showing total absence of the endothelial layer. L: lumen; EL: internal elastic lamina; M: media; A: adventitia. (H + E stain × 200)

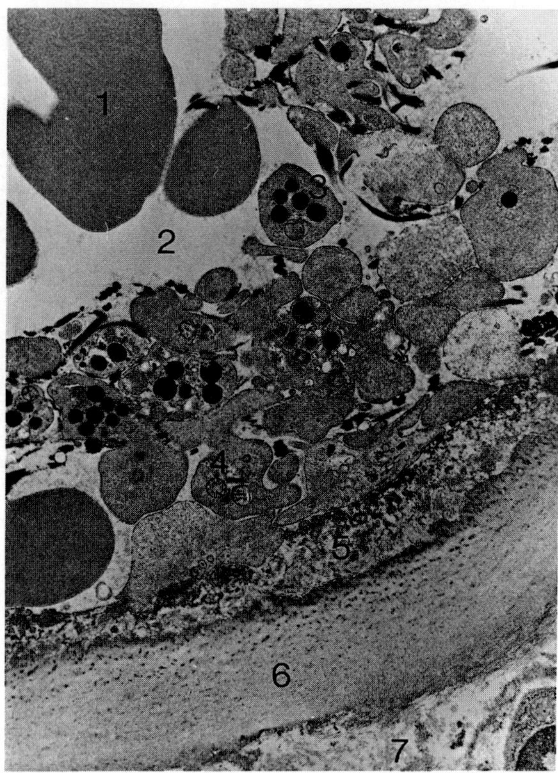

Fig. 3. Electronmicrograph of rabbit aorta 24 hours after endothelial denudation demonstrating protein debris and a carpet of platelets adherent to the internal elastic lamina. 1: red blood cell; 2: lumen; 3: platelet; 4: degranulated platelet; 5: protein debris; 6: internal elastic lamina; 7: media. (×950)

development of intimal hyperplasia.[10,11] The technique is based on that initially described by Fogarty in clinical practice.

A balloon catheter is inflated and withdrawn several times resulting in complete removal of the endothelium (Fig. 2). The external elastic lamina is now exposed to the bloodstream and, being thrombogenic, platelets immediately accumulate and form a covering layer together with fibrin and protein debris from the desquamated endothelium. Within 24 hours the platelets have formed aggregates (Fig. 3) which are mixed with erythrocytes, polymorphonuclear leucocytes and monocytes in a network of fibrin. Three to five days after the procedure the first evidence of a neo-intima is seen with vascular SMCs on the luminal side of the internal elastic lamina. By 8 days there are layers of SMCs (Fig. 4) and the increase in this smooth muscle mass is the predominant feature until maximal neo-intimal thickening occurs after approximately 4 weeks (Fig. 5). It is not until this stage that normal endothelial cells begin to appear. Whether this neo-intima persists or regresses with time is totally unpredictable.

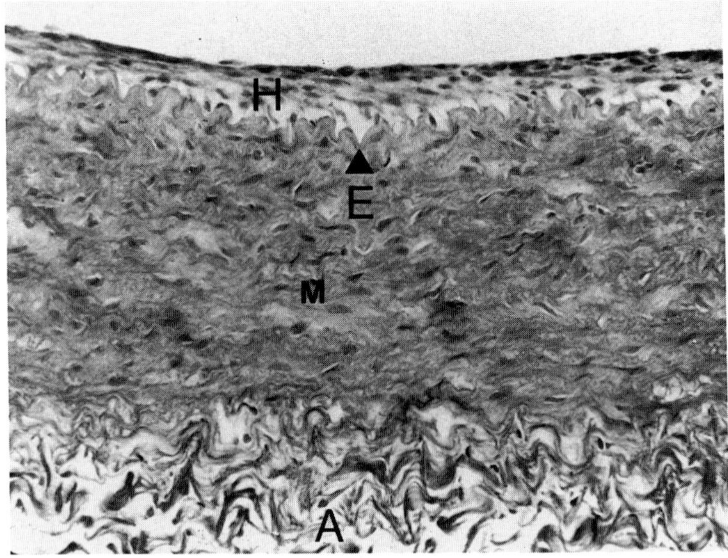

Fig. 4. Photomicrograph of rabbit aorta 8 days following endothelial denudation demonstrating the early appearance of intimal hyperplasia. H: intimal hyperplasia; E: internal elastic lamina; M: media; A: adventitia. (H + E × 200)

PATHOGENESIS OF INTIMAL HYPERPLASIA

In a series of important publications over the last 20 years Ross' group have investigated the role of the platelet in the aetiology of intimal hyperplasia.[12–14] They formulated the 'response to injury' hypothesis which centred on the platelet and its growth factor—platelet derived growth factor (PDGF). This hypothesis suggested that endothelial trauma exposed the underlying internal elastic lamina with subsequent platelet aggregation and adherence. This is followed by release of PDGF from the platelet granules (Fig. 3) and under the influence of this growth factor the vascular SMCs of the media are stimulated to migrate across the internal elastic lamina and then proliferate to form the neo-intima.

However, it is now apparent that the process is a little more complex. Endothelial cells, SMCs and macrophages can also produce PDGF and SMCs from intimal hyperplasia lesions can elaborate a PDGF-like mitogen.[15] These observations suggest a possible feedback mechanism for SMC proliferation involving PDGF. But there are other candidates which may at least contribute to the formation of intimal hyperplasia. Other factors which are produced by the same cells include transforming growth factor-alpha and beta, fibroblast growth factor (FGF) and interleukin-1 all of which induce SMC proliferation under the appropriate circumstances.

It is of some interest that SMC proliferation continues long after platelet aggregation has ceased suggesting that while PDGF might have an initiating role, other factors must be responsible for maintaining the development of intimal hyperplasia. Monocytes appear early at the site of endothelial denudation and this is probably part of the 'inflammatory response'. PDGF has been shown to be chemotactic for monocytes but monocyte involvement continues several weeks (Fig. 6) after the

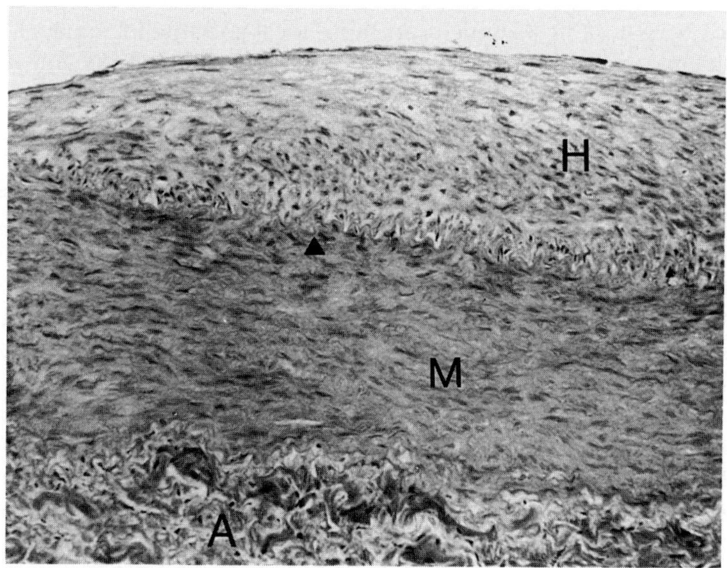

Fig. 5. Photomicrograph of rabbit aorta 28 days following endothelial denudation. H: intimal hyperplasia; M: media; A: adventitia; arrow to internal elastic lamina. (H + E × 200)

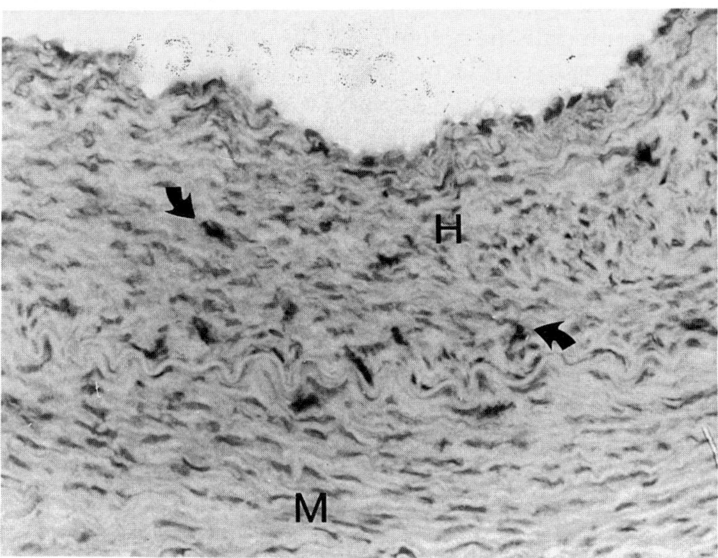

Fig. 6. Photomicrograph of rabbit aorta 14 days following endothelial denudation showing monocytes (arrowed). They are seen in both the media and the hyperplastic intima. H: intimal hyperplasia; M: media. (cholinesterase stain × 200)

vessel wall is no longer thrombogenic.[16] Activated tissue macrophages have been shown to produce macrophage derived growth factor (MDGF) which has many similarities to PDGF and is also capable of stimulating SMC proliferation.[17] Macrophages may also be mediators of intimal hyperplasia through the byproducts of their metabolism. Oxygen metabolism within macrophages results in the production of oxygen radicals which can cause local endothelial injury. Macrophages also produce leukotriene B4 which is chemotactic for neutrophils and may increase their production of oxygen radicals.[18]

It is also likely that there is a balance between stimulatory factors and inhibitory factors. Clowes and Karnovsky demonstrated the ability of heparin to reduce SMC proliferation[19] and it is known that the vessel wall cells can synthesize their own heparin. PGE1 and interferon gamma are also inhibitors of SMC proliferation and a reduction in any of these inhibitors will increase the capacity for the stimulatory factors to take effect.

Already it is apparent that the multiplicity of factors involved in the aetiology of SMC proliferation produces a series of events which makes it extremely difficult to pinpoint the significance of any one element. When it is also considered that changes in vessel wall compliance and tensile strength (as at an anastomosis) and alterations in flow rates may encourage the development of intimal hyperplasia, and that certain lipids (e.g. fish oils) may be regulators of growth factor secretion, it is not surprising that we have yet to fully elucidate the pathways involved in the development of intimal hyperplasia.

PATHOPHYSIOLOGY OF INTIMAL HYPERPLASIA

Given the imposing list of possible agents involved in the aetiology of intimal hyperplasia it is easy to appreciate the potential for disarray in the physiology of the vessel wall once it has become hyperplastic. There is little doubt that the SMCs have been transformed from a quiescent to a proliferative state and it is not surprising that there is corresponding alteration in many functions of these cells.

While it is apparent that the vessel wall is immediately covered by a layer of platelets following endothelial denudation, evidence is accumulating to suggest that these vessels may continue to have increased clotting activity. Brody *et al.* have shown reduced amounts of the naturally occurring anticoagulants, tissue plasminogen activator and thrombomodulin, in aortocoronary vein grafts.[20] There is also experimental evidence that low flow in vein grafts is associated with an increase in fibrinogen concentration[21] and an increase in intimal hyperplasia.[22] Confirmatory clinical evidence of these findings has been provided by the group at Charing Cross where the plasma fibrinogen concentration was shown to be a very important variable predicting femoropopliteal graft failure, along with continued cigarette smoking,[23] and is summarized by Powell (p. 87).

Clowes *et al.* have demonstrated still further alteration in the coagulation process during the development of intimal hyperplasia[24] and Kohler and Clowes discuss this further (p. 15). They have shown that plasminogen activation following endothelial denudation is increased and differentially regulated with urokinase-type plasminogen activator present during proliferation of vascular SMCs and tissue type plasminogen activator present during the migration phase. This might suggest that these plasminogen activators could have specific functions related to SMC proliferation and migration.

Connective tissue production is increased during the development of intimal hyperplasia with greater accumulation of type I collagen which may contribute to the formation of atherosclerotic fibrotic plaques and vessel occlusion. A correlation between the increase in cell mass, seen during vascular SMC proliferation, and an increase in elastin has also been reported.[25]

Further derangement in vessel function is evident from a series of reports investigating vasoreactivity after endothelial denudation and during the subsequent intimal thickening. Rabbit aorta develops increased vasoreactivity with a 12-fold increase in response to noradrenaline (Fig. 7) and this has also been demonstrated *in vivo* in a canine model.[26,27] This alteration in contractility is associated with an increase in alpha1 receptor affinity for noradrenaline and an associated increase in intracellular metabolism.[28] On the other hand vasodilatation in response to acetylcholine becomes increasingly less as the degree of intimal thickening increases.[29] Recent studies on pieces of vein grafts have confirmed similar changes in vasoreactivity in humans.[30]

THE PREVENTION OF INTIMAL HYPERPLASIA

Given the foregoing account of the development of intimal hyperplasia and its pathophysiology it can be readily appreciated that it is unlikely that no one measure is likely to result in the prevention of intimal hyperplasia. Many of the technical considerations and the introduction of newer techniques are discussed in detail in other chapters. The role of compliance mismatch, laser recanalization and mechanical atherectomy, continued smoking, surgical technique and surveillance programmes are given particular consideration. The following is an attempt to provide an overview of the experimental and clinical evidence that pharmacological prophylaxis can reduce the development of intimal hyperplasia.

ANTIPLATELET DRUGS

Given the longstanding attention that has been paid to the platelet it is no surprise that there is so much data on antiplatelet therapy. However, the results of many

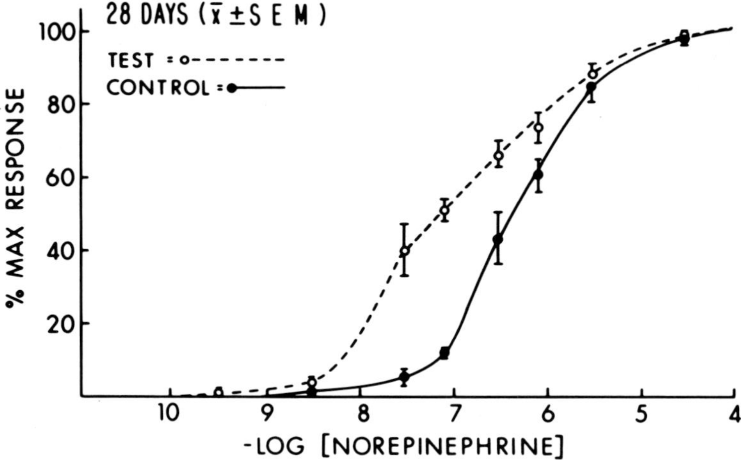

Fig. 7. Standardized dose-response curves (x ± SD) in rabbit aorta to demonstrate increased sensitivity to noradrenaline 28 days after endothelial denudation ($p = 0.002$).

of these studies have been equivocal or contradictory and appear to be species dependent. Hagen *et al.*[31] and McCann *et al.*[32] have shown a reduction in intimal hyperplasia in primates with peripheral bypasses while Metke *et al.*[33] had similar findings in canine coronary grafts. However, antiplatelet therapy in the rabbit or canine peripheral bypasses has either no benefit[34,35] or actually increases the amount of intimal hyperplasia.[36] In humans the evidence for antiplatelet therapy is also confusing. Cheesebro *et al.* have demonstrated increased patency of coronary grafts[37] and Meek *et al.* showed that antiplatelet therapy was beneficial following carotid endarterectomy.[38] However, the benefit of antiplatelet therapy for peripheral vein bypass grafts is unproven.[39,40] These contradictory results are probably related to many factors such as dosage, the introduction of treatment before or after surgery and platelet function and response to aspirin in different species.

It should not be forgotten that other antiplatelet agents have been investigated. The use of ticlopidine following both peripheral vein bypasses[41] and coronary angioplasty[42] has been studied but it has not been shown to be of significant benefit. Thromboxane synthetase inhibitors (including ibuprofen) have been investigated in experimental models with similar findings.[43,44]

Because populations that have a high dietary intake of fish oils have a reduced incidence of atherosclerosis, dietary supplements of fish oils have been given to patients undergoing coronary angioplasty. One study showed a restenosis rate of 16% compared to 36% in a placebo treated group.[45] It has also proved to be beneficial in reducing intimal hyperplasia in a canine model of peripheral vein bypass grafts.[46] The active agent is eicosapentaenoic acid which reduces platelet aggregation and total platelet counts. However, the case for fish oils is not yet proven as not all the reported studies support these findings. The topic of antiplatelet therapy is dealt with in detail by Edwards and McCollum (p. 69).

ANTICOAGULANTS

It is 14 years since Clowes and Karnovsky demonstrated that heparin inhibits injury-induced intimal hyperplasia.[19] Heparin inhibits both proliferation and migration of the SMC[47] but does not interfere with endothelial cell regeneration. It is now apparent that both endothelial and vascular SMCs can synthesize and secrete a heparin like inhibitor of proliferation but only when the cells are quiescent.[48] It would appear that this function is lost when the cells are transformed into a proliferative state. However, while heparin can inhibit SMC migration and proliferation it is obvious that intimal hyperplasia will still occur in its presence as very few vascular procedures do not include heparin in the protocol. It is far less clear whether there is a role for Warfarin in reducing intimal hyperplasia.

STEROIDS

Because of the prominence of inflammatory cells during the development of intimal hyperplasia and atherosclerosis, corticosteroids have been investigated. In experimental studies steroids have reduced the development of atherosclerosis.[49,50]

However, a large multicentre placebo-controlled study on restenosis after coronary angioplasty showed an incidence of 40% at 6 months in the placebo and prednisolone treated group.[51]

CARDIOVASCULAR AGENTS

Because of the suggestion that vasospasm may be associated with restenosis, calcium antagonists have been used prophylactically. However, once again, the experimental data are favourable but this is not borne out by the clinical experience. Verapamil reduces intimal hyperplasia in the rabbit aorta[52] but nifedipine had no effect on recurrent stenosis after coronary angioplasty.[53]

There has been recent interest in another group of drugs, the angiotensin converting enzyme (ACE) inhibitors, as a result of a report suggesting that intimal hyperplasia following rabbit aorta denudation could be decreased by 80%.[54] This has been supported by similar findings in rabbit vein bypass grafts but the reduction was less dramatic.[55] Clinical studies with this group of drugs are awaited.

Yet another antihypertensive agent, the alpha1 adrenergic antagonist prazosin hydrochloride, has been studied for its effect on SMC proliferation. This agent reduces intimal hyperplasia by 40% in a rabbit model of endothelial denudation.[56] Prazosin is thought to reduce the turnover of the phosphatidylinositol cycle through which various growth factors, including PDGF, induce mitogenesis.

SUMMARY

In conclusion, intimal hyperplasia is a universal and predictable response to endothelial denudation. It should be thought of as 'healing' by the vessel wall but unfortunately this is often uncontrolled and is a common cause of restenosis. It is apparent that this failure is due to a multiplicity of factors rather than just mechanical stenosis. The transformation of the vascular SMC from a quiescent to a proliferative cell produces many changes in the normal physiology including increased thrombogenicity and connective tissue production, the appearance of inflammatory cells and increased vasoconstriction. As each of these aspects has been identified new approaches have been tried with the appropriate pharmacological agent to reduce the development of intimal hyperplasia. Given the wide range of factors involved it is not surprising that these studies have usually been only partly successful in experimental models and have been less than convincing in human studies. However, we must continue trying to identify the pathways involved in the pathogenesis of intimal hyperplasia so that we can alter our surgical technique and materials as required and so we can get closer to pharmacological control of SMC proliferation. If we do manage to control this process we would not only improve the results of our current techniques but we would also greatly improve the likelihood of the new minimally invasive techniques being of value.

REFERENCES

1. Carrel A: Resultats eloignes de la transplantation des veines sur les arteres. Rev De Chir 41:987, 1910
2. Carrel A, Guthrie CC: Results of the biterminal transplantation of veins. Am J Med Sci 132:415–422, 1906
3. Roubin GS, King SB, Douglas JS: Restenosis after percutaneous transluminal coronary angioplasty: the Emory University Hospital experience. Am J Cardiol 60:39B–43B, 1987
4. Szilagyi DE, Elliot JP, Hageman JH, Smith RF, Dall'Olmo CA: Biologic fate of autogenous vein implants as arterial substitutes: clinical, angiographic and histopathologic observations in femoro-popliteal operations for atherosclerosis. Ann Surg 197:232–244, 1973
5. Whittemore AD, Mannick JA: The ischaemic leg. Adv Surg 15:293–316, 1981
6. Towne JB: Role of fibrointimal hyperplasia in vein graft failure. J Vasc Surg 10:583–585, 1989
7. Grondin CM: Late results of coronary artery grafting: is there a flag on the field? J Thorac Cardiovasc Surg 87:161, 1984
8. Aldoori MI, Baird RN: Prospective assessment of carotid endarterectomy by clinical and ultrasound methods. Br J Surg 74:926–929, 1987
9. Baumgartner HR, Studer A: Geizielte uberdehnung der aorta abdominalis am normal- und hypercholesterinaeam-ischen kannichen. Pathol Microbiol (Basel) 26:129–148, 1963
10. Spaet TH, Stemerman MB, Veith FJ, Lejnieks I: Intimal injury and regrowth in the rabbit aorta. Circ Res 36:58–70, 1975
11. Schwartz SM, Stemerman MB, Benditt EP: The aortic intima. II. Repair of the aortic lining after mechanical denudation. Am J Pathol 81:15–42, 1975
12. Ross R, Glomset JA: Atherosclerosis and the arterial smooth muscle cell. Science 180:1332–1339, 1973
13. Ross R: Atherosclerosis—a problem of the biology of arterial wall cells and their interaction with blood components. Arteriosclerosis 1:293–311, 1981
14. Ross R: The pathogenesis of atherosclerosis—an update. N Engl J Med 314:488–500, 1986
15. Birinyi LK, Warner SJC, Salomon RN, Callow AD, Libby P: Observation on smooth muscle cell cultures from hyperplastic lesion of prosthetic bypass grafts: production of platelet-derived growth factor-like mitogen and expression of a gene for a PDGF-receptor, a preliminary study. J Vasc Surg 10:157–165, 1989
16. Lucas JF, Makhoul RG, Cole CW *et al*: Mononuclear cells adhere to sites of vascular balloon catheter injury. Curr Surg 43:112–115, 1986
17. Shimokado K, Raines EW, Madtes DK *et al*: A significant part of macrophage-derived growth factor consists of at least two forms of PDGF. Cell 43:277–285, 1985
18. Greisler HP: The role of the macrophage in intimal hyperplasia. J Vasc Surg 10:566–568, 1989
19. Clowes AW, Karnovsky MJ: Suppression by heparin of smooth muscle cell proliferation in injured arteries. Nature 265:625–626, 1977
20. Brody JI, Pickering NJ, Fink GB: Immunocytochemical features of obstructed saphenous vein-coronary artery by-pass grafts. J Clin Pathol 42:477–483, 1989
21. Kuroki M, Okadome K, Inokuchi K, Sugimachi K: Intimal hyperplasia: The permeation of serum-derived substance into the arterial autovein graft under abnormal blood flow. Jap J Surg 18:300–307, 1988
22. Dobrin PB, Littooy FN, Endean ED: Mechanical factors predisposing to intimal hyperplasia and medial thickening in autogenous vein grafts. Surgery 105:393–400, 1989
23. Wiseman S, Kenchington G, Dain R *et al*: Influence of smoking and plasma factors on patency of femoropopliteal vein grafts. Br Med J 299:643–646, 1989
24. Clowes AW, Clowes MM, Au YPT, Reidy MA, Belin D: Smooth muscle cells express urokinase during mitogenesis and tissue type plasminogen activator during migration in injured rat carotid artery. Circ Res 67:61–67, 1990
25. Boyd CD, Kniep AC, Pierce RA *et al*: Increased elastin mRNA levels associated with surgically induced intimal injury. Conn Tiss Res 18:65–78, 1988
26. O'Malley MK, Hagen P-O, Mikat EM *et al*: Increased vascular contraction and sensitivity to norepinephrine following endothelial denudation is inhibited by prazosin. Surgery 99:36–44, 1986

27. O'Malley MK, Morris JJ, Makhoul RG *et al*: Norepinephrine-induced vasoconstriction is increased in intimal hyperplastic arteries of the dog. Surgery 2:217–223, 1987
28. O'Malley MK, Cotecchia S, Hagen P-O: Increased receptor agonist affinity and responsiveness of phosphatidylinositol turnover: a possible mechanism for catecholamine supersensitivity in rabbit aortic intimal hyperplasia. J Surg Res 1991 (in press)
29. Weidinger FF, McLenachan JM, Cybulsky MI *et al*: Persistent dysfunction of regenerated endothelium after balloon angioplasty of rabbit iliac artery. Circulation 81:1667–1679, 1990
30. Cross KS, El-Sanadiki MN, Murray JJ *et al*: Functional abnormalities of experimental autogenous vein graft neoendothelium. Ann Surg 208:631–638, 1988
31. Hagen P-O, Wang ZG, Mikat EM, Hackel DB: Antiplatelet therapy reduces aortic intimal hyperplasia distal to small diameter vascular prosthesis (PTFE) in non-human primates. Ann Surg 195:328–335, 1982
32. McCann RL, Hagen P-O, Fuchs JCA: Aspirin and dipyridamole decrease intimal hyperplasia in experimental vein grafts. Ann Surg 191:238–243, 1980
33. Metke MP, Lie JT, Fuster V, Josa M, Kaye MP: Reduction of intimal thickening in canine coronary by-pass vein grafts with dipyridamole and aspirin. Am J Cardiol 43:1144–1148, 1979
34. Radic ZS, O'Malley MK, Mikat EM *et al*: The role of aspirin and dipyridamole on vascular DNA synthesis and intimal hyperplasia following deendothelialisation. J Surg Res 41:84–91, 1986
35. DeCampli WM, Kosek JC, Mitchell RS, Handen CE, Miller DC: Effects of aspirin, dipyridamole and cod liver oil on accelerated myointimal proliferation in canine veno-arterial allografts. Ann Surg 208:746–754, 1988
36. Murday AJ, Gershlick AH, Syndercombe-Court YD, Mills P, Lewis CT: Intimal thickening in autogenous vein graft in rabbits: influence of aspirin and dipyridamole. Thorax 39:457–461, 1984
37. Chesebro JH, Fuster V, Elveback LR *et al*: Effect of dipyridamole and aspirin on late vein graft patency after coronary bypass operations. N Engl J Med 310:209–214, 1984
38. Meek AC, Chidlow A, Lane IF, Greenhalgh R, McCollum CN: Platelet kinetics following carotid endarterectomy; the effect of aspirin and patch angioplasty. Eur J Vasc Surg 2:99–104, 1988
39. McCollum C, Kenchington G, Alexander C, Franks P, Greenhalgh R: Antiplatelet drugs in femoropopliteal bypass: A multicentre trial. J Vasc Surg 1991 (in press)
40. Kohler JK, Kaufman JL, Kacoyanin G *et al*: Effect of aspirin and dipyridamole on the patency of lower extremity bypass grafts. Surgery 96:462–467, 1984
41. Shionoya S, Sakurai T, Ueyama T *et al*: Effect of Ticlopidine on graft patency following arterial reconstructive surgery in the lower extremity: a multicenter three year prospective study. Vasc Surg 20:541–547, 1990
42. White CW, Knudson M, Schmidt D *et al*: Neither ticlopidine nor aspirin-dipyridamole prevents restenosis post PTCA: results from a randomised placebo-controlled multicenter trial (Abstract). Circulation 76:(Suppl. IV):IV-213, 1987
43. McCready RA, Price MA, Kryscio RJ *et al*: Failure of antiplatelet therapy with ibuprofen (Motrin) to prevent neointimal fibrous hyperplasia. J Vasc Surg 2:205–213, 1985
44. Graham LM, Brothers TE, Darvishian D *et al*: Effects of thromboxane synthetase inhibition on patency and anastamotic hyperplasia of vascular grafts. J Surg Res 46:611–615, 1989
45. Dehmer GJ, Popma JJ, Van den Berg EK *et al*: Reduction in the rate of early restenosis after coronary angioplasty by a diet supplemented with n-3 fatty acids. N Engl J Med 319:733–740, 1988
46. Landymore RW, Kinley CE, Cooper JH *et al*: Cod-liver oil in the prevention of intimal hyperplasia in autogenous vein grafts used for arterial bypass. J Thorac Cardiovasc Surg 89:351–357, 1985
47. Clowes AW, Clowes MM: Kinetics of cellular proliferation after arterial injury. IV. Heparin inhibits rat smooth muscle mitogenesis and migration. Circ Res 58:839–845, 1986
48. Fritze LMS, Reilly CF, Rosenberg RD: An antiproliferative heparin sulfate species produced by post confluent smooth muscle cells. J Cell Biol 100:1041–1049, 1985

49. Dury A: Influence of cortisone on lipid distribution and atherogenesis. Ann NY Acad Sci 72:870–884, 1959
50. Bailey JM, Butler J: Pathology: influence of anti-inflammatory agents on experimental atherosclerosis. Nature 212:731–732, 1966
51. Pepine CJ, Hirshfield JW, Macdonald RG *et al*: A controlled trial of corticosteroids to prevent restenosis after coronary angioplasty. Circulation 81:1753–1761, 1990
52. El-Sanadiki MN, Cross KS, Mikat EM, Hagen P-O: Verapamil therapy reduces intimal hyperplasia in balloon injured rabbit aorta. Circulation 76:314, 1987
53. Whitworth HB, Roubin GS, Hollman J *et al*: Effect of nifedipine on recurrent stenosis after percutaneous coronary angioplasty. J Am Coll Cardiol 8:1271–1276, 1986
54. Powell SJ, Clozel J-P, Muller RK *et al*: Inhibitors of angiotensin-converting enzyme prevent myointimal proliferation after vascular injury. Science 245:186–188, 1989
55. O'Donohoe MK, Schwartz LB, Radic ZS *et al*: Reduction of intimal hyperplasia in experimental vein grafts by the angiotensin converting enzyme inhibitor captopril. Surg Forum XLI:317–318, 1990
56. O'Malley MK, McDermott EWM, Mehigan D, O'Higgins NJ: Role for Prazosin in reducing the development of rabbit intimal hyperplasia after endothelial denudation. Br J Surg 76:936–938, 1989

Regulation of Intimal Hyperplasia After Vascular Reconstruction

Ted R. Kohler and Alexander W. Clowes

All forms of arterial reconstruction are plagued by restenosis and failure in the first several months due to intimal hyperplasia. This process, which consists of smooth muscle cell (SMC) proliferation and matrix deposition, is a universal response of the vessel wall to injury. It occurs after any of the current methods of reconstruction including bypass, endarterectomy, atherectomy, or angioplasty. It is critical that this process be thoroughly understood if long-term patency is to be improved. The key question is what regulates the proliferative response. Two forces may be at work, an initial response to the injury that occurs at the time of reconstruction and a long-term adaptation to haemodynamic changes.

THE ACUTE RESPONSE TO INJURY

The acute response has been studied in a variety of animal models. In the rat model using balloon catheter injury of the common carotid artery,[1] the endothelium, an extremely delicate structure, is removed easily (Fig. 1). Platelets adhere immediately to the subendothelium, but this process is limited to approximately 24 hours following injury. After this time platelets no longer adhere in large numbers for reasons that are not well understood but are likely to be related to coating of the exposed surface with fibrin or other proteins. Attached platelets spread and then release their granules, which contain many factors that are both mitogenic and chemotactic for SMCs and white blood cells (among these are transforming growth factor beta, platelet-derived growth factor [PDGF], and epidermal growth factor).

The injured surface is repopulated by the ingrowth of endothelium from the adjacent, uninjured artery and from the orifices of uninjured branch vessels. In the rat, this process is limited to approximately 10 mm. There are distinct species variations in the extent to which the endothelium will grow in over an injured segment. While it is not known to what extent endothelium can repopulate injured segments in man, it is likely that this process is limited to 1–2 cm since this is the distance that endothelium typically grows out from the adjacent artery onto the surface of polytetrafluoroethylene (PTFE) grafts. It is not known how endothelial regrowth is regulated. The cells are capable of replication when reinjured and therefore are not senescent.[2] Recent work has demonstrated that it is possible to stimulate further cell growth and obtain complete coverage of extensive denuded surfaces by adding basic fibroblast growth factor (FGF).[3] Replacement of a normal endothelial surface may be important not only to reduce thrombogenicity of the vessel but also to limit the proliferation of underlying SMCs. Smooth muscle cell proliferation and matrix deposition cease in re-endothelialized areas of

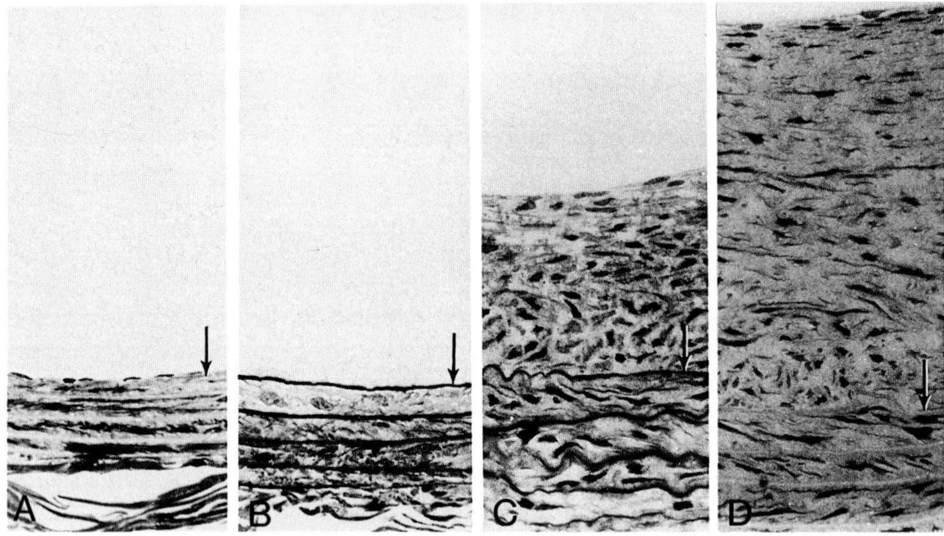

Fig. 1. Histologic cross-sections of rat carotid artery injured by the passage of a balloon embolectomy catheter. A. Normal artery; B. Acutely denuded artery with endothelium missing; C. and D. Thickened artery at 2 and 12 weeks. Matrix accumulation accounts for the increase in intimal thickening between 2 and 12 weeks. Arrow marks the internal elastic lamina. Reprinted with permission from Laboratory Investigation 49:327–333, 1983.

balloon-injured rat carotid arteries. This may be due to release of growth inhibitors by the endothelium. *In vitro,* endothelial cells produce a heparin-like factor that is inhibitory for SMC growth.[4]

Smooth muscle cells respond almost immediately to the injury. In the first week 20–40% of medial SMCs enter the replication cycle and continue to proliferate at a high rate.[5,6] Soon after injury some, but not all, of these cells migrate from the media into the intima, where proliferation continues. It has long been thought that growth factors released by platelets are largely responsible for SMC proliferation. In an early study using balloon injury of rabbit arteries, thrombocytopenic animals were found to have less intimal thickening than controls.[7] On the other hand, thrombocytopenia has little effect on SMC proliferation in injured rat carotid artery, but it does cause a marked reduction in migration.[8] These data support the view that platelets play a role not in the initiation of proliferation but in the movement of cells between tissue compartments. Hence, proliferation and migration may be under separate control.

If platelets are not the major source of growth promoting activity, what is? Cell culture studies indicate that SMC proliferation might be stimulated by production of growth factors from any of the various cell types in the wall including macrophages and the SMC themselves.[9] Recent evidence from animal experiments suggests that SMC proliferation is triggered mainly by injury to the cells in the media (Fig. 2). The role of direct injury to the media is suggested by the observation that endothelial denudation by a fine wire which does not damage the wall also does not cause SMC proliferation; in contrast, acute distension causing medial tearing without

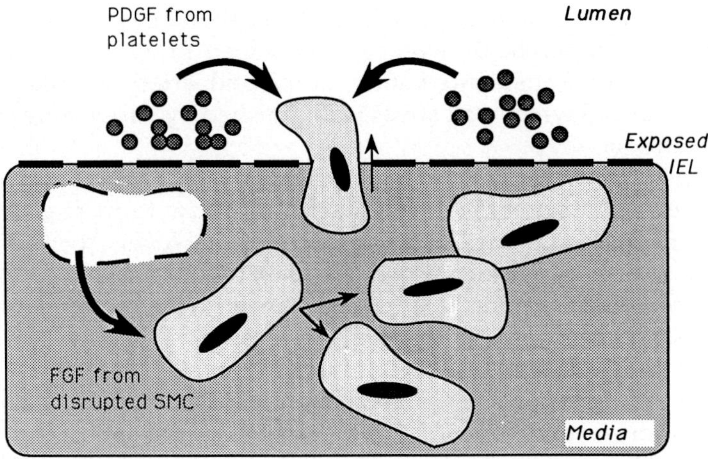

Fig. 2. Diagram depicts how basic fibroblast growth factor (FGF) from disrupted smooth muscle cells (SMC) might stimulate the initial wave of proliferation. Platelet-derived growth factors (PDGF) would then accelerate migration of the SMC from the media to the intima.

significant endothelial damage does induce SMC proliferation.[10] Basic FGF is released when cells are disrupted and might be present in the injured artery. That FGF is stimulating SMC growth is suggested by experiments demonstrating inhibition of the first wave of proliferation by anti-FGF antibodies (M. A. Reidy, personal communication). In addition, an infusion of recombinant FGF causes a substantial increase in SMC proliferation. Platelet factors (e.g. platelet derived growth factor: PDGF) might perform other tasks such as the regulation of SMC migration. The data defining a role for PDGF come from studies showing that infusion of the growth factor (in its BB isoform) following rat balloon injury results in a significant but relatively small increase in SMC proliferation,[11] but it causes a substantial increase in intimal thickening at 1 week (unpublished observations). These data suggest that this growth factor stimulates migration much more than proliferation.

SMC replication declines to near normal levels by 12 weeks except at the surface of denuded areas. Although the SMC number does not increase appreciably between 2 and 12 weeks, intimal thickening continues due to increased matrix deposition by these cells. Thus, intimal hyperplasia is a result of early SMC proliferation and migration into the intima and subsequent matrix deposition.

LONG-TERM ADAPTATION TO HAEMODYNAMIC CHANGES

Haemodynamic factors that may affect wall structure in the long-term include pressure and shear. These forces are particularly important when a vessel that normally carries flow at low pressure, such as a vein, is placed into the arterial circulation. The early work of Carrel and Guthrie[12,13] first demonstrated wall thickening in vein grafts, which was interpreted as adaptation to the arterial circulation. Increased pressure results in increased wall stress, and thickening of the vein graft wall then reduces the wall stress to relatively normal levels. It may also result in luminal narrowing.[14] The importance of increased stress in producing wall thickening is supported by work we performed in a rabbit model using the external jugular vein transplanted into the carotid artery circulation.[15] Intimal hyperplasia is reduced when wall stress is diminished by supporting the vein graft with a rigid external wrap.

It has long been known that blood flow (and therefore shear rate) is an important regulator of vessel diameter. Arteries dilate in response to increased flow due to arteriovenous fistulas until shear is reduced to normal levels.[16,17] Aortorenal vein bypass grafts, which carry high flow, are particularly prone to dilatation and aneurysm formation.[18] Conversely, arterial diameter is reduced by flow reduction.[19] Intimal hyperplasia also appears to be regulated in part by shear rate. Wall thickening is increased in both vein and PTFE grafts when shear is decreased.[20–24]. We now have evidence that increased flow reduces intimal thickening in a baboon model using a highly porous experimental PTFE graft that forms a complete endothelial lining by ingrowth of capillaries through the graft matrix.[20] We also have data to suggest that intimal hyperplasia following balloon injury in the rat carotid artery is reduced by increased shear, even though endothelium is absent in this model.[25]

METHODS OF CONTROLLING INTIMAL HYPERPLASIA

How might intimal hyperplasia be modified to reduce failures of arterial reconstruction? Several approaches are possible including drugs to inhibit proliferation of SMCs or encourage regrowth of endothelium, biologic methods to provide a normal endothelium, and improved techniques to reduce wall injury or stent vessels.

Many classes of drugs affect the vessel wall. Antiplatelet agents can reduce initial platelet adherence and therefore may prevent some short-term failure due to early thrombosis. Clinical trials have demonstrated that these agents can improve stress of coronary artery bypass grafts if they are given in the immediate operative period,[26] but they have not been found to improve patency rates of lower extremity bypass grafts when started the day following surgery.[27] These findings are consistent with the data mentioned above suggesting that in animal models of balloon injury, platelets are not necessary for SMC proliferation, although they may play an important part in migration of these cells into the intima.

Calcium channel blockers can reduce intimal hyperplasia following balloon injury and diminish atherosclerotic changes in animal models, probably through inhibition of early SMC proliferation.[28–31] Clinical trials with these agents are limited at the time of this writing and have not yet demonstrated a clear effect in preventing restenosis following coronary angioplasty.

Heparin inhibits both SMC proliferation and migration and is effective in reducing intimal hyperplasia in the rat balloon injury model.[32,33] It does so without affecting endothelial regeneration. Heparin is active after the first few hours following injury and has no increased effect if continued for more than 7 days. It affects matrix production, causing decreased deposition of elastin and collagen and increased accumulation of proteoglycan. Some subfragments of heparin have only mild anticoagulant properties but are still potent inhibitors of intimal hyperplasia. Clinical trials with these agents will be underway soon.

The angiotensin system may act locally in the vessel wall to modify its structure. Angiotensin II can stimulate SMC proliferation, and angiotensin converting enzyme (ACE) inhibitors can reduce intimal hyperplasia following balloon catheter injury.[34] Further support for the role of this enzyme in regulating wall structure comes from work demonstrating that ACE activity is present in the endothelium-denuded aorta.[35] We have preliminary data suggesting that the combination of heparin plus an ACE inhibitor is more effective than either agent alone in reducing intimal hyperplasia following rat carotid artery injury.

Other drugs that are known to inhibit growth have been used in an effort to reduce intimal hyperplasia. Cytotoxic agents may reduce proliferation, but they have systemic effects that generally limit their applicability. There is some suggestion that steroids can reduce intimal hyperplasia in an animal model of balloon injury,[36] but there are no clinical data supporting use of these agents. Beta blockers have been tried without success, and fish oils have been ineffective in reducing restenosis following coronary angioplasty, although these agents inhibit platelet aggregation and enhance fibrinolysis and vasodilatation.

Techniques of revascularization can be modified to reduce injury to the vessel wall. Since the original work with vein grafting by Carrel and Guthrie, vascular surgeons have tried to minimize trauma to the vein to decrease wall thickening. When venous segments are handled roughly and dilated vigorously before implantation, they lose much of their endothelium and develop pronounced thickening in comparison with carefully-handled veins.[37] Reduced endothelial damage is often viewed as one reason why the *in situ* technique results in improved vein graft patency. Since increased blood flow appears to reduce intimal hyperplasia, increasing flow by treatment of distal obstructive lesions or creation of an arteriovenous fistula may also improve long-term success rates of arterial reconstructions.

Providing synthetic bypass grafts with an endothelial lining should reduce thrombogenicity and may reduce intimal thickening by inhibiting proliferation of underlying SMC. One approach is to seed the graft with autogenous endothelial cells. This method has been used in human grafts, with some preliminary evidence that endothelial-lined grafts are less thrombogenic.[38–40] Whether or not this technique can provide a durable endothelial surface and improve patency rates remains to be determined. An endothelial lining may also result from capillary ingrowth through the graft matrix. If grafts are made with a sufficiently large pore size, capillaries can grow in through them and reach the luminal surface where they then change from a tubular morphology and spread to cover the surface. This phenomenon has been observed in Dacron grafts and highly porous (60 micron (μm) internodal distance) PTFE grafts.[20,41–43] Dacron grafts do not appear to endothelialize by this mechanism in humans[44–46] and recent evidence suggests that wrapped porous PTFE may not as well (unpublished data).

Perhaps the most dramatic method of controlling intimal hyperplasia is to introduce genes with specific growth promoters or inhibitors directly into the cells of the vessel wall. Several investigators have reported successful transfer of genes into both endothelial cells and SMC in animal models.[47–49] Another group has inserted a plasminogen activator gene into endothelial cells used to cover a fibronectin-coated metal stent, thus presumably making it less thrombogenic.[50] These methods have great promise not only for direct control of intimal hyperplasia at the cellular and molecular level, but in treatment of systemic disorders, for example by providing insulin-producing cells in the arterial intima of diabetic patients.

In summary, intimal hyperplasia is a universal response to vessel injury in which SMC proliferation and matrix deposition causes thickening of the wall and narrowing of the lumen. Direct damage to the wall stimulates SMC proliferation while other factors, such as PDGF released from platelets, cause migration of these cells into the intima. A host of growth factors produced by platelets, SMC, endothelial cells, and white blood cells in the vessel wall work in a complex interaction that determines the extent of this proliferative process. In the long term, haemodynamic factors are also important. Decreased shear and increased pressure increase intimal thickening. Possible methods of controlling this process include reduction of the initial injury, use of various drugs to reduce the proliferative response, and biologic methods to provide a new endothelial surface or to introduce genes for factors that can regulate this process.

REFERENCES

1. Clowes AW, Reidy MA, Clowes MM: Mechanisms of stenosis after arterial injury. Lab Invest 49:208–215, 1983
2. Reidy MA, Clowes AW, Schwartz SM: Endothelial regeneration. V. Inhibition of endothelial regrowth in arteries of rat and rabbit. Lab Invest 49:569–575, 1983
3. Lindner V, Majack RA, Reidy MA: Basic fibroblast factor stimulates endothelial regrowth and proliferation in denuded arteries. J Clin Invest 85:2004–2008, 1990
4. Castellot JJ, Addonizio ML, Rosenberg R, Karnovsky MJ: Cultured endothelial cells produce a Heparinlike inhibitor of smoooth muscle cell growth. J Cell Biol 90:372–379, 1981
5. Majesky MW, Schwartz SM, Clowes MM, Clowes AW: Heparin regulates smooth muscle S phase entry in the injured rat carotid artery. Circ Res 61: 296–300, 1987
6. Clowes AW, Schwartz SM: Significance of quiescent smooth muscle migration in the injured rat carotid artery. Circ Res 56: 139–145, 1985
7. Friedman RJ, Stemerman MB, Wenz B, Moore S, Gauldie J: The effect of thrombocytopenia on experimental arteriosclerotic lesion formation in rabbits: Smooth muscle cell proliferation and re-endothelialization. J Clin Invest 60:1191–1201, 1977
8. Fingerle J, Johnson R, Clowes AW, Majesky MW, Reidy MA: Role of platelets in smooth muscle cell proliferation and migration after vascular injury in rat carotid artery. Proc Natl Acad Sci USA 86:8412–8416, 1989
9. Walker LM, Bowen-Pope DF, Ross R, Reidy MA: Production of platelet-derived growth factor-like molecules by cultured arterial smooth muscle cells accompanies proliferation after arterial injury. Proc Natl Acad Sci USA 83:7311–7315, 1986
10. Clowes MM, Fingerle J, Reidy MA: Kinetics of cellular proliferation after arterial injury. V. Role of acute distension in the induction of smooth muscle proliferation. Lab Invest 60:360–364, 1989
11. Jawien A, Lindner V, Bowen-Pope DF, Schwartz SM *et al*: Platelet-derived growth factor (PDGF) stimulates arterial smooth muscle cell proliferation *in vivo*. FASEB J 4:A342 (Abstract), 1990
12. Carrel A, Guthrie CC: Results of the biterminal transplantation of veins. Am J Med Sci 132:415–422, 1906
13. Carrel A, Guthrie CC: Uniterminal and biterminal venous transplantations. Surg Gynecol Obstet 2:266–286, 1906
14. Zwolak RM, Adams MC, Clowes AW: Kinetics of vein graft hyperplasia: Association with tangential stress. J Vasc Surg 5:126–136, 1987
15. Kohler TR, Kirkman TR, Clowes AW: The effect of rigid external support on vein graft adaptation to the arterial circulation. J Vasc Surg 9:277–285, 1989

16. Kamiya A, Togawa T: Adaptive regulation of wall shear stress to flow change in the canine carotid artery. Am J Physiol 239:14–21, 1980
17. Zarins CK, Zatina MA, Giddens DP, Ku DN, Glagov S: Shear stress regulation of artery lumen diameter in experimental atherogenesis. J Vasc Surg 5:413–420, 1987
18. Stanley JC, Ernst CB, Fry WJ: Fate of 100 aortorenal vein grafts, Characteristics of late graft expansion; aneurysmal dilatation; and stenosis. Surgery 74:931–944, 1973
19. Langille BL, O'Donnell F: Reductions in arterial diameter produced by chronic decreases in blood flow are endothelium-dependent. Science 231:405–407, 1986
20. Kohler TR, Kirkman TR, Clowes AW: Intimal hyperplasia in polytetrafluorethylene grafts is reduced by increased flow. FASEB J 4:A1153 (Abstract), 1990
21. Berguer R, Higgins RF, Reddy DJ: Intimal hyperplasia. Arch Surg 115:332–335, 1980
22. Rittgers SE, Karayannacos PE, Guy JF: Velocity distribution and intimal proliferation in autologous vein grafts in dogs. Circ Res 42:792–801, 1978
23. Morinaga K, Okadome K, Kuroki M, Miyazaki T, Muto Y: Effect of wall shear stress on intimal thickening of arterially transplanted autogenous veins in dogs. J Vasc Surg 2:430–433, 1985
24. Mii S, Okadome K, Onohara T, Yamamura S, Sugimachi K: Intimal thickening and permeability of arterial autogenous vein graft in a canine poor-runoff model: Transmission electron microscopic evidence. Surgery 108:81–89, 1990
25. Kohler TR, Jawien A, Clowes AW: Effect of shear on intimal hyperplasia following arterial injury in rats. Circulation 82 (Suppl 3):400, 1990
26. Goldman S, Copeland J, Moritz T *et al*: Saphenous vein graft patency 1 year after coronary artery bypass surgery and effects of antiplatelet therapy: Results of a Veterans Administration Cooperative Study. Circulation 80:1190–1197, 1989
27. Kohler TR, Kaufman MD, Kacoyanis G *et al*: Effect of aspirin and dipyridamole on the patency of lower extremity bypass grafts. Surgery 96:462–466, 1984
28. Jackson CL, Bush RC, Bowyer DE: Mechanism of antiatherogenic action of calcium antagonists. Atherosclerosis 80:17–26, 1989
29. Jackson CL, Bush RC, Bowyer DE: Inhibitory effect of calcium antagonists on balloon catheter-induced arterial smooth muscle cell proliferation and lesion size. Atherosclerosis 69:115–122, 1988
30. Lichtlen PR, Hugenholtz PG, Rafflenbeul W *et al*: Nifedipine trial. Lancet 335:1109–1113, 1990
31. El-Sanadiki MN, Cross KS, Murray JJ *et al*: Reduction of intimal hyperplasia and enhanced reactivity of experimental vein bypass grafts with verapamil treatment. Ann Surg 212:87–96, 1990
32. Kohler TR, Kirkman TR, Clowes AW: Effect of heparin on adaptation of vein grafts to arterial circulation. Arteriosclerosis 9:523–528, 1989
33. Clowes AW, Clowes MM: Kinetics of cellular proliferation after arterial injury. II Inhibition of smooth muscle growth by heparin. Lab Invest 52:611–616, 1985
34. Powell JS, Clozel JP, Muler RKM *et al*: Inhibitors of angiotensin-converting enzyme prevent myointimal proliferation after vascular injury. Science 245:186–188, 1989
35. Pipili E, Manolopoulos VG, Catravas JD, Maragoudakis ME: Angiotensin converting enzyme activity is present in the endothelium-denuded aorta. Br J Pharmacol 98:333–335, 1989
36. Chervu A, Moore WS, Quinones-Baldrich WJ, Henderson T: Efficacy of corticosteroids in suppression of intimal hyperplasia. J Vasc Surg 10:129–134, 1989
37. LoGerfo FW, Quist WC, Cantelmo NL, Haudenschild CC: Integrity of vein grafts as a function of initial intimal and medial preservation. Circulation 68II:117–124, 1983
38. Ortenwall P, Wadenvik H, Risberg B: Reduced platelet deposition on seeded versus unseeded segments of expanded polytetrafluoroethylene grafts: Clinical observations after a 6-month follow-up. J Vasc Surg 10:374–380, 1989
39. Fasol R, Zilla P, Deutsch M, Fischlein T, Laufer G: Human endothelial cell seeding: Evaluation of its effectiveness by platelet parameters after one year, J Vasc Surg 9:432–436, 1989

40. Ortenwall P, Wadenvik H, Kutti J, Risberg B: Endothelial cell seeding reduced thrombogenicity of Dacron grafts in humans. J Vasc Surg 11:403–410, 1990
41. Sauvage LR, Berger KE, Wood SJ *et al*: Interspecies healing of porous arterial prostheses. Arch Surg 109:698–705, 1974
42. Clowes AW, Zacharias RK, Kirkman TR: Early endothelial coverage of synthetic arterial grafts—porosity revisited. Am J Surg 153:501–504, 1987
43. Zacharias RK, Kirkman TR, Clowes AW: Mechanisms of healing in synthetic grafts. J Vasc Surg 6:429–436, 1987
44. Sauvage LR, Berger K, Beilin LB *et al*: Presence of endothelium in an axillary-femoral graft of knitted Dacron with an external velour surface. Ann Surg 182:749–753, 1975
45. Szilagyi DE, Smith RF, Elliott JP, Allen HM: Long-term behavior of a Dacron arterial substitute. Ann Surg 162:453–477, 1965
46. Wesolowski SA, Fries CC, Hennigan G *et al*: Factors contributing to long-term failures in human vascular prosthetic grafts. J Cardiovasc Surg 5:544–567, 1964
47. Wilson JM, Birinyi LK, Salomon RN *et al*: Implantation of vascular grafts lined with genetically modified endothelial cells. Science 244:1344–1346, 1989
48. Nabel EG, Plautz B, Boyce FM, Stanley JC, Nabel J: Recombinant gene expression in vivo within endothelial cells of the arterial wall. Science 244:1342–1344, 1989
49. Nabel EG, Plautz G, Nabel GJ: Site-specific gene expression *in vivo* by direct gene transfer into the arterial wall. Science 249:1285–1288, 1990
50. Dichek DA, Neville RF, Zwiebel JA *et al*: Seeding of intravascular stents with genetically engineered endothelial cells. Circulation 80:1347–1353, 1989

Compliance: A Critical Parameter for Maintenance of Arterial Reconstruction?

Thomas Schmitz-Rixen and George Hamilton

The widespread use of graft replacement material led with increasing frequency to complications arising from these prostheses. It should be kept in mind that the true incidence of failure of arterial grafts is believed to be higher than that reported in the literature.[1,2] The discussion is still open on identifying those inherent features of vascular grafting that could contribute to long-term success or short-term failure. Also, the history of arterial graft development reflects the need for their improvement. The search has been prompted for better arterial substitutes, among others, for repair particularly of lesions of smaller arteries. An 'ideal' graft for any arterial replacement should be a blood conduit that is easily integrated biologically into the host tissues and able to maintain its patency indefinitely. The analysis of characteristics inherent in graft material and their interplay with those of the host should provide a closer focus on biologic behaviour of the inner surface with the media. It appears that in the long run host factors may be more difficult to overcome than the problem of achieving an ideal graft. Although improved grafts with a rapid flow surface and nonthrombogenic lining are approaching the criteria of an ideal arterial conduit, the overriding questions still concern the nonideal host vessels or the nonideal condition the host vessel is exposed to. Thus, the present clinical studies have not fulfilled the hope of an ideal new endothelial lining of these grafts.[3–6]

Unfortunately in prosthetic, biologic and autogenous vein grafts there are healing limitations in humans in contrast to the healing ability in some experimental animals. Regardless of these healing differences, all of the current grafts may develop morphologic alterations, more or less severe, that could lead to stenosis or complete occlusion. Recent experience[7] has shown that neither expanded polytetrafluoroethylene (ePTFE) nor human umbilical vein give satisfactory results in lower limb revascularization operations if the distal anastomosis is below the knee or beyond. The seriousness of this lack of a suitable reconstruction material is made more apparent by the fact that surgeons' technical capabilities have improved vastly since 1980. With satisfactory graft material, i.e. *in situ* saphenous vein, limb salvage results have increased, but even the saphenous vein itself is not a perfect arterial substitute as we know from cardiovascular experience with aortic coronary bypass surgery.

The ideal graft should have a blood compatible flow surface with fixed endothelium and basement membrane and physiological mechanical properties. There are a number of biological and plastic materials competing for these goals. Aneurysm formation and high infection rates in biological prostheses has led to a trend away from biologic grafts in favour of plastic materials.[8,9] However, no plastic graft material has been identified as entirely blood compatible, as the complications with the artificial heart revealed, and all plastic materials studied in clinical trials so far stimulate an uncontrollable proliferative response in host arteries at the distal anastomosis; thus causing failure of grafts when of small calibre, even though they are generally successful when used to interpose larger diameter vessels. This distal anastomotic subintimal hyperplasia (SIH) is an ubiquitous pathologic entity in late graft occlusion.[10] The cause of SIH has been the subject of much investigation. The role of compliance mismatch between host artery and vascular grafts in the development of SIH is discussed in this chapter. While compliance may, in fact, be an important parameter in determining the results of bypass grafting, the dominant influence of haemodynamic and thrombogenic factors has continued to mask what is probably a very subtle effect.

The nature of compliance mismatch is complex, as it is determined by the compliance of host artery, anastomosis, graft, and the occasional presence of a perianastomotic hypercompliant zone[11] The theoretic haemodynamic consequences of an artery–graft compliance mismatch include increased impedance to flow and decreased distal perfusion[12] and disturbed flow or turbulence, which could lead to graft thrombosis.[13] A compliance mismatch also produces pulsatile mechanical stresses at the anastomoses[14] which have been theoretically linked to suture line disruption and to the development of false aneurysm formation[14] as well as to the development of SIH near anastomoses[15–17] the major cause of late graft failure.

HISTORICAL BACKGROUND

William Harvey (Fig. 1) who began the modern approach to arterial physiology[18] published in 1628 his famous treatise *Exercitatio anatomica de motu cordis et sanguinis in animalibus*. Harvey demonstrated that arteries carry blood and not blood and air as previously thought. Hales[19] in 1773 deduced that the elastic reservoir of the arterial system smooths the sharply pulsatile output of the heart. A translation of Hales's work into German introduced the quaint term *Windkessel* to the subject. Prior to the last war all fire engines were fitted with an air reservoir (in German the Windkessel) to damp

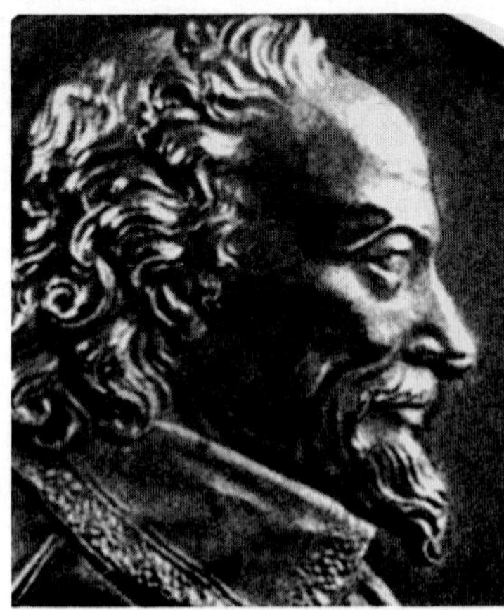

Fig. 1. William Harvey.

the sharp pulsations from the pistons. The elasticity of the air is analogous to that of the arterial wall. After Hales most progress was made in fields related to arterial physiology. By the turn of the century it was possible to record arterial pressure and flow waveforms with reasonable accuracy and this allowed Frank[20] to advance arterial physiology by applying the Windkessel theory by adding standard wave transmission theory. Taylor[21] perpetuated this approach and advanced our understanding of wave reflection. Cox[22] developed a different mathematical model for the arterial tree. Theoretical progress is now slowed by problems of measurement and at present we do not know which model is correct. Fortunately, even without a mathematical model of the circulation in which all parameters have been experimentally verified it is possible to describe the behaviour of a segment of an artery.

DEFINITION OF COMPLIANCE

Arterial compliance, which depends on, and is an expression of, the structural properties of the vessel wall, is defined as the fractional change in diameter in response to a unit change in pressure.[23] It can be measured without knowledge of the wall thickness and can thus be obtained relatively noninvasively. Because of the nonlinear response of blood vessel diameter to pressure, compliance must be specified with reference to a certain value of pressure (e.g. mean pressure—or diastolic pressure in a few publications). Compliance can be calculated from either excursions of diameter and pressure during a cardiac cycle (dynamic compliance, $\partial l)/1)/\partial P$) or the slope of the pressure diameter curve generated by slow inflation/deflation of the blood vessel (quasistatic compliance, $\partial D/\partial P \times 1/D$). Both of these can be measured *in vitro* or *in vivo*, allowing for studies of native vessels and arterial prostheses.

$$\text{Compliance} = \frac{\partial D}{D \times \partial P} \times 100$$

While not strictly correct, compliance can be thought of as the reciprocal of the slope of the pressure-diameter curve of a vessel. Examples of such curves for artery, vein, rubber, polytetrafluoroethylene (PTFE), polyurethane (PUR) and knitted Dacron, obtained *in vitro* by slow pressurization, are given in Fig. 2. The difference in shape between the curves for synthetic and biological materials reflects their linear and nonlinear elastic properties, respectively, discussed in greater detail below.

For convenience in comparing different vessels, a standard reporting mean pressure of 100 mmHg has been adopted (Fig. 2). When the thickness of a vessel is much less than its diameter, it makes little difference whether the external or internal diameter is used in calculating the compliance. However, when thickness is equivalent to a major fraction of the external diameter ($t > 0.06$, $R = 0.12\,D$), as with many vessels of interest, the distinction becomes critical. It is extremely important, therefore, to specify which diameter was used in calculating compliance. Unless otherwise noted, values of compliance will reflect measurements of outer vessel diameter.

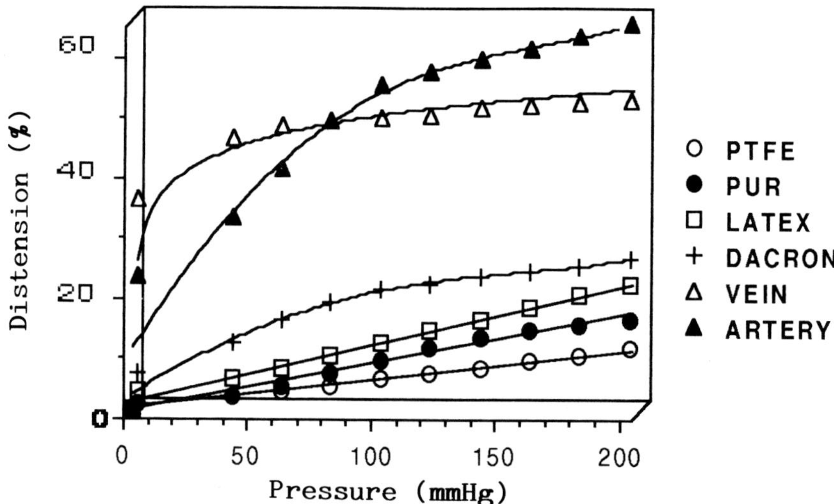

Fig. 2. Distension of biologic and synthetic material under static conditions. PTFE = 6 mm ePTFE standard wall graft, PUR = 6 mm polyurethane graft of low porosity, LATEX = Latex rubber, DACRON = 8 mm knitted Dacron graft.

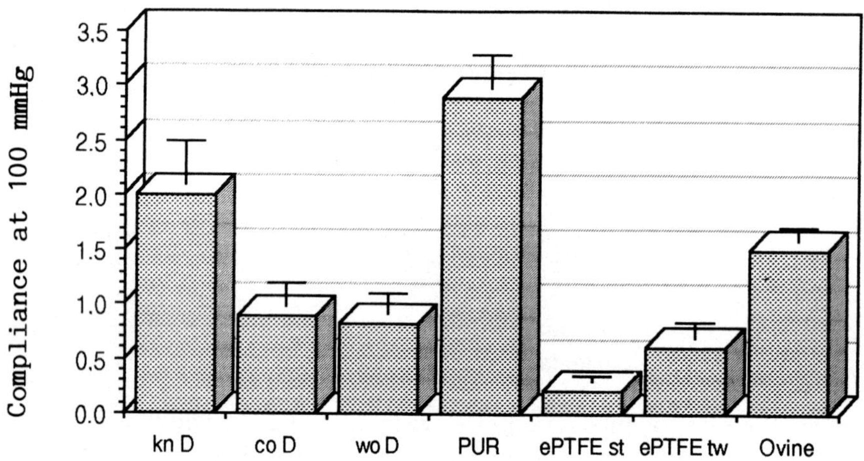

Fig. 3. Compliance values of different graft materials at 100 mmHg (knD = knitted Dacron; coD = gelatine coated Dacron; woD = woven Dacron; PUR = polyurethane of median porosity; ePTFE st = standard wall ePTFE graft; ePTFE tw = thin wall ePTFE graft; Ovine = ovine graft with Dacron mesh—2nd generation).

Due to the nonlinear elastic nature of the arterial wall, arterial compliance varies strongly with intraluminal pressure. Compliance cannot, therefore, be characterized by a single value, representative of the entire range of pressure over which an artery functions. When arterial compliance is measured over a range of pressures, a curve

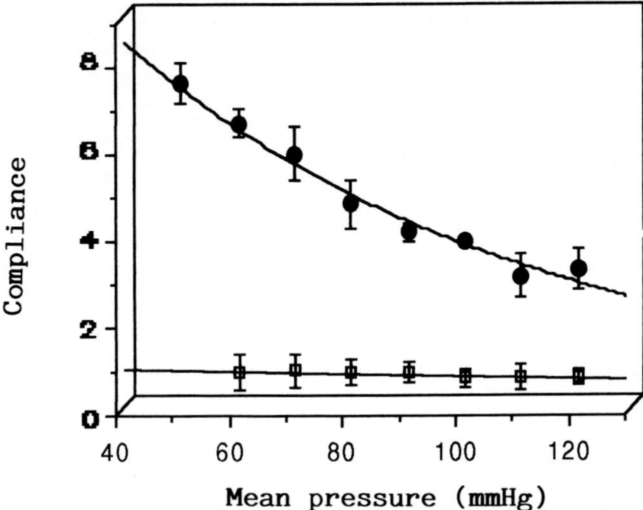

Fig. 4. Compliance-pressure curve of the superficial femoral artery of a 35-year-old male (●) (SFA 35 m: measured at five different locations: $y = 14.371 * 10^{(-5.9013e\text{-}3X)}$ $R^2 = 0.968$) compared with the compliance-pressure curve of a 6 mm ePTFE graft (□) (ePTFE: average and standard deviation of five grafts measured: $y = 0.94895 - 2.5877e\text{-}3X$ $R^2 = 0.716$).

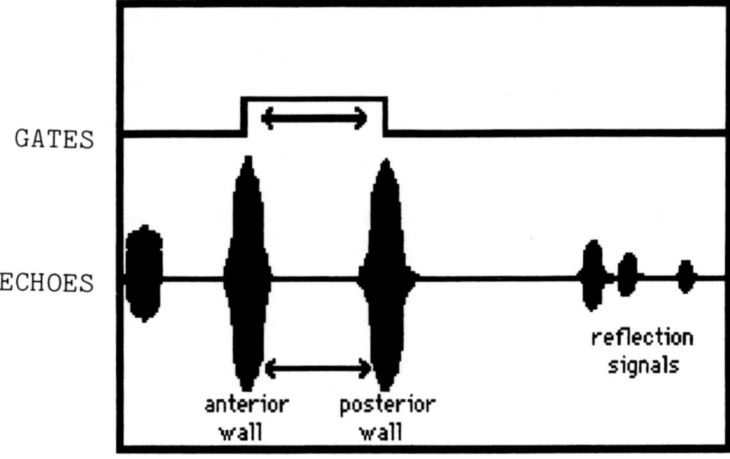

Fig. 5. Oscilloscope output of the ultrasonic echotracker. Electronic gates are aligned with the echoes corresponding to the anterior and posterior wall of a blood vessel or graft.

of compliance vs pressure can be obtained; this characterization of compliance–pressure relationships can enable different vessels to be compared more meaningfully[1] (Fig. 4).

TECHNIQUE

Compliance is calculated from measured values of pressure and diameter. Pressure is usually measured via catheter or manometer probe as close to the site of interest as possible. Diameter can be measured by a number of techniques, including phase-locked echotracking ultrasound[24] which has the advantage of not requiring surgery to study vessels up to 3 cm below the surface of the skin. We have used the echotracking method to examine the reciprocal influence of compliance on arterial graft function and behaviour and of the grafting procedure on the compliance of the host arteries (Fig. 5). Inherent in the measurement of compliance is the ability to quantitate accurately changes in vessel diameter during a cardiac cycle. Various instruments have been used to measure diameter, such as circumferential disposed mercury in silastic strain gauges,[14,15] diametrically opposed piezoelectric crystals,[25] cantilever transducers,[26,27] pressure and flow waveform analysis,[28] high speed video motion analysis[29] and most recently a helium–neon laser[30] and a photographic technique using a stroboscope flash[29]

PHYSIOLOGY AND PATHOLOGY

Studies of arterial wall mechanisms over the last three decades have clearly established the anisotropic nature of arteries; i.e. the nonlinear response of diameter changes to blood pressure alterations.[22,31] The compliance of arteries varies depending on their anatomic location and size, age and state of health. Compliance also depends on smooth muscle tone and thus on drugs that can affect tone, as well as the degree to which a vessel may have been surgically manipulated. Studies performed in animals and with human tissue show that compliance tends to decrease with distance from the heart, increasing age, and atherosclerosis, but there are few data that qualitatively relate compliance to the severity of disease.[32] With medial

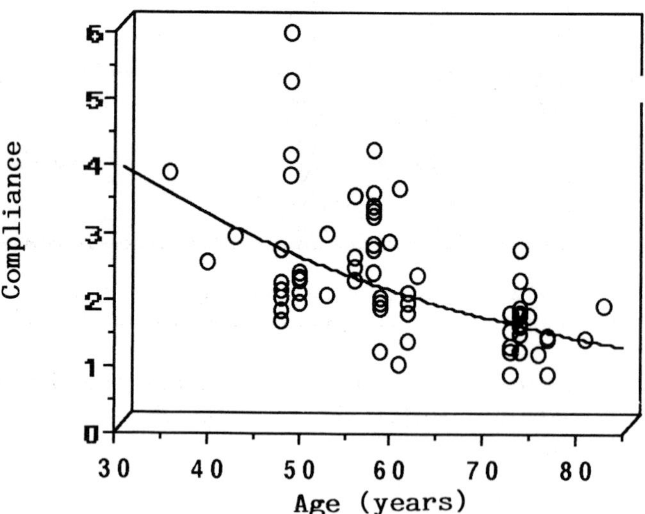

Fig. 6. Tendency of correlation of compliance (○) (at 100 mmHg mean pressure) with increasing age on human pathology specimens without calcification and major plaque formation (intimal thickness <0.1 mm) ($y = 7.5358 * 10^{(-9.7910e\text{-}3X)}$ $R^2 = 0.355$) ($n = 73$).

calcification, as occurs in many diabetic patients, or increasing age, arterial compliance can be reduced dramatically.

In an artificial circulation (the artificial dog) dynamic compliance[33] was measured on 149 human pathology specimens of the superficial femoral artery. Compliance was calculated from measured values of pressure and diameter. Pressure was measured via catheter as close to the site of interest as possible. Diameter and diameter change were identified by phase-locked echotracking ultrasound. The measured sections of the superficial femoral arteries were subsequently fixed in formalin. On HE stains wall thickness was measured using an image analysis system on a personal computer. On these 149 specimens, obtained from pathology between 18 and 28 h postmortem, there was no correlation at all of compliance values with increasing age. Only when counting specimens without calcification and no compromised residual lumen ($n=73$) was there a tendency of loss of compliance with increasing age (Fig. 6). A strong correlation of loss of compliance was found with increasing intimal thickness (Fig. 7) and concomitant decreasing medial thickness. However, in no case was there loss of quality of compliance as demonstrated in the nonlinear response to a range of different pressure values, as in the compliance-pressure curves of a 76-year-old male and a 52-year-old diabetic female with given calcification (Fig. 8).

Balloon dilatation of 60 additional specimens with a residual lumen of less than 50% of diameter to at least 75% could increase compliance (Fig. 9). The message we found is that severity of disease is correlated with loss of compliance in quantity but not in quality. Even severely diseased arteries do not lose nonlinear response to the variation of pressure values. This is provided by still functioning parts of the media as the balloon dilatation data suggest.

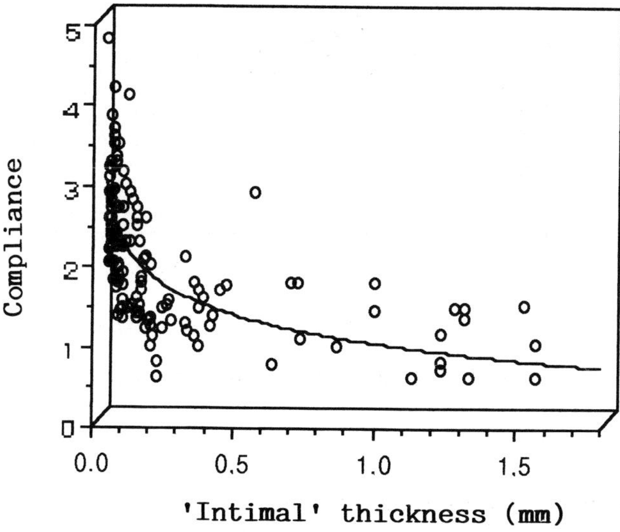

Fig. 7. Correlation of thickening of the subendothelial layer with compliance (○) (at 100 mmHg mean pressure) in human pathology specimen ($y=0.90911+-1.1357*\log(x)$ $R^2=0.465$) ($n=149$).

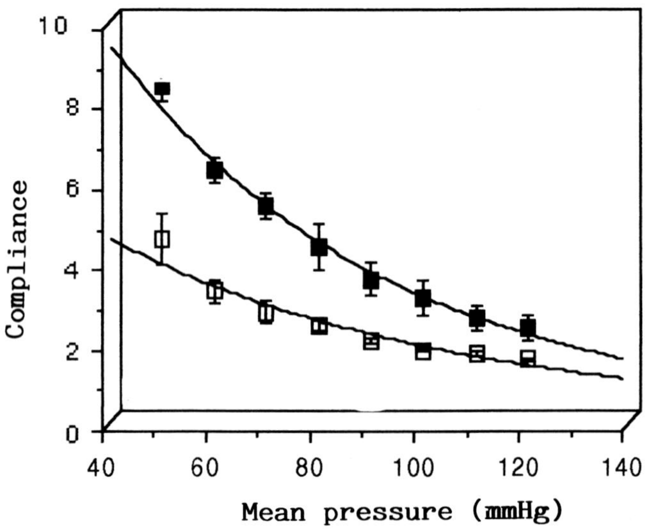

Fig. 8. Compliance-pressure curves of the superficial femoral artery of a 76-year-old male (■) (SFA 76 m: $y = 19.415 * 10^{(-7.9751e\text{-}3x)}$ $R^2 = 0.990$) and a 52-year-old diabetic female with severe calcification (□) (SFA 52 f: $y = 8.2186 * 10^{(-6.4819e-3x)}$ $R^2 = 0.947$).

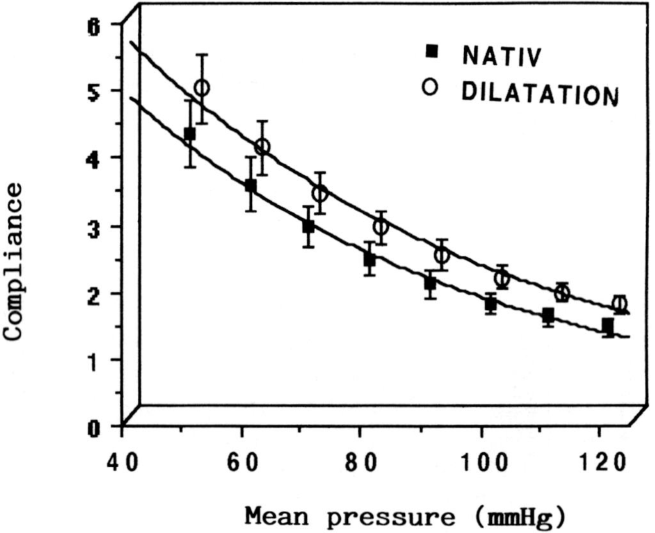

Fig. 9. Balloon dilatation of SFA specimens increased compliance (pooled data) ($n = 60$).

EFFECT ON PATENCY

Over 30 years ago it was noted that the distensibility of a bypass graft is often less than that of the host artery and that this property may change during the period of implantation,[34] but this phenomenon received very little attention until about 15 years ago.[35-37] In 1976 Baird and Abbott hypothesized that a difference in circumferential compliance of a small diameter graft and its host artery is detrimental to graft performance and can result in lower patency rates.[12] A number of experimental studies supported this hypothesis, but they were either inadequately controlled[38,39] or provided only circumstantial evidence.[40–42] Because thrombogenic events can occur in any case, regardless of compliance mismatch, it was very difficult to isolate a true effect of compliance. Previous studies that supported the compliance hypothesis, in fact, compared grafts that differed in more than biomechanical properties. Studies of human femoropopliteal grafts[41] and canine femoral grafts,[40] in which patency appeared to be related to compliance, were simultaneously comparing synthetic with biologic grafts with different flow surfaces and thrombogenic properties. Polyurethane grafts, in which maximum patency was obtained by matching arterial compliance[38,39] also differed in porosity, which will influence platelet deposition and thus patency.

It was in 1986 that Abbott[43] was able to present an experimental study to support the compliance theory conclusively. Biomechanical properties of canine autografts served as isolated variables providing match and mismatch in circumferential compliance. The following criteria were fulfilled: 1. graft compliance either matched the host artery or was substantially lower; 2. grafts differed only in circumferential compliance; 3. blood compatibility of the grafts' flow surfaces was identical; 4. compliant and stiff grafts were implanted in a bilateral model in which each animal serves as its own control. This hypothesis was tested in 14 dogs by implanting paired arterial autografts, prepared with differential glutaraldehyde fixation of carotid arteries in the femoral arteries of the same dog. Briefly, a segment of one carotid artery was excised and divided. The first portion (compliant graft) was filled with 0.025% buffered glutaraldehyde at 100 mmHg and immersed in normal saline solution externally for 30 min. The second portion (stiff graft) was equally filled but was immersed instead in 10% glutaraldehyde for 1 h. Thus the luminal flow surfaces of both graft types were exposed to identical concentrations of glutaraldehyde. These grafts differed only in circumferential compliance: they were 100% (compliant) vs 40% (stiff) as compliant as the host artery. There was also a match/mismatch in the quality of compliance (i.e. nonlinear response to blood pressure variation). Compliance mismatch was significant for the tubular and anastomotic type. The flow surfaces were identical as determined by physicochemical measurements (critical surface tension, infrared reflectance spectroscopy, water porosity, glutaraldehyde cytotoxicity assay, tissue culture for endothelial cells) and scanning electron microscopy. Both graft types lacked viable cells, as shown by *in vitro* cell culture. In 14 dogs, eight stiff and two compliant grafts clotted within 3 months, the latter doing so within 24 h of their contralateral counterparts. Cumulative patencies by life table were 85% and 37% for compliant and stiff grafts, respectively ($p<0.05$) (Fig. 10). Exclusion bilateral failures further increased the significance of this difference ($p<0.01$).

Two recent studies oppose the compliance theory.[44,45] Both authors worked with polyurethane grafts of different compliance covered in one study with crosslinked gelatin. These studies did not show any positive effect of graft compliance. However, they failed to show whether the compliant grafts were not only matching the arterial system at 100 mmHg but also matching compliance in quality, which is a major fact as demonstrated below. There was also no control for the absorption rate of the gelatin.

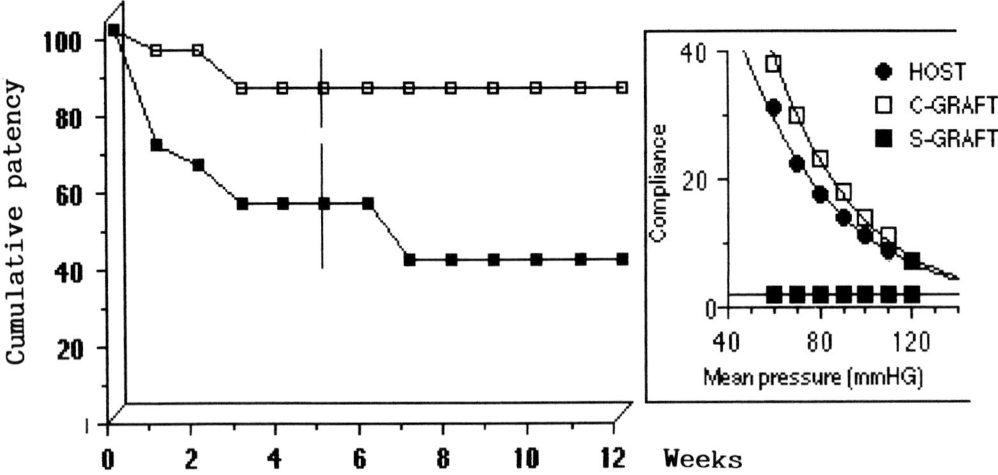

Fig. 10. Patency vs implantation time in 14 compliant (□) and 14 stiff (■) autografts in a canine experiment ($p < 0.05$ according to log rank test). The insert represents compliance-pressure curves of host artery (●), compliant and stiff graft.

ANASTOMOTIC COMPLIANCE

The creation of an end-to-end arterial anastomosis always generates a focal decrease in diameter of at least 10–20%,[11] depending on whether continuous or interrupted sutures are used. It also depends on the surgeon's experience. This diameter drop causes a concomitant drop in compliance, to a degree again determined by anastomotic technique and suture material. More elastic suture material (Novafil® from Davis & Geck) compared to standard material (Prolene® from Ethicon) was able to diminish the anastomotic compliance mismatch (Fig. 11). However, the change in compliance from distant host artery to anastomosis is not monotonic; there is often a paradoxical increase in compliance, averaging 50%, with a peak located 3–5 mm from the anastomosis. Abbott *et al.*[46,47] have termed this compliance profile the 'paraanastomotic hypercompliance zone' or PHZ[48] (Fig. 12). It also is seen in arteries anastomosed to grafts of autogenous vein and ePTFE. PHZ is also seen more frequently with continuous vs interrupted anastomoses and gives a new dimension to the concept of compliance mismatch between an artery and a graft: it may now be necessary to consider differences in compliance between the PHZ's peak and low values centred in the anastomosis, rather than the less dramatic 'tubular' mismatch determined by the nominal difference between artery and graft. Thus suture, or anastomotic, 'compliance' may have as much effect on the arterial wall and the healing response as does the compliance of a graft itself. An inelastic suture or snare placed around an intact artery to create an incompliant anastomosis-like diameter reduction also creates PHZ. The location and shape of the PHZ profile, together with data from other laboratories[10,17,49] on the profile of subintimal thickening near anastomoses, led to the hypothesis that PHZ, with its local increase in motion of the arterial wall, may be responsible for the smooth muscle cell proliferation or the deposition of connective tissue. Subintimal hyperplasia has been

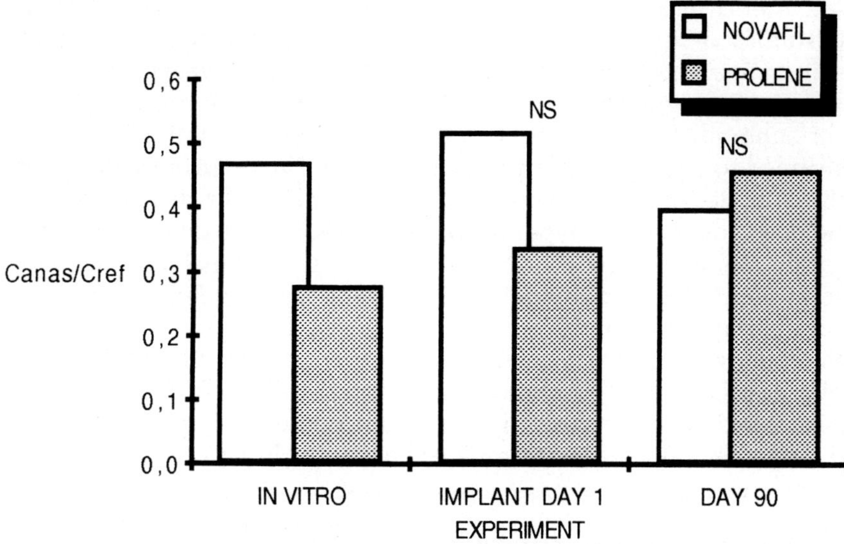

Fig. 11. Anastomotic compliance mismatch with different sutures. Use of more compliant suture material (Novafil®) could demonstrate a diminished compliance mismatch in an *in vitro* experiment compared with standard inelastic suture material (Prolene®). This was reproducible in a canine experiment implanting autologous vein grafts at the time of implantation; 90 days after implantation there was no difference, but mismatch was lower in general ($p<0.01$).

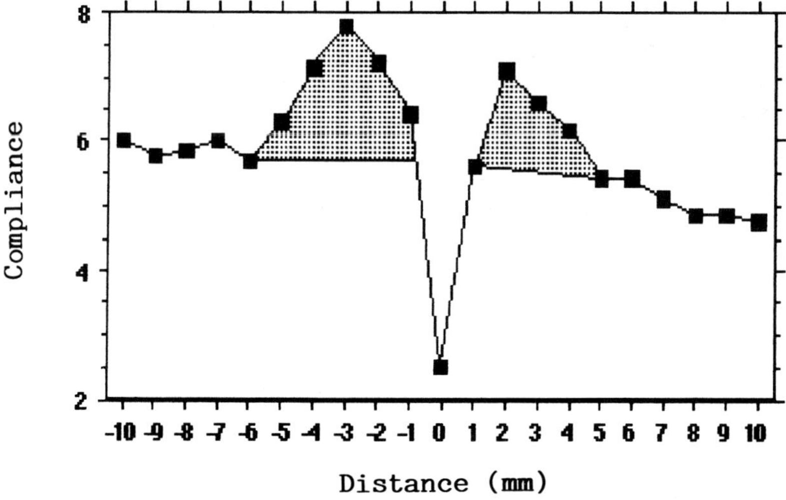

Fig. 12. Para-anastomotic hypercompliant zone (PHZ). Typical compliance profile of a continuous anastomosis: Compliance vs distance. Anastomosis is at 0 mm. Shaded areas denotes PHZ.

seen in the arteries proximal and distal to grafts in studies by others. This led to extensive studies of numerous grafts of synthetic or biologic origin that were implanted in canine femoral arteries. Although PHZ was present and compliant grafts had a significantly higher patency rate than stiff ones, none of the grafts failed because of subintimal hyperplasia[43]. Rabbit and canine arteries had then been balloon stripped to induce a hyperplastic response. The occurrence of hyperplasia even in these models has been inconsistent, especially in the dog, suggesting that PHZ alone does not ensure a hyperplastic response. On the other hand, increased cellular proliferation in canine arteries, which was maximal in PHZ, could be confirmed. Nevertheless, up to now, there is still a 'missing link' in the cause and effect of intimal hyperplasia.[46]

An anastomotic compliance mismatch can also theoretically induce disturbed flow that may be associated with increased activation or deposition of platelets or other thrombosis-related events, which in turn could promote a hyperplastic response. As mentioned above, increased thrombosis occurred in less compliant grafts.

LONG-TERM IMPLANTATION STUDIES

It has recently been learned that graft compliance and the presence of compliance mismatch at the host/graft anastomoses may influence graft patency[43] through haemodynamic factors which contribute directly to platelet activation and thrombus deposition, or through the stimulation of intimal hyperplasia.[36] This led to the preferential use, by some, of biological grafts whose compliance more nearly matches that of human arteries in the lower extremities.[50] However, the problem of structural degeneration in long-term clinical implants[8,9,51–54] has now prompted the re-evaluation of biologically derived prostheses.

The current chemical treatment of biologic material allows retention of mechanical properties, such as compliance, in terms of quantity as well as quality. Some plastic grafts have been designed to a numerical compliance value similar to that of a normal healthy vessel; but none has normal quality. Biological materials which possess mechanical properties in terms of quality (i.e. nonlinear response to increasing pressure) were investigated in a long-term canine study[55] because clinically implanted biological prostheses of biological origin have recently been shown to develop aneurysms within several years. However, grafts of biological origin may have an advantage, in that they inherently possess compliance characteristics closer to those of artery, which can, in theory at least, be preserved while stabilizing their structure through collagen crosslinking.[56,57] To study the behaviour of biomechanical properties after implantation, bovine heterografts ('Solco-P', Solco-Basel AG, Birsfelden, CH), derived from carotid arteries that were ficin-digested and chemically treated to crosslink collagen, and implanted in canine iliofemoral arteries for 27–45 months, were studied *in vivo* and *in vitro*. A number of different agents has been used to crosslink the collagen of biological prostheses, most notably dialdehyde starch (Johnson and Johnson's bovine carotid artery. 'Artegraft'[58]) and glutaraldehyde (Meadox Medical's human umbilical vein: 'Biograft'[59]) both of which have had clinical use. Both have also been found to undergo structural changes after implantation, including calcification of the vessel wall and/or aneurysmal degeneration, either of which may cause a loss of compliance.[60] It appears, therefore, that these common crosslinking agents provide insufficient protection to the prosthetic implant when it is exposed to attack by the host's defence mechanisms. In this study, a novel crosslinking process based on the use of adipyl dichloride has been applied to bovine carotid arteries,[61] resulting in a conduit with compliance similar to that of human saphenous vein. This graft has been the subject of several investigations, including canine[62] and clinical studies, and attempts to develop an *in vitro* assay of a biological graft's potential for aneurysm formation.[60] In one of these studies, patency and histological results were reported after 12 months of implantation.[61] In this same study, seven grafts survived for up to 44 months and were extensively evaluated on explantation.[56] Seven of seven grafts were patent with only one showing evidence of focal aneurysm. Measurements of mechanical properties, including water permeability, compliance, and burst pressure, and of heat shrink temperature and dry weight were obtained before and after a period of controlled exposure to bacterial collagenase; all data suggested that much of the original graft had been replaced with host tissue. However, enzyme susceptibility was less than that of fresh bovine arteries, indicating that at least in some of the grafts crosslinked collagen was preserved. The compliance of these explants was similar to that reported for autogenous vein and also retained mechanical properties in a qualitative manner (Fig. 13). Histological examination of the graft wall revealed a central zone devoid of cellular infiltration, despite encapsulation by cellular 'intimal' and adventitial zones containing host-generated collagen. It had been thought that, for a biologically derived prosthesis to be successful, it must be able to resist totally degradation by the host. While this may still be desirable, the results suggest that a successful graft can well tolerate a controlled rate of resorption, when matched by a similar rate of new collagen formation. In fact, graft replacement by host collagen may be the most desirable occurrence, as this process would ultimately reduce any

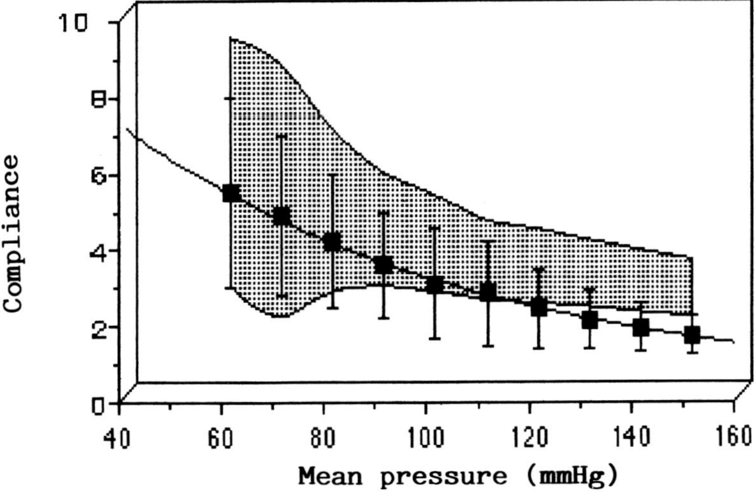

Fig. 13. Dynamic compliance of seven explanted bovine grafts 27–45 months after implantation (averaged data). Shaded region represents the 95% confidence band of compliance for 10 similar, unimplanted controls ($y = 12.074 + 10^{(-6.1043e\text{-}3x)}$ $R^2 = 0.997$).

potential for immunological or inflammatory attack. In this regard, the biological graft is not unlike grafts made from bio-absorbable synthetics, which may act as a scaffold for the development of a living graft or 'pseudo-artery'.[63–66]

The concept of the biological prosthesis as a resorbable scaffold for arterial remodelling clearly needs further study, as does the potential usefulness of *in vitro* tests of explanted materials. Similarly, whether our results from canine studies have application for the most stringent of models—clinical implantation—must still be determined.

A compliant synthetic graft, similar in quantity, was also tested in a long-term implantation study.[67] A recently developed microporous, microfibrous vascular prostheses from PUR has proved to be comparably compliant to human host artery. To study the process of tissue incorporation and the behaviour of biomechanical properties, 24 PUR grafts and 24 ePTFE grafts of two different brands were implanted in the femoral and carotid arteries of dogs in random fashion. Biomechanical properties were obtained *in vivo* after implantation with a 40-month follow-up. There was significant difference in compliance between unimplanted controls of PUR vs ePTFE grafts (Fig. 14) ($p<0.001$). However, it should be noted that both graft types display a linear response to the alteration of blood pressure. After implantation there was significant loss of compliance of the PUR grafts correlated with the implantation time (Fig. 15) ($p=0.003$, $R^2=0.883$); PTFE grafts also stiffened after implantation. There was no difference in patency after 40 months (PUR 26±9.71%, PTFE 39±10.81%, $x^2=0.4$, $p=0.6$). Collagenase treatment improved compliance of explanted PUR grafts to the value of unimplanted controls but did not do so in ePTFE grafts. The conclusion is that host tissue incorporation failed to preserve compliance in PUR grafts.

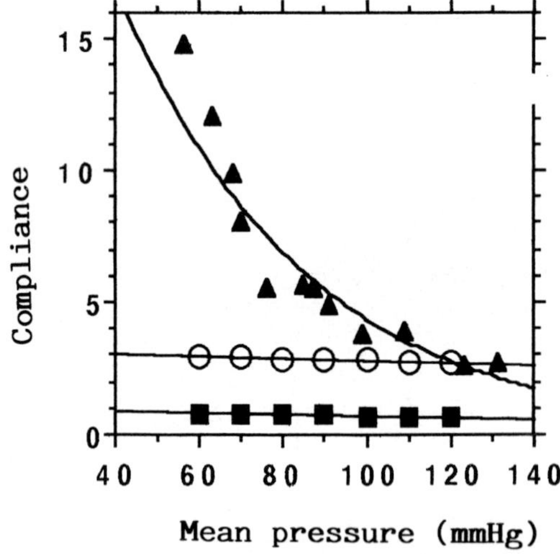

Fig. 14. Comparative drawing of compliance-pressure curves of PUR (○) and ePTFE (■) grafts and an *in vivo* compliance-pressure curve of the common femoral artery of a mongrel dog (FA) (▲), demonstrating the mismatch of compliance between ePTFE-grafts and the canine artery and the match of compliance between PUR-grafts and the canine artery at higher pressure levels but still mismatch in compliance at the critical lower pressure level. Note the nonlinear regression curve of the host artery ($y=42.032*10^{(-9.8351e\text{-}3x)}$ $R^2=0.916$).

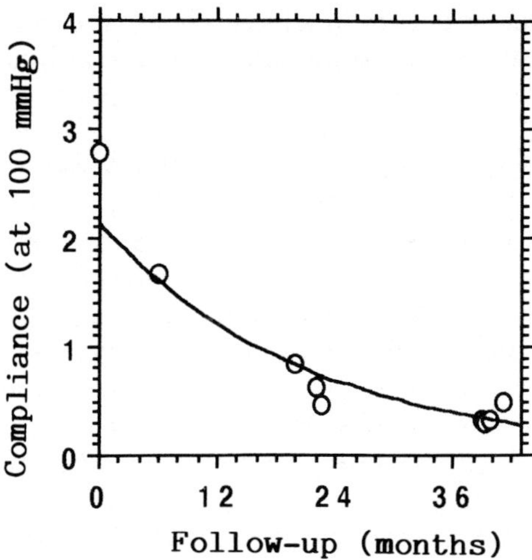

Fig. 15. After implantation there was significant loss of compliance of the PUR-grafts correlated with implantation time ($y = 2.1379 * 10^{(-2.0563e\text{-}2x)}$ $R^2 = 0.883$).

The control of properties as a function of time is of particular importance since the initial compliance mismatch increases with time, due to the growth of firm, fibrous tissue into graft, as has also been verified on knitted Dacron grafts,[68] a phenomenon which further reduces graft compliance to approximately one-third of its original value. This is particularly disturbing since tissue ingrowth is a desirable feature because the body must heal the prosthetic grafts. These apparently contradictory requirements must be met.

It is very intriguing to notice, however, that when autogenous vein grafts are implanted, the tissue ingrowth does not alter the compliance to such a high degree. Vein graft thickening in the arterial circulation is an adaptive process described first by Carrel and Guthrie in 1906[69] and may be of central importance to the development of pathologic subintimal hyperplasia.[70] Experimental and clinical data[71] demonstrate the development of subintimal hyperplasia in the first 6 months after implantation regardless of whether the *in situ* or the reversed technique was used. There was no decrease in compliance over time whereas vein grafts were found less compliant than previously suspected. The superior performance of vein grafts could not be due to absolute values of compliance which are surprisingly low but to the quality which is nonlinear in response to pressure alterations. However, one can as well advocate, that it seems much more likely that the superiority of veins has more to do with their being of living tissue and providing an intact endothelial surface when prepared properly, and less to do with being compliant.

The host artery itself exhibits, apart from the natural variability in compliance, changes of biomechanical properties. Compliance decreases significantly, for example, when the vessel is surgically exposed.[72] This is caused by arterial spasm, because it can be minimized by protecting the vessel in a warm, moist environment, such as ultrasonic gel. After simple exposure of the artery and wound closure, compliance diminished to approximately 50% of its initial value by 2 weeks.[73] At 4 weeks, in some cases, there was a partial reversal of this decreased compliance.

Whether reversal ultimately occurs in all vessels, or if compliance ever returns to initial levels, is not known because the studies were not carried further.

HEALING RESPONSE AND SUBINTIMAL HYPERPLASIA

From the perspective of arterial grafting the significance of mismatch in compliance reduces flow and increases the probability for thrombotic failure. The influence of wall motion (or lack thereof) is detrimental to the healing response of the host artery. This latter effect is evidenced probably in the occurrence of subintimal hyperplasia at anastomotic junctions and in vein grafts but may also influence the incorporation of a graft by host tissue and the development of the graft pseudo(neo)intima.

Wall motion associated with a compliant vessel can affect the growth, orientation and synthetic activity of smooth muscle and endothelial cells.[74–76] *In vitro* studies have shown that pulsation increases the production of collagen[74] and prostacyclin,[77] events related to hyperplasia and patency. Studies on growing rabbits and rats with bioresorbable aortic prostheses demonstrate an increased production of elastin in vessels with greater wall motion.[65,74] Similarly, studies on the growing spontaneously hypertensive rat demonstrate that cells of some arteries respond to higher pressure by producing a thicker extracellular matrix.[78] Furthermore, the secretion by endothelial cells of growth and relaxing factors that influence smooth muscle cell behaviour may depend on motion-related stresses to which they are exposed.[10,79,80] Also, flow separation and shear stress induced by even less ideal end-to-side anastomoses enhance subintimal hyperplasia by endothelial injury which exposes myoblasts and myofibroblasts to the influence of blood-borne substances

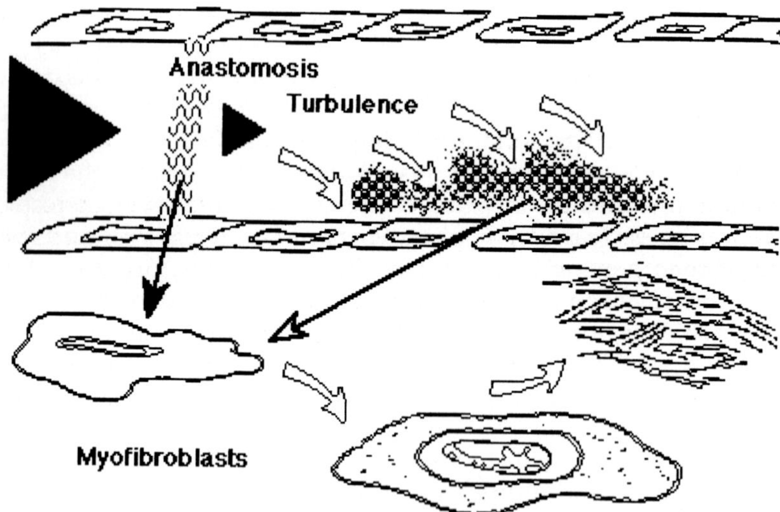

Fig. 16. The development of subintimal hyperplasia. Schematic representation of interaction of endothelial and medial cells due to disturbed flow caused by an anastomosis displaying compliance mismatch. Haemodynamic (flow disturbance), biomechanical (compliance mismatch, PHZ) and endothelial (open gap junctions) parameters influence the morphogenesis of subintimal hyperplasia.

(platelets, platelet-derived growth factors, complement, monocytes) (Fig. 16).[80] Thus luminal surface cells, which are subject to interactions with blood, also influence the behaviour of medial cells, which in turn assure wall compliance. Compliance probably also influences the healing of arterial grafts, defined as host incorporation and endothelialization of its surface. Little is known about the interrelationship between cells of the arterial wall and surface and of their interactions with grafts.

SUMMARY

Summarizing the results of the studies it is likely that match or mismatch between the anisotropic behaviour of the host artery and the linear or nonlinear response to varying blood pressure of the graft influences patency results. Any mismatch in tubular compliance in a quantitative manner will contribute to the long-term results but in a lesser degree. Disturbance of the biomechanical properties of the arterial tree due to vascular anastomosis seems to be of upmost importance to the outcome, but up to now we have not been able to demonstrate a link conclusively between compliance mismatch and the occurrence of subintimal hyperplasia. The present results imply a major impact on future graft design and the development of better anastomotic techniques, because compliance is a critical parameter for maintenance of arterial reconstructions.

The potential importance of compliance mismatch raises a number of questions:

1. How much compliance mismatch (in quantity, in quality, tubular, anastomotic?) can be tolerated, and how does surface thrombogenicity influence this parameter?
2. How will healing modify arterial compliance and must graft compliance parallel these changes?
3. Given the nonlinear elasticity of arteries, should a graft or stent mimic this behaviour?
4. Is there compelling evidence that anastomotic compliance is a major component of overall compliance mismatch?
5. Should more attention be directed to the development of a more compliant suture material (including absorbable suture material) or anastomotic technique?
6. How can compliance and nonlinear elasticity of a future graft be preserved?
7. Should future graft design include the potential of the body to rebuild a blood vessel—and what are the limitations of this potential?
8. Finally, should a graft's compliance match that of normal artery or that of diseased vessels?

ACKNOWLEDGEMENTS

We recognize the efforts of a number of investigators who contributed substantively, through many years of research, to the development of the methods used in this article: W. M. Abbott, J. Megerman, G. I. Italien, D. F. Warnock, J. E. Hasson,

R. D. Maloney, R. N. Baird, I. G. Kidson, D. Bouchier-Hayes, R. Walden, K. H. Hanel, R. P. Cambria, V. Sciacca, B. Seifert, K. Skevas and B. Klein. The presented work was done in the Vascular Research Laboratory (Figs 10, 11, 12, 13) of the Massachusetts General Hospital, Harvard Medical School, Boston, USA (Directors: W. M. Abbott MD and J. Megerman PhD) and the Gerhard-Hess Laboratory (Figs 2, 3, 4, 6, 7, 8, 9, 13, 14, 15) (Head: Dr.med.Th.Schmitz-Rixen) in the Department of Surgery, University of Cologne, FRG (Director: Prof.Dr.Dr.H. Pichlmaier). All animal procedures were carried out under full sterile protocol, and in compliance with the FRG Law for the Prevention of Cruelty to Animals (BGBl. 1 S. 1277, 1972).

REFERENCES

1. DeWeese JA, Blaisdell FW, Foster JH: Report of the Intersociety Commission for Heart Disease Resources: Optimal resources for vascular surgery. Arch Surg 105:948–955, 1972
2. Pourdeylrini B, Wagner D: On the correlation between the failure of vascular grafts and their structural and material properties: A critical analysis. J Biomed Mat Res 20:375–409, 1986
3. Hollier LH, Fowl RJ, Pennell RC *et al*: Are seeded endothelial cells the origin of neointima on prosthetic vascular grafts? J Vasc Surg 3:65–73, 1986
4. Zilla P, Siedler S, Fasol R, Sharefkin JB: Reduced reproductive capacity of freshly harvested endothelial cells in smokers: a possible shortcoming in the success of seeding? J Vasc Surg 10:143–148, 1989
5. Kent KC, Shindo S, Ikemoto T, Whittemore AD: Species variation and the success of endothelial cell seeding. J Vasc Surg 9:271–276, 1989
6. Callow AD: Endothelial cell seeding: problems and expectations. J Vasc Surg 6:318–319, 1987
7. Quinones-Baldrich WJ, Busuttil RW, Baker JD *et al*: Is the preferential use of polytetrafluoroethylene grafts for femoropopliteal bypass justified? J Vasc Surg 8:219–228, 1988
8. Giordano JM, Keshishian JM: Aneurysm formation in human umbilical vein grafts. Surgery 91:443–445, 1982
9. Broyn T, Christensen O, Fossdal JE *et al*: Early complications with a new bovine arterial graft (Solcograft P). Acta Chir Scand 152:263–266, 1986.
10. Sottiurai VS, Yao JST, Batson R *et al*: Distal anastomosis intimal hyperplasia: histopathologic character and biogenesis. Ann Vasc Surg 1:26–33, 1989
11. Hasson JE, Megerman J, Abbott WM: Suture technique and para-anastomotic compliance. J Vasc Surg 3:591–598, 1986
12. Baird RN, Abbott WM: Pulsatile blood flow in arterial grafts. Lancet ii:948, 1976
13. LoGerfo FW, Quist WC, Nowak MD: Downstream anastomotic hyperplasia: A mechanism of failure in Dacron arterial grafts. Ann Surg 197:479, 1983
14. Kinley CE, Paasche PE, MacDonald AS *et al*: Stress at vascular anastomosis in relation to host artery: Synthetic graft diameter. Surgery 75:28, 1974
15. Kinley CE, Marble AB: Compliance: A continuing problem with vascular grafts. J Cardiovasc Surg 21:163, 1980
16. Madras P, Ward C, Johnson W, Singh P: Anastomotic hyperplasia. Surgery 90:922, 1981
17. Sottiurai VS, Fry WJ, Stanley JC: Ultrastructure of medial smooth muscle and myofibroblasts in human arterial dysplasia. Arch Surg 113:1280–1288, 1978
18. Harvey W: De motu cordis. Keynes G. (Ed.). London: Nonesuch Press, 1628
19. Hales S: Statical essays. History of Medicine Series, Library of the New York Academy of Medicine. New York: Hafner Publishing, p. 22, 1733
20. Frank O: Die Grundform des arteriellen Pulses. Z Biol 37:483–526, 1899
21. Taylor MG: An approach to the analysis of the arterial pulse wave. Phys Med Biol 1:258–269, 321–329, 1957

22. Cox RH: Blood flow and pressure propagation in the canine femoral artery. J Biomech 3:131–49, 1970
23. Megerman J, Abbott WM: Compliance in vascular grafts. *In* Vascular Grafting, Wright C (Ed.). Boston: John Wright-PSB, pp. 344–364, 1983
24. Hokanson DE, Mozersky DJ, Summer DS, Strandness DE Jr: A phase-locked echo tracking system for recording arterial diameter changes *in vivo*. J Appl Physiol 32:728–733, 1972
25. Pagani M, Mirsky I, Baig H *et al*: Effect of age on aortic pressure-diameter and elastic stiffness-stress relationships in unanesthetized sheep. Circ Res 44:420, 1979
26. Kidson IG: The effect of wall mechanical properties on patency of arterial grats. Ann R Coll Surg (Engl) 65:24–29, 1983
27. Murgo JP, Cox RH, Peterson LH: Cantilever transducer for continuous measurement of arterial diameter *in vivo*. J Appl Physiol 31:948, 1971
28. Drues ME, Young DF: Prediction of arterial compliance from pressure and flow waveform. Biomed Sci Instrum 25:233–238, 1989
29. Schmitz-Rixen Th: Unpublished developments.
30. Brant AM, Rodgers VGJ, Borovetz HS: Measurement *in vitro* of pulsatile arterial diameter using a helium-neon laser. J Appl Phys 62(2):679–683, 1987
31. Dobrin PB: Mechanical properties of arteries. Physiol Rev 58:397–449, 1978
32. Megerman J, Abbott WM: Clinical importance of the compliant conduit. *In* Vascular Dynamics. Westerhof N, Gross DR (Eds). New York: Plenum Publishing Corp. pp. 263–276, 1989
33. Schmitz-Rixen Th, Wolff M, Ersami H, Pichlmaier H: Compliance of atherosclerotic arteries, presented at the annual VIIIth postgraduate meeting: Association of International Vascular Surgeons in Madonna di Campiglio, (Finnlandia Prize). 1991 (in prep).
34. Newton WT, Stokes JM, Butcher HR: Changes in the elasticity of arterial substitutes following implantation. Surgery 46:579–588, 1959
35. Waddell W, Vogelfanger I, Bose M *et al*: Changes in contractility, compliance, and elasticity in experimental arterial vein autografts. Can J Surg 16:252, 1973
36. Lye CR, Sumner DS, Hokanson DE: The transcutaneous measurement of the distal properties of the human saphenous vein femoral-popliteal bypass graft. Surg Gynecol Obstet 141:891–895, 1975
37. Hokanson DE, Strandness DE: Stress-strain characteristics of various arterial grafts. Surg Gynecol Obst 127:57–60, 1968
38. Annis D, Bornat A, Edwards R: An elastomeric vascular prosthesis. Trans Am Soc Artif Intern Organs 24:209, 1978
39. Seifert KB, Albo D, Knowlton H, Lyman DJ: Effect of elasticity of prosthetic wall on patency of small-diameter arterial prostheses. Surg Forum 30:206, 1979
40. Kidson IG, Abbott WM: Low compliance and arterial graft occlusion. Circulation 58(Suppl. I): 1, 1978
41. Walden R, L'Italien GJ, Megerman J, Abbott WM: Matched elastic properties and successful arterial grafting. Arch Surg 115:1166–1169, 1980
42. Baird R, Abbott W: Elasticity and compliance of canine femoral and jugular vein segments. Am J Physiol 233:H15–H21, 1977
43. Abbott WM, Megerman JM, Hasson JE, L'Italien G, Warnock D: Effect of compliance mismatched upon vascular graft patency. J Vasc Surg 5:376–382, 1987
44. Uchida N, Emoto H, Kambic H *et al*: Compliance effect on patency of small diameter vascular grafts. ASAIO Trans 35:556–558, 1989
45. Fisher AC, How TV, deCossart L, Annis D: The longer term patency of a compliant small diameter arterial prosthesis. Trans Am Soc Artif Intern Organs 31:324–328, 1985
46. Abbott WM, Megerman J: Adaptives responses of arteries to grafting. J Vasc Surg 9:377–378, 1989
47. Hasson J, Megerman J, Abbott W: Increased compliance near vascular anastomoses. J Vasc Surg 2:419–423, 1985
48. Hamilton G, Schmitz-Rixen Th, Megerman J *et al*: Comparison of anastomotic compliance of different suture materials. Eur J Vasc Surg (submitted for publication)

49. Batson RC, Sottiurai VS, Craighead CC: Linton patch angioplasty: An adjunct to distal bypass with polytetrafluorethylene grafts. Ann Surg 199:684–693, 1984
50. Abbott WM, Bouchier-Hayes DJ: The role of mechanical properties in graft design. *In* Graft Materials in Vascular Surgery, Miami H, Dardik H (Eds). Symposia Specialists, pp. 59–78, 1978
51. Layer ET, King RJ, Jamieson CW: Early aneurysmal degeneration of human umbilical vein bypass grafts. Br J Surg 71:709–710, 1984
52. Dardik H, Ibrahim IM, Sussman B *et al*: Biodegradation and aneurysm formation in umbilical vein grafts: observations and a realistic strategy. Ann Surg 199:61–68, 1984
53. Hasson JE, Newton WD, Waltman MD *et al*: Mural degeneration in the glutaraldehyd-tanned umbilical vein graft: incidence and implications. J Vasc Surg 4:243–50, 1985
54. Schroeder A, Imig H, Peiper U *et al*: Results of a bovine collagen vascular graft (Solcograft P) in infrainguinal positions. Eur J Vasc Surg 2:315–321, 1988
55. Schmitz-Rixen Th, Megerman J, Anderson J *et al*: Longterm study of a compliant biological vascular graft. Eur J Vasc Surg 1991 (in press)
56. Barker WF, Crawford ES, Mannick JA, Wylie FJ: The current status of femoropopliteal bypass for arteriosclerotic occlusive disease: a panel discussion. Surgery 79:30–36, 1976
57. Abbott W, Cambria R: Control of physical characteristics (elasticity and compliance) of vascular grafts. Biol Synth Vasc Prostheses 189–220, 1982
58. Dale WA, Lewis MR: Further experiences with bovine arterial grafts. Surgery 80:711–721, 1976
59. Dardik H, Baier RE, Mennaghan M *et al*: Morphologic and biophysical assessment of long-term human umbilical cord vein implants used as vascular conduits. Surg Gynecol Obstet 154:17–26, 1982
60. Hamilton G, Megerman J, L'Italien GJ *et al*: Prediction of aneurysm formation in vascular grafts of biologic origin. J Vasc Surg 7:400–408, 1988
61. Geroulanos S, von Meiss U, Walter P *et al*: A new vascular prosthesis for small diameter vessel replacement. Trans Am Soc Artif Intern Organs 28:200–204, 1982
62. Erasmi H, Horsch S, Müller J *et al*: Gefäßersatz bei kleinkalibrigen Arterien—eine neue bovine Kollagenprothese. Langenbecks, Arch Chir 360:97–107, 1983
63. Greisler HP, Ellinger J, Schwarcz Th *et al*: Arterial regeneration over polydioxanone prostheses in the rabbit. Arch Surg 122:715–721, 1987
64. van der Lei B, Wildevuur C, Nieuwenhuis P: Compliance and biodegradation of vascular grafts stimulate the regeneration of elastic laminae in neoarterial tissue: An experimental study in rats. Surgery 99:45–52, 1986
65. Galletti PM, Aebischer P, Sasken HF, Goddard MB, Chiu T: Experience with fully resorbable aortic grafts in the dog. Surgery 103:231–241, 1988
66. van der Lei B, Nieuwenhuis P, Molenaar I, Wildevuur CRH: Long term biologic fate of neoarteries regenerated in microporous, compliant, biodegradable, small caliber vascular grafts in rats. Surgery 101:459–469, 1987
67. Schmitz-Rixen Th, Skevas K, Lehnhardt FJ, Erasmi H, Braun B: Compliance changes in microporous polyesterurethan grafts. Abstract Band: ESVS '90 (European Society for Vascular Surgery—IV Annual Meeting), 60, 1990. EIVS accepted for publication.
68. Sawyer PN, Srinivasan S: The role of electromechanical surface properties in thrombosis at vascular interfaces: Cumulative experience of studies in animal and man. Bull N Y Acad Med 48:235–256, 1972
69. Carrel A, Guthrie C: Uniterminal and biterminal venous transplantations. Surg Gynecol Obstet 2:266, 1906
70. Zwolak RM, Adams MC, Clowes AW: Kinetics of vein graft hyperplasia: Association with tangential stress. J Vasc Surg 5:126–136, 1987
71. Cambria RP, Megerman J, Abbott WM: Endothelial preservation in reversed and *in situ* autogenous vein grafts. Ann Surg 202:50–55, 1985
72. Megerman J, Hasson J, Warnock D, L'Italien G, Abbott W: Noninvasive measurements of nonlinear arterial elasticity. Am J Physiol 250:H181–188, 1986
73. Hasson JE, Megerman J, Abbott WM: Postsurgical changes in arterial compliance. Arch Surg 119:788–791, 1984

74. Leung DY, Glagov S, Mathews MB: Cyclic stretching stimulates synthesis of matrix components by arterial smooth muscle cells *in vitro*. Science 191:475–477, 1976
75. Sumpio BE, Banes AJ, Levin LG, Johnson G Jr: Mechanical stress stimulates aortic endothelial cells to proliferate. J Vasc Surg 3:253–256, 1987
76. Eskin SG, Ives CL, McIntire LV, Navarro LT: Response to cultured endothelial cells to steady flow. Microvasc Res 28:87–94, 1984
77. Frangos JA, Eskin SG, McIntire LV, Ives Cl: Flow effects on prostacyclin production by cultured human endothelial cells. Science 227:1477–1479, 1985
78. McGuire PG, Brocks D, Killen PD, Orkin RW: Increased deposition of basement membrane macromolecules in specific vessels of spontaneously hypertensive rat. Am J Path 135:291–299, 1989
79. Sottiurai VS, Kollros P, Glagov S, Zarins CK, Mathews MB: Morphologic alteration of cultured arterial smooth muscle cells by cyclic stretching. J Surg Res 35:490–497, 1983
80. Sottiurai VS, Batson RC: Role of myofibroblasts in pseudointima formation. Surgery 94:792–801, 1983

Vein Collars Make Femorocrural ePTFE Grafts Worthwhile

Mark R. Tyrrell and John H. N. Wolfe

Arterial operations have been possible for the last hundred years[1] and femoropopliteal bypasses for 84 years.[2] Nevertheless, the principles commonly applied to arterial bypass surgery are essentially those derived from plumbing—the simple shunting of blood around an area of occlusion. While the tolerance allowed by the passage of large volumes of blood through large calibre vessels is reasonably successful in the case of aortic and iliac reconstructions, the dismal results reported for prosthetic reconstructions to crural vessels are an indicator of our failure to appreciate the complexities of the biology of the living arterial wall and pulsatile blood flow.

In general, the more proximal the disease and reconstruction, the greater the chances of long-term success. In the case of reconstruction to arteries below the knee, average patency rates of 68.4% at 5 years follow-up have been reported, but only where the conduit is vein.[3] Prosthetic bypass (principally using expanded polytetrafluoroethylene—ePTFE) of the same segment is associated with a considerably poorer outcome (mean average patency at 5 years 26.6%).[3] Some have reported reasonable results using prosthesis to a single calf vessel—in the region of 40%—but figures vary widely. Many surgeons will admit that their patency rates and limb salvage rates using ePTFE to an isolated crural vessel are so poor that primary amputation might be considered a better option if no adequate vein is available.[4] This was also our personal experience and we had abysmal patency rates using direct anastomosis of ePTFE to an isolated crural vessel in the lower third of the calf.

Miller *et al.*[5] then published his results using a vein collar at the distal anastomosis. At the same time Taylor *et al.* were experimenting with the use of a vein patch at the lower anastomosis in order to broaden and lengthen the anastomosis[6] (Figs 1a and 1b). Both these authors have reported outstanding results[7,8] and we have used the Miller collar to improve our results dramatically for a group of patients in whom primary amputation was the only alternative.[9]

It must, of course, be accepted that early enthusiasts often publish better results than those of later series. Clearly there are pitfalls in comparing different series since surgical technique, the technician, and also poorly defined factors such as disease severity and underlying systemic disorders affecting blood flow and coagulability, will undoubtedly affect outcome. Nevertheless, as each of these techniques appears to offer some benefit in circumstances widely believed to be hopeless (namely prosthetic reconstruction to single calf vessels) they deserve consideration. An analysis of their structure and consequent theoretical haemodynamic advantages in the light of our understanding of the causes of prosthetic graft occlusion holds the potential for the design of better surgical approaches to this difficult and increasingly common clinical problem.

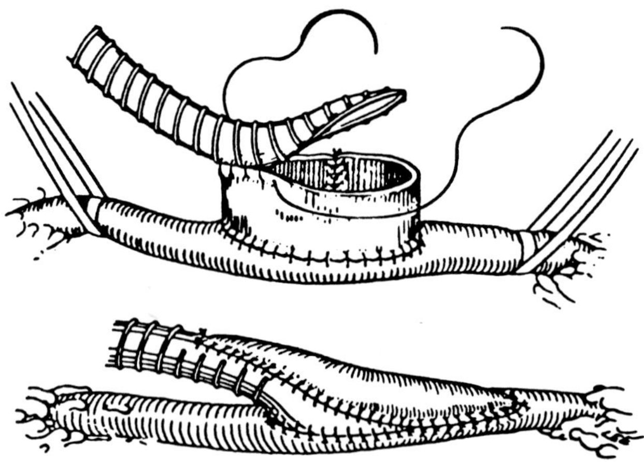

Fig. 1a & 1b. Two methods of juxtaposing vein between PTFE and artery at the distal anastomosis. a (Upper): The Miller collar. b (Lower): The Taylor patch. (Reproduced with permission from Eur J Vasc Surg.)

IS VEIN ALWAYS AVAILABLE?

As a backlash from the lazy abuse of ePTFE instead of vein there have been many surgeons who have suggested that veins are always available for grafts from groin to distal crural vessels at the ankle. At St Mary's Hospital this is not the case and we assume that other surgeons encounter similar problems to ourselves. An increasing number of patients have previously undergone cardiac surgery or peripheral arterial reconstruction and have iatrogenically induced arm thrombophlebitis. When this has been associated with venepuncture in the anticubital fossa and harvesting of the saphenous veins there may be few further sources of autogenous vein. Under these circumstances we would have previously resorted to primary amputation in patients with only a short segment of crural vessel patent, but our results using a vein collar are sufficiently encouraging for us to revascularize the legs of these patients with severe end-stage arterial disease.

MECHANISMS OF GRAFT FAILURE

The ultimate event in graft failure is graft thrombosis. As long ago as the 1840s Virchow identified the causes of thrombosis within the vascular system, to paraphrase: an abnormal vessel wall; slow flow; and an excessive coagulability of the blood.[10] Although blood coagulability is evidently of considerable importance the first two are the principal technical concern to the vascular surgeon.

The importance of vessel wall thrombogenicity is widely recognized. Dacron is highly thrombogenic, but yields good patency rates when used in the proximal vascular system where flow rates are high. Expanded polytetrafluoroethylene (ePTFE) is one of the least thrombogenic materials yet devised but nevertheless has patency rates that are poor when it is used for femorodistal reconstruction. This illustrates the sensitivity of the interaction between rate of flow and vessel wall thrombogenicity. It is clear that a highly thrombogenic surface will not cause graft failure if flow rates are high, but that a relatively nonthrombogenic one will result in thrombosis if flow is sluggish. It is therefore necessary to examine the reasons for slow graft flow.

Clearly the resistance to flow imposed by the size of the outflow vessel and recipient arterial bed is very important. In health this contribution to resistance to flow is ultimately dictated by the state of dilatation of the precapillary arterioles in the recipient arterial bed. In disease, however, stenosis of arteries proximal to the precapillary arterioles may result in a greater degree of resistance to flow than that imposed by the precapillary sphincters. In this instance the resistance to flow is fixed and may be beyond the physiological tolerances for slow flow—a virtually nonthrombogenic graft may then thrombose. As already indicated, the presence of an abnormally thrombogenic arterial graft wall considerably increases the risk of thrombosis. Therefore, under conditions where flow is sluggish because of limitations in the size of the recipient arterial bed venous grafts are less likely to occlude than prosthetic ones. The importance of a living endothelial cell lining has prompted a great deal of research into methods of seeding a lining onto prosthetic materials—to date this research has not yielded a clinically useful result.

The development of peri-graft or graft stenoses during the first year is also a critically important consideration—these may be in the mobilized donor or recipient arteries, the graft itself, or at the anastomoses. Once again, venous grafts with stenoses are less likely to suffer the final disaster of thrombosis than prosthetic ones since patency can be maintained at very slow flow rates. Furthermore, myo-intimal hyperplasia, the major curse of arterial surgery, appears to be more common at the distal anastomosis of prosthetic grafts than in vein grafts.

Early graft failures (up to 30 days) are usually attributed to errors of technique or patient selection and they account for 20% of graft failures. Occlusions occurring 2 years after the insertion of the graft can usually be blamed on progression of the underlying atheromatous process.[11] But, those grafts that occlude between a month and 2 years are often related to graft-related stenoses and many of these can be ascribed to myo-intimal hyperplasia (see chapter by Wolfe *et al.*, p. 119).

Assuming a technically satisfactory result, where good graft flow is achieved, then intimal hyperplasia assumes primary importance as a cause for prosthetic graft failure. Unfortunately, the prevention of the accumulation of this material is difficult to address—mainly because its mechanisms of deposition are not well understood. Current theories suggest that platelets have a key role to play. It is thought that their subintimal accumulation and their subsequent release of various factors triggers smooth muscle cell growth.[12,13] The subintimal accumulation of platelets may well be a result of haemodynamic phenomena, but these are poorly understood. Most theorists implicate the lifting of endothelial cells (which overlap like fish scales) by turbulent eddies or low shear stress with a consequent exposure of subintimal tissue to platelets.

Graft-arterial compliance mismatch has been suggested as a cause for abnormal near-wall flow that may result in intimal hyperplasia.[14–17] The static, distorting consequences of an anastomotic compliance mismatch have already been alluded to, but there is also evidence accumulating to suggest a dynamic problem that may accelerate peri-anastomotic deposition of intimal hyperplasia. The mechanisms by which compliance changes exert their effects are not clear, but abrupt changes in vessel wall mechanical characteristics may lead to changes in near-wall flow (shear stress) in a pulsatile system.[18] The potential haemodynamic consequences of an abrupt compliance mismatch have been summarized by Kidson.[17] However, the importance of a compliance mismatch is difficult to assess directly. It is difficult to measure *in vivo* and its haemodynamic relevance is difficult to quantify. In addition, the arterial distortion that arises as a consequence of direct ePTFE-artery anastomoses may directly influence the deposition of intimal hyerplasia.[19,20]

ADVANTAGES OF A COMPLEX ePTFE/VEIN/ARTERIAL ANASTOMOSIS

There are several potential explanations for the apparent success of the Miller collar and Taylor patch. Before attributing success to either the technique or technicians concerned, it is important to consider the question of selection. Selection of patients for referral to centres with special interests may affect results adversely by concentrating patients with extremely difficult distal vessels, or favourably by concentrating patients in whom a reconstruction is more favourable (since the particularly difficult patients are not even referred). To our surprise, we have found that some patients in whom an unsuccessful previous reconstruction has been performed may have excellent distal vessels. Ironically, patients in whom an ill-judged, injudicious attempt at bypass has been attempted may have a more favourable prognosis following a distal reconstruction than those in whom it is a primary procedure since the degree of underlying arterial disease is less. For these reasons we do not believe that it is worthwhile or legitimate to put too much weight on comparisons between results from different surgeons and centres. We must each seek to improve our own results.

Advantages in the immediate stage

The first potential advantage of a vein interposition technique is purely technical. Indeed, Miller originally devised the technique in order to simplify the distal anastomosis and place his sutures more accurately. It is both easier and more aesthetic to anastomose vein to a 1–2 mm artery than to attempt the same anastomosis with ePTFE. We have performed some experiments that support this contention:

By making casts of the internal anatomy of anastomoses of ePTFE to cadaveric internal mammary artery we have been able to compare direct ePTFE to artery anastomoses with the Miller collar and Taylor patch techniques. Ten anastomoses of each type were inflated at 100 mmHg pressure with a silicone based polymer (Dow Corning Hansil Ltd). The polymer was allowed to cure for 24 hours before removing the ePTFE, artery and vein from the cast. Each cast was then examined both intact and by inspection of serial transverse sections. To assess the cross-sections in the immediate vicinity of the anastomotic heel and toe for distortion, we divided their maximal and minimal diameters (as measured using the PCB inspection glass). The

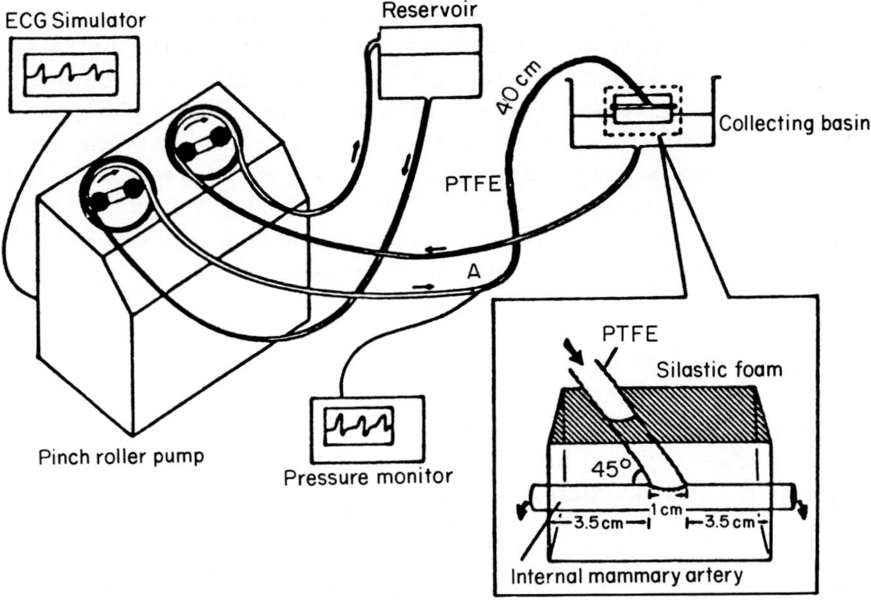

Fig. 2. A schematic representation of the perfusion circuit. This comprised a pinch-roller pump with the capacity to simulate pulsatile flow triggered by a simulated ECG, a pressure monitoring device inserted at the junction of the pump tubing and PTFE, and (enlargement) an anastomosis embedded in silastic foam with standardized geometry. The second pinch-roller pump, collecting vessel and reservoir allowed for continuous perfusion of the anastomoses. Flow estimation was by timed collection. (Reproduced with permission from Eur J Vasc Surg.)

more closely the resulting figure approached 1 the more nearly round was the specimen.

Three of the direct anastomoses showed naked eye evidence of distortion of the recipient artery in the immediate vicinity of the anastomotic toe. Neither of the other techniques showed similar deformity in any of the specimens studied. In the region of the anastomotic toe, the medium 'roundness' (Dmax-min %) was less for the direct anastomoses (81%) than either the Miller collar (92%, $p=0.001$) or the Taylor patch anastomoses (93.5%, $p=0.001$).

This evidence was supported by flow studies (Fig. 2). Anastomoses were constructed using ePTFE and cadaveric internal mammary artery and perfused with time expired blood. The circuit consisted of a Stockert double-headed pinch roller pump (Shiley Ltd) which was able to simulate pulsatile flow triggered by a simulated ECG, a pressure measuring device (Datascope PA2000 pressure monitor and a Gould P50 Transducer, Datascope Ltd), and a Sarns water circulator (Biomedical Ltd) to ensure a constant (37°C) perfusion temperature. All specimens examined were perfused with ABO compatible packed red cells diluted with haemaccel to a haematocrit of 38–42% and anticoagulated with sodium heparin.

To summarize the results: we showed that flow was similar under standard conditions whichever method of anastomosis was used. We then went on to correlate flow with internal mammary artery diameter. One would therefore expect a good correlation between flow and diameter providing there was no resistance at the anastomosis. There was good correlation for all anastomoses at the heel and the correlation was also good for the toe of both the Miller collar ($r=0.84$, $p<0.01$) and the Taylor patch ($r=0.92$, $p=0.005$) but in the case of flow from the toe of direct ePTFE-arterial anastomoses there was no correlation between flow and vessel diameter ($r=0.04$). It is therefore evident that there was resistance to flow at the toe of direct ePTFE-artery anastomoses and it would be logical to assume that this flow limiting area might be the cause of early graft failure.

Advantages in the intermediate stage

There is also some evidence to suggest that these techniques reduce graft occlusion in the intermediate period (1 month to 2 years). The cross-sectional area of the vessel developing myointimal hyperplasia is of great importance: The effects will be more disastrous in a 1-mm artery than a 5-mm graft. The proponents of the composite prosthetic/vein graft consider this to be similar to the two vein collar/patch techniques. But if a segment of small calibre vein is anastomosed end-to-end to the ePTFE it is unlikely that the surgeon will produce a 2-cm distal anastomosis between vein and artery. A 2-cm anastomosis is an easy, almost inevitable outcome of the vein collar/patch techniques.

Despite the many deficiencies in our understanding, it is worth examining the possible advantages of vein interposition in the reduction of graft-arterial compliance mismatch. Although the overall compliance mismatch persists, its transience is reduced. In particular, as the difference in compliance is greater between ePTFE and vein than between vein and artery the accumulation of intimal hyperplasia is, in theory, likely to develop at the interface between ePTFE and vein (where the

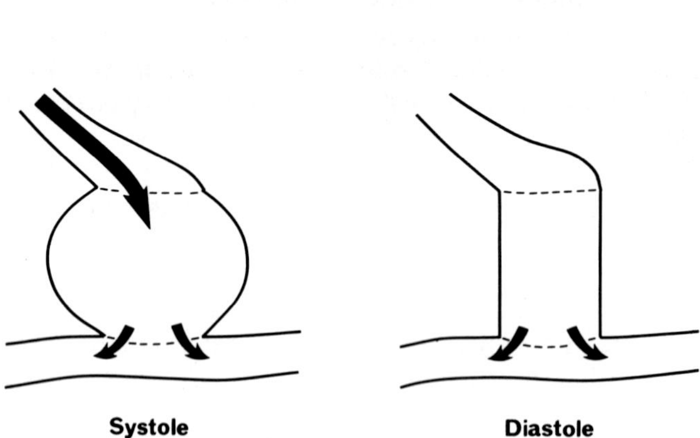

Fig. 3. The *incorrect* peripheral heart theory. During systole the compliant vein collar fills with blood that is discharged during diastole. Our experiment did *not* support this theory.

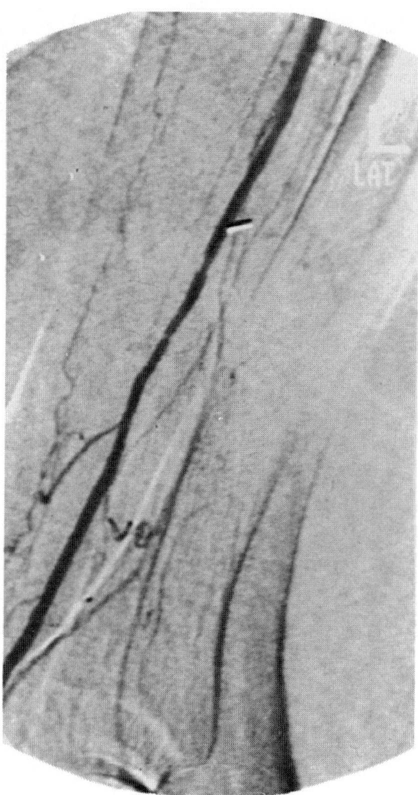

Fig. 4. PTFE/vein collar graft occlusion at 1 year. The ligaclip marks the site of anastomosis — note that the posterior tibial artery has been spared.

diameter is large) rather than at the outflow tract into the small calibre artery. In a canine model Suggs *et al.*[21] produced results that suggested that the vein cuff prevented juxta-anastomotic myointimal hyperplasia in the short term. We have looked at the anastomoses of patients whose grafts finally failed and found that the intimal hyperplasia, as expected, was at the junction between the ePTFE and vein collar and there was relative sparing of the host artery. This sparing was sometimes dramatic (Fig. 4), and allowed successful further reconstruction in a patient who would otherwise have required amputation.

We have some evidence to suggest that by turning the vein through 90° before performing the collar the compliant characteristics of the vein are maximized. We examined the venous elastic properties of 16 specimens of normal vein and nine specimens of vein containing short interposed segments of re-orientated vein. In order to assess the wall elastic properties, we measured strain as a function of distending pressure. This was achieved using the apparatus shown in Fig. 5. This comprised two pressure reservoirs which instantly deliver a preset pressure at the switch of a three-way tap, and an 'in line' pressure measuring device to monitor pressure in the specimen and the pressure reservoirs individually, and a camera and tripod to record dimensional changes.

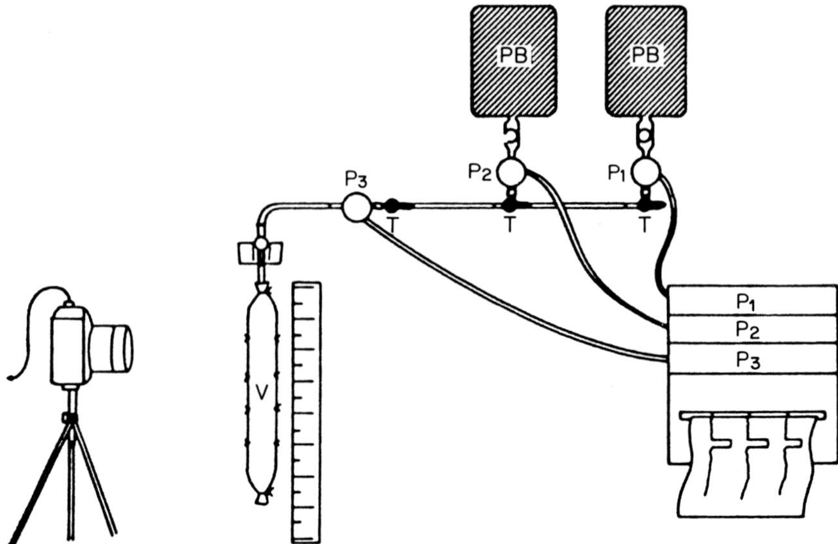

Fig. 5. The vein wall mechanical properties were stressed by the application of two distending pressures (10 mmHg and 150 mmHg). The pressures were preset by the use of pressure bags (PB). Abrupt, accurate changes in pressure were achieved by switching the three-way taps (T). Five minutes after pressurization, a photograph was taken of the vein specimen (V). Changes in dimension were measured directly from the photographs. (Reproduced with permission from Eur J Vasc Surg.)

The measurements for circumferential and longitudinal strain were then compared and longitudinal strain was, on average, $\times 7.2$ the circumferential strain produced by the increase in distending pressure ($p<0.002$). This showed conclusively that human vein, like artery, is anisotropic. In the segments of vein that had a re-orientated segment the strain in that segment was $\times 1.95$ that of the normally orientated segment ($p<0.005$). These results show that the 'compliance' of a vein is greater in its longitudinal length than circumferentially. However, these properties may have been lost when the vein was slit open to form a sheet and we therefore had to perform the second experiment to see how the re-orientated segment of vein performed. Although the differences were less marked they remained significant and we attribute this reduced difference to the suture lines. A further suggested advantage of a compliant venous chamber at the end of the ePTFE graft has been coined the peripheral heart hypothesis (Fig. 3). This theory proposes there is increased flow during diastole due to the discharge of blood from the compliant vein collar—thus reducing the risk of thrombosis. However, this theory is incorrect. The wall elastic characteristics of human long saphenous vein have been investigated *in vitro*[22] and it appears most unlikely that even relatively large venous chambers would significantly increase graft flow.

The oval distortion, however, that we found with direct ePTFE to artery anastomoses, may have an intermediate deleterious effect on graft patency. This oval distortion increases resistance (an oval has a smaller cross-sectional area than a circle of the same circumference) and sheer stresses are redistributed.

Both these mechanisms might accelerate the accumulation of intimal hyperplasia in an area where a small amount of thickening will produce dramatic percentage changes in cross-sectional area. Madras has observed a greater deposition of myointimal hyperplasia on distorted arterial wall which he ascribes to an increase in transmural stress rather than a haemodynamic phenomenon.[19]

Whatever the mechanism there is accumulating evidence to support the impression that the Miller collar reduces arterial stenosis due to intimal hyperplasia and this may be a true reduction or redistribution of the myointimal hyperplasia to an area where luminal narrowing is less critical.

CONCLUSIONS

There is encouraging clinical evidence (Fig. 6) to support our continuing policy of using ePTFE with a vein collar when no autologous arm or leg vein is available for femorocrural grafts. We have attempted to review some of the experimental evidence that might explain why these vein segments are effective. In the immediate

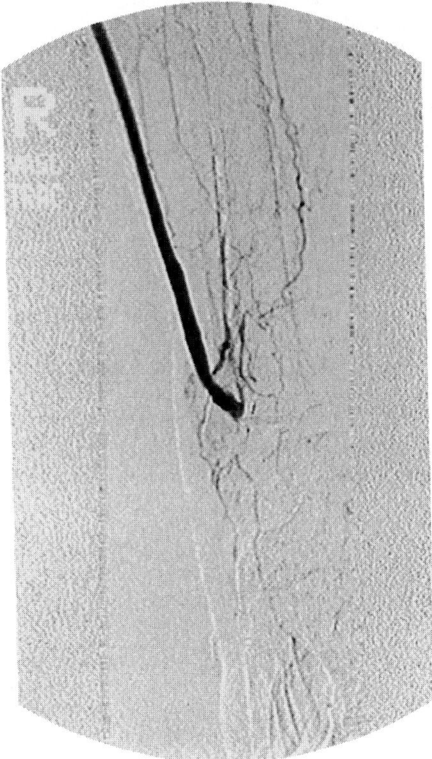

Fig. 6. DSA performed 3 years after a PTFE/vein collar graft was anastomosed to the anterior tibial artery at the ankle. The graft continues to function despite poor run-off vessels.

postoperative phase the advantages might relate to improved technique, the length of the anastomosis and less anastomotic distortion. The intermediate results may be improved by altering the site of intimal hyperplasia thus sparing the small calibre distal artery. Furthermore, this process may be dampened by the interposition of a compliant vein collar.

We then have to consider the two popular techniques—the Miller collar and the Taylor patch. The Miller collar has the disadvantage of an ugly vertical well that produces considerable turbulence when reviewed by duplex. The Taylor patch is haemodynamically more aesthetic but has the disadvantage that there is a considerable area of direct ePTFE-to-artery anastomosis. This area of direct anastomosis may be the source of myointimal hyperplasia and arterial damage. We have sought to embrace the advantages of both these techniques to produce a simple vein collar with no direct anastomosis between ePTFE and artery and a tapering toe. Twenty-one grafts have been inserted with this modified collar and are under review.

REFERENCES

1. Gluck T: Die moderne chirurgie des cirkulationsapparates. Berl Klinik 1:120, 1898 *In* Fundamentals of Vascular Grafting, Wesolowski SA, Dennis C (Eds). New York: McGraw-Hill, 1963
2. Goyanes J: Nuevos trabajos de chirurgica vascular, substuction plastica de las arterias por las venas o arterioplastica venosa, applicada como nuevo metodo, al tratamiento de los aneurysmas. El Siglo Med 53:446, 1906
3. Michaels JA: Choice of material for above-knee femoropopliteal bypass graft. Br J Surg 76:7–14, 1989
4. Bell PRF: Are distal vascular procedures worthwhile? Br J Surg 72:335, 1985
5. Miller JH, Foreman RK, Ferguson L, Faris I: Interposition vein cuff for anastomosis of prosthesis to small artery. Aust NZ J Surg 54:283–285, 1984
6. McFarland RJ, Taylor RS: Une amelioration technique d'anastomose des prostheses arterielles femoro-distales. Phebologie 41:229–233, 1988
7. Taylor RS, McFarland RJ, Cox MI: An investigation into the causes of failure of PTFE grafts. Eur J Vasc Surg 1:335–343, 1987
8. Miller JH, Foreman RK, Ferguson L, Faris I: Interposition vein cuff for anastomoses of prosthesis to small artery. Aust NZ J Surg 54:283–285, 1984
9. Tyrrell MR, Grigg MJ, Wolfe JHN: Is arterial reconstruction to the ankle worthwhile in the absence of autologous vein? Eur J Vasc Surg 3:429–434, 1989
10. Haeger K: The Illustrated History of Surgery. London: Harold Starke, 1989
11. Whittemore AD, Clowes AW, Couch NP, Mannik JA: Secondary femoropopliteal reconstruction. Ann Surg 193:35–42, 1980
12. DeWeese JA: Anastomotic intimal hyperplasia. *In* Vascular Grafts, Sawyer PN, Kaplutt MJ (Eds). New York: Appleton-Century-Crofts, pp. 147–152, 1978
13. Clowes AW, Reidy MA, Clowes MM: Mechanisms of stenosis after arterial injury. Lab Invest 49:208–215, 1983
14. Christenson JT, Elkof B, Ah-Huneidi W, Owunwanne A: Elastic and thrombogenic properties for different vascular grafts and their influence on patency. Int Angiology 6:81–87, 1987
15. Clarke RE, Apostolou S, Kardos JL: Mismatch of mechanical properties as a cause of arterial prosthesis thrombosis. Surg Forum XXVII:208–210, 1976
16. Hasson JE, Abbott WM: Complications of artery-graft compliance mismatch. *In* Complications in Vascular Surgery. London: Grune & Stratton, pp. 549–559, 1985
17. Kidson IG: The effect of wall mechanical properties on patency of arterial grafts. Ann Royal Coll Surg (Engl) 65:24–29, 1983

18. Caro CG, Fitz-Gerald JM, Schruter RO: Arterial wall shear and distribution of early atheroma in man. Nature 223:1159–1161, 1969
19. Bolduc ME, Simpson MA, Espanola C, Petschek HE, Madras FN: The extent and morphology of intimal hyperplasia with the use of arterial patches. J Cardiovasc Surg 30 (Suppl):89–90, 1989
20. Tyrrell MR, Chester JF, Vipond MN *et al*: Experimental evidence of support the use of interposition vein collars/patches in distal PTFE anastomoses. Eur J Vasc Surg 4:95–101, 1990
21. Suggs WD, Henriques HF, DePalma RG: Vein cuff interposition prevents juxta-anastomotic neointimal hyperplasia. Ann Surg 207:717–723, 1988
22. Tyrrell MR, Clark GH, Wolfe JHN: Consideration of the mechanical properties at the distal anastomosis of PTFE grafts may improve patency rates. J Cardiovasc Surg 30 (Suppl):91, 1989

Endothelial Cell Linings of Grafts

M. G. Walker, H. M. H. Carr, M. Welch and R. Vohra

Ever since Herring *et al.* first described the clinical application of endothelial cell seeding for prosthetic grafts in 1978, there has remained an optimism that this technique may ultimately improve patency of small diameter grafts particularly when used for infra-inguinal reconstruction.[1] When a prosthetic graft is implanted in humans, pannus ingrowth of native endothelium is limited to 2–3 mm only,[2] complete endothelialization never being achieved. Why this is so remains unanswered. However, knowledge of endothelial cell physiology has gathered such momentum that its myriad functions are now much clearer (Table 1), in particular the complex mechanism of coagulation in health and disease involving pro- and anticoagulant functions (Table 2).

HARVESTING, CELL SOURCE AND LABELLING OF ENDOTHELIAL CELLS

Whilst successful mechanical harvesting of endothelial cells from veins has been reported,[3] this technique has had limited success[4] and has largely been replaced by enzymatic harvesting using commercially available crude collagenase.[5–8] Sharefkin *et al.* comparing crude and purified collagenases showed no significant difference in mean harvest efficiency between the two, although the latter caused less degradation of fibronectin.[9] Herring *et al.*[10] have suggested a ratio of venous area to graft area of 0.425 in their animal experiments in order to yield sufficient endothelial cells to line an arterial prosthesis.

Two types of endothelial cells may be obtained for use: macrovascular adult human endothelial cells from autogenous vein;[5,6] and microvascular adult human endothelial cells from adipose tissue.[11] Human umbilical vein also provides a source of macrovascular endothelial cells.[5,12] In theory adipose tissue as a source of endothelial cells is very attractive because of abundant cell yield, but to date pure isolates have been impossible to obtain. A variety of methods exist for endothelial cell identification such as a typical morphology, angiotensin converting enzyme activity, prostacyclin synthesis and Ulex staining, the most reliable being their positivity for Factor VIII related antigen.[11,13]

Labelling of endothelial cells with indium-111-oxine first described by Sharefkin *et al.*[14] has proved to be a simple and reliable method for studying cell attachment and retention on vascular grafts. Successful labelling of these cells in suspension, both freshly harvested and cultured, as well as those growing on grafts has been reported.[15–17] Most spontaneous leakage of this isotope occurs in the first 30 min after labelling.[13] It is nontoxic up to 18 h beyond which its toxicity remains unknown.[18]

Table 1. Endothelial cell functions

1. Anti- and procoagulant balance
2. Balance of expression of activities that promote or inhibit the growth of smooth cells and fibroblasts
3. Leucocyte adhesion
4. Cytokine production
5. Expression of histocompatibility antigens

Table 2. Endothelial cell products related to thrombosis

Anticoagulant	*Procoagulant*
1. Heparin-like glycosaminoglycans	Tissue factor
2. Prostacyclin	Von Willebrand factor
3. Plasminogen activator	Plasminogen activator inhibitor
4. Thrombomodulin	Thrombospondin
5. Endothelial derived relaxing factor (EDRF)	Collagens
6. 13-hydroxy-octadecadienoic acid (13-HODE)	

SEEDING TECHNIQUES

Three methods exist whereby endothelial cells may be used to line a prosthetic graft. The first involves enzymatic harvesting of macrovascular endothelial cells in the operating room and seeding the graft immediately prior to implantation. The second is to culture endothelial cells on the graft in laboratory to achieve a confluent lining. The third is to 'sod' the graft with supra-confluent microvascular endothelial cells obtained from adipose tissue.

Although immediate seeding can be performed in the operating room as a single-stage procedure, the graft remains vulnerable during the critical 2–3 weeks after implantation until confluence is achieved. On the other hand, a graft implanted with a confluent endothelial cell monolayer offers immediate protection during the critical period when thrombosis is most likely. Set against this are the disadvantages of patients requiring two operative procedures associated with an increased risk of sepsis. Whilst 'sodding' lends itself largely to the use of microvascular endothelial cells, Zilla *et al*. have reported an *in situ* technique of endothelial cell harvesting using collagenase along with low density plating giving 14 million first passage cells 26 days after harvest.[19]

COATING OF GRAFTS WITH PROTEIN MATRICES

Endothelial cell seeding of uncoated ePTFE and Dacron has met with universal failure.[20–24] In order to enhance cell adherence, precoating of these grafts with either preclot, fibronectin or collagen has been used in our laboratory.[25] Preclot matrix was obtained by filling the graft segment with blood and leaving it for 90 min. At the end of this period the graft was washed gently with phosphate buffer saline leaving the graft coated with preclot matrix ready for seeding. Fibronectin coating was achieved by incubating the graft with the required concentration of fibronectin at 37 °C for 60–90 min. Collagen IV coating was obtained by incubating the graft at room temperature for 90 min.

Although several authors have studied the effect of fibronectin coating on endothelial cell adherence to vascular prosthetic grafts,[18,26,27] the optimum concentration of fibronectin as well as time of incubation has not been previously determined, differing concentrations varying from 10 to 1000 μg/ml being used.[26,27] To address this issue, we studied the adsorption of I^{125} labelled fibronectin to ePTFE quantitating the amount attached in relation to concentration and time of incubation. The number of molecules bound per cm^2 of graft was estimated e.g. at a concentration of 50 μg/ml at 90 min, there were 4.0×10^{11} molecules of fibronectin/cm^2. Fibronectin binding increased with a rise in its concentration though not on a linear basis. In addition the actual percentage of fibronectin attached to the graft decreased as concentration rose. This was $19.3 \pm 1.7\%$ at 10 μg/ml compared to $6.2 \pm 0.9\%$ at 250 μg/ml. Fibronectin binding increased significantly with longer incubation. At a concentration of 50 μg/ml fibronectin coated on ePTFE resisted shear stress of flow satisfactorily with 70% retention at 120 min.[28]

Endothelial cell adherence to grafts coated with different concentrations of fibronectin was also compared. Excessive fibronectin was not found necessary for endothelial cell adherence. A concentration of 50 μg/ml was selected as cell adherence at this concentration was no different than 150 and 250 μg/ml and better than 25 and 10 μg/ml.[28]

ENDOTHELIAL CELL ADHERENCE TO GRAFTS COATED WITH DIFFERENT MATRICES

Although Dacron and ePTFE have been successfully seeded with endothelial cells *in vitro* as well as *in vivo*,[7,8,20,23,26,29,30,31] a direct comparison with or without different matrices has not been previously described. Endothelial cell adherence to these grafts and gelatin impregnated Dacron (Gelseal) de novo or coated with preclot, collagen and fibronectin was compared.[25]

Comparison of matrices

Laminin has been found unsuitable as a matrix for endothelial cell seeding.[20,23] Anderson *et al.*[20] used collagen I on ePTFE and found significantly better adherence when compared to fibrin or fibronectin, whereas Pratt *et al.*[21] found a mixture of collagen I and III helpful. In our laboratory, collagen IV was found to be inferior to fibronectin and preclot.[25]

Fibronectin's ability to enhance cell adherence to ePTFE has been extensively investigated.[18,24] Kesler *et al.*[18] found 89.9% cell attachment to ePTFE coated with fibronectin compared to 62.6% with preclot. Our experiments have shown cell adherence to fibronectin coated ePTFE and Dacron $82.5 \pm 3.5\%$ and $82.0 \pm 3.5\%$

respectively, though surprisingly, endothelial cell adherence to Gelseal coated with fibronectin was lower compared with Dacron coated with fibronectin, a greater adherence being expected because of fibronectin's binding sites for gelatin.[25]

Cell adherence to ePTFE, Dacron and Gelseal coated with preclot matrix was 86.6±3.2%, 89.8±3.9% and 83.4±7.8% respectively which was significantly better than fibronectin and collagen IV.[25]

Comparison of grafts

Cell attachment to Dacron and ePTFE was significantly greater than Gelseal when coated with any of the three matrices although uncoated Gelseal had a significantly better cell adherence than ePTFE and Dacron.[25]

Comparison of incubation times

Whilst Anderson *et al.*[20] observed cells adhering to ePTFE within 15 min, most endothelial cells in our studies were noted to adhere within 30 min, there being no statistically significant difference between cell adherence at 30, 60 and 90 min.[25]

ENDOTHELIAL CELL KINETICS

Endothelial cell monolayers must be able to resist the shear stress of flowing blood. Studies in an animal model by Rosenman *et al.*[31] showed 19% initial cell attachment of which 70% were retained 30 min after implantation of the seeded graft. Lundgren *et al.*[32] showed better cell retention after flow with adult venous endothelial cells compared to umbilical venous endothelial cells. On the other hand, Schneider *et al.*[12] successfully achieved confluent and durable monolayers of umbilical venous endothelial cells on ePTFE.

Whilst Sentissi *et al.*[16] performed flow studies on grafts with endothelial cell monolayers grown over a 2-week period, Kesler *et al.*[18] using endothelial cells in high densities incubated the graft for 18 hours before flow. In our studies adult human endothelial cells grown in culture were acutely attached prior to flow.

Flows of 49-236 ml/min have been measured in saphenous vein grafts in humans.[33–36] The yield stress of endothelial cells is 350–400 dynes/cm^2 and can only be achieved in a 6 mm graft with a flow rate of 13 l/min.[37] Physiological shear stress akin to that in a femoropopliteal graft was simulated by selecting flows up to 300 ml/min in an artificial circuit.[38] Endothelial cells were labelled with indium-111-oxine for quantitative analysis. As leakage of isotope is negligible, the reduction in counts over the graft during flow represented cell loss. Initial losses were due to rapid detachment of those endothelial cells which were still rounded and minimally attached. In all experiments irrespective of the matrix, flow rate or graft, cell loss decreased after 30 min.

Comparison of matrices

The ability of fibronectin and preclot to support newly formed endothelial cell monolayers in response to shear stress of flow was compared.[38] Both matrices supported endothelial cell monolayers equally well when exposed to 300 ml/min with 2-h cell retentions of $58.3 \pm 15.5\%$ and $56.5 \pm 15.2\%$ respectively (Fig. 1). On the other hand, results with preclot were better at lower flows up to 200 ml/min. Kesler *et al.*[18] in their studies found 61.6% retention on ePTFE coated with fibronectin compared to 25.8% with preclot. Endothelial cell retention described by Schneider *et al.*[12] with bovine dermal collagen was equivalent to that with preclot in our study.

Comparison of grafts

Kinetics characteristics of endothelial cells on fibronectin coated ePTFE and Gelseal were compared. Although initial cell adherence with Gelseal was poor compared to ePTFE, once cells attached they resisted shear stress of flow better at 200 ml/min and equally well at 300 ml/min with 2-h retention of $69.0 \pm 6.0\%$ and $66.5 \pm 5.5\%$ respectively (Fig. 2).[39]

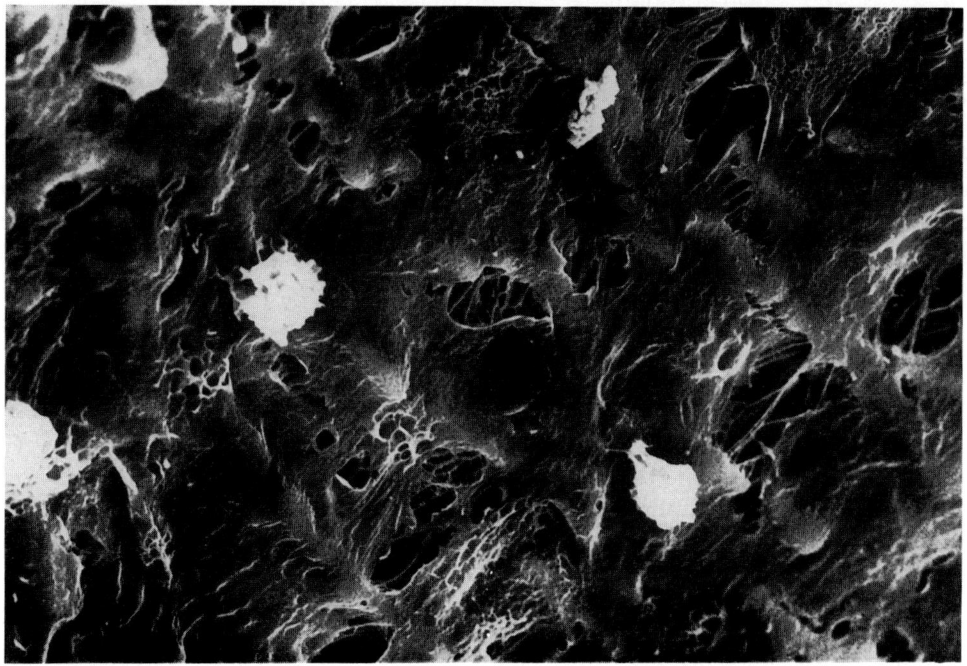

Fig. 1. SEM of retained endothelial cells on ePTFE coated with fibronectin after exposure to a flow of 300 ml/min for 120 min. Tight intercellular junctions and exposed graft are seen. (Scale: 50 μm = 48 mm.)

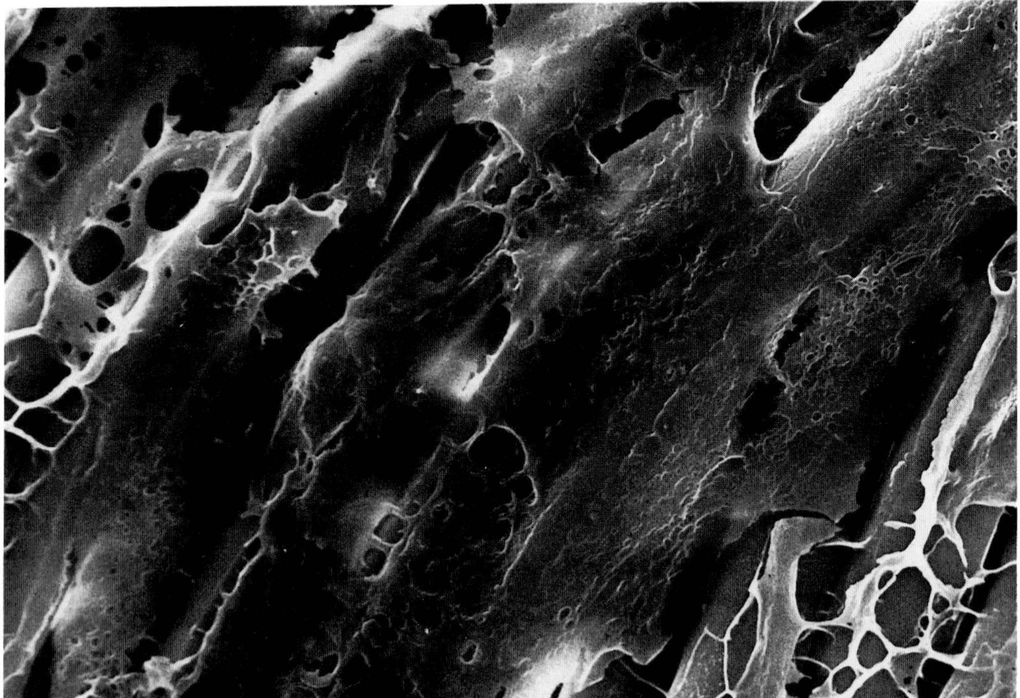

Fig. 2. SEM of retained endothelial cells on Gelseal graft coated with fibronectin after exposure to a flow of 300 ml/min for 120 min. (Scale 20 μm = 25 mm.)

Comparison of incubation periods

A comparison of endothelial cell kinetics after 30 and 90 min of endothelial cell seeding on fibronectin coated grafts was performed. Although seeding efficiency at 30 min was lower, cell retention after 2 h of flow was marginally better being 62.1±6.6% compared to 55.4±12.9% at 90 min incubation (Fig. 3). This difference was not statistically significant.[13]

CELL CHARACTERISTICS ON GRAFTS

Characteristics of endothelial cells on ePTFE and Dacron were studied using scanning electron microscopy (SEM), cell to cell relationship and ultrastructure studies with transmission electron microscopy.[5,13,25,26,40,41] Endothelial cells attached to Dacron appeared thinned and stretched out whilst on ePTFE appeared regular. Cells were seen growing in the crevices amongst the Dacron fibres. Selective attachment to the nodes of ePTFE was usual (Fig. 4) although occasionally in an atypical environment anchoring to the internodular fibrils with pseudopodia was seen.

HUMAN CLINICAL STUDIES

The first clinical seeding trial was reported by Herring *et al.*[42] using mechanically derived endothelial cells in a variety of arterial reconstructions using Dacron. Only

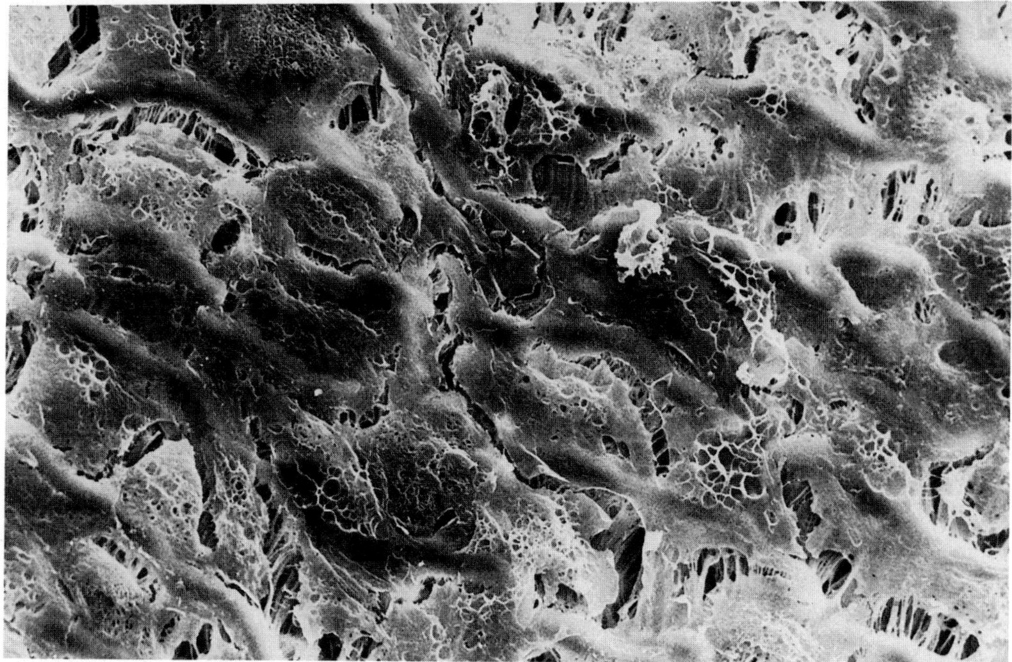

Fig. 3. SEM of retained endothelial cells on ePTFE coated with fibronectin after exposure to a flow of 200 ml/min for 120 min. Incubation period of endothelial seeding was 30 min. (Scale: 50 μm = 30 mm.)

nonsmokers with seeded femoropopliteal grafts showed better patency than those unseeded. Walker *et al.*[43] also using a mechanical method of harvesting compared 13 seeded with 20 unseeded ePTFE grafts implanted in patients undergoing surgery for severe arterial disease. The cumulative patency rates at 9 months for seeded and unseeded groups were 78.8% and 60.8% respectively. Whilst indium platelet scans showed a reduction in uptake in the seeded group at 3 months, this was not statistically significant. Herring *et al.*[44] further reported improved patency of ePTFE in a series of 17 seeded and 14 unseeded grafts, cumulative patency at 1 year being 81.6 ± 12.3% and 30.8 ± 18.7% respectively. Zilla *et al.*[45] showed that even after 14 weeks, endothelialization did not occur although platelet function, uptake and survival favoured the seeded group. Ortenwall *et al.*[46] studied 22 patients in whom one limb of a Dacron bifurcation prosthesis was seeded with endothelial cells, the other limb being sham-seeded with culture medium. Indium-111-oxine platelet labelling was employed to study the grafts at 1, 4 and 12 months postsurgery. The seeded limbs exhibited significantly less deposition of radiolabelled platelets than the controls.

CURRENT STATUS

After more than a decade of intense interest and research on the subject, there has been relatively little progress in the clinical field where several major issues require

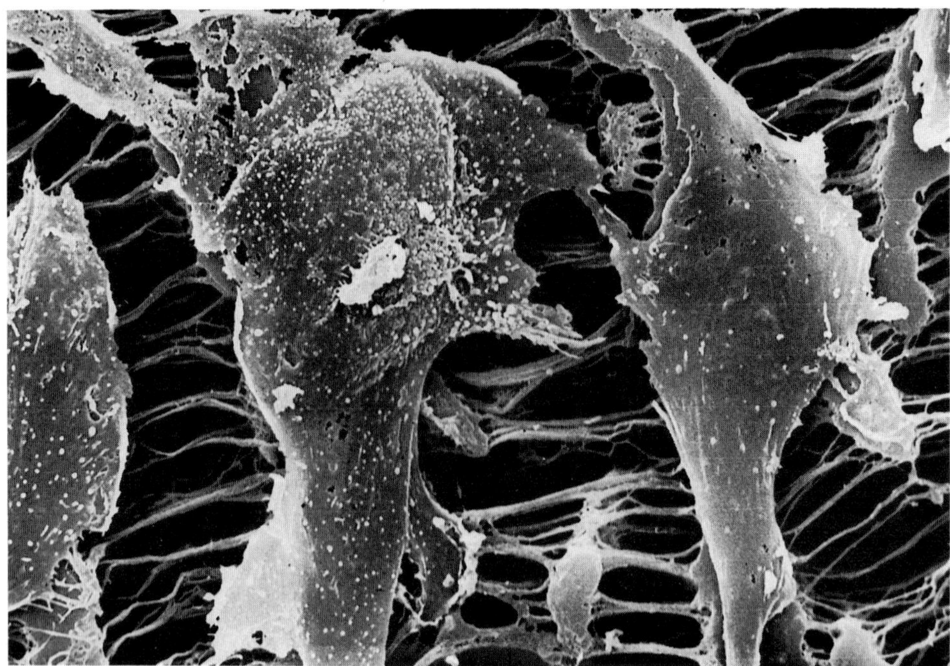

Fig. 4. SEM showing selective attachment of endothelial cells to nodes of ePTFE coated with collagen IV. (Scale: 20 μm = 36 mm.)

resolution. In particular the ability to harvest cells and endothelialize the graft in the operating room in a short time demands simple techniques. Whether cell function is significantly altered by harvesting remains largely unanswered as does the question of the ability of such seeded cells to resist the shear stress of flowing blood. There has been considerable debate regarding smooth muscle cell contamination at the time of harvesting, since it is known that when such cells are seeded as a mixture, there is a tendency to realignment which may not be detrimental.[47] To date the only method of identifying seeded endothelial cells on grafts in humans requires the indirect indium labelled platelet scanning technique which is observer-dependent. Although gene transfer technology has confirmed the origin of endothelial cell on grafts as the seeded cell or its progeny in animal experiments,[48] application of this technique to humans has yet to be established.

REFERENCES

1. Herring M, Gardener A, Glover J: A single-staged technique for seeding vascular grafts with autogenous endothelium. Surgery 84:498–504, 1978
2. Clowes AW, Gown AM, Hanson SR, Reidy MA: Mechanisms of arterial graft failure I: Role of cellular proliferation in early healing of PTFE prostheses. Am J Pathol 118:43–54, 1985
3. Ryan US, White LA: Varicose veins as a source of adult human endothelial cells. Tissue & Cell 17(2):171–176, 1985
4. Thomson GJL: A cellular lining for ePTFE vascular grafts. Studies using adult human endothelial and mesothelial cells. MD Thesis, University of Glasgow, Scotland, 1989

5. Zilla P, Fasol R, Preiss P *et al*: Use of fibrin glue as a substrate for *in vitro* endothelialization of PTFE vascular grafts. Surgery 105:515–522, 1990
6. Herring M, Dilley R, Cullison T, Gardner A, Glover G: Seeding endothelium on canine arterial prostheses—the size of the inoculum. J Surg Res 28:35–38, 1980
7. Schmidt SP, Hunter TJ, Hirko M *et al*: Small-diameter vascular prostheses: Two designs of PTFE and endothelial cell-seeded and nonseeded Dacron. J Vasc Surg 2:292–297, 1985
8. Kempczinski RF, Rosenman JE, Pearce WH *et al*: Endothelial seeding of a new PTFE vascular prosthesis. J Vasc Surg 2:424–429, 1985
9. Sharefkin JB, Van Wart HE, Cruess DF, Albus RA, Levine EM: Adult human endothelial cell harvesting. Estimates of efficiency and comparison of crude and partially purified bacterial collagenase preparations by replicate microwell culture and fibronectin degradation measured for enzyme-linked immunosorbent assay. J Vasc Surg 4:567–577, 1986
10. Herring M, Dilley R, Cullison T, Gardener A, Glover J: Seeding endothelium on canine arterial prostheses—the size of the inoculum. J Surg Res 28:35–38, 1980
11. Jarrell BE, Williams SK, Stokes G *et al*: Use of freshly isolated capillary endothelial cells for the immediate establishment of a monolayer on a vascular graft at surgery. Surgery 100:392–399, 1986
12. Schneider PA, Hanson SR, Price TM, Harker LA: Durability of confluent endothelial cell monolayers on small-caliber vascular prostheses *in vitro*. Surgery 103:456–462, 1988
13. Vohra RK, Thomson GJL, Carr HMH, Sharma H, Walker MG: The response of rapidly formed adult human endothelial monolayers to shear stress of flow: A comparison of fibronectin coated teflon and gelatin impregnated Dacron grafts. Surgery 1991 (in press)
14. Sharefkin JB, Latker C, Smith M, Rich NM: Endothelial cell labelling with indium-111-oxine as a marker of cell attachment to bioprosthetic surfaces. J Biomed Mat Res 17:345–357, 1983
15. Ortenwall P, Wadenvik H, Kutti J, Risberg B: Reduction in deposition of indium 111-labelled platelets after autologous endothelial cell seeding of Dacron aortic bifurcation grafts in humans: A prelminary report. J Vasc Surg 6:17–25, 1987
16. Sentissi JM, Ramberg K, O'Donnell TF, Connolly RJ, Callow AD: The effect of flow on vascular endothelial cells grown in tissue culture on polytetrafluoroethylene grafts. Surgery 99:337–342, 1986
17. Thomson GJL, Vohra R, Walker MG: Cellular seeding of ePTFE vascular grafts: a comparison between adult human endothelial and mesothelial cells. Ann Vasc Surg 3:140–145, 1989
18. Kesler KA, Herring MB, Arnold MP *et al*: Enhanced strength of endothelial attachment on polyester elastomer and polytetrafluoroethylene graft surfaces with fibronectin substrate. J Vasc Surg 3:58–64, 1986
19. Zilla P, Fasol R, Dudeck U *et al*: *In situ* cannulation, microgrid follow-up and low density plating provide first passage endothelial cell masscultures for *in vitro* lining. J Vasc Surg 12:180–189, 1990
20. Anderson JM, Abbuhl MF, Herring T, Johnston KH: Immunohistochemical identification of components in the healing response of human vascular grafts. J Am Soc Artif Intern Organs 8:79–85, 1984
21. Pratt KJ, Jarrell BE, Williams SK: Kinetics of endothelial cell-surface attachment forces. J Vasc Surg 7:591–599, 1988
22. Thomson GJL, Vohra R, Carr HMH, Walker MG: Adult human endothelial cell seeding using expanded polytetrafluoroethylene (ePTFE) vascular grafts—A comparison of four substrates. Surgery 1991 (in press)
23. Hasson JE, Wiebe DH, Sharefkin JB, D'Amore PA, Abbott WA: Use of tritiated thymidine as a marker to compare the effects of matrix proteins on adult human vascular endothelial cell attachment: Implications for seeding of vascular prostheses. Surgery 100:884–892, 1986
24. Ramalanjaona G, Kempczinski RF, Rosenman JE, Douville E, Silberstein EB: The effect of fibronectin coating on endothelial cell kinetics in polytetrafluoroethylene grafts. J Vasc Surg 3:264–272, 1986
25. Vohra RK, Thomson GJL, Carr HMH, Sharma H, Walker MG: A comparison of different vascular prostheses and matrices in relation to endothelial seeding. Br J Surg 1991 (in press)

26. Foxall TL, Auger KR, Callow AD, Libby P: Adult human endothelial cell coverage of small-caliber Dacron and polytetrafluoroethylene vascular prostheses *in vitro*. J Surg Res 41:158–172, 1986
27. Lindblad B, Wright SW, Sell RL *et al*: Alternative techniques of seeding cultured endothelial cells to ePTFE grafts of different diameters, porosities, and surfaces. J Biomed Mat Res 21:1013–1022, 1987
28. Vohra R, Thomson GJL, Carr HMH, Sharma H, Walker MG: The role of fibronectin in endothelial seeding of vascular prostheses. Artif Organs 14(1):41–45, 1990
29. Graham LM, Burkel WE, Ford JW: Immediate seeding of enzymatically derived endothelium on Dacron vascular grafts. Arch Surg 115:1289–1294, 1980
30. Stanley JC, Burkel WE, Graham LM, Lindblad B: Endothelial cell seeding of synthetic vascular prostheses. Acta Chir Scand Suppl 529:17–28, 1985
31. Rosenman JE, Kempczinski RF, Pearce WH, Silberstein EB: Kinetics of endothelial cell seeding. J Vasc Surg 2:778–784, 1985
32. Lundgren CH, Herring MB, Arnold MP, Glover JL, Bendick PJ: Fluid shear disruption of cultured endothelium: The effect of cell species, fibronectin cross-linking and supporting polymer. Trans Am Soc Artif Intern Organs 32:334–338, 1986
33. Mannick JA, Jackson BT: Haemodynamics of arterial surgery in atherosclerotic limbs. I. Direct measurement of blood flow before and after vein grafts. Surgery 59:713–720, 1966
34. Bernhard VM, Ashmore CS, Rodgers RE, Evans WE: Operative blood flow in femoro-popliteal and femoro-tibial grafts for lower extremity ischaemia. Arch Surg 103:595–599, 1971
35. Cronestrand R, Ekestrom S: Blood flow after peripheral arterial reconstruction. I. Measurements after ilial-femoro-popliteal arterial reconstructions with the electro-magnetic flowmeter and implanted flow probes during operation and in the early postoperative periods. Scand J Thorac Cardiovasc Surg 4:159–171, 1970
36. Harris PL, Campbell H: Adjuvant distal arteriovenous shunt with femorotibial bypass for critical ischaemia. Br J Surg 70:377–380, 1983
37. Strandness DE, Sumner SA: Grafts and grafting. *In* Haemodynamics for Surgeons, Strandness DE, Sumner SA (Eds). New York: Grune & Stratton, pp. 342–395, 1975
38. Vohra R, Thomson GJL, Carr HMH, Sharma H, Walker MG: Effect of shear stress imposed by flow on endothelial cell monolayers on ePTFE comparing preclot and fibronectin matrices. Eur J Vasc Surg 4:33–41, 1990
39. Vohra R, Carr HMH, Thomson GJL *et al*: In-vitro adherence and kinetics studies of adult human endothelial cell seeded polytetrafluoroethylene (ePTFE) and gelatin impregnated Dacron (Gelseal) grafts. Eur J Vasc Surg 1991 (in press)
40. Kachler J, Zilla P, Fasol R, Deutsch M, Kadletz M: Precoating substrate and surface configuration determine adherence and spreading of seeded endothelial cells on polytetrafluoroethylene grafts. J Vasc Surg 9:535–541, 1989
41. Herring M, Baughman S, Kesler K *et al*: Endothelial seeding of Dacron and Polytetrafluoroethylene grafts: the cellular events of healing. Surgery 96:745–754, 1984
42. Herring M, Gardener A, Glover J: Seeding human arterial prostheses with mechanically derived endothelium. The detrimental effect of smoking. J Vasc Surg 1:279–289, 1984
43. Walker MG, Thomson GJL, Shaw JW: Endothelial cell seeded versus non-seeded ePTFE grafts in patients with severe peripheral vascular disease. *In* Endothelialization of Vascular Grafts, Zilla P, Fasol RD, Deutsch M (Eds). Basel, Switzerland: Karger, pp. 245–248, 1987
44. Herring MB, Compton RS, LeGrand DR *et al*: Endothelial seeding of polytetrafluoro-ethylene popliteal bypasses: A preliminary report. J Vasc Surg 6:114–118, 1987
45. Zilla P, Fasol R, Deutsch M *et al*: Endothelial cell seeding of polytetrafluoroethylene vascular grafts in humans: A preliminary report. J Vasc Surg 6:535–541, 1987
46. Ortenwall P, Wadenvik H, Kutti J, Risberg B: Endothelial cell seeding reduces thrombogenicity of Dacron grafts in humans. J Vasc Surg 11:403–410, 1990
47. Wang Z, Du W, Guang-di L, Li-qun P, Sharefkin J: Rapid cellular luminal coverage of Dacron inferior vena cava prostheses in dogs by immediate seeding of autogenous endothelial cells derived from omental tissue: results of a preliminary trial. J Vasc Surg 12:168–179, 1990
48. Callow AD: The vascular endothelial cell as a vehicle for gene therapy. J Vasc Surg 11:793–798, 1990

FACTORS PROLONGING PATENCY

Platelet Inhibitory Therapy

Allen Edwards and Charles McCollum

Vascular surgery has progressed rapidly in the last half-century with the introduction of prosthetic materials for arterial bypass or replacement. Vorhees *et al*. (1952) were the first to show that large calibre arteries could be safely replaced with a seamed graft made of Vinyon N (sailcloth) and DeBakey (1953) followed soon after with the first use of Dacron.[1] These early uses of prosthetic materials met with considerable success, failures being due to mechanical problems, in particular aneurysmal dilatation at the suture line. Graft design in these early days concentrated on methods of improving the physical characteristics of graft materials: in particular, increasing mechanical strength, reducing compliance mis-match between graft and vessel, and improving the handling characteristics. When used to replace large calibre vessels such as the aorta and the iliac arteries these crude materials performed well with few thrombotic complications.

It was not until vascular surgeons attempted to bypass small and medium sized arteries such as those below the level of the inguinal ligament and the coronary arteries that the problem of graft thrombogenicity became apparent. For femoropopliteal bypass few surgeons can achieve patency rates with prosthetic materials to match those of autogenous vein[2,3] and when prosthetics are used in aortocoronary bypass, failure is almost universal. Thus, when the saphenous vein is unavailable or inadequate, the need for drug therapy to improve patency in prosthetic bypass is most apparent.

The platelet in graft failure

If we are to improve patency in arterial bypass we must first understand the reasons for failure. There has been considerable research into the physical properties of grafts such as durability, elasticity and compliance, yet the fundamental difference between a prosthesis and autogenous vein is the luminal surface. Whenever blood passes over a foreign surface platelets will adhere and undergo their release reaction. Normal blood vessels are lined by a confluent endothelium which is nonthrombogenic due to the secretion of various inhibitors of platelet function such as prostacyclin and fibrinolytic substances. The platelet appears to be of prime importance in bringing about graft failure and platelet adhesion to prosthetic surfaces may lead to the formation of laminated thrombus (Fig. 1). This appears to be the main cause of graft failure within the first 6 months following surgery; later failures being due to myo-intimal hyperplasia near to the anastomoses. This phenomenon may also be platelet mediated through the release of platelet derived growth factors.[4] Platelet inhibition therefore may represent an attractive way to improve arterial bypass patency.

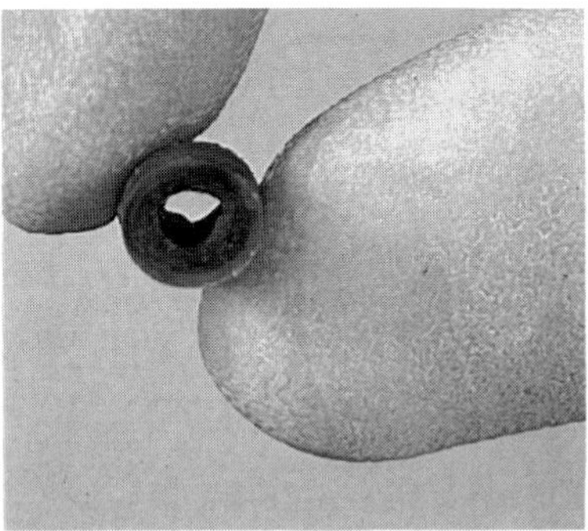
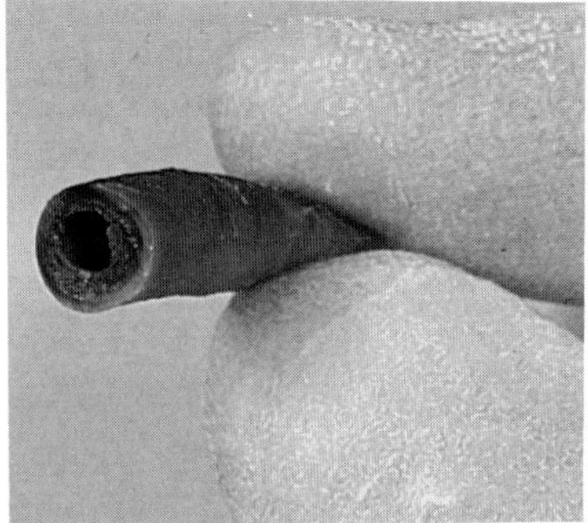

Fig. 1. Laminated thrombus within a 6-mm PTFE arterial graft.

THROMBOSIS IN VEIN BYPASS

The endothelial layer in autogenous vein is lost following implantation in the arterial circulation, whether by a reversed or *in situ* technique.[5] Repair resembles that following endarterectomy where the intima is replaced by fibrosis and myo-intimal cells migrate from the muscle layer to form a confluent luminal surface.[6] The endothelium recovers, but intimal thickening leads to progressive luminal narrowing and an appearance not unlike rapidly progressing atherosclerosis.[7] Thus vein graft failure appears to occur in two ways:

1. Thrombosis during the period of endothelial loss.
2. Intimal hyperplasia which occurs over a period of months to years.[8]

THROMBOSIS IN PROSTHETIC GRAFTS

When prosthetic material is exposed to flowing blood fibrinogen is adsorbed onto its luminal surface leading to platelet adhesion.[9] This is initially reversible but becomes stabilized by fibrin into a laminated thrombus. In the months following implantation of aortobifemoral grafts there is an increase in fibrinogen consumption which returns to normal by 6–9 months.[10] However, studies in man using platelets radiolabelled with the isotope ^{111}Indium show that platelets continue to adhere to the surface of Dacron grafts for many years following surgery and in all probability these grafts remain thrombogenic indefinitely.[11,12] Porosity and double velour, which are features of modern graft design appear to have no effect on early thrombogenicity or on the rate at which thrombogenicity improves with time and graft maturation.[13]

Physical factors remain important in graft occlusion. A 1-mm layer of pseudo-intima in a 10-mm graft increases resistance to blood flow by 144%, yet the same thickness of thrombus in a 6-mm graft would increase resistance by 406%. Resistance and turbulence promote platelet deposition by disrupting the cell stream in laminar flow. This explains greater pseudo-intimal thickness at bifurcations, anastomoses and sites of kinking which are all causes of turbulence. In long grafts, thrombotic substances and platelet release factors accumulate in blood as it flows along the graft, increasing blood cell reactivity in the distal graft. This explains the occlusions that develop in the distal anastomosis and the higher failure rates of prosthetic grafts which extend below the knee.

PLATELET INHIBITORY THERAPY IN VEIN BYPASS

Evidence in favour of platelet inhibitory therapy in vein bypass has largely been based on studies in patients undergoing aortocoronary bypass[14]. However, the British multicentre femoropopliteal bypass trial initiated in October 1984 offers an opportunity to assess the role of platelet inhibitory therapy in patients undergoing bypass with autogenous vein.[15] Patients were randomized to receive either aspirin (300 mg) in combination with dipyridamole (150 mg twice daily) or placebo started 2 days prior to surgery. Graft patency was assessed independently by trial co-ordinators using objective criteria and other cardiovascular events (myocardial infarction or stroke) recorded. Randomization of 549 patients produced comparable groups of 286 patients on aspirin and dipyridamole (ASA + DPM) and 263 on placebo. The indications for surgery were rest pain or gangrene in 60% of patients. There was no significant difference in bleeding complications between the two groups but there was a higher incidence of reoperation for bleeding in patients on ASA + DPM. Cumulative graft patency on placebo was 72%, 62% and 60% at 1, 2 and 3 years respectively and 78%, 70% and 61% on ASA + DPM (Fig. 2). These differences failed to reach statistical significance. However, this trial was analysed on an intention to treat basis and may have been influenced substantially by both poor compliance

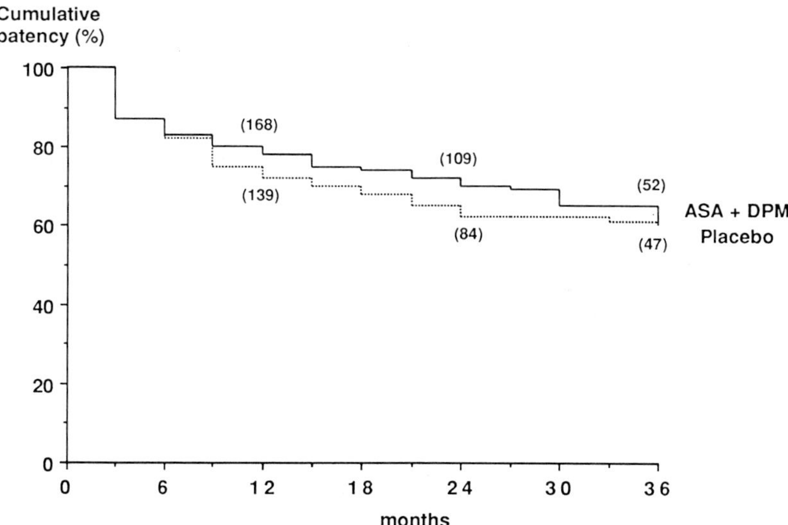

Fig. 2. Graft patency plotted using life table methods comparing patients randomized to aspirin plus dipyridamole (ASA + DPM) and placebo. An apparent improvement in patency by 2 years is lost by 3 years and the overall difference fails to reach statistical significance ($p = 0.43$).

Table. 1. Cardiovascular events and graft failure (rate/1000 patient-years of therapy)

	Placebo (n=263)		ASA+DPM (n=286)		
	n	rate	n	rate	p
Myocardial infarct	34	84.4	19	39.7	0.006
Stroke	19	47.1	16	33.5	0.30
Graft failure	86	213.4	86	179.9	0.211
Total	139	344.9	121	253.1	0.003

in the ASA+DPM patients and inappropriate aspirin consumption by patients on placebo.

The main result and conclusion of this study was on the effects of antiplatelet agents on other cardiovascular events such as myocardial infarction and stroke (Table 1). At an average follow-up of 34 months there were 53 (132/1000 patient-years of follow-up) cardiovascular events in the placebo group compared with 35 (73/1000 patient-years) in those on aspirin and dipyridamole ($p=0.04$). The main advantage in treating patients undergoing peripheral arterial bypass would appear to be the effect on all cardiovascular events rather than any perceived benefit in the prevention of graft thrombosis. The effect has already been recognized in patients treated with antiplatelet agents following myocardial infarction and stroke.[16–18]

PLATELET INHIBITORY THERAPY IN PROSTHETIC BYPASS

A number of platelet inhibitory drugs have been studied in experimental models of prosthetic arterial bypass.[19–21] Aspirin is the standard against which other drugs have been compared, and the combination of aspirin and dipyridamole is still widely prescribed although the role of dipyridamole is increasingly in doubt. This combination has been shown to reduce the incidence of pseudo-intimal hyperplasia and myo-intimal hyperplasia in experimental models of arterial bypass.[20,21] In another study ^{111}Indium-platelet deposition and pseudo-intimal hyperplasia were both reduced by cyclo-oxygenase inhibition.[22]

In femoropopliteal bypass the rate of platelet deposition on the graft lumen has been measured using radiolabelled platelets.[23] The rate of accumulation of ^{111}Indium-platelets in the week following surgery was found to be a sensitive indicator of subsequent graft thrombosis. Grafts which accumulated platelets at a rate in the upper half of the range were more than twice as likely to fail than grafts in the lower half of the range. This platelet deposition was inhibited by aspirin and dipyridamole and the cumulative patency by life table improved from 36% at 12 months on placebo to 67% on aspirin and dipyridamole. There are surprisingly few properly conducted clinical trials of antiplatelet therapy in patients with peripheral vascular disease. What studies there have been, have all demonstrated a clear benefit in favour of antiplatelet therapy in prosthetic bypass. This benefit applies to femoropopliteal bypass with either Dacron or polytetrafluoroethylene (PTFE).[24–26]

Further evidence for the use of antiplatelet therapy in femoropopliteal bypass comes from the UK femoropopliteal bypass trial. Patients undergoing prosthetic

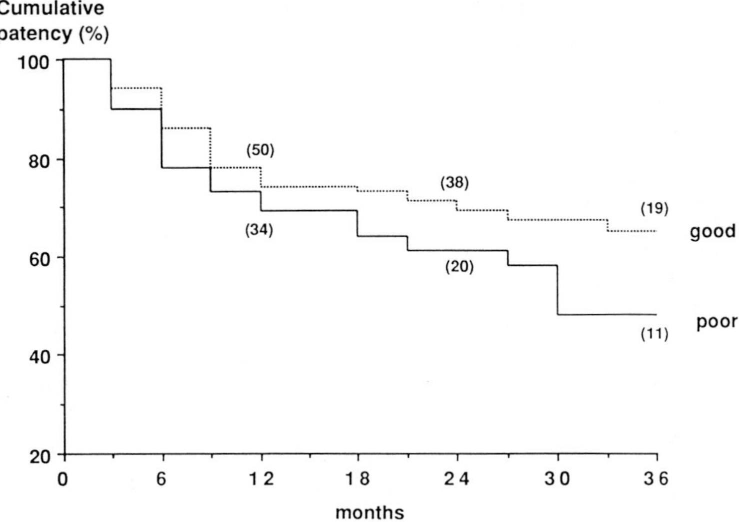

Fig. 3. Cumulative patency in prosthetic femoropopliteal bypass was reduced in patients who fail to take antiplatelet medication. 'Poor compliance' is defined as failing to take more than 10 tablets per month (<90% compliance) ($p<0.05$).

bypass with either PTFE or human umbilical vein were all given ASA+DPM. However, those patients who failed to comply with this treatment had a higher rate of graft failure than patients who took their medication regularly (Fig. 3). A poor complier was defined as someone who failed to take more than 10 tablets a month. In practice, most patients either took their medication reliably or discontinued treatment completely. The cumulative patency at 2 and 3 years in those who continued antiplatelet therapy was 69% and 65% respectively compared with 61% and 48% in patients who did not take their medication regularly ($p<0.05$).

The role of anticoagulants in maintaining graft patency has never been adequately studied in this country and will be discussed further, in the chapter by Kretschemer *et al.* (p. 77).

CONCLUSIONS

As prosthetic materials perform well in the aorto-iliac region with few thrombotic complications the risks of long-term antiplatelet therapy cannot be justified merely to improve graft patency. The effect of platelet inhibitory therapy on patency in femorofemoral and axillofemoral grafts has never been studied. For those with prosthetic femoropopliteal bypasses antiplatelet therapy is indicated; our current choice of antiplatelet agents being the combination of aspirin and dipyridamole. Hopefully, the development of more selective agents with less side-effects such as thromboxane antagonists will become available in the near future. Although ASA+DPM did not improve patency in vein bypass, they did reduce the rate of other cardiovascular events, in particular myocardial infarction. As this is the case, many vascular surgeons will feel that all their patients undergoing arterial bypass;

of whatever type, would benefit from the prescription of antiplatelet therapy for the protection it confers against other cardiovascular events.

REFERENCES

1. Sauvage LR, Berger K, Barros D'Sa AAB *et al*: Dacron arterial prostheses. *In* Graft Materials in Vascular Surgery, Dardik H (Ed.). Chicago: Yearbook Medical Publishers, 1978
2. Bergan JJ, Yao ST, Flinn WR, Graham LM: Prosthetic grafts for the treatment of lower limb ischaemia. Br J Surg 69:S34–S37, 1982
3. Callow AD: Current status of vascular grafts. Surg Clin N Am 62:501–513, 1982
4. Clowes AW, Adams MC: Smooth muscle proliferation and arterial graft failure. *In* Reoperative Arterial Surgery, Bergan Y (Ed.). Orlando, London: Grune & Stratton, 1986
5. Ramos JR, Berger K, Mansfield PB, Sauvage LR: Histological fate and endothelial changes of distended and non-distended vein grafts. Ann Surg 183:205–228, 1976
6. Landymore RW, Kinley CE, Cameron CA: Intimal hyperplasia in autogenous vein grafts for arterial bypass: a canine model. Cardiovasc Res 19:589, 1985
7. Imparato AM: Intimal and neointimal hyperplasia. *In* Femoro-distal Bypass, Greenhalgh RM (Ed.). London: Pitman Medical, 1990
8. Sladen JG, Gilmour JL: Vein graft stenosis: Characteristics and effect of treatment. Am J Surg 141:549, 1981
9. Salzman EW, Lindon J, Brier D *et al*: Surface-induced platelet adhesion, aggregation and release. Ann NY Acad Sci 283:114–27, 1977
10. McCollum CN, Kester R, Rajah SM, Learoyd P, Pepper M: Arterial graft maturation: The duration of thrombotic activity in Dacron aortobifemoral measured by platelet survival and fibrinogen kinetics. Br J Surg 68:61–64, 1981
11. Goldman M, Norcott HC, Hawker RJ *et al*: Platelet accumulation on mature Dacron grafts in man. Br J Surg 69:S38–S40, 1982
12. Ritchie JL, Stratton JR, Hamilton GW *et al*: Indium[111] platelet imaging for detection of platelet deposition in abdominal aortic aneurysms and prosthetic arterial grafts. Am J Cardiol 47:882–889, 1981
13. Goldman M, McCollum CN, Hawker RJ, Drolc Z, Slaney G: Dacron arterial grafts: the influence of porosity, velour and maturity on thrombogenicity. Surgery 92:947–952, 1982
14. Chesbro JH, Fuster V, Elveback LR *et al*: Effect of dipyridamole and aspirin on late vein-graft patency after coronary bypass operations. N Engl J Med 310:209, 1984
15. McCollum CN, Alexander CE, Kenchington G, Franks PJ, Greenhalgh RM: Anti-platelet drugs in femoro-popliteal vein bypass: a multicentre trial. J Vasc Surg 1991 (in press)
16. Anti-platelet trialists' collaboration. Secondary prevention of vascular disease by prolonged anti-platelet treatment. Br Med J 296:320–331, 1988
17. UK-TIA Study Group. United Kingdom transient ischaemic attack (UK-TIA) aspirin trial: interim results. Br Med J 296:316–320, 1988
18. Hennekens CH, Buring JE, Sandercock P, Collins R, Peto R: Aspirin and other anti-platelet agents in the secondary and primary prevention of cardiovascular disease. Circulation 80:749–756, 1989
19. McCollum CN, Crow MJ, Rajah SM, Kester RC: Anti-thrombotic therapy for vascular prostheses; An experimental model testing platelet inhibitory drugs. Surgery 87:668–676, 1980
20. Hagen PO, Wang ZG, Mikat EM, Hackel DB: Antiplatelet therapy reduces aortic intimal hyperplasia distal to small diameter vascular prostheses (PTFE) in non-human primates. Ann Surg 195:328–339, 1982
21. Oblath RW, Buckley FO, Green RM, Schwartz SI, DeWeese JA: Prevention of platelet aggregation and adherence to prosthetic vascular grafts by aspirin and dipyridamole. Surgery 84:37–43, 1978
22. Lane IF, Irwin JTC, Jennings SA, McCollum CN: Effect of the cyclo-oxygenase inhibitor Indobufen on platelet accumulation in prosthetic vascular grafts. Br J Surg 1986:73, 563–565

23. Goldman M, Hall C, Bykes J, Hawker RJ, McCollum CN: Does ^{111}Indium-labelled platelet deposition predict patency in prosthetic arterial grafts? Br J Surg 70: 635–638, 1983
24. Donaldson DR, Salter MCP, Kester RC *et al*: The influence of platelet inhibition on the patency of femoro-popliteal Dacron bypass grafts. Vasc Surg 19:224, 1985
25. Clyne CAC, Archer TJ, Atuhaire LK *et al*: Randomize control trial of a short course of aspirin and dipyridamole (Persantin) for femoro-distal grafts. Br J Surg 74:246, 1987
26. Green RM, Roedesheimer LR, DeWeese JA: Effects of aspirin and dipyridamole on expanded polytetrafluoroethylene graft patency. Surgery 92:1016–1026, 1982

The Role of Oral Anticoagulation

G. Kretschmer, Gabriela A. Berlakovich, F. Herbst,
M. Prager, Th. Sautner and M. Schemper

Bypass surgery using the autologous saphenous vein as a vascular substitute is the treatment of choice in patients with atherosclerotic arterial disease in the femoropopliteal level.[1–4] Patency rates after 5 years (more than 60%)[1–3] and after 10 years (40%)[5] are at hand. During the last decade immense efforts were seen to refine the technique and to render more and more distally situated vascular parts of the vascular tree accessible for reopening procedures. Quickly it became obvious that pharmacological interventions are needed to maintain patency once achieved in high risk patients, in particular in those with compromised run-off segments.[6] For long-term success it is only logical to consider antiplatelet drugs or oral anticoagulants.[7] Since we have failed to show an effect using antiplatelet drugs,[8] we analysed our clinical series and conducted a prospective clinical trial using oral anticoagulants in an attempt to improve results after vein bypass surgery.

PATIENTS AND METHODS

Analysis of the clinical series

All patients, who underwent elective vein grafting for femoropopliteal atherosclerosis from 1970–90, were eligible for evaluation. The results were obtained in the usual manner on an outpatient basis performing clinical examination, pulse palpation, calculation of the systolic ankle brachial pressure index (Doppler ultrasound), and in still inconclusive cases an arteriogram was obtained. Postoperative pharmacological intervention was started during the second week after surgery and as a rule continued throughout the life of the graft but mostly until death of the patients. The final decision to use oral anticoagulants (phenprocoumon tablets, 3 mg each) was the surgeon's and exclusion criteria are described below.

The clinial trial

During the years 1979–88 175 consecutive patients were seen with chronic obliterative arterial disease in the femoropopliteal level. Patients were staged preoperatively according to the Fontaine classification. A classical venous bypass was carried out using the autologous saphenous vein; the proximal anastomosis was positioned at the common femoral artery, the distal anastomosis was situated above or below the knee. To demonstrate a technically satisfactory result, completion and/or postoperative arteriography was performed.

Exclusion criteria for using the trial drugs were a history of, or the endoscopically confirmed diagnosis of, gastroduodenal ulceration, need for or contra-indications to anticoagulants or platelet inhibitoring drugs, age over 75 years and unwillingness to comply with the requirements of the trial.

Finally during the second postoperative week 130 patients were randomly allocated either to the therapy ($n = 66$; started as phenprocoumon) or the control group, which remained without any anticoagulant treatment ($n = 64$).

Computer assisted follow-up examinations were performed every 3 months during the first postoperative year and therefore at semi-annual or—if felt indicated—shorter intervals. Special care was taken that both treatment and control group received equal scrutiny in detecting graft reocclusion; all reocclusions were confirmed by arteriography. In addition major amputation during observation was recorded. Particular attention was paid to compliance with treatment and satisfactory stabilization of coagulation by monitoring prothrombin time (Quick value or Hepatoquick® [Boehringer, Ingelheim, FRG] or Thrombotest [Nycomed®, Immuno AG, Vienna, Austria]) results and modifying treatment accordingly. The goals were 15–25% for Quick value, 10–20% for Hepatoquick and 5–12% for Thrombotest. The intention was to check the anticoagulant treatment at every outpatient appointment. The staff in the outpatients department did know all the vascular patients on oral anticoagulants, since patients in Austria are supposed to carry an 'anticoagulation' chart, which is to be produced on request. Altogether the staff controlled 311 patients on oral anticoagulants for bypass procedures below the inguinal ligament but was not able to recognize the participants of the trial. The medication was prescribed for the whole observation period during graft patency, limb salvage and finally until the patients' death.

STATISTICAL METHODS

The documentation system of the Austrian Society of Vascular Surgery was used to enter details of all surgical treatment procedures into the main frame IBM 4381 computer at the faculty of Medicine (180 variables per surgical intervention, more than 8000 operations since 1965). Data were stored on line and retrieved with Statistical Analysis System (SAS) software.[9] The use of SAS and Biomedical Dixon Program BMDP-1L (life) facilitated patency analysis.[10]

Patients were assigned to the groups by adaptive randomization.[11] Prognostic factors considered were sex, age, diabetes mellitus, blood pressure and clinical status prior to surgery. The patency curves were analysed by the Kaplan–Meier method,[12] differences were checked with Breslow's[13] and Mantel's[14] tests in a bitailed manner.

In six patients, anticoagulant treatment was discontinued for various reasons (epistaxis: one; gastrointestinal haemorrhage: three; unknown cause: one; suspected cerebral stroke: one). Nevertheless for evaluation these patients remained in the group, to which they had been assigned originally (intention to treat principle).[15] Two patients randomized to the control group were treated with phenprocoumon for cardiac reasons and for autologous vein bypass surgery respectively and both were excluded from that date on.

The primary end points were graft re-occlusion and major limb loss respectively.

RESULTS

Analysis of the clinical series

The functional status of all femoropopliteal autologous vein grafts done electively was analysed ($n=658$) and Kaplan–Meier estimates were obtained: 163 patients were treated with oral anticoagulants and 360 remained without postoperative pharmacological intervention, whereas 135 receiving antiplatelet drugs as well as patients with immediate occlusions were excluded from analysis. The treatment influenced the primary probability of function in a statistically significant way in favour of oral anticoagulants ($p \leqslant 0.002$ Breslow, $p \leqslant 0.007$ Mantel) as shown in Fig. 1. The median graft patency was 68.2 ± 23.6 (SE) months in the untreated group and 90.1 ± 12.7 (SE) months in the treatment group.

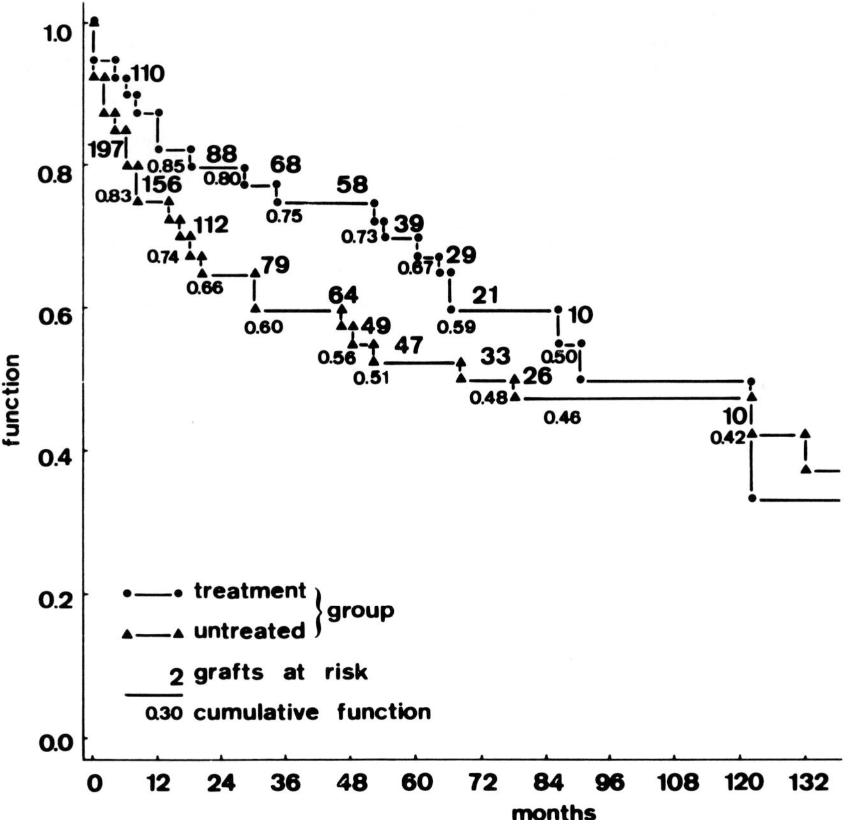

Fig. 1. Femoropopliteal vein grafts. Analysis of the clinical series; probability of graft patency (Kaplan–Meier function) treated vs untreated group; numbers above the curve indicate grafts at risk; numbers below give the cumulative proportion functioning.

The prospective trial

The median duration of primary function for the treated patients was more than 120 months, whereas only 93.0 months in the control group; 13 patients reoccluded their graft in the treated and 23 in the untreated group. Thus the therapy group had a higher probability of function ($p \leqslant 0.006$ Breslow, $p \leqslant 0.013$ Mantel; Fig. 2).

The median duration of limb salvage was more than 120 months in the therapy group, whereas it was 100 months in the control group. During the observation period three patients lost their limb in the therapy and 13 in the control group, again the difference being significant ($p \leqslant 0.007$ Breslow, $p \leqslant 0.004$ Mantel; Fig. 3).

In the treated group 27 patients died and 37 died in the untreated group making a total of 64. Causes of death were malignancies in three, gastrointestinal haemorrhage due to anticoagulant treatment in one patient (after 68 months of treatment) and the underlying cardiovascular disease in the remaining patients.

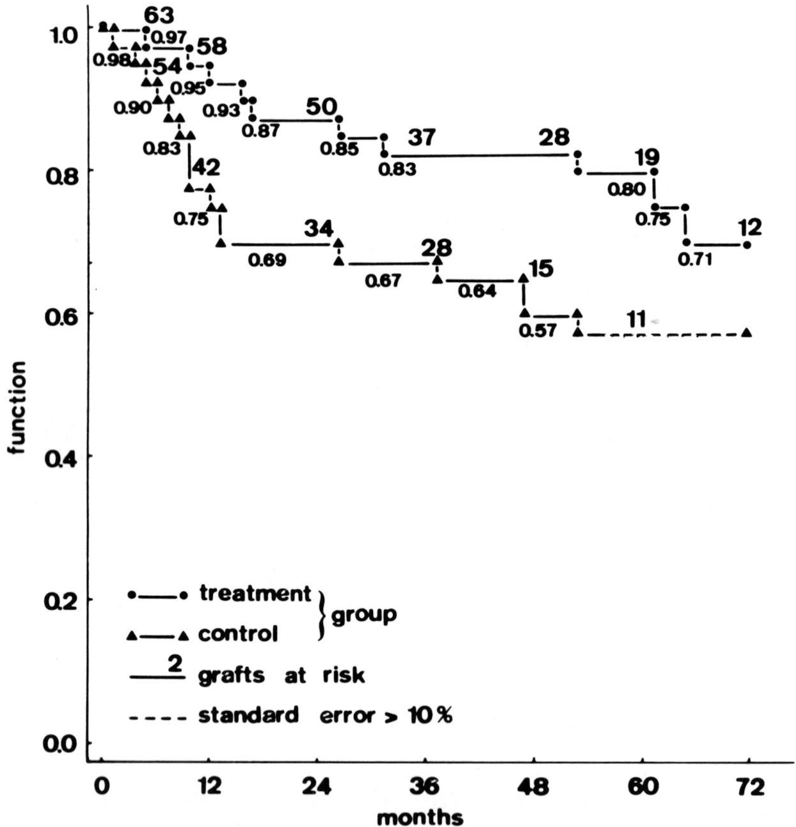

Fig. 2. The prospective trial; probability of graft patency (Kaplan–Meier function), treated vs untreated controls; numbers above the curve indicate grafts at risk; numbers below give the cumulative proportion functioning. Interrupted lines show the interval, when the standard error exceeds 10%.

Table 1 summarizes the risk factors in both groups and confirms their even balance.

Altogether 1432 single prothrombin time estimations were carried out, in general in monthly intervals. Over the years of follow-up between 75–81% of the estimations were safe within therapeutical limits, 3–5% were below the limit of treatment and in the remaining samples above the margin of anticoagulation.

The graphical design of the Kaplan–Meier curves followed the recommendations established by the Ad Hoc Committee On Reporting Standards of the Society For Cardiovascular Surgery and the North American Chapter of the International Society For Cardiovascular Surgery respectively.[16]

DISCUSSION

We have demonstrated that an oral anticoagulant drug regimen was effective at the femoropoliteal level in preventing autologous saphenous vein bypass reocclusion

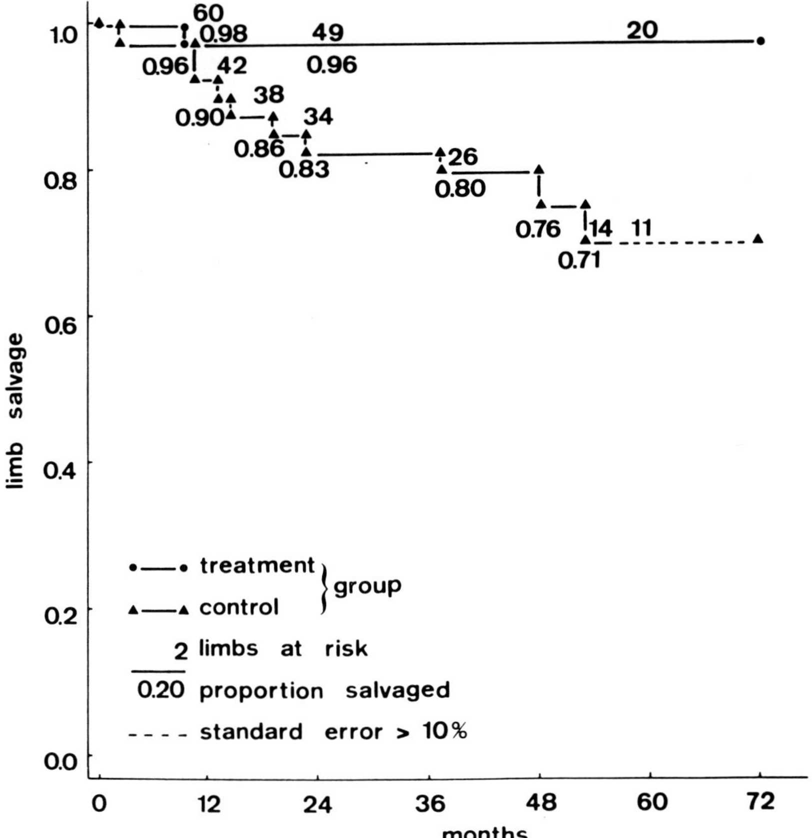

Fig. 3. The prospective trial; probability of limb salvage; numbers above the curve indicate limbs at risk; numbers below give the cumulative proportion of limbs salvaged. Interrupted lines show the interval, when the standard error exceeds 10%.

Table 1. Balancing of risk factors in the treatment (TG) group vs the control (0) group

Variable	*TG*	*0*
$n = 130$	66	64
Sex		
male $n = 102$	52	50
female $n = 28$	14	14
Age		
mean ± SEM (years)	62.5 ± 8.3	62.3 ± 8.9
< 55 years	12	13
55–65 years	27	23
> 65 years	27	28
Diabetic state		
0	43	41
diabetes mellitus	19	17
insulin dependent	4	6
Blood pressure		
< 160/90 mmHg	48	47
> 160/90 mmHg	18	17
Cardiac pathology		
0	38	38
ischaemic myocardiopathy	3	3
history of myoc. infarction	14	13
arrhythmia	11	10
Smoking habits		
0	12	14
< 10	7	5
10–20 cigarettes/day	23	19
> 20	24	26
*Clinical status prior to surgery**		
St. II, II–III	32	30
St. III, IV	34	34
Distal anastomotic site		
above knee	28	28
below knee	38	36
Ankle–brachial pressure index		
< 0.3	21	24
0.3–0.4	17	13
0.4–0.5	13	20
> 0.5	15	7

*according to the Fontaine classification.

and influenced the incidence of subsequent limb loss. The initial information concerning graft patency was derived from an analysis of the clinical series followed up as long as 11 years. Based on that information the results were reproduced in a randomized clinical trial followed up for 7 years.

Efficacy of treatment

There was a marked difference between groups untreated and treated during the first 18 months both in the analysis and the trial (88% vs 60% of grafts patent at 18 months). Later in the course the curves seemed to parallel each other, but probably show a second decline after approximately 60 months of treatment. Fibrous hyperplasia of the intima, myo-intimal proliferation, stenosis of the valvular rings, suture line stenosis and aneurysmatic dilatation are the changes made responsible for early graft reocclusion, whereas progression of the underlying atherosclerotic arterial disease is said to be the cause of late graft failure.[17,18] Considering these reasons on one hand and the mode of action of antiplatelet drugs on the other their prescription during early and long-term follow-up seemed justified.

Much of the current enthusiasm to use antiplatelet drugs originates from the classical paper by Chesebro *et al.*[19] Later, antiplatelet drugs as well as oral anticoagulants were shown to be equally effective in preventing aortocoronary graft reocclusion,[20] but aspirin was less cumbersome to use, although the optimal dose, possible combinations of drugs and the importance of side-effects such as gastrointestinal intolerance are still open to intensive debate. Two trials (one in Switzerland[21] and one in the Netherlands[22]) seemed to show a beneficial effect of oral anticoagulants in peripheral vascular disease and following vascular repair. The Dutch trial enrolled patients with atherosclerotic disease managed operatively and nonoperatively, testing oral anticoagulants versus placebo in a double-blind setting.

It is tempting to speculate that following bypass surgery oral anticoagulants might act in preventing stagnation thrombosis in long and small calibre grafts with compromised run-off. It has been shown that critical flow rates exist, below which, as in vein grafts bridging long distances, the incidence of thrombosis rises markedly.[23] Because surgeons are reluctant to start phenprocoumon immediately after surgery, the medication was initiated during the second postoperative week, in general following postoperative arteriography. As soon as a satisfactory technical result was obtained, the treatment assignment was done and the therapy was adjusted accordingly.

Safety of treatment

The prothrombin time levels showed to be within safe therapeutic limits of anticoagulation in 75–81% of estimations. There were several bleeding complications, but the most dangerous possible event, i.e. intracranial haemorrhage, never occurred. Nevertheless one patient was lost after 5.5 years of treatment due to gastrointestinal bleeding related to the medication.

Duration of treatment

The therapy was continued throughout the whole observation period at least in the trial. Since the most striking difference between the groups became obvious in the first 2 years, the medication might be cancelled beyond 2 years following surgery. Cancellation of anticoagulants once commenced may induce cardiac events, at least in the elderly patient with a history of coronary artery disease.[24] Oral anticoagulants have shown to be of value in prolonging the life of vascular patients by preventing vascular events in general and cardiac events in particular.[25,26] Furthermore long-term therapy seemed to reduce the incidence of major amputations.

Study limitations

Although restricted by the number of patients involved, this is a single centre study reporting a series of patients with uniform assessment, management and follow-up. In the trial no patient was lost to follow-up.

This is a randomized but not placebo controlled trial, because it was felt unacceptable to justify regular blood sampling and adjustment of placebo over years and finally hand out 'blinded' anticoagulation charts, which patients are supposed to carry and to produce in case of medical emergency.

Obviously these difficulties are the reason, why only a few placebo controlled trials administering oral anticoagulants where conducted and continued over several years.[20,22,24,26,27] Of course the participants in the trial were invited to outpatient visits with equal frequency implemented by the BMDP program. Graft re-occlusion and limb loss were used as hard primary end points.

Clinical implications

The analysis suspected and the trial confirmed the efficacy of oral anticoagulant treatment in the prevention of vein graft occlusion. During long-term therapy one severe complication occurred. The therapy successfully improved limb salvage rate, therefore oral anticoagulants should be continued for many years following vein bypass surgery.

REFERENCES

1. De Weese JA, Rob ChG: Autologous venous bypass grafts five years later. Ann Surg 174:346–365, 1971
2. Reichle FA, Rankin KP, Tyson R, Finestone A, Shuman CH: Long term results of 474 arterial reconstructions for severely ischemic limbs: a fourteen year follow up. Surgery 85:93–102, 1979
3. Grimley RP, Obeid ML, Ashton F, Slaney G: Long term results of autogenous vein bypass grafts in femoropopliteal arterial occlusion. Br J Surg 66:723–726, 1979
4. Kretschmer G, Huk I, Polterauer P *et al*: Der autologe Venenbypass in der Therapie der arteriellen Verschlußkrankheit der femoro-poplitealen Etage. Wr Klin Wschr 98:830–838, 1986

5. De Weese JA, Rob ChG: Autogenous venous grafts ten years later. Surgery 82:775–784, 1977
6. Dormandy J: Surgical pharmacotherapy. Eur J Vasc Surg 3:379–380, 1989
7. Berquist D: Pharmacological intervention to increase patency; the problem. In: Pharmacological Intervention to Increase Patency after Arterial Reconstruction. Berquist D, Lindblatt B (Eds). Malmö: ICM AB, pp. 11–18, 1989
8. Kretschmer G, Rossmann E, Piza F *et al*: Is antiplatelet therapy of value following repair of iliaco-femoro-popliteal occlusion? Evaluation of a clinical trial. Br J Surg 77:A 346, 1990
9. SAS/STAT User's Guide, Cary, Version 6, North Carolina, USA: SAS-Institute 1990
10. Dixon WJ, Brown MD, Engleman L: BMPD statistical software manual. Berkeley, USA: University of California Press 1990
11. Pocock SJ, Simon R: Sequential treatment assignment with balancing for prognostic factors in the controlled clinical trial. Biometrics 31:103–115, 1975
12. Kaplan EL, Meier P: Nonparametric estimation from incomplete observations. J Am Statist Assoc 53:457–481, 1958
13. Breslow N: A generalised Kruskal–Wallis Test for comparing K-samples subject to unequal patterns of censorship. Biometrika 57:579–582, 1970
14. Mantel N: Evaluation of survival data and two new rank order statistic arising in its consideration. Cancer Chemother Rep 50: 163–165, 1965
15. Pocock SJ: Clinical Trials. New York: Wiley, pp. 176–184, 1984
16. Ad Hoc Committee on Reporting Standards: Society for Vascular Surgery/North American Chapter International Society for Cardiovascular Surgery. Suggested standards for reports dealing with lower extremity ischemia. J Vasc Surg 4:80–94, 1988
17. Whittemore AD, Clowes AW, Couch NP, Mannick JA: Secondary femoro-popliteal reconstruction. Ann Surg 193:35–42, 1981
18. Li Calzi LK, Stansel HC. Failure of autogenous reversed saphenous vein femoro-popliteal grafting; pathophysiology and prevention. Surgery 91:352–361, 1982
19. Chesebro JH, Fuster V, Elvenback LR *et al*: Effect of dipyrimadole and aspirin on late graft patency after coronary bypass operations. N Engl J Med 310:209–214, 1984
20. Pfisterer M, Burkart F, Jockers G *et al*: Trial of low dose aspirin plus dipyridamole versus anticoagulants for prevention of aortocoronary vein graft occlusion. Lancet ii:1–7, 1989
21. Schneider E, Brunner U, Bollinger A: Medikamentöse Rezidivprophylaxe nach femoro-poplitealer Arterienrekonstruktion. Angio 2:73–77, 1979
22. De Smit P, Van Urk H: The effects of long term treatment with oral anticoagulants in patients with peripheral vascular disease. *In* 30. Hamburger Symposium über Blutgerinnung, Basel, Tilsner V, Matthias FR (Eds). Editiones 'Roche', pp. 211-216, 1988
23. Sonnenfeldt T, Cronestrand R: Factors determining the outcome of reversed saphenous vein femoro-popliteal bypass grafts. Br J Surg 67:642–648, 1980
24. Sixty Plus Reinfarction Study Research Group: A double blind trial to assess long term oral anticoagulant therapy in elderly patients after myocardial infarction. Lancet ii:989–993, 1980
25. Kretschmer G, Wenzl E, Schemper M *et al*: Influence of postoperative anticoagulant treatment on patient survival after femoro-popliteal vein bypass surgery. Lancet i:797–799, 1988
26. Smith P, Arnesen H, Holme I *et al*: The effect of warfarin on mortality and reinfarction after myocardial infarction. N Engl J Med 323:147–152, 1990
27. Loeliger EAA, Hensen F, Kroes L *et al*: A double blind trial of long term anticoagulant treatment after myocardial infarction. Acta Med Scand 182:549–566, 1967

The Patients' Contribution to Graft Patency

Janet T. Powell

Arterial reconstruction is costly but often rewarded by limb salvage. The secrets of successful reconstruction include a good surgeon, a good graft and a good patient. Here I will focus on how a good patient improves the success of femoropopliteal bypass grafting.

The indications for femoropopliteal bypass grafting include disabling claudication, critical ischaemia and gangrene, the triad of ischaemic leg disease. Large epidemiological studies have demonstrated an array of risk factors for ischaemic heart disease including raised cholesterol, raised fibrinogen, smoking and positive family history.[1–4] Such studies are lacking for ischaemic leg disease. There are many indications that smoking is a particularly potent risk factor for ischaemic leg disease, both for development and progression of disease.[5–7] How smoking influences the development and progression of ischaemic leg disease is not understood. Smoking influences platelet function,[8,9] increases the permeability of the endothelium,[10] increases plasma fibrinogen and plasma viscosity[11] and promotes vasoconstriction and vasoconstrictive thromboxane synthesis.[12,13] Smoking is considered a bad thing and all surgeons encourage their patients to stop smoking. Until recently, however, we had little firm evidence with which to confront the patient undergoing vascular reconstruction. Nearly all patients undergoing femoropopliteal bypass grafting have a long smoking history. Nicotine is a powerfully addictive substance. Giving up smoking is difficult, patients wish to be co-operative and may deceive the clinician about their inability to give up smoking.[14] There have been many studies which have investigated the effect of smoking on vascular reconstruction. When these have relied on the patient self reporting, smoking does not emerge as a significant risk factor for graft failure.[15–17] A small study listing carboxyhaemoglobin as an index of smoking did find that smoking was associated with graft failure, the patients having a variety of different grafts: vein, prosthetic, aortic and distal.[18]

Previous trials have indicated the efficacy of antiplatelet drugs in prosthetic bypass[19] and aspirin has proved beneficial in the primary and secondary prevention of cardiovascular disease.[20,21] Whilst aspirin appears to have little influence on vein graft patency, using an intention to treat basis, it does influence cardiovascular morbidity and mortality in these patients.[22] The purpose of femoropopliteal vein grafting is to keep legs on and keep patients walking. Exercise could improve the development of collaterals but its role in influencing graft patency has not been investigated.

The establishment of a multicentre trial of antithrombotic drugs and graft materials for femoropopliteal bypass provided a large pool of patients for investigation. Where saphenous vein was available patients were randomized to receive aspirin and persantin or placebo[22] and if vein was not available patients were randomized to receive either a PTFE or a human umbilical vein graft.[23] The patients were independently monitored for graft patency by trial co-ordinators, who obtained blood

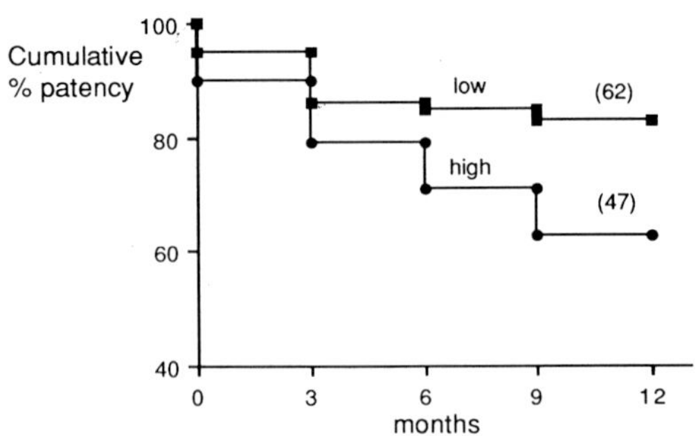

Fig. 1. Vein graft patency in smokers and nonsmokers. Patients with thiocyanate <70 μmol/l (nonsmokers) had a significantly improved patency rate at 1 year, 84%, compared with patients with thiocyanate >70 μmol/l (smokers), 63%: $p<0.02$. The number of patients is given in parentheses.

samples at 6 months after bypass. These blood samples (vein grafts $n=189$, prosthetic grafts $n=93$) were analysed for the smoking markers, carboxyhaemoglobin thiocyanate, lipids, fibrinogen and salicylate. The results were analysed using life tables.

On direct questioning by the trial co-ordinators only 20% of patients with a vein bypass continued to smoke 6 months after reconstruction. Smoking markers indicated that 45% of all patients continued to smoke 6 months following arterial reconstruction. There are rewards for the 55% who have stopped smoking. Graft patency in patients with thiocyanate levels <70 μmol/l (nonsmokers) was significantly higher at 12 months, 84%, compared with smokers (thiocyanate >70 μmol/l) where patency was only 63% after 1 year, $p<0.02$ (Fig. 1). The life table for prosthetic grafts has a similar appearance, patients with lower thiocyanate concentrations had a graft patency at 1 year of 85% compared with only 66% in smokers, $p<0.05$ (Fig. 2). The use of smoking markers has removed the ambiguity of deception (Fig. 3) and clearly demonstrates that graft patency depends on stopping smoking.

Most vein graft failures occur in the first few months after femoropopliteal bypass suggesting that graft thrombosis may contribute to graft failure. Smoking increases

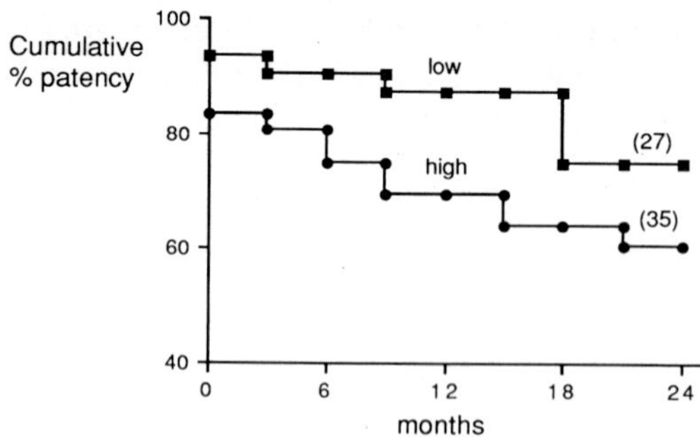

Fig. 2. Prosthetic graft patency in smokers and nonsmokers. Patients with thiocyanate <70 μmol/l (nonsmokers) had a significantly higher patency rate at 1 year, 85%, compared with patients with thiocyanate >70 μmol/l (smokers), 66%: $p<0.05$. The number of patients is given in parentheses.

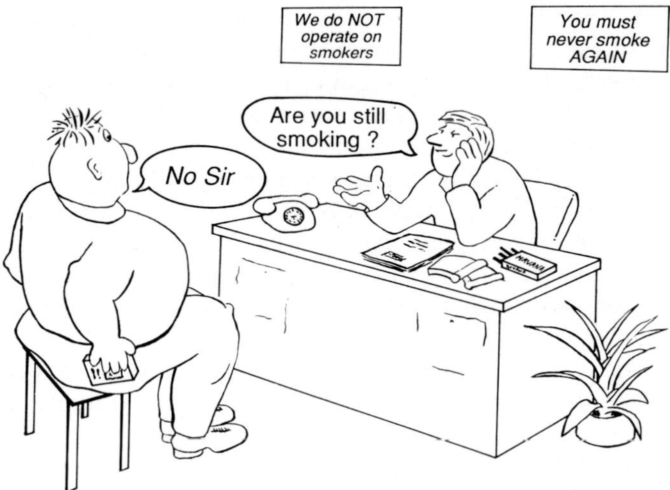

Fig. 3. Deception amongst smokers.

plasma fibrinogen,[9,11] the principal protein found in thrombus, as fibrin. Increased plasma fibrinogen levels are also a powerful predictor of vein and prosthetic graft failure.[24,25] For vein grafts patients with below median fibrinogen levels had a 1-year patency rate of 90% compared with only 57% in patients with above median fibrinogen levels, $p<0.0002$ (Fig. 4). For prosthetic grafts, patients with below median fibrinogen levels had a significantly improved patency (84%) at 2 years compared with a patency of only 51% in patients with above median fibrinogen levels, $p<0.025$.[25] Fibrinogen and smoking were the two principal factors that adversely affected both vein and prosthetic graft patency.

Smoking is mostly an all-or-nothing phenomenon. A patient continues smoking or a patient stops smoking. Stopping smoking will gradually effect a 5–10% reduction in plasma fibrinogen.[11] Other factors recognized to increase plasma fibrinogen levels include ageing, obesity, the acute phase response, diabetes and genetic background. The patient can do little about ageing but age itself was not a poor prognostic indicator in the Femoropopliteal Bypass Trial. Obesity is within the control

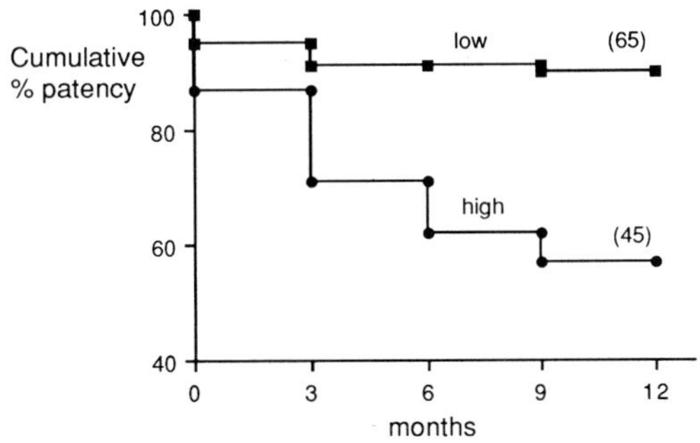

Fig. 4. Vein graft patency and plasma fibrinogen. Patients with concentrations < median (●); patients with concentrations > median (■), numbers of patients with patent grafts is given in parentheses.

of the patient and weight loss can effect rapid reductions in fibronogen level of 5–10%. The acute phase response will cause fibrinogen levels to double within 4–5 days of an acute event, elective or emergency surgery being one such event. This unwanted increase of fibronogen levels secondary to the bypass surgery must contribute to early graft failure from thrombosis. The acute phase response wanes within 14 days. It has also been suggested that there is a strong genetic contribution to the plasma fibrinogen level,[26] with subjects homozygous for a polymorphic variant of the beta-fibrinogen gene having the highest fibrinogen levels. The association has been demonstrated in healthy nonsmokers but it has not been found in patients with peripheral arterial disease.[27] In these patients heavy smoking appears to be the most powerful influence on fibrinogen levels.

Thrombosis is balanced by fibrinolysis. Two variables associated with fibrinolysis were also studied in patients undergoing vein grafting: D-dimer is a fibrinolytic cleavage product of crosslinked fibrin and plasminogen activator inhibitor (PAI-1) is an endogenous inhibitor of tissue plasminogen activator, secreted by the liver, platelets and endothelial cells. Whilst both these variables were increased in patients, compared with a healthy control population, neither variable was associated with graft failure (Table 1). In contrast lipoprotein (a), a homologue of plasminogen, considered to antagonize the action of plasminogen at the endothelial surface[28] was associated with vein graft failure (Table 1). Active fibrinolysis, which can be promoted by exercise, may be a further controllable factor helping to maintain graft patency.

Since thrombosis is likely to contribute to vein graft failure the important purpose of the Femoropopliteal Bypass Trial was to investigate the efficacy of antiplatelet drugs on vein grafts. The vein graft patency in patients randomized to aspirin and persantin was not significantly different from patients randomized to placebo.[22] I have already indicated that about one-quarter of all patients appear to be untruthful about their smoking habits. A similar proportion (28/80, 35%) appeared to be noncompliant with the active aspirin–persantin tablets. Interestingly about one-quarter of patients on placebo (18/65, 26%) had salicylate in their serum sample taken at 6 months after bypass. Some of these had been prescribed aspirin by their general practitioner, who must have overlooked or forgotten the letter asking him or her not to prescribe aspirin, other patients may have used compound medications, such as Beecham Powders, not realising that they contained aspirin. When graft patency

Table 1. Thrombotic and fibrinolytic risk factors and 1-year vein graft patency in 157 patients

	Patent grafts (n = *113)*	*Occluded grafts* (n = *44)*
Mean age (years)	67.0	65.5
% Male	70	75
Diabetes (%)	19	16
Fibrinogen (g/l)	3.9 (2.8–5.4)	**4.8 (3.3–8.0)
D-Dimer (mg/l)	280 (60–460)	170 (70–580)
PAI-1 U/ml	13.3 (3–24.2)	15.5 (5.6–29.8)
Lipoprotein (a) (mg/l)	10.7 (7.2–12.2)	*11.8 (7.8–13.0)

The figures for plasma variables are given as median (10–90 centiles).
Significant difference *$p<0.05$, **$p<0.001$.

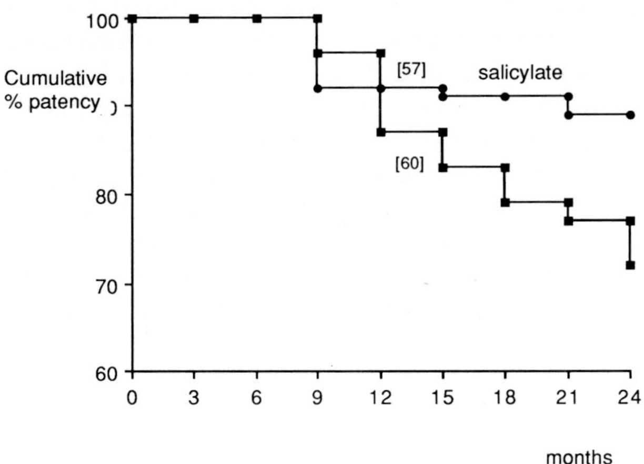

Fig. 5. Vein graft patency and serum salicylate. Of patients with vein grafts patent at 6 months after bypass, those with salicylate present in their serum, had a higher patency rate at 1 year, 92%, compared with those not taking aspirin or other salicylates, 87%, $p<0.05$. The number of patients is given in parentheses.

was analysed on the basis of serum salicylate in patients with patent grafts 6 months after bypass those taking aspirin had a significantly improved graft patency at 1 year, 92%, compared with those not taking aspirin, patency 87%, $p<0.05$ (Fig. 5).

These results indicate that there are good patients and patients. The good patients stop smoking and take their aspirin. The good patient probably looks after himself in other ways, takes exercise to improve his circulation. Indeed the maxim of stop smoking, keep walking given to claudicants[29] can equally be applied to the patient after distal vascular reconstruction. Stopping smoking helps decrease plasma

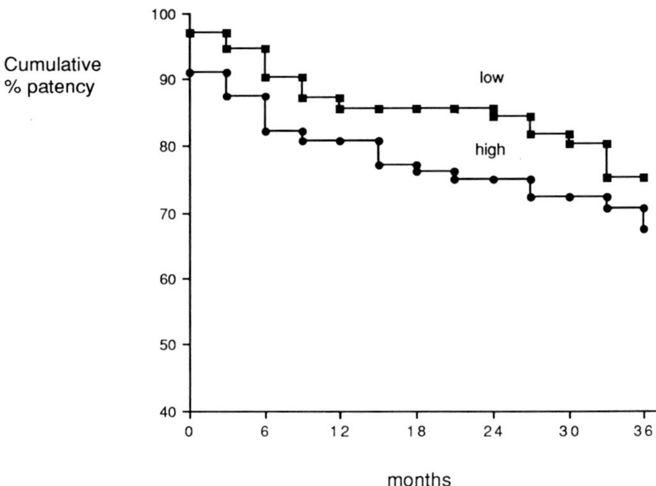

Fig. 6. Vein graft patency and body mass index. The more obese patients, those with body mass index above median, had a lower graft patency, 76%, at 3 years than patients with below median body mass index, 68%. The number of patients is given in parentheses.

fibrinogen and keeping walking promotes fibrinolysis.[30,31] The good patient, whether through diet or exercise is not overweight. Increased body mass index also may adversely influence graft patency (Fig. 6). The good patient does well and provides satisfying results for the surgeon. How can we help the other patients who would appear to prefer an amputation to quitting smoking? Breaking the nicotine habit requires help. These other patients and their families need counselling. There is also evidence that nicotine chewing gum facilitates quitting smoking in hospital patients.[29] This is an area where we could be more helpful and all patients who have smoked until reconstruction should be offered the opportunity of nicotine chewing gum to help them quit the smoking habit. The prescription of low dose aspirin to all vein graft patients could also be considered. Such measures must be more cost-effective than secondary reconstruction or amputation.

ACKNOWLEDGEMENTS

I would like to thank all the participants of the Femoropopliteal Bypass Trial for permission to study their patients. The Femoropopliteal Bypass Trial was supported by the Medical Research Council by grants to C. N. McCollum and R. M. Greenhalgh. The laboratory studies were supported by a grant from the British Heart Foundation to R. M. Greenhalgh and J. T. Powell.

REFERENCES

1. Kannel WB, McGee D, Gordon T: A general cardiovascular risk profile. The Framingham Studies. Am J Cardiol 38:46–51, 1976
2. Gordon T, Kannel WB, Castelli WB, Dawber TR: Lipoproteins, cardiovascular disease and death. The Framingham Studies. Arch Intern Med 141:1128–1131, 1981
3. Meade TW, Brozovic M, Chakrabarti RR *et al*: Haemostatic function and ischaemic heart disease. Principal results of the Northwick Park Heart Study. Lancet ii:533–537, 1986
4. Durrington PN, Hunt L, Ishola M, Arrol S: Apolipoprotein (a), AI and B and parental history in men with early onset ischaemic heart disease. Lancet i:1070–1073, 1988
5. Kannel WB, Shurtleff D: The Framingham Study. Cigarettes and the development of intermittent claudication. Geriatrics 28:61–68, 1973
6. Strong JP, Richards ML: Cigarette smoking and atherosclerosis in autopsied men. Atherosclerosis 23:451–476, 1976
7. Hughson WG, Mann JI, Tubbs DV, Woods HF, Walton I: Intermittent claudication: factors determining outcome. Br Med J i:1377–1379, 1978
8. Schmidt KG, Rassmusen JW: Acute platelet activation induced by smoking. *In vivo* and *ex vivo* studies in humans. Thromb Haemostas 51:279–282, 1984
9. Nowak J, Murray JJ, Oates JA, Fitzgerald GA: Biochemical evidence of a chronic abnormality in platelet and vascular function in healthy individuals who smoke cigarettes. Circulation 76:6–14, 1987
10. Allen DR, Browse NL, Rutt DL, Butler L, Fletcher C: The effects of cigarette smoke, nicotine and carbon monoxide on the permeability of the arterial wall. J Vasc Surg 7:139–152, 1988
11. Meade TW, Iveson J, Stirling J: Effects of changes in smoking and other characteristics on clotting factors and the risk of ischaemic heart disease. Lancet ii:986–988, 1987
12. Winniford MD, Jansen D, Reynolds GA *et al*: Cigarette smoking induced vasoconstriction in atherosclerotic coronary artery disease and prevention by calcium antagonists and nitroglycerin. Am J Cardiol 59:203–207, 1987

13. Lassila R, Seyberth HW, Haapanen A *et al*: Vasoactive and atherogenic effects of cigarette smoking: a study of monozygotic twins discordant for smoking. Br Med J 297:955–957, 1988
14. Sillett RW, Wilson MB, Malcolm RE, Ball KP: Deception amongst smokers. Br Med J ii:1185–1186, 1978
15. Green RM, Ouriel K, Ricotta JJ, DeWeese JA: Revision of failed infrainguinal bypass graft: principles of management. Surgery 100:646–653, 1986
16. Kretschmer G, Wenzl E, Piza E *et al*: The influence of anticoagulant treatment on the probability of function in femoropopliteal vein bypass surgery. Surgery 1–2:453–459, 1987
17. Rutherford RB, Jones DN, Bergentz S-E *et al*: Factors affecting the patency of infrainguinal bypass. J Vasc Surg 8:236–246, 1988
18. Greenhalgh RM, Laing SP, Cole PV, Taylor CTW: Smoking and arterial reconstruction. Br J Surg 68:605–607, 1981
19. Green RM, Roedersheimer LR, DeWeese JA: Effects of aspirin and dipyridamole on the patency of lower extremity bypass grafts. Surgery 92:462–466, 1985
20. Hennekens C, Peto R, Hutchinson GB, Doll R: An overview of the British and American aspirin studies. N Engl J Med 308:923–924, 1988
21. Antiplatelet Trialists Collaboration: Secondary prevention of vascular disease by prolonged antiplatelet treatment. Br Med J 296:320–331, 1988
22. McCollum CN, Alexander C, Kenchington G, Franks PJ, Greenhalgh RM: Antiplatelet drugs in femoropopliteal bypass: A multicentre trial. J Vasc Surg 11:1991 (in press)
23. McCollum CN, Kenchington G, Alexander C, Franks PJ, Greenhalgh RM: PTFE or HUV for femoropopliteal bypass: a multicentre trial. Eur J Vasc Surg 1991 (in press)
24. Wiseman SA, Kenchington G, Dain R *et al*: Influence of smoking and plasma factors on patency of femoropopliteal vein grafts. Br Med J 299:643–646, 1989
25. Wiseman S, Powell JT, Greenhalgh RM *et al*: The influence of smoking and plasma factors on prosthetic graft patency. Eur J Vasc Surg 4:57–61, 1990
26. Humphries SE, Dubowitz M, Cook M, Stirling J, Meade TW: Role of genetic variation at the fibrinogen locus in determination of plasma fibrinogen concentrations. Lancet i:1452–1454, 1987
27. Wiseman SA, Jaye PD, Powell JT *et al*: Frequency of DNA polymorphisms of the apolipoprotein B and fibrinogen genes in young patients with peripheral arterial disease. Appl Cardiovasc Biol i:118–124, 1989
28. Miles LA, Fless GM, Levin EG *et al*: A potential basis for the thrombotic risks associated with lipoprotein (a). Nature 339:301–302, 1989
29. Housley E: Treating claudication in five words. Br Med J 296:1483–1484, 1988
30. Ferguson EW, Bernier LL, Banta GR *et al*: Effects of exercise and conditioning on clotting and fibrinolytic activity in men. J Appl Physiol 62:1416–1421, 1987
31. Drygas WK: Changes in blood platelet function, coagulation and fibrinolytic activity in response to moderate, exhaustive and prolonged exercise. Int J Sports Med 9:67–72, 1988
32. Lan W, Sacks HS, Sze PC, Chalmers TC. Metaanalysis of randomized controlled trials of nicotine chewing gum. Lancet ii:27–30, 1987

The Choice of Prosthetic Material for Femoropopliteal Bypass

Peter J. Franks

Although saphenous vein has been used for femoropopliteal bypass for many years it has remained the treatment of choice for patients undergoing femoropopliteal bypass. However, in a substantial number of patients saphenous vein is not available for various reasons, so alternative materials have had to be developed for these patients.

In 1951 Dacron was first used as an arterial conduit.[1] Since then there have been a number of series reported of patients undergoing femoropopliteal bypass with a range of reported cumulative patencies. Stephen *et al.*[2] reported a 50% 1-year patency with Dacron, whilst Smits *et al.*[3] produced a 4-year patency of 80% above knee, and 54% below knee. Further advances in the manufacturing process improved 4-year patency in one study from 56% using external velour Dacron to 78% using noncrimped Dacron.[4]

Since the introduction of Dacron other types of prosthetic material have become widely available. A Teflon based product polytetrafluorethylene (PTFE) was designed, manufactured and used in arterial surgery in 1973.[5] Several reports have been published of graft patency for this material over different periods of follow-up. As with Dacron, the reported patency appears to dependent on the level of the distal anastamosis, with one study reporting 3-year patency of 82% above knee compared with 45% below knee.[6] However, in a study published in the same year Veith *et al.* found a 3-year patency of 79% above knee which was higher in the below knee anastamosis at 86%.[7]

In 1976 Dardik described the use of gluteraldehyde tanned human umbilical vein (HUV) for arterial reconstruction in the baboon.[8] Four years later they reported a series of 183 femoropopliteal reconstructions using this material.[9] At 1 year, 84% patency was achieved which dropped to 76% at 3 years.

Although these initial series are interesting the results have demonstrated wide differences in reported patency rates. This probably reflects more the skill of the individual surgeons and patient selection rather than results from which useful comparisons of the prosthetic materials can be drawn. Other series have been published which attempt to compare different prosthetic materials in patients who were operated on by the same surgeon. In 1981 Weisel *et al.* reported their experience of using HUV, PTFE and autologous vein grafts.[10] They found a 3-year patency of 34% in HUV and 33% in PTFE compared with 75% in saphenous vein. Conversely Cranley *et al.* found higher 5-year patency rates for patients with claudication when using HUV compared with PTFE (81% vs 65%) and in patients undergoing limb salvage (74% vs 41%).[11] A retrospective review comparing Dacron and PTFE grafts produced poorer 2-year patency for PTFE in patients with claudication (90% vs 78%) and for limb salvage (55% vs 21%).[12] Clifford compared Dacron and HUV grafts and found the 1-year patency difference was wide (80% vs 48% respectively) with both dropping at 2 years (57% vs 39%).[13]

Despite the number of published series it is still difficult to prove any benefit of one prosthetic graft over another. Although the groups of patients receiving different prosthetic types may be similar, graft selection for particular patients may make the results misleading. Moreover, many clinics may have introduced a second prosthetic at a different time. This may influence the results as operative and postoperative procedures change over the years.

RANDOMIZED TRIALS OF PROSTHETIC MATERIALS

To test whether a particular graft performs better than another it is not sufficient to compare the experience of large series with different grafts. The randomized controlled trial is the internationally accepted method for testing the efficacy of drugs and other treatments in medical science. This method can and has been equally applied to surgery, with randomization between different graft types.

Prior to the UK femoropoliteal bypass trial there were only two previously reported randomized trials of HUV vs PTFE. Eickhoff *et al.*[14] reported a series of 105 patients who underwent below knee femoropopliteal bypass over a 4-year follow-up. At 1 year the patency rates were 53% for PTFE compared with 74% for HUV. At 4 years the results were 22% and 42% respectively, a statistically significant difference in patency over the follow-up period. A major problem with this trial was the lack of standardization of antithrombotic therapy which is known to improve graft patency rates in patients with PTFE grafts.[15,16] Similarly, in patients with above knee grafts there was no standardization of antithrombotic therapy, making the results difficult to interpret.[17]

One of the major thrusts of the UK femoropopliteal trial was to determine whether the insertion of one particular graft conferred an advantage in primary patency over and above the other provided that antiplatelet drugs were standardized between the two groups. This would provide definitive evidence of a difference rather than relying on the nonrandomized observational studies of previous reports.

THE UK FEMOROPOPLITEAL BYPASS TRIAL

The trial was a collaboration between 47 vascular surgeons co-ordinated through two centres in London and Birmingham. For patients who received a saphenous vein graft the aim was to determine whether antiplatelet therapy (aspirin 300 mg + dipyridamole 150 mg twice daily) improved primary graft patency, the results of which are reported in Chapter 6. For the patients who received a prosthetic graft the aim was to determine whether the use of PTFE was significantly different from HUV with respect to graft patency, with both treatment groups receiving antiplatelet therapy.[18] The analysis was based on an 'Intention to treat' basis for the centres randomizing patients. Aspirin (600 mg per day) and dipyridamole (300 mg per day) were given to all patients who received a prosthetic graft in line with previously published randomized placebo controlled trials of these drugs in prosthetic graft patency.[15,16] Objective testing of grafts was made by two trial co-ordinators using hand-held Doppler probes and measuring ankle brachial pressure indices. Failure was confirmed by either duplex imaging, digital subtraction angiography or isotope angiography. It was anticipated that 200 patients would be entered into this trial, which would be capable of detecting a 20% difference in failure rate assuming a background failure rate of 50% (5% level of significance 80% power).

MAIN RESULTS OF TRIAL

After 5 years a total of 252 prosthetic grafts had been inserted, with an average follow-up of 35 months. Of these, 191 came from centres who were randomizing patients to either prosthetic material. The remainder either received Dacron grafts ($n=20$) or were receiving nonrandomized HUV or PTFE grafts ($n=41$).

Over the follow-up period 101/252 grafts failed. Most failures occurred early, with a failure rate of 52/1000 patient-months over the first 3 months, reducing to 21/1000 by 6–12 months and 10/1000 in subsequent years. As expected, there was a significantly poorer patency rate in below knee prosthetics compared with above knee at 3 years (35% vs 65% $p<0.0001$), Fig. 1.

For the patients coming from the randomizing centres, the cumulative patency for PTFE grafts at 1, 2 and 3 years was 61%, 56% and 48% compared with 68%, 63% and 57% with HUV (Fig. 2). This difference failed to achieve statistical significance ($p=0.270$).[18]

SECONDARY PATENCY AS AN INDICATOR OF SUCCESS

In 1980 Veith *et al.* reported on 175 PTFE grafts.[19] In this series nine thrombosed within 1 month and 22 between 1 and 23 months. Of the early failures four were

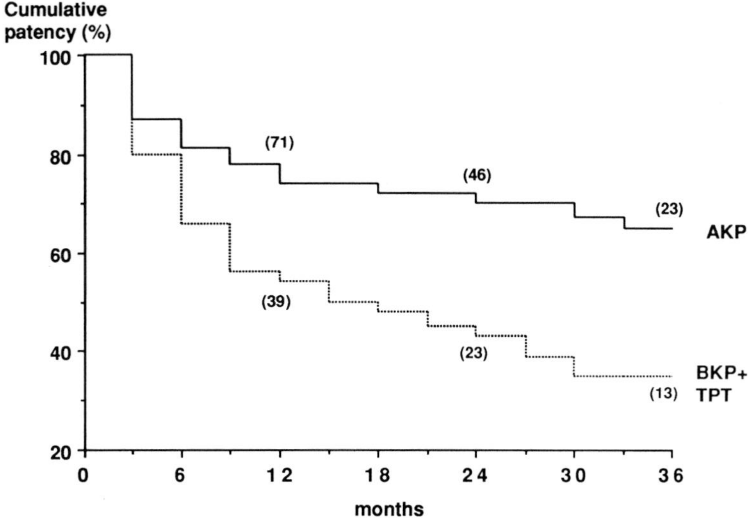

Fig. 1. Comparison between above knee and below knee primary patency in all patients who received a prosthetic graft. There was a significantly higher patency in the above knee group (logrank $p<0.0001$).

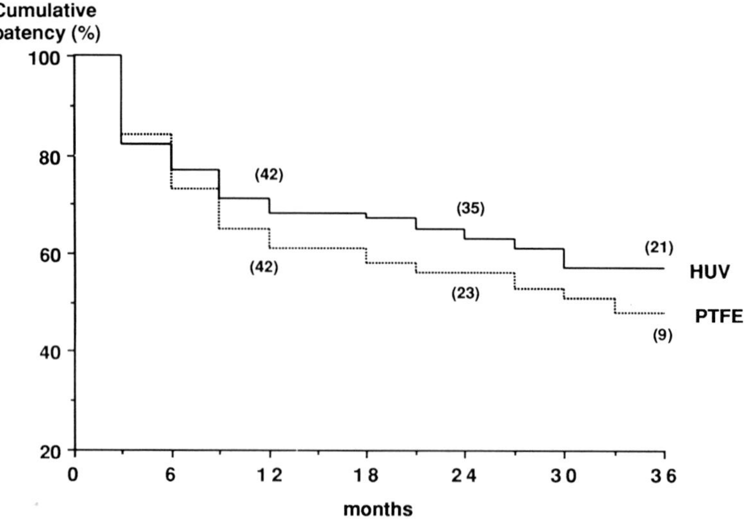

Fig. 2. Primary patency in patients randomized to receive either PTFE or HUV grafts. There was no statistically significant difference over the follow-up period ($p = 0.270$).

by thrombectomy and five with graft extensions. All of these grafts were patent at last follow-up ranging from 3 to 27 months. Of the 22 late failures, 25% were due to intimal hyperplasia and treated with incision and patch angioplasty, 42% had graft extensions and 33% underwent thrombectomy. Similarly, Eickhoff *et al.* attempted thrombectomy in 14 cases, though it was successful in four out of nine PTFE grafts and two out of five HUV grafts.[14]

Although the UK trial found no significant difference between prosthetic types for primary failure, data were available on patients who underwent thrombectomy to determine whether this improved patency rates in any direction. There were 19 out of 79 primary graft failures in whom a thrombectomy was attempted.

Of these, 12 were HUV and seven PTFE grafts. When analysing by this secondary patency the results were significantly better in patients who were randomized to HUV compared with PTFE ($p = 0.050$). However, the trial was designed to detect primary patency as the main end-point with no definite policy on attempts to recanalate the graft. Although this number of thrombectomies was small the improved patency in HUV grafts was sufficient to make the result statistically significant. Care must be employed when drawing conclusions from these results, since there was no policy on thromectomy, with only four centres performing more than one secondary procedure. Bias may be introduced by centres selecting to operate only on one type of graft, but on the data available, HUV had improved secondary patency.

LIMB SALVAGE

Of greater importance to the patient is whether the insertion of a graft prevents the need for amputation. Data were collected on patients whose grafts had failed, to determine amputation postfailure. In all, 12 patients who had a HUV graft and 23 patients with a PTFE graft underwent major amputation. When analysed by life table the cumulative limb salvage rate was 85% at 2 and 3 years for HUV and 74% and 69% respectively for PTFE ($p=0.077$), Fig. 3.

LONG-TERM FOLLOW-UP

Although the results of this trial have revealed some useful data on the two prosthetic types there is still a need for information on long-term follow-up. Of the patients entered into this trial, average follow-up was only 35 months. Clearly, in order to determine the full extent of the comparison of the grafts a longer follow-up period must be considered, particularly with late failure which may be dependent on factors other than those for early failure. This may be particularly important for HUV grafts which may become aneurysmal necessitating further surgery.[20,21]

THE FUTURE OF RANDOMIZED TRIALS OF PROSTHETIC MATERIALS

Although the trials so far performed on prosthetic materials have produced useful results, there is scope for further trials as new materials are introduced. The application of organized randomized trials has been established in surgery. There must always be an attempt to estimate the clinical benefit required for a trial to be successful in order that realistic estimates of sample size can be produced before the trial starts. Wrong conclusions may be drawn from nonsignificant results purely because the numbers entered into a trial may be too small. Similarly, incorrect

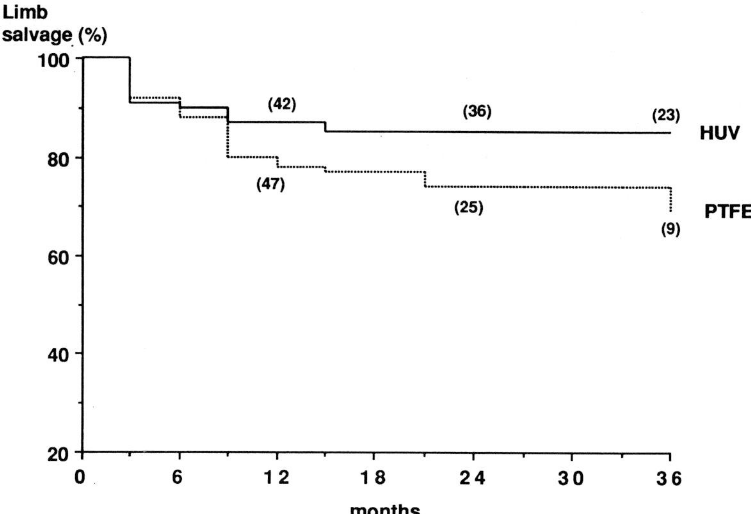

Fig. 3. Limb salvage in patients randomized to receive either PTFE or HUV grafts. The difference between graft types (23 PTFE 12 HUV amputations) failed to achieve statistical significance by the logrank method ($p=0.077$).

conclusions may be drawn from over analysing the data to generate significant results.

To generate the large numbers necessary for a trial there is great value in collaboration between centres performing similar surgical techniques in multicentre trials. Although this will mix individual skills of surgeons this must be employed to determine the overall benefit of a prosthetic material as it is used country wide, not single centre results which may be biased.

CONCLUSION

In the past the choice of prosthetic material in patients undergoing femoropopliteal bypass has to a large extent been based on personal preference of the surgeon and nonrandomized observational studies of different graft types. There is a great need for randomized trials using standardized inclusion and exclusion criteria and standard drug treatment which may influence the end points of the trial. Only the scientific approach of a randomized trial can demonstrate true benefits which may occur in one graft type compared with another. The requirement of large numbers of patients and long follow-up make this work difficult to achieve in single units.

Collaboration in multicentre trials of the type discussed, using the specialist skills of co-ordinators and statisticians will make the work of an acceptable scientific standard from which useful conclusions can be drawn.

REFERENCES

1. Vorhees AB, Jaretski A, Blakemore AH: Uses of tubes constructed from Vinyon-N cloth in bridging arterial defects. Ann Surg 135:332, 1952
2. Stephen M, Loewenthal J, Little JM *et al*: Autogenous veins and velour Dacron in femoropopliteal arterial bypass. Surgery 81:314, 1977
3. Smits PJH, Brands LC: Four years experience with dacron velour vascular prostheses in the femoro-popliteal region. J Cardiovasc Surg 21:53, 1980
4. Kenney DA, Sauvage LR, Wood SJ: Comparison of non crimped, externally supported EXS and crimped non-supported Dacron prostheses for axillofemoral and above knee femoro-popliteal bypass. Surgery 92:931, 1982
5. Matsumoto H, Hasegawa T, Fuse K: A new vascular prosthesis for small caliber artery. Surgery 74:519–522, 1973
6. Christensen JT, Broome A, Eklof B, Norgren L: Revascularization of popliteal and below knee arteries with expanded PTFE graft: Long term results of 196 reconstructions. J Cardiovasc Surg 22:461, 1981
7. Veith FJ, Gupta SK, Daly V: Femoropopliteal bypass to the isolated popliteal segment: Is polytetrafluorethylene graft acceptable? Surgery 89:296, 1981
8. Dardik H, Dardik H: Successful arterial substitution with modified human umbilical vein. Ann Surg 182:252–258, 1976
9. Dardik H, Ibrahim IM, Jarrah M, Sussman BC, Dardik H: Three year experience with glutaraldehyde-stabilized human umbilical vein for limb salvage. Br J Surg 67:229–232, 1980
10. Weisel RD, Johnstone KW, Baird RJ, Drezner AD: Comparison of conduits for leg revascularization. Surgery 89:8–15, 1981
11. Cranley JJ, Hafner CD: Revascularization of the femoropopliteal arteries using saphenous vein, polytetrafluorethylene and umbilical vein grafts. Five and six year results. Arch Surg 117:1543, 1982

12. Brands LC, Van Bockel JH, Jorning PJG, Smits PJH: A retrospective study of autogenous saphenous vein, Dacron velour and PTFE in femoropopliteal bypass grafting. *In* International Symposium on Arterial Reconstruction of the Lower Limb, Suy R, Shaw HL (Eds). Oxford: Medical Education Services, pp. 21–31, 1980
13. Clifford PC, Gazzard V, Lawrance RJ, Clyne CAC, Webster JHH: Below knee femoropopliteal bypass in severe ischaemia; results using EXS Dacron and human umbilical vein. Ann Roy Coll Surg (Eng) 68:319–322, 1986
14. Eickhoff JH, Broome A, Ericsson BF *et al*: Four years' results of a prospective, randomized clinical trial comparing polytetrafluorethylene and modified human umbilical vein for below-knee femoropopliteal bypass. J Vasc Surg 6:506–511, 1987
15. Green RM, Roedersheimer LR, DeWeese JA: Effects of aspirin and dipyridamole on expanded polytetrafluorethylene graft patency. Surgery 92:1016–1026, 1982
16. Goldman M, Hall C, Dykes J, Hawker RJ, McCollum CN: Does III indium platelet deposition predict patency in prosthetic arterial grafts? Br J Surg 70:635–638, 1983
17. Aalders GJ, van Vroonhoven TJMV, Lobach HJC, Wijffels CCSM: PTFE versus human umbilical vein in above knee femoro-popliteal bypass. Early results of a randomized clinical trial. J Cardiovasc Surg 229:186–190, 1988
18. McCollum C, Kenchington G, Alexander C, Franks P, Greenhalgh M: PTFE or HUV for femoropopliteal bypass: A multicentre trial. Eur J Vasc Surg 1991 (in press)
19. Veith FJ, Gupta S, Daly V: Management of early and late thrombosis of expanded polytetrafluorethylene (PTFE) femoropopliteal bypass grafts: Favourable prognosis with appropriate reoperation. Surgery 87:581–587, 1980
20. Dardik H, Ibrahim IM, Sussman B *et al*: Biodegradation and aneurysm formation in umbilical vein grafts. Observation and a realistic strategy. Ann Surg 199:61–68, 1984
21. Boontje AH: Aneurysm formation in human umbilical vein grafts used as arterial substitutes. J Vasc Surg 2:524–529, 1985

SURVEILLANCE OF ARTERIAL RECONSTRUCTION

Can Colour Duplex Surveillance of Femorodistal Vein Bypasses Result in Reduction of Graft Failures?

Jaap Buth, Ben Disselhoff, Ellie Truyen and Leo Stam

Postimplantation problems in femorodistal bypasses such as the development of stenoses have been recognized as a significant factor in vein graft failure in the first 2 years.[1–4] Methodical follow-up should primarily aim at the prevention of recurrent ischaemic symptoms. However, regular history-taking and pulse palpation at postoperative follow-up often fails to indicate impending graft failure. In addition it has been recognized that only few grafts can ultimately be saved by thrombectomy or thrombolytic therapy once complete graft thrombosis has occurred.[5–7] As a result periodic surveillance of femorodistal bypasses with a noninvasive screening method to detect pre-occlusive stenotic lesions has become well accepted.

Although it seems a rational approach to screen vein grafts for anatomic abnormalities several questions have remained unanswered. The natural history of graft stenosis has not been completely elucidated in that the proportion of stenoses that actually progress to the point of graft thrombosis is unknown. Which noninvasive method is to be employed to reliably detect graft stenoses against reasonable cost?

Methods suitable for periodic graft examination that have been evaluated in recent years are Doppler ankle pressures and duplex scanning. Doppler ankle pressure measurement is the method most widely employed for evaluating graft function at follow-up and this method is attractive because of its simplicity and low cost. Duplex methods seem valuable in that they are sensitive for haemodynamically nonsignificant stenosis and they may alert the vascular surgeon in good time to a graft at risk for thrombosis.[8] Also colour-duplex (C-duplex) has been applied successfully for the follow-up surveillance of peripheral bypass grafts.[9–11] Advantages of the colour system include enhanced imaging which facilitates the detection of artery- and graft stenoses. In addition examination time is markedly reduced compared to conventional grey-scale duplex.[10]

The necessity of these advanced screening methods in the assessment of the severity of graftstenosis however is uncertain. Doubts about the benefit of searching and repairing early graft lesions have been expressed.[12] In addition it is not settled what duplex criteria are the best indicators for pre-occlusive stenosis. Finally studies evaluating graft surveillance rarely compare the results with nonscreened control series. The beneficial effect of surveillance programs and long-term graft patency, is therefore not indisputably demonstrated. The purpose of this chapter is to review findings that may justify the set-up of a surveillance protocol. In addition a recently accomplished study of a clinical series is presented.

ANKLE BLOOD PRESSURE MEASUREMENTS FOR DETECTING GRAFT STENOSES

Ankle pressure indices (API) as an indicator for significant stenoses in femorodistal grafts or adjacent inflow and run-off arteries have extensively been investigated. In an earlier series of 77 grafts from our institution that were screened with C-duplex and API 13 severe graft or anastomotic stenoses were identified during the follow-up period.[9] Compared to the API in the early postoperative period a decrease of more than 0.15, which was considered to indicate a significant obstruction, was observed in only four limbs. All 13 stenotic lesions were revised using patch plasty. Following this procedure an increase of more than 0.15 was observed in seven. As a diagnostic parameter ankle pressures were only useful in 31%. This may in part be a result of the fact that stenotic lesions in some cases may be unnoticed at the time of the operation and are first identified at a follow-up C-duplex examination.

The little diagnostic value of API had been established previously by others. Wolfe *et al.* found that a decrease of API indicated a significant graftstenosis in 50% and Bandyk *et al.* found that 36% of stenotic lesions were missed by API determination.[13,14]

A decrease of API in our experience often coincided with the return of symptoms a fact that detracts even more from its usefulness as a tool in detecting stenoses that otherwise would not be identified. In a large retrospective study evaluating 232 bypasses followed over a 5-year period a decrease of API of more than 0.20 at any interval of the follow-up did not herald impending graft failure.[12] In this report it was emphasized that resting API was insensitive even for significant angiographic abnormalities. In another study it was found that adding postexercise measurements of API improved the sensitivity for identifying graft stenosis.[15] However, in the relative large proportion of patients that have either noncompressible arteries or cannot perform a treadmill test API or postexercise API can not be used.

Despite its little diagnostic value in detecting stenotic lesions ankle blood pressures will undoubtly remain part of follow-up examinations. This measurement is suitable for documenting graft occlusions and severe outflow obstruction in all cases when footpulses are not palpable. In addition ankle blood pressure measurements are used by some to supplement a duplex surveillance protocol in that respect that grafts with evidence of stenoses are being followed with frequent intervals until symptoms or a drop in API develop.[16,17] This would, however, not be our own policy as will be described hereafter.

INSTRUMENTATION AND METHODS IN C-DUPLEX GRAFT SURVEILLANCE

Grigg *et al.* demonstrated a wide observer variability in mean volume flow measurements performed with duplex and these workers pointed out that an increase in peak systolic velocity (PSV) over the site of a stenotic lesion in a graft or an artery was a more reliable parameter for its diagnosis.[18] A drawback of the conventional grey-scale B-mode duplex is that several pulsed Doppler flow samplings along the entire length of the graft are needed to search for stenotic lesions. This method is therefore rather time consuming.

Because of its unique properties C-duplex appears particularly suited for mapping peripheral blood vessels and femorodistal bypasses for the purpose of detecting and localizing stenotic lesions. Quantitative pulsed Doppler velocity data can be obtained from a given point within the arterial lumen and velocity measurements can be performed as in conventional duplex scanning.

During C-duplex examination, the entire length of the graft from the groin to the host artery well below the distal anastomosis is traced with a 7.5 MHz transducer unless the artery is deep when a 5 MHz transducer is used. The patient lies in the supine position for scanning the femoral and above knee popliteal segment as well as the crural vessels, while the below knee popliteal artery is best assessed with the patient in the prone position. Anastomotic areas at the posterior tibial and anterior tibial arteries are visualized from the medial and anterior approach respectively. The peroneal artery is sometimes difficult to examine. Scanning from the lateral and medial site both usually have to be attempted to find the optimal flow signal. Stenotic segments can be identified by locally increased peak velocities and poststenotic turbulence characterized by colour coded forward and reversed currents. Diameter changes are measured and recorded.

Following graft imaging, midstream pulsed Doppler signals are recorded over normal and diseased vascular segments. The degree of spectral broadening and increase of PSV is classified according to the criteria as described by Jäger *et al.* for the evaluation of peripheral arteries.[19] Graft stenoses are categorized in normal: less than 30% reduction of diameter; mild: 30–50%; and significant: more than 50%, according to velocity and turbulence criteria combined with the findings at imaging (Figs 1, 2).

PRESENT STUDY

Recently we reviewed the records of 147 patients who underwent a femorodistal bypass procedure between January 1987 and April 1990. In these patients 155 bypasses were performed with autologous vein used in all of them. Only patients with open grafts following the first postoperative month were considered. Symptoms were intermittent claudication in 53, ischaemic rest pain in 61, gangrene or ulceration in 37 and aneurysmal disease in four. In 97 the *in situ* technique was used while *ex situ* veins from different locations were used in 58. Femoropopliteal grafts were used in 75 and femorocrural bypasses in 80 cases.

The follow-up graft surveillance protocol comprised a C-duplex scan every 3 months during the first year and every 6 months during the second year. This protocol was followed in 116 grafts (group A), while 39 patients for various reasons did not undergo C-duplex graft surveillance (group B). In this latter group follow-up was limited to assessment of conventional parameters as the return of symptoms, diminished or absent graft or distal artery pulsations and a decreased API. The proportion of diabetics, distribution of ischaemic stages, type and extent of grafts were comparable in the two groups as was the average age of the patients. During the study period it was the policy of the department to request an intra-arterial DSA examination when a significant stenosis was suspected on the basis of duplex criteria or conventional parameters. For this review the diameter reduction was determined by DSA or when this was not performed by C-duplex imaging.

In 48 grafts stenoses were identified which were significant (more than 50% diameter reduction) in 41 (26%) and mild (30–50% stenosis) in seven (4%). A second stenosis was simultaneously identified in 11 grafts. Of all stenoses 37 were located in adjacent inflow arteries, the proximal anastomosis or the above knee graft segment. In 22 cases the stenosis was in the below knee graft segment, the distal anastomosis or the adjacent run-off arteries. The time of onset of the 48 primary

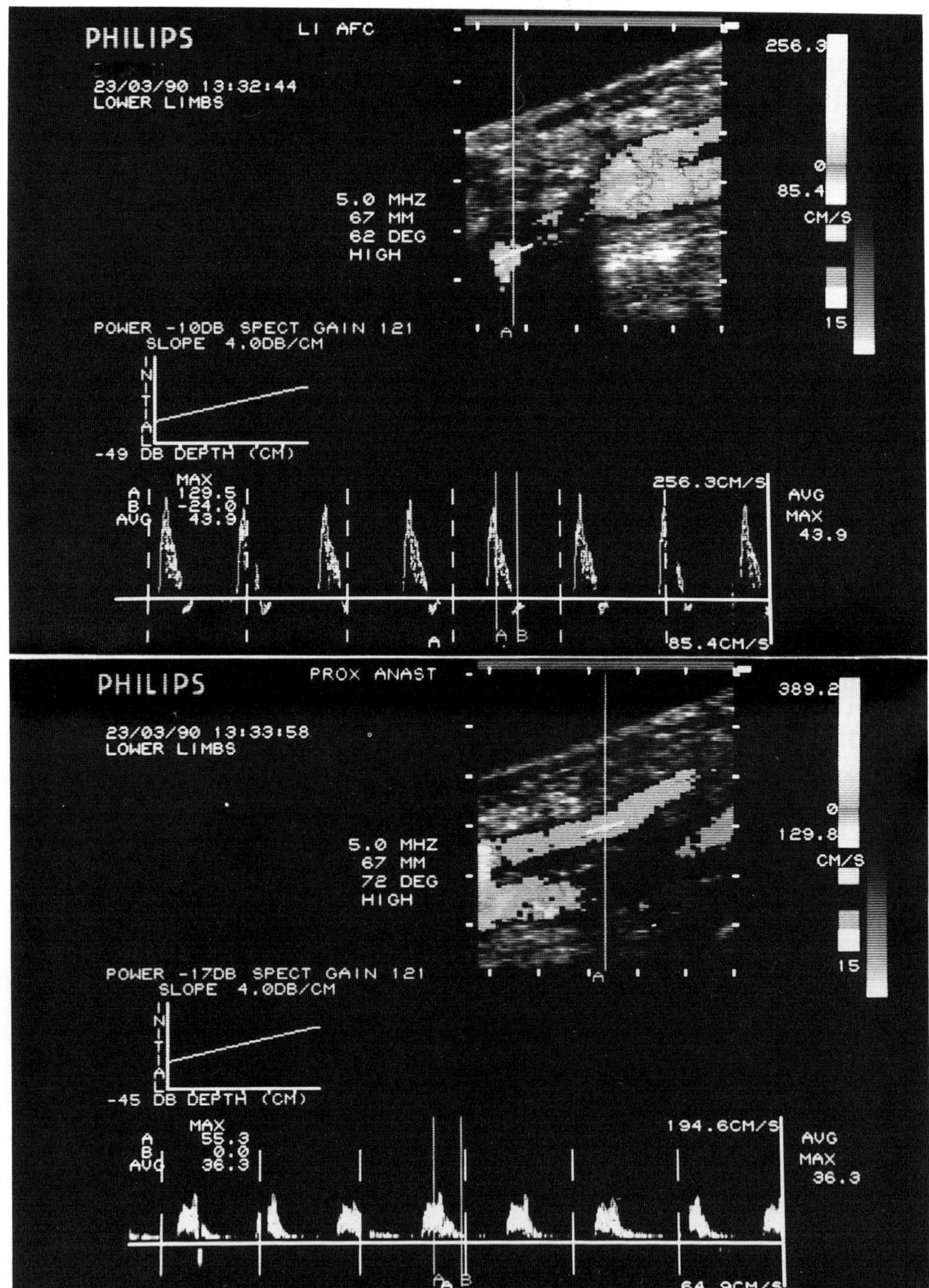

Figs 1a, b. Grey-scale reproduction of C-duplex findings in the above-knee portion of a bypass. a (Upper): Stenosis (40% as measured at arteriography) just proximal from the anastomosis at the common femoral artery with moderately increased PSV (129.5 cm/s). Calcification causes acoustic shadow precluding diameter measurement from C-duplex image. b (Lower): Monophasic flow pattern in the graft with normal PSV (55.3 cm/s).

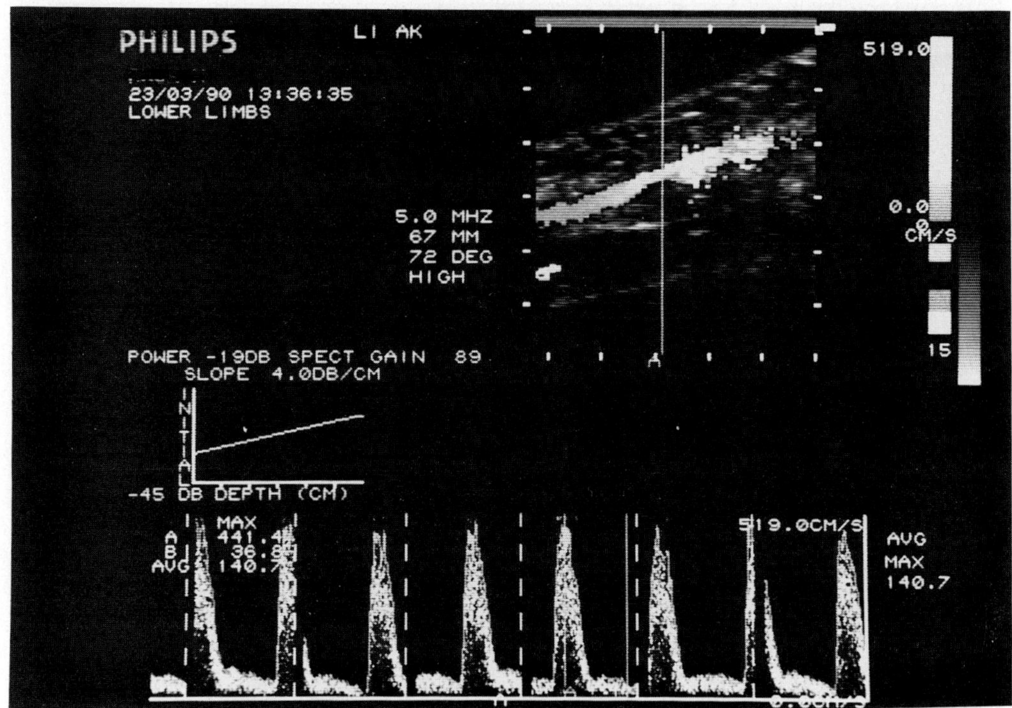

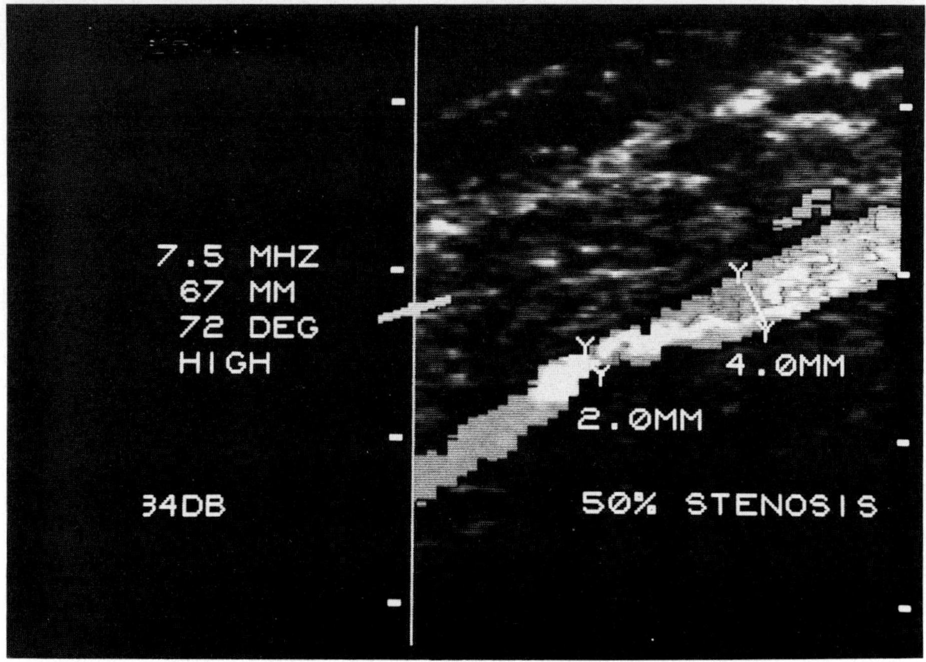

Figs 1c, d. Grey-scale reproduction of C-duplex findings in the above knee portion of a bypass: 50% measured stenosis in the mid-thigh portion of the vein graft with markedly increased PSV (441.4 cm/s).

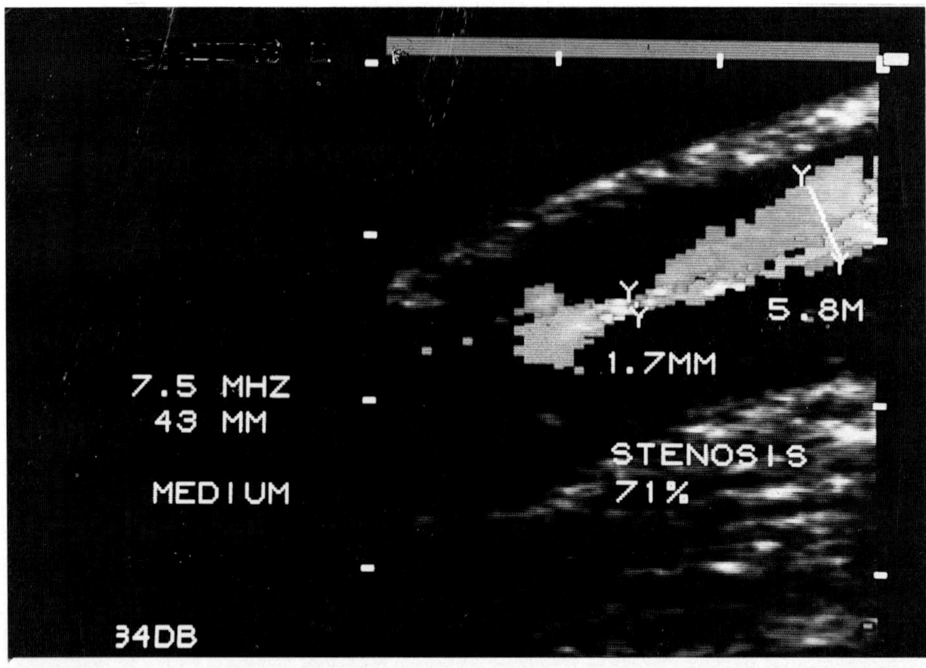

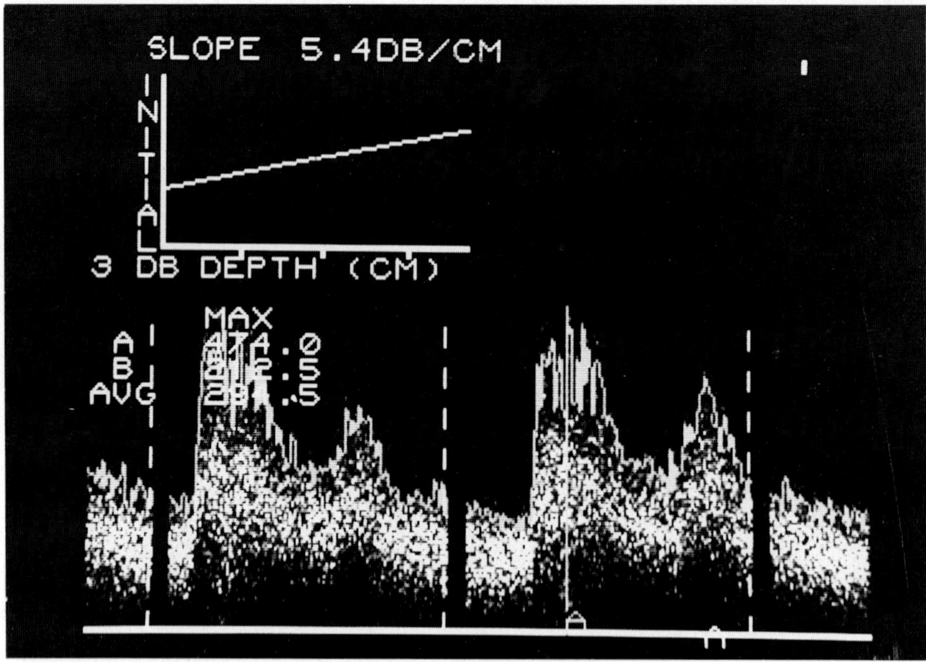

Fig. 2a, b. Grey-scale reproduction of stenosis with a measured 70% diameter reduction. PSV is markedly increased (474.0 cm/s) and intensive spectrum broadening of flow signal is present.

stenotic lesions was in 40 grafts in the first year following the bypass procedure, while 8 developed stenoses between 12 and 36 months (Fig. 3). It is of interest that all seven mild stenoses were first detected longer than 6 months after the operation.

The incidence of stenoses was significantly higher in group A with C-duplex surveillance (43 grafts, 37%) as compared with group B that had follow-up using conventional criteria (five grafts, 13%). Secondary patency rates (including patency maintained by revisions of stenotic lesions) were calculated for both groups. Group A had a significantly better three-year patency (91%) as compared to group B (64%) (Fig. 4). It must be reiterated that grafts that occluded in the first month were excluded from this analysis.

Although no uniform policy was followed by the different responsible surgeons, most severe stenoses, over 50% diameter reduction, came to a revision. Therefore the better patency in group A can be ascribed to the more frequent employment of secondary procedures for graft or adjacent artery stenosis.

Often historic controls or literature data are used to compare the patency as obtained in duplex surveillance studies.[4,20] The present series represents a comparison with a conventionally screened group with similar characteristics operated in the same period in the same institution. Reasons for not having C-duplex screening were in approximately half of the cases due to judgement of the surgeon and in half from lack of compliance to the follow-up of the patients.

From our experience as well as from a report from Moody *et al.*[20] a significantly higher patency rate in the group with duplex surveillance could be observed. The question whether duplex surveillance is an absolute necessity will first be answered after a randomized prospective study comparing groups with and without periodic duplex screening has been accomplished. Until the results of such a study are known an approach of active search for stenotic lesions following bypass grafting is justified by results as currently reported by different workers in this field.

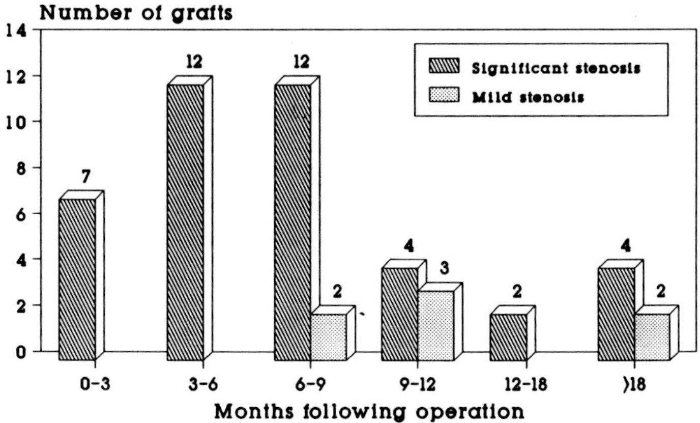

Fig. 3. Temporal distribution of the onset of graft stenosis.

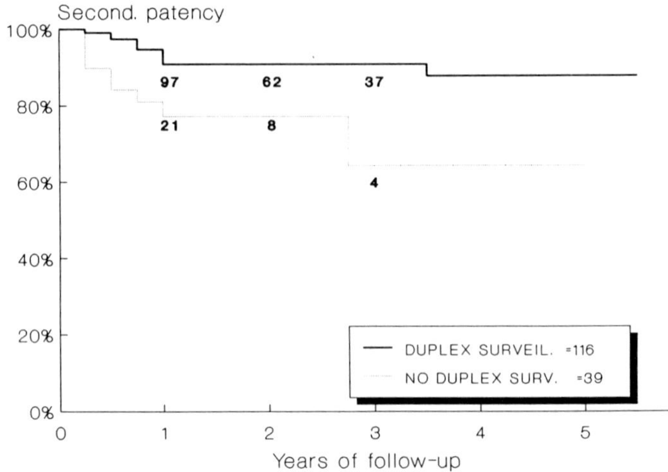

Fig. 4. Cumulative secondary patency rates in Group A (grafts with C-duplex surveillance) and Group B (grafts with follow-up using conventional criteria for stenotic changes); $p = 0.00528$ (logrank).

C-DUPLEX CRITERIA AND ASSESSMENT OF SEVERITY OF GRAFT STENOSIS

From the start of our study we have combined the Doppler velocity spectrum criteria of Jäger *et al.*[19] with diameter measurements as enabled by the colour image. In patients where a stenosis of more than 30% was suspected these findings could in most cases be compared with available DSA studies. All other patients were assumed not to have a stenosis.

For all patients the duplex peak systolic velocity index (PSV-index) was assessed. This is the ratio of the PSV within a normal segment and the PSV within the narrowest part of the stenosis. For normal grafts a PSV-index was assessed by dividing the value obtained at a proximal and at a distal point of the graft. Normal grafts have an index close to 1. Stenotic grafts are characterized by lower PSV-indices indicating locally increased blood flow velocity.

A graphic representation shows that there is a weak correlation between the API and the PSV-index (Fig. 5). It is clear that only the latter variable can be used to discriminate bypasses with and without a stenosis. A PSV-index of 0.65 separates these categories with a sensitivity of 86%, a specificity of 97% and a kappa-corrected accuracy of 0.85. Most of the significant graft stenoses and five of the seven grafts with mild stenoses had a PSV-index lower than 0.65.

Similarly PSV as measured at the site of the stenosis was compared for grafts with and without stenoses and a slightly less discriminating value was observed. A PSV higher than 110 cm/s usually indicated a significant stenosis (sensitivity 89%, specificity 94% and kappa 0.83).

Our findings are in complete agreement with the previous findings of Grigg *et al.* in that 'high velocity criteria' provide an accurate indicator for significant, although most often not-pressure-reducing, stenosis.[8] In fact our criterium of an index value of less than 0.65 parallels their criterium, that was a local PSV increase of more than 50%.

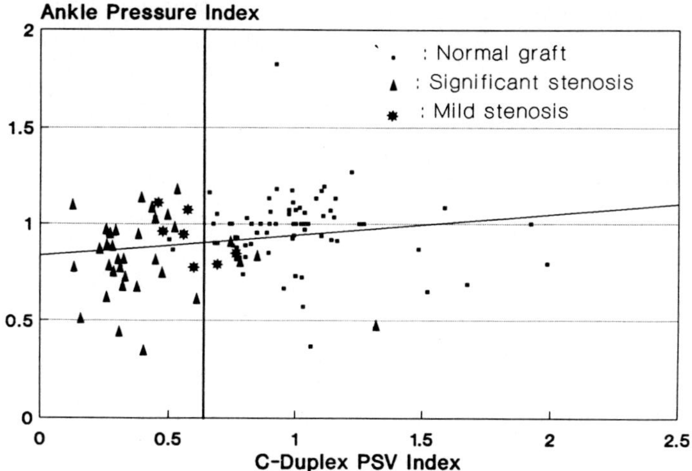

Fig. 5. Correlation of PSV-index and ankle pressure index for patients with and without graft stenosis; $p = 0.0021$, $r = 0.289$.

In addition a decrease of the PSV along the entire length of the femorodistal bypass to less than 45 cm/s has been documented to reflect a critical stenosis and a graft at risk for occlusion.[4,14,16] When our data were correlated according to this criterium we found a sensitivity as low as 12% and a specificity of 98%. Only five patients with identified stenoses fulfilled this 'low velocity criterium'. In these patients there was one with inflow stenosis, one with run-off disease and three cases with multiple graft stenoses. Only one patient without an identified stenosis had a graft PSV lower than 45 cm/s and this patient occluded his graft after 2½ years. From this, one may conclude that the low velocity criterium may be particularly useful in identifying inflow and run-off disease as well as multiple graft stenoses. Also Taylor *et al.*[21] have observed that an average PSV lower than 45 cm/s is more often associated with a native artery stenosis.

C-Duplex parameters were correlated to the angiographically determined degree of stenoses. The image-measured diameter reduction correlated not very well with the severity of the stenosis (Fig. 6a). It seems that C-duplex image often underestimates the degree of stenosis. This may be due to acoustic scattering and enhancement at the site of a stenosis represented by coloured pixels outside the vessel lumen.

A better agreement was shown by the PSV-index and the degree of stenosis as determined by arteriography (Fig. 6b). Of 19 grafts with stenoses of 75% or more 15 had a PSV-index less than 0.40. However two of the grafts with a PSV-index in the normal range, that is higher than 0.65, had an average graft PSV lower than 45 cm/s. This illustrates that both high and low velocity criteria should be considered in graft evaluation.

DOES THE PRESENCE OF A STENOSIS INFLUENCE GRAFT PATENCY?

Bandyk reported in 1989 comparable four-year patency in grafts without a stenotic lesion and grafts with revised stenoses.[22] In our material secondary procedures for

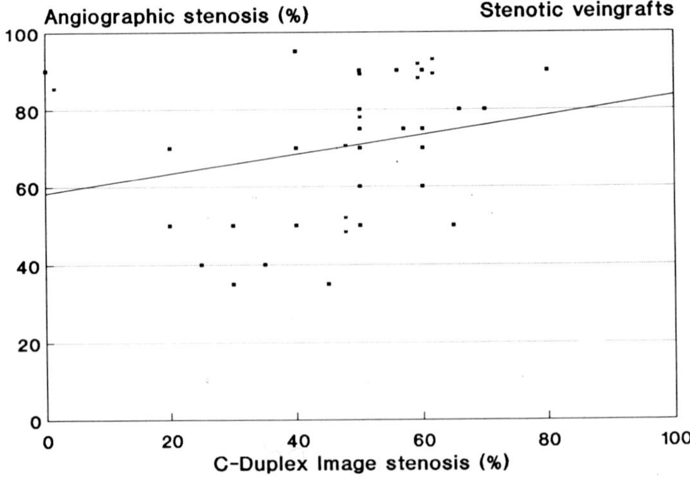

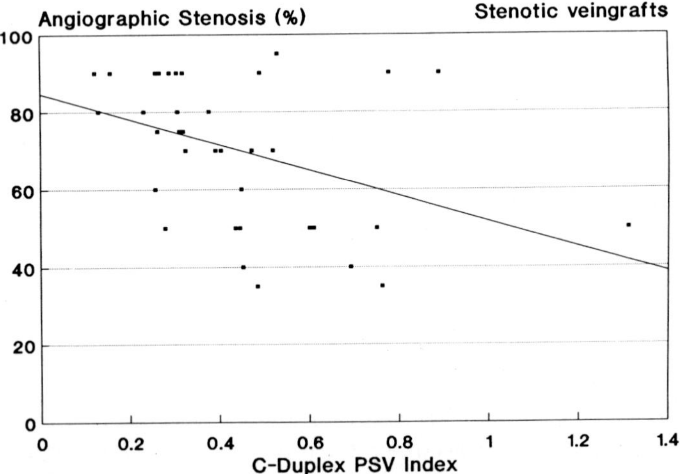

Fig. 6a, b. Correlation of severity of stenosis as determined by intraarterial DSA with a (Upper): C-duplex image measured diameter reduction; $p = 0.020$, $r = 0.380$. b (Lower): PSV-index; $p = 0.0013$; $r = -0.404$.

stenoses were performed in 33 grafts (Fig. 7); 15 grafts did not undergo a revisional procedure. The reasons for this were a stenosis less than 50%, delay in admission for an interventional procedure, failure of patients to return in time for a next follow-up visit and in some cases a deliberate conservative attitude elected by the responsible surgeon. A Kaplan–Meier life table analysis was performed to compare patency rates of the stenotic grafts with and without revision (Fig. 8). A significant difference was observed. The secondary 3-year patency in revised grafts was 93% as opposed to 53% in nonrevised grafts.

The fact that grafts with noncorrected stenoses tend to fail has been reported by most other authors although no life table data were provided. In addition our data do

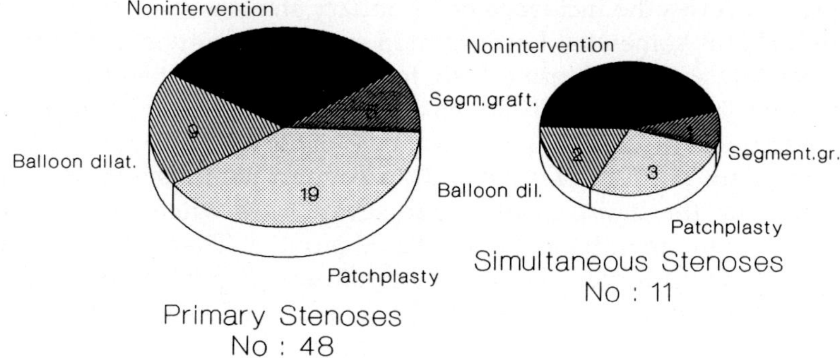

Fig. 7. Managment of all identified stenotic lesions.

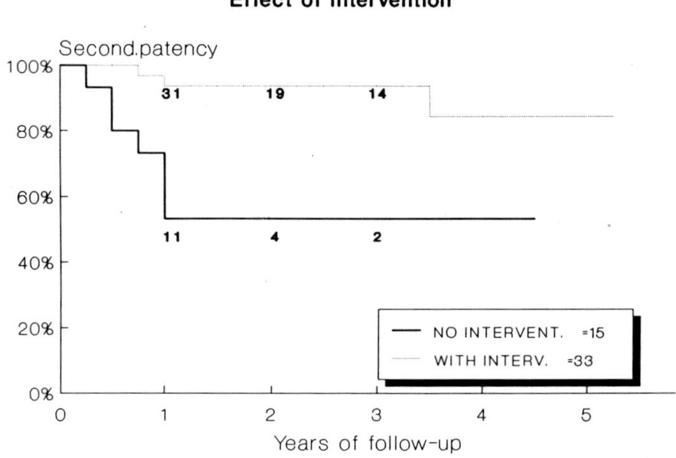

Fig. 8. Cumulative secondary patency rates in grafts with revised stenoses and stenotic grafts without re-intervention; $p = 0.00145$ (logrank).

suggest that when a severe stenotic lesion is diagnosed it is better not to wait until a next follow-up visit and not consider the patient as a waiting list case. Several of our grafts occluded shortly after an admission had been scheduled. In fact only one of these grafts has remained open without revising its 60% stenosis.

None of the seven mild stenoses were revised. At continued C-duplex follow-up all mild stenoses have remained stable for periods from 2 to 13 months.

RESTENOSIS AFTER GRAFTREVISION

After a secondary procedure for a stenotic lesion vein graft or anastomotic area restenosis has been observed in 23–29% of grafts.[7,23,24] In addition it has been demonstrated that PTA is more often followed by a restenosis as a surgical revision.[25]

In the present series the incidence of secondary stenosis (>50%) was 19% (nine of 48 grafts) what is somewhat lower than in some other reports. In all nine grafts tertiary procedures were performed, six for true recurrent stenosis and three for secondary stenosis at different locations as the initial stenosis. Because of the low number of restenoses we could not demonstrate a higher incidence after PTA compared to surgical revision. The time of onset of the secondary stenosis was after an interval 6–24 months after the initial procedure in seven cases while one restenosis was detected in the first 6 months and one after 27 months. These observations would suggest that follow-up surveillance is to be continued for periods longer than 1 year after a secondary procedure. It should be emphasized that in these continued noninvasive screenings the duplex examination should not be confined to the area of the intial stenosis because three of nine secondary stenoses developed in remote segments.

CONCLUSIONS

A duplex surveillance protocol appears valuable in detecting stenoses in approximately 25% of femorodistal veingrafts. Progression to occlusion can effectively be prevented by timely revision. Although a randomized prospective study demonstrating the advantages of a surveillance protocol both in terms of limb salvage and improved cost benefit ratio has to be performed, at present duplex screening especially within the first year seems justified. As most stenoses start early after the operation we now start as suggested by others C-duplex screening not later than after the sixth postoperative week.[24] Mild stenosis in our experience has a late onset, usually after 6 months, and does not show a tendency to progress rapidly.

Our policy remains to interfere in all stenoses greater than 50% (PSV-index less than 0.65). When a stenosis with a diameter reduction of more than 75% is suspected on the basis of a PSV-index lower than 0.40 (high velocity criterium) or an average graft PSV less than 45 cm/s (low velocity criterium) the patient should be scheduled for intervention urgently. Once a stenosis is dilated or treated surgically there is approximately a 20% chance of recurrence and for that reason graft surveillance should be continued after a secondary procedure for a 2-year period.

REFERENCES

1. Szilagy DE, Elliot JP, Hageman JH, Smith RF, Dallolmo CA: Biological fate of autologous vein implants as arterial substitutes. Ann Surg 178:232–246, 1973
2. Whittemore AD, Clowes AW, Couch NP, Mannick JA: Secondary femoropopliteal reconstruction. Ann Surg 193:34–42, 1981
3. Sladen JD, Gilmour JL: Vein graft stenosis. Characteristics and effect of treatment. Am J Surg 141:549–553, 1981
4. Bandyk DF, Kaebnick HW, Stewart GW, Towne JB: Durability of the *in situ* saphenous vein arterial bypass: A comparison of primary and secondary patency. J Vasc Surg 5:256–268, 1987
5. Cohen JR, Mannick JA, Couch NP, Whittemore AD: Recognition and management of impending vein-graft failure. Arch Surg 121:758–759, 1986
6. Belkin M, Donaldson MC, Whittemore AD *et al*: Observation of the use of thrombolytic agents for thrombotic occlusion of infrainguinal vein grafts. J Vasc Surg 11:289–296, 1990

7. Berkowitz HD, Greenstein S, Barker CF, Perloff LJ: Late failure of reversed vein bypass grafts. Ann Surg 210:782–786, 1989
8. Grigg MJ, Nicolaides AN, Wolfe JHN: Detection and grading of femorodistal vein graft stenoses: Duplex velocity measurements compared with angiography. J Vasc Surg 8:661–666, 1988
9. Disselhoff B, Buth J, Jakimowicz J: Early detection of stenosis of femoro-distal grafts. A surveillance study using colour-duplex scanning. Eur J Vasc Surg 3:43–48, 1989
10. Sladen JG, Reid JDS, Cooperberg PL *et al*: Color flow duplex screening of infrainguinal grafts combining low- and high-velocity criteria. Am J Surg 158:107–112, 1989
11. Londrey GL, Hodgson KJ, Spandone DP, Ramsey DE, Barkmeier LD, Sumner DS: Initial experience with color-flow duplex scanning of intrainguinal bypass grafts. J Vasc Surg 12:284–290, 1990
12. Barnes RW, Thompson BW, MacDonald CM *et al*: Serial noninvasive studies do not herald postoperative failure of femoropopliteal or femorotibial bypass grafts. Ann Surg 210:486–494, 1989
13. Wolfe JHN, Thomas LN, Jamieson CW, Browse NL, Burnand KG, Rutt DL: Early diagnosis of femorodistal graft stenoses. Br J Surg 74:268–270, 1987
14. Bandyk DF, Seabrook GR, Moldenhauer P *et al*: Hemodynamics of vein graft stenosis. J Vasc Surg 8:688–695, 1988
15. Brennan JA, Walsh AKM, Beard JD, Bell PRF: The role of simple non-invasive testing in vein graft surveillance. Europ Soc Vasc Surg, Rome, September 1990
16. Bandyk DF: Postoperative surveillance of infrainguinal bypass. Surg Clin North Am 70:71–85, 1990
17. Green RM, McNamara J, Ouriel K, DeWeese JA: Comparison of infrainguinal graft surveillance techniques. J Vasc Surg 11:207–215, 1990
18. Grigg MJ, Wolfe JHN, Tovar A, Nicolaides AN: The reliability of duplex derived haemodynamic measurements in the assessment of femoro-distal grafts. Eur J Vasc Surg 2:177–181, 1988
19. Jäger KA, Phillips DJ, Martin RL *et al*: Noninvasive mapping of lower limb arterial lesions. Ultrasound Med Biol 11:515–521, 1985
20. Moody P, Gould DA, Harris PL: Vein grafts surveillance improves patency in femoropopliteal bypass. Eur J Vasc Surg 4:117–121, 1990
21. Taylor PR, Tyrrell MR, Crofton M *et al*: Prediction of femoro-distal grafts at risk of occlusion using colour flow imaging: improved criteria. Europ Soc Vasc Surg, Rome, September 1990
22. Bandyk DF, Schmitt DD, Seabrook GR, Adams MB, Towne JB: Monitoring functional patency of in situ saphenous vein bypasses: The impact of a surveillance protocol and elective revision. J Vasc Surg 9:286–296, 1989
23. Bandyk DF, Bergamini TM, Towne JB, Schmitt DD, Seabrook GR: Durability of vein graft revision: A comparison of surgical techniques. SVS/ICVS. Los Angeles, June 1990
24. Taylor PR, Wolfe JHN, Tyrell MR: Graft stenosis: Justification of 1-year surveillance. Br J Surg 77:1125–1128, 1990
25. Thompson JF, McShane MD, Gazzard V, Clifford PC, Chant DB: Limitations of percutaneous transluminal angioplasty in the treatment of femoro-distal graft stenoses. Eur J Vasc Surg 3:209–211, 1989

Graft Surveillance — A Biased Overview

J. H. N. Wolfe, P. R. Taylor and N. J. Cheshire

The failure of arterial bypass grafts for lower limb ischaemia continues to be a significant problem for the vascular surgeon. Reported 5-year failure rates vary from 20–75%,[1–4] and the vast majority of these occur within the first two postoperative years.[5]

The reasons for graft thrombosis have been the subject of many papers in the literature, but Szilagyi and his associates were probably the first to recognize the significance of graft related stenoses and their implications for graft patency.[6]

Many centres have now adopted surveillance programmes to identify and treat these stenoses, but their justification is not universally accepted. In this chapter we discuss the current controversies and their implications for clinical practice.

IS GRAFT SURVEILLANCE JUSTIFIED?

During the last two decades the indications for performing reconstructive arterial surgery for lower limb ischaemia have changed. Whereas previously many grafts were inserted for relatively long distance claudication, this proportion has steadily decreased. One reason for this change is the marked clinical deterioration that may be associated with early graft failure. The patient who presents for further reconstructive surgery, after graft thrombosis, with less accessible residual vessels, compounds this problem. The majority of grafts, therefore, are now inserted for incapacitating claudication or critical ischaemia. The failure of these grafts is associated with a critical leg that cannot always be salvaged.

It is now generally accepted that the causes of graft failure can be divided into three groups depending upon the postoperative time interval[7] (Fig. 1). First, those that fail within the first month are due to either technical failures or poor judgement in the selection of patients. Technical failures can be decreased by using intra-operative techniques such as Doppler,[26] duplex, angiography or the measurement of peripheral resistance.[27,28] Approximately 10–15% of graft failures occur in this period.

Grafts which fail after 2 years usually do so due to progression of underlying atherosclerosis. Measures which may be of benefit to this group include the cessation of smoking, adequate control of diabetes, hypertension and hyperlipidaemia. Approximately 2–3% of grafts per annum fail late.

From 1 month to 2 years, grafts are at risk of thrombosis from graft related stenoses. This group accounts for the vast majority of failures (75–85%). The biggest impact on long-term graft survival would therefore come from the identification and treatment of these graft-related stenoses. There is little doubt that procedures performed on a haemodynamically compromised graft which is still patent, are associated with a much higher salvage rate than procedures undertaken for thrombosed grafts.[2,7]

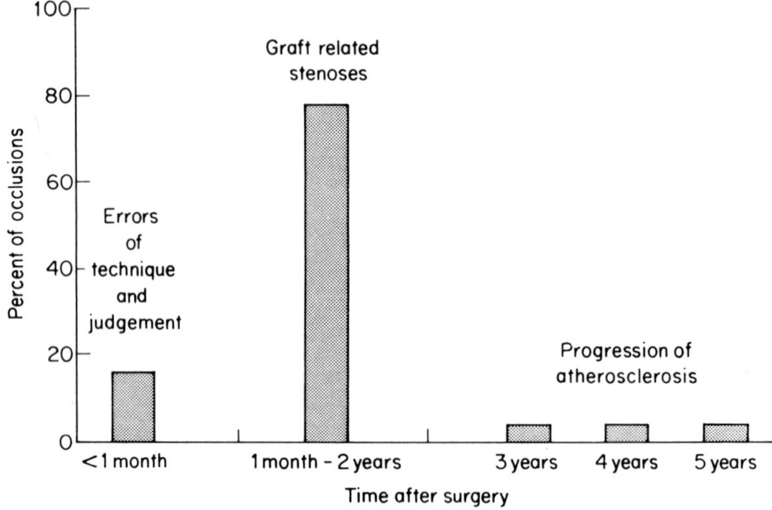

Fig. 1. Graph showing causes and percentage of graft thromboses in relation to postoperative time period. (Derived from Brewster *et al.*)

For these reasons we believe that surveillance is justified. It must be recognized, however, that the evidence relating graft stenoses to thrombosis is circumstantial. There are studies which show an increased graft failure rate if these stenoses are not treated, but to date the number of patients is small.[6–8] There is a need for a randomized control trial to investigate the natural history of graft-related stenoses and the results of intervention.

WHICH TECHNIQUE SHOULD BE USED TO DIAGNOSE GRAFT-RELATED STENOSES?

There are several techniques which can be used to assess graft patency, but not all these can detect tight localized stenoses. It is this confusion which has bedevilled discussions on the relative merits of each technique.

Clinical palpation

The presence of a pulse in a graft indicates merely that a pressure wave is passing along its length, and does not indicate flow. The presence or absence of a pulse gives no indication of impending thrombosis. Clinical palpation, therefore, has a very limited place in graft surveillance.

Doppler treadmill

A Doppler probe detects flow within vein grafts, and is a useful test to ascertain graft patency. If this is combined with recording the Doppler ankle pressures before and after exercise useful information concerning graft function can be obtained. Early workers found this a useful screening method.[23,24] Unfortunately, treadmill postexercise ankle Doppler pressures are relatively insensitive since differences of 0.15 in the ankle brachial systolic pressure index are within the limitations of the test.[9] This is likely to be a major reason why half of graft-related stenoses are missed using this technique.[2,10,17,19,23] The advantages of the technique are simplicity and low cost but lack of sensitivity means that graft stenoses will be missed. We believe that Doppler treadmill studies are therefore of limited use in graft surveillance but others disagree.[25]

Angiography

This remains the yardstick against which other methods are measured. When digital subtraction angiography (DSA) became available, intravenous imaging (IVDSA) became practical for the first time and could be performed on an outpatient basis. Prior to this follow-up arteriography was difficult to justify, particularly for asymptomatic patients. We, therefore, embarked on a prospective study to compare clinical assessment, ankle Doppler pressure assessment and arteriography in the detection of graft stenoses,[17] which revealed that up to one half of angiographic stenoses were not being detected by the other modalities. Although IVDSA is a sensitive test it is expensive and time consuming. Furthermore, the 'flushed' feeling during the contrast infusion is uncomfortable and patient compliance dwindles with repeated investigations. In addition, good left ventricular function is required for high standard intravenous images. Because of this some centres are now using intra-arterial DSA through a fine bore needle in the groin.

These studies in the early 1980s revealed a 20% graft stenosis rate. At that time this figure was considered to be due to poor operative technique, but as other units corroborated these results this high rate of stenosis development became accepted. It is now well established that 15–25% of patients develop a graft-related stenosis.

DUPLEX

At the same time some centres began using Doppler flow analysis combined with real time B-mode ultrasound imaging.[13] This has proved to be a very powerful tool in assessing grafts postoperatively. The ultrasound scan is used to identify the graft, after which the cursor may be accurately placed to measure the frequency change (Doppler shift) caused by the movement of blood within the lumen. If the angle between the Doppler beam and the graft is continuously measured then the velocity of blood flow in the graft can be calculated from the frequency change. Several units were able to predict graft stenosis by a single reading of graft velocity or flow. We were unable to reproduce this accuracy and found little correlation with the stenoses shown on angiography (Fig. 2).

This was disappointing since duplex assessment has clear advantages over angiography in relation to time, expense and the patient's comfort. Bandyk *et al.*[13] relied on an average peak systolic velocity of less than 45 cm/s. This has the advantage of simplicity but we contend that graft threatening stenoses are missed by this method.

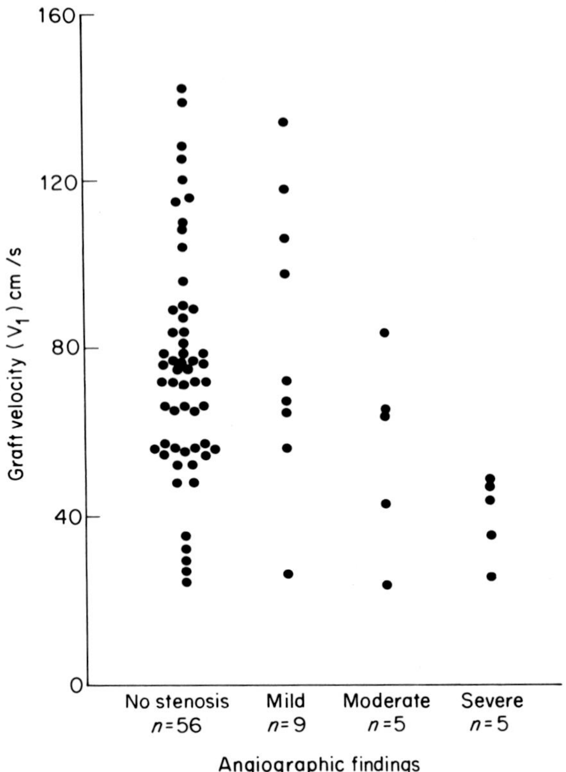

Fig. 2. Scattergram showing overlap of duplex derived velocity findings in grafts shown to be normal or stenosed on angiography. (Reproduced with kind permission of J Vasc Surg.)

Furthermore, if there is a very low flow it is likely that simple methods, such as a history of a recent onset of further claudication or a reduction in ankle systolic pressure, will alert the clinician to further investigation.

The concept of measuring the change in velocity across the stenosis was then developed.[29] Inaccuracies are compounded by the difficulty of measuring graft diameter but this can be negated by measuring the velocity ratios.

Grafts have no branches, therefore flow at any one point in the graft is equal to that at any other point (Fig. 3). Flow is a product of velocity and cross-sectional area, therefore any reduction in area will be associated with a proportional increase in velocity. Any localized increase in velocity is indicative of a stenosis and the degree of stenosis is directly proportional to the increase in velocity.[11] Changes greater than 100% within a 2 cm portion of the graft indicate a significant stenosis (V2 : V1 ratio >2). Velocity is a much more reliable indicator of stenosis than flow, which is prone to change with the patient's cardiac output and also with peripheral resistance. We found a high incidence of interobserver error in the measurement of flow.[12]

A series of 75 patients were studied prospectively using intravenous angiography and duplex scanning[29] comparing both the change in velocity and average peak

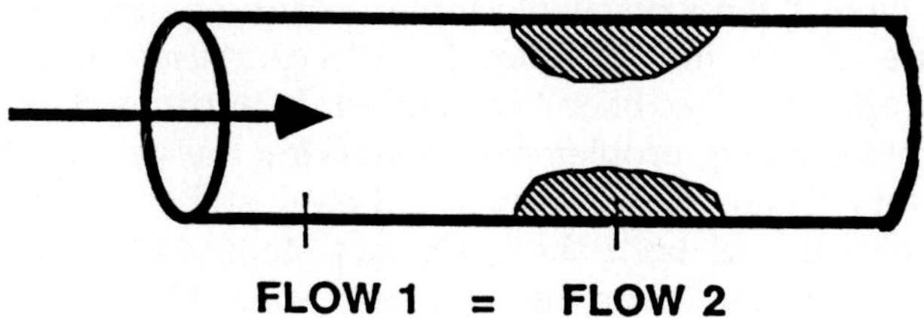

Fig. 3. Diagram showing effect of stenosis on velocity. Flow is a product of cross-sectional (CS) area and velocity and is equal at points 1 and 2. (Reproduced with kind permission of Br J Surg.)

systolic velocity. The results show that a change in velocity of greater than 100% (V2 :V1 ratio greater than 2) identified all graft related stenoses as detected by DSA. However, it did not detect stenoses in the distal native arteries since these are small and difficult to image accurately. Average peak systolic flow velocity failed to detect half of the graft-related stenoses but identified all distal stenoses in the native vessels.[14] A combination of both of these criteria therefore seems to identify all grafts at risk of thrombosis (Fig. 4).

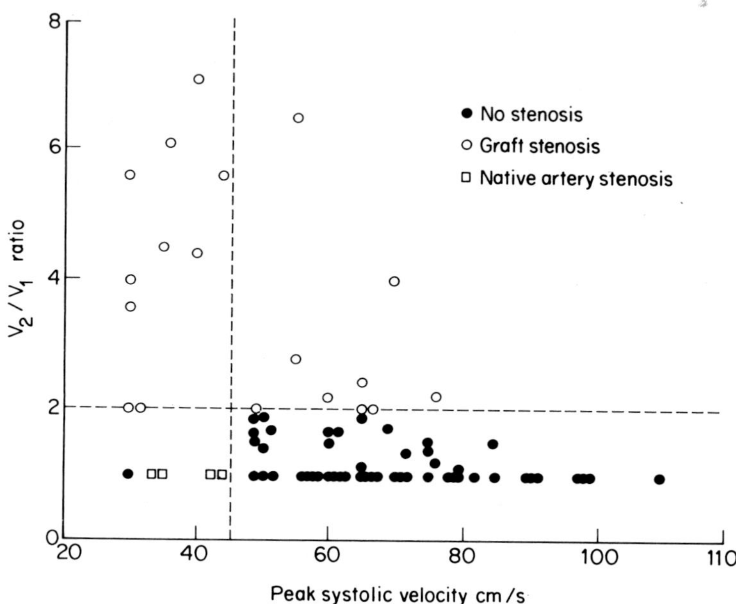

Fig. 4. $V_2 : V_1$ ratio findings compared with peak systolic velocity in grafts which are normal and stenosed on angiography. $V_2 : V_1$ ratio detects all stenoses within grafts but misses four patients with native vessel stenosis who were detected by a peak systolic velocity less than 45 cm. (Reproduced with kind permission of Eur J Vasc Surg.)

Some centres have been critical of duplex scanning. In particular, the time consuming nature of the investigation (which decreases in proportion to the experience of the operator) has been highlighted. In addition there are areas, such as the popliteal fossa, where problems of identifying the vessel have disillusioned some potential users. Colour flow Doppler, although still expensive, allows quicker and easier identification of both the graft and stenoses,[14,15] and may improve acceptance of the technique over the next few years. Other workers have been sceptical of the value of V2 : V1 ratio measurement, pointing out that vein grafts often change calibre at the site of large branches. We believe this criticism is invalid if the velocity change can be shown to revert to the prestenosis velocity at a distal site in the graft.

IMPEDANCE ANALYSIS

An exciting and simple technique has been developed in Bristol using computer calculated impedance analysis to detect stenoses in both the grafts and distal native vessels.[16] The early results are encouraging and further studies by other centres are necessary to critically evaluate this technique with regard to identification of grafts at risk of thrombosis. Such a technique could prove a useful adjunct to the presently available surveillance modalities but we have no experience of its use at present.

ARE SURVEILLANCE PROGRAMMES COST EFFECTIVE?

Graft surveillance programmes are time consuming and expensive, so that the results of intervention must be justified. Also the time limit at which the detection rate does not justify the expense must be identified.

We have recently completed a prospective study of 412 femoropopliteal and femorocrural grafts which were assessed at 6 weeks, 3, 6, 9, and 12 months and then at 6-monthly intervals using both duplex scanning and IVDSA.[10] The overall incidence of stenoses was 17%, and was higher in femorocrural grafts (20%) than femoropopliteal grafts (15%). The majority of stenoses appeared within 6 months of operation, and no new stenoses were detected after 1 year (Fig. 5). Others have reported late stenoses but none of their studies were prospective so that it is uncertain when the stenoses initially developed.

Our results suggest that surveillance programmes should be intensive for the first 6 months, and the grafts should be further assessed at 1 year. After this period, the stenosis occurrence rate is too low to justify continued intensive surveillance except in those grafts which have been shown to have a stenosis which is being observed for progression.

The cost effectiveness of such a surveillance programme has been calculated. A duplex scanner has an initial capital cost of approximately £45 000, and many district general hospitals already own such machines. Maintenance costs are free for the first year and are then approximately 10% of the purchase price annually. The cost, therefore, over a 5-year period is £18 000. The cost of a technician to operate the

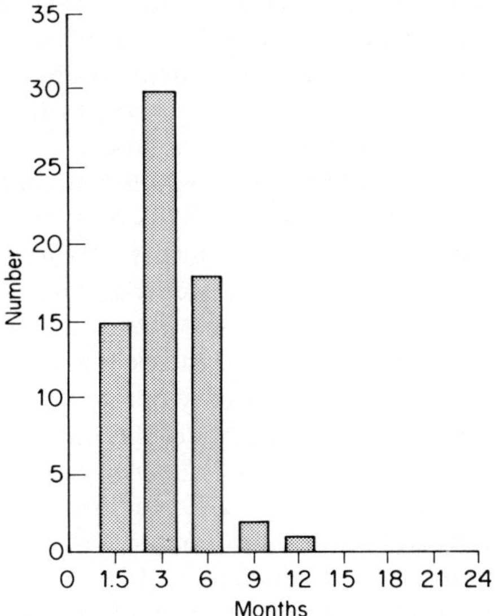

Fig. 5. Numbers of stenoses detected shown with postoperative time. (Reproduced with kind permission of Br J Surg.)

machine is approximately £15 000 per annum, so that over a 5-year period the total cost of purchasing and operating a duplex scanner amounts to £138 000 or about £30 000 per annum. In our own hospital, approximately one-third of the time of the scanner is used for graft surveillance (i.e. £10 000 per annum). One hundred grafts are performed each year and each is scanned six times in the first postoperative year. Each scan, therefore, costs about £20. The incidence of graft stenosis approaches 20%, therefore the cost of detecting each stenosis is £500. Most of the stenoses detected are corrected, so that the cost of repair needs to be brought into the calculation. Hospitalization and repair is estimated at £2000 per patient. The total cost for the surveillance of 100 grafts for 1 year, the detection and repair of 20 stenoses is approximated at £50 000. The cost of an amputation in the UK has been estimated to be more than £25 000, therefore limb loss has to be prevented in only 2% of patients for the programme to be cost effective.

TREATMENT OF GRAFT-RELATED STENOSES

Graft-related stenoses can be treated by either balloon dilatation or surgery. Balloon dilatation is a relatively simple and quick method of treatment but the results have been variable.[10,18,19] Some poor initial results were due to technical failures. The pressures needed to dilate short web stenoses are very high—of the order of 12–15 atmospheres. We have recently amalgamated the data from three centres in the UK with widely varying results to try to deduce which stenoses are suitable for balloon dilatation.[20] The site of the stenosis within the graft, type of graft and number of stenoses had no significant effect on patency after balloon dilatation. The length of the stenosis, however, was critical; those less than 1 cm long were associated with a patency rate of 80% at a mean follow-up of 2 years. Stenoses which were longer than 2 cm were associated with very poor long-term patency (33% at a mean 2-year follow-up). The numbers were small, but there seems little doubt that balloon dilatation should only be used for short web stenoses.

Surgery is associated with consistently better results than balloon dilatation[2,5,7,10,18] and should be performed for longer stenoses. This may be either in the form of a patch angioplasty or a jump graft.[21] We use jump grafts for long stenoses and for those close to the anastomosis, where dissection may be difficult and hazardous.

By intervening in grafts which have been shown to have graft-related stenoses, secondary patency rates may be improved. Bandyk has shown that in a group of femoropopliteal *in situ* vein bypass grafts, primary patency rates of 48% are improved to 89% at 36 months with treatment. The comparable figures for femorotibial *in situ* vein grafts were 58% and 80% at 36 months.[22] Harris[8] has also shown a change in patency rates following the introduction of a surveillance programme. Both these series are open to the criticism that other improvements in technique or management may have influenced their success. Nevertheless, this suggests that intervention is associated with higher long-term graft patency, which in turn seems to justify graft surveillance programmes. The ultimate proof would be a prospective randomized control trial to compare the results of intervention with conservative treatment in patients with proven graft related stenoses. This is, however, becoming increasingly difficult as the circumstantial evidence mounts.

CONCLUSIONS

We believe that graft surveillance programmes are justified for the first postoperative year. Clinical examination, hand-held Doppler and treadmill are insufficient to identify all grafts at risk of thrombosis. Duplex scanning using both average peak systolic flow velocity and localized changes in velocity greater than 100% will identify all grafts at risk of thrombosis. Angiography can then be used prior to surgery or balloon dilatation.

REFERENCES

1. Whitney DG, Khan EM, Estes JW: Vascular occlusion of the arterialised saphenous vein. Ann Surg 42:879–886, 1976
2. Cohen JR, Mannick JA, Couch NP, Whittemore AD: Recognition and management of impending vein graft failure. Arch Surg 121:758–759, 1986
3. Harris PL, Jones D, How T: A prospective randomised clinical trial to compare *in situ* and reversed vein grafts for femoro-popliteal bypass. Br J Surg 74:252–255, 1987
4. Rutherford RB, Jones DN, Bergentz SE *et al*: Factors affecting the patency of infra-inguinal bypass. J Vasc Surg 8:236–246, 1988
5. Brewster JC, LaSalle AJ, Robison JG, Strahorn EC, Darling RC: Femoro-popliteal graft failures: Clinical consequences and success of secondary reconstructions. Arch Surg 118:1043–1047, 1983
6. Szilagyi DE, Elliott JP, Hageman JH, Smith RF, Dallolmo CA: Biological fate of autogenous vein implants as arterial substitutes. Ann Surg 178:232–246, 1973

7. Whittemore AD, Clowes AW, Couch NP, Mannick JA: Secondary femoro-popliteal reconstruction. Ann Surg 193:35–42, 1981
8. Moody P, Harris PL: Vein graft surveillance improves patency in femoro-popliteal bypass. Eur J Vasc Surg 4:117–121, 1990
9. Ouriel K, Zairns CK: Doppler ankle pressure—an evaluation of three months of expression. Arch Surg 177:1297–1300, 1982
10. Taylor PR, Wolfe JHN, Tyrrell MR, Mansfield AO, Nicolaides AN, Houston RE: Graft stenosis—justification of a single year of surveillance. Br J Surg 77:1125–1128, 1990
11. Grigg MJ, Nicolaides AN, Wolfe JHN: Femoro-distal vein bypass graft stenoses. Br J Surg 75:737–740, 1988
12. Grigg MJ, Wolfe JHN, Tovar A, Nicolaides AN: The reliability of duplex derived haemodynamic measurements in the assessment of femoro-distal grafts. Eur J Vasc Surg 2:177–181, 1988
13. Bandyk DF, Cato RF, Towne JB: A low flow velocity predicts failure of femoro-popliteal and femoro-tibial bypass grafts. Surgery 98:799–809, 1985
14. Taylor PR, Tyrrell MR, Bassan B, Nicolaides AN, Wolfe JHN: Prediction of femoro-distal grafts at risk of occlusion using colour flow imaging; improved criteria. Eur J Vasc Surg (in press)
15. Disselhoff B, Buth J, Jakimovicz J: Early detection of stenosis of femoro-distal grafts. A surveillance using colour duplex scanning. Eur J Vas Surg 2:43–48, 1989
16. Wyatt MG, Tennant WG, Baird RN, Horrocks M: Can immediate analysis predict outcome following femoro-popliteal/distal (FPD) bypass. Br J Surg (in press)
17. Wolfe JHN, Lea Thomas M, Jamieson CW *et al*: Early diagnosis of femoro-distal graft stenoses. Br J Surg 74:268–270, 1987
18. Veith FJ, Weister RK, Gupta *et al*: Diagnosis and management of failing lower extremity reconstructions prior to graft occlusion. J Cardiovasc Surg 25:381–384, 1984
19. Thompson JF, McShane MD, Gazzard V, Clifford PC, Chant ADB: Limitations of percutaneous transluminal angioplasty in the treatment of femoro-distal graft stenoses. Eur J Vasc Surg 3:209–211, 1989
20. Taylor PR, Gould D, Harris P, Al-Kutoubi A, Wolfe JHN: Balloon dilatation of graft stenoses—why do they fail? Tripartite Meeting of the British and Irish, Canadian and Dutch Vascular Surgical Societies, London Nov 1990
21. Wolfe JHN, Taylor PR: Repair of the failing femoro-distal graft. *In* Vascular Surgical Techniques: An atlas, 2nd edn, Greenhalgh RM (Ed.). London, Philadelphia: WB Saunders, pp. 287–293, 1989
22. Bandyk DF, Kaebnick HW, Stewart GW, Towne JB: Durability of the in situ saphenous vein arterial bypass; A comparison of primary and secondary patency rates. J Vasc Surg 5:256–268, 1987
23. Berkowitz H, Hobbs C, Roberts C *et al*: Value of routine vascular laboratory studies to identify vein graft stenosis. Surgery 90:971–997, 1981
24. Taylor RS, Fox ND: Ultrasonic prediction of graft failure. J Cardiovasc Surg 18:309–316, 1977
25. Brennan J, Walsh AK, Beard J, Bell PRF: The role of simple non invasive testing in vein graft surveillance. Presented at European Society for Vascular Surgery Annual Meeting Rome Sept 1990
26. Tyrrell MR, Halliday A, Taylor P, Wolfe JHN: Pre-operative graft assessment is simple and inexpensive. Presented at the Vascular Surgical Society Annual Meeting Dundee Nov 1989
27. Parvin S, Bell PR: The use of peripheral resistance measurements in the assessment of severe peripheral vascular disease. Br J Surg 71:311–312, 1984
28. Scott D, Vowden P, Beard J, Horrocks M: Non-invasive estimation of peripheral resistance using PGR before femoro-distal bypass. Br J Surg 77:391–395, 1990
29. Grigg M, Nicolaides A, Wolfe JHN: Detection and grading of femoro-distal vein graft stenoses: Duplex velocity measurements compared with angiography. J Vasc Surg 18:661–666, 1988

Duplex Surveillance of *in situ* Vein Grafts

Mary Paula Colgan, Edmond J. Prendiville, Maria C. Grouden,
Martin P. Molloy, Dermot J. Moore and Gregor D. Shanik

Saphenous vein bypass grafting for occlusive disease of the lower extremity arterial tree was first performed by Goyanes in 1906.[1] Kunlin reported the initial results using reversed saphenous vein to bypass an occlusion of the superficial femoral artery in 1949.[2] The first successful bypass to the infrapopliteal arterial tree was performed by Palma in 1960[3] and Baird reported results of bypass to the malleolar level 6 years later.[4] Limb salvage of 71 and 51% at 1 and 3 years respectively was reported by Riechle in 1980[5] in a group of patients undergoing reversed vein bypass to the tibial vessels for impending limb failure. These results lent impetus to the continuing search for the optimal conduit for arterial reconstruction.

Hall[6] reported the use of the *in situ* saphenous vein for limb salvage using an open technique for valve ablation. Leather and co-workers[7] using refined techniques for valve ablation reported superior results for infra-inguinal bypass and encouraged renewed interest in the technique.

The theoretical and practical advantages of *in situ* grafting include 1) less traumatization of the conduit with possible resultant reduced thrombogenicity, 2) greater vein utilization and 3) easier anastomotic techniques due to the comparable vessel sizes. There are however inherent problems some of which are exclusive to the technique. These include 1) the development of arteriovenous (AV) fistulae, 2) stenosis secondary to valve cusp retention or inadequate ablation and 3) anastomotic or body graft stenosis, which occur as frequently in reversed vein as in *in situ* vein grafts.

Because of these associated problems many authors have recommended routine postoperative surveillance with duplex scanning. The results of Whittemore and colleagues emphasize the importance of detecting graft stenoses[8] as 5-year patency rates were in excess of 80% when stenoses were repaired prior to graft failure and were $<40\%$ when stenoses were repaired in conjunction with thrombectomy.

In 1986 we reported our early findings of graft surveillance[9] using duplex imaging. A total of 49 grafts were followed and three AV fistulae were identified and localized and subsequently repaired under local anaesthesia. Eleven graft stenoses in five grafts were identified and all except one had a significant drop in the corresponding ankle brachial index (ABI). In this study we chose the presence of a peak systolic frequency of $\geqslant 6000$ Hz as indicative of an haemodynamically significant stenosis. Grigg and co-workers use a duplex derived velocity ratio to define and quantify graft stenosis.[10] They studied 75 grafts at 3-monthly intervals using ABIs, duplex imaging and intravenous digital subtraction angiography (IVDSA). The peak systolic velocity at any point within the graft was defined as V_2 and the peak systolic velocity at any point within 2 cm of V_2 was defined as V_1. Percent stenosis was then defined as follows:

$$\%\ \text{stenosis} = 100\ (1 - \sqrt{V_1/V_2})$$

Within 1 year of surgery 25% of all grafts were found to have a stenosis on angiography and in only one instance was there a corresponding drop in ABI. Nineteen were considered not to be haemodynamically significant; however, five progressed over the first year to become haemodynamically significant while three occluded without warning. An additional four of the 56 nonstenosed grafts occluded. In a more recent report from the same unit[11] the authors report the results of surveillance of 412 femorodistal procedures. Sixty-six stenoses occurred, 24 non-haemodynamic and 42 haemodynamic; 63% occurred within the first 6 months and none were detected after 1 year. The authors conclude that with careful surveillance within the first year of surgery continued surveillance beyond this time is not necessary.

To study if this holds true for *in situ* grafts to the tibial vessels we followed 29 patients who had undergone *in situ* bypass grafting up to 5 years previously (mean follow-up 3.2 years). From June 1984 to June 1989 a total of 129 *in situ* bypass grafts were performed in this unit and, of these patients, 56 had died in the intervening time. In an additional 34 instances graft failure had occurred leaving 39 grafts available for study. Six patients were unable to travel and four refused arteriography leaving 29 patients in whom study was complete. Over the same period a total of 322 grafts surveillance studies had been performed. All 29 patients had normal 1-year surveillance studies. Patients underwent the following procedures:

1. Estimation of ankle brachial indices
2. Duplex scanning of the graft
3. Triplex scanning of the graft
4. Intra-arterial DSA.

All studies were performed blindly.

ANKLE BRACHIAL INDICES

Using a continuous-wave Doppler flowmeter systolic pressures were recorded from all three tibial vessels and the highest value used to calculate the ankle brachial index.

DUPLEX IMAGING*

(Model 518, Hoffrel Instruments Inc;, S. Norwalk Connecticut, USA)

Doppler spectral information and B-mode images were obtained along the entire length of the graft. A peak systolic velocity of >6000 Hz was considered indicative of an haemodynamically significant stenosis.

TRIPLEX SCANNING

(Ultramark 9, ATL Inc., Bothell, Washington, USA)

Diagnosis was based mainly on the colour profile and spectral information only sought when this was abnormal. Peak systolic velocity measurements were used

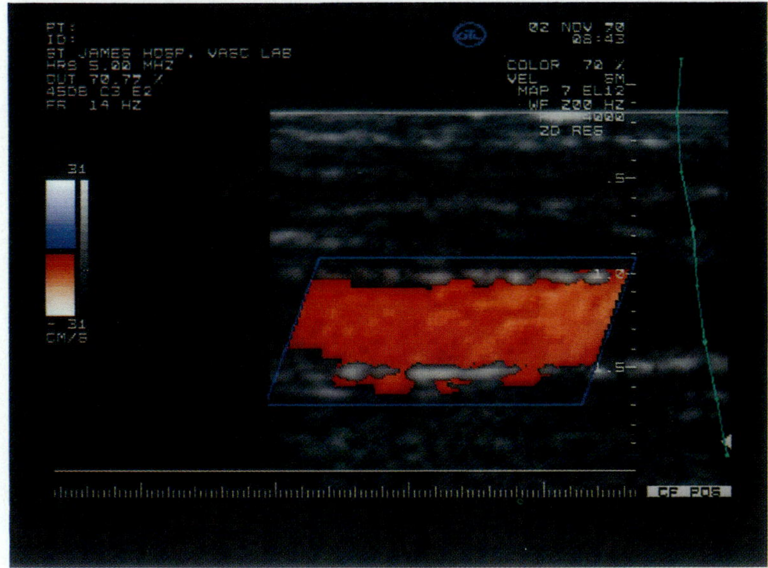

Fig. 1. Triplex scan of a normal *in situ* graft.

rather than frequency values. Figure 1 illustrates a normal *in situ* graft and Fig. 2 a haemodynamically significant graft stenosis and the corresponding spectral displays are illustrated in Figs 3 and 4.

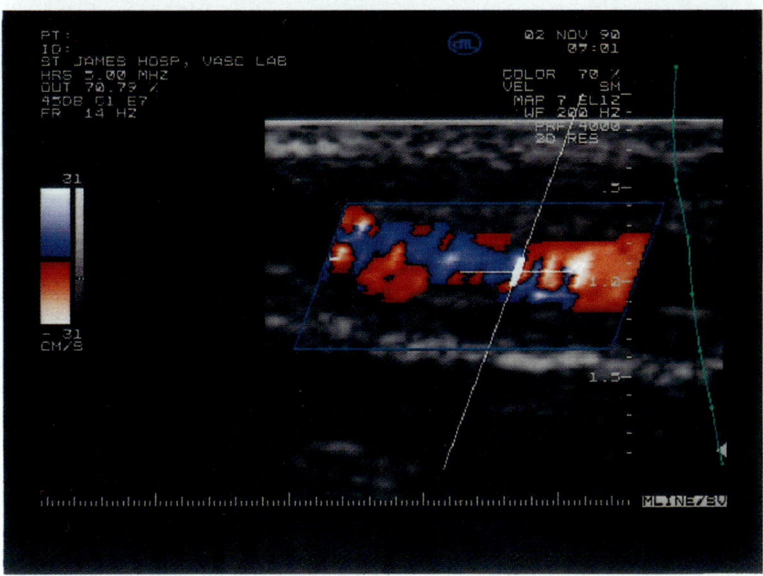

Fig. 2. Triplex scan of a graft stenosis showing increased colour saturation and poststenotic turbulence.

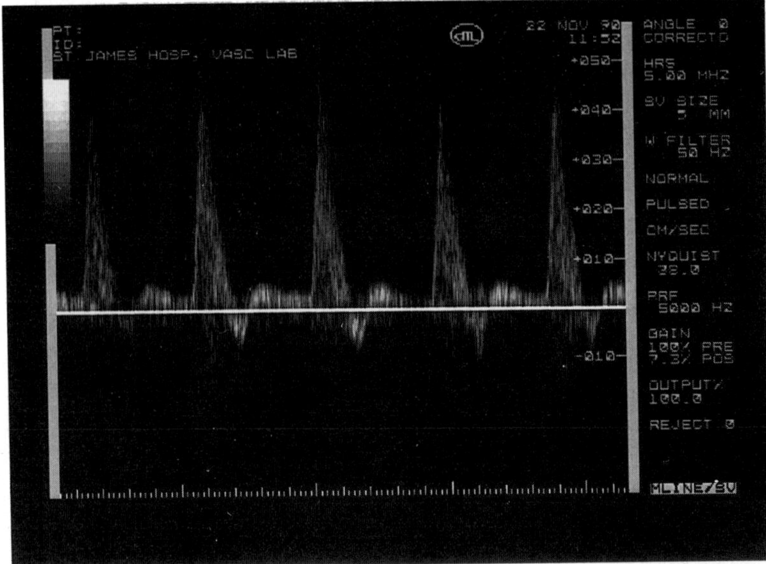

Fig. 3. Normal spectral analysis.

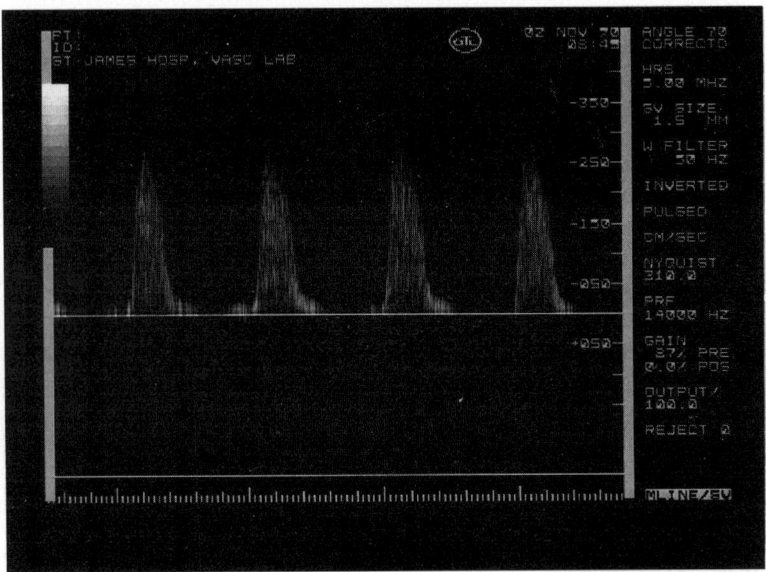

Fig. 4. Spectrum analysis from graft stenosis showing an increased peak systolic velocity.

INTRA-ARTERIAL DIGITAL SUBTRACTION ANGIOGRAPHY (IADSA)

All studies were performed and read by a consultant radiologist on an outpatient basis. The radiologist was unaware of the results of the noninvasive studies.

The overall results are illustrated in Tables 1–3. A total of nine grafts problems were identified on arteriography and two additional stenoses were identified,

Table 1. Sensitivity and specificity of ABIs in detecting graft stenoses

ABI	*Normal*	*Angiography* *<50%*	*>50%*	*Occlusion*
Normal	18	4	2	—
Abnormal	—	—	—	3

Specificity = 100% Sensitivity = 33%

Table 2. Sensitivity and specificity of duplex scanning in detecting graft stenoses

Duplex	*Normal*	*Angiography* *<50%*	*>50%*	*Occlusion*
Normal	16	2	2	—
<50%	2	2	—	—
>50%	—	—	2	—
Occlusion	—	—	—	3

Specificity = 88% Sensitivity = 64%
Perfect agreement 79% Kappa 0.61 ± 0.14

Table 3. Sensitivity and specificity of triplex scanning in detecting graft stenoses

Triplex	*Normal*	*Angiography* *<50%*	*>50%*	*Occlusion*
Normal	18	1	2	—
<50%	—	3	—	—
>50%	—	—	2	—
Occlusion	—	—	—	3

Specificity = 100% Sensitivity = 73%
Perfect agreement 89% Kappa 0.80 ± 0.11

one in an iliac artery and the other in the proximal common femoral artery. Of the nine graft problems three were occlusions, four a stenosis <50% and the remaining two >50% stenosis. All three occlusions had a significant reduction in ankle brachial indices and were correctly identified on duplex and triplex scanning. The two proximal stenoses were also associated with a reduced ABI and neither lesion was identified on imaging. The ABI was normal in the remaining cases of graft stenosis and four and five lesions were correctly identified by both duplex and triplex imaging respectively. The overall sensitivity and specificity of duplex and triplex was 64% and 88% and 73% and 100% respectively. Two additional <50% lesions were diagnosed by duplex; however, they were not confirmed by angiography.

The time interval from surgery to detection graft problems varied greatly. The occlusions occurred 2, 3 and 4 years postoperatively, the inflow disease at 14 months and at 4 years. One each of the <50% and >50% stenoses occurred at 14 months, three at 3 years and the final lesion (<50%) at 4 years.

These findings again confirm those of others in emphasizing the unreliability of ABI measurements and the sensitivity of duplex scanning in detecting inherent graft problems.[9,10,12,13] Our findings with triplex scanning showed an improvement in both sensitivity and specificity and additionally the time required for performing the scan was reduced due to the ease of following the colour profile.

Five graft stenoses (18%) were identified in this patient group and inflow/outflow lesions in two (7%). This emphasizes the importance of continued graft surveillance beyond 1 year.

Duplex/triplex scanning are highly sensitive in detecting graft problems. We recommend patient review 3-monthly for the first year and then every 9 months thereafter with angiography for those patients with a reduction in ABI or a lesion noted on imaging.

REFERENCES

1. Goyanes DJ: Nuevos trabajos de arugia vascular: substitucion plastica de las arterias por las venas, o arterioplastica venosa, aplicada, como nuevo metodo, al tratamiento. Siglo Med 53:561–564, 1906
2. Kunlin J: le traitment de l'arterite obliterante par la greffe veineuse. Arch Chir Mal Coeur 42:371–372, 1949
3. Palma EC: Treatment of arteritis of the lower limbs by autogenous vein grafts. Estratto da Minerva cardioangiologica Europea. Minerva Med 8:36–49, 1960
4. Baird RJ, Tutassaura H, Hiyagishima RT: Saphenous vein bypass graft to arteries of the ankle and foot. Ann Surg 172:1059–1063, 1970
5. Reichle FA, Martinson MW, Rankin KP: Infrapopliteal arterial reconstruction in the severely ischemic lower extremity: A comparison of long-term results of peroneal and tibial bypasses. Ann Surg 191:59–66, 1980
6. Hall KV: The great saphenous vein used "in-situ" as an arterial shunt after extirpation of the vein valves. Surgery 51:492–495, 1962
7. Leather RP, Shah DM, Karmody AM: Infrapopliteal arterial bypass for limb salvage: Increased patency and utilization of the saphenous vein used "in-situ". Surgery 90:1000–1008, 1981
8. Whittemore AD, Clowes AW, Couch JNP: Secondary femoro-popliteal reconstruction. Ann Surg 193:35–42, 1981
9. Cullen PJ, Leahy AL, Ryan SB *et al*: The influence of duplex scanning on early patency rates of in situ bypass to the tibial vessels. Ann Vasc Surg 1:340–346, 1986
10. Grigg MJ, Nicholaides AN, Wolfe JHN: Detection and grading of femorodistal vein graft stenoses: Duplex velocity measurements compared with angiography. J Vasc Surg 8:661–666, 1988
11. Taylor PR, Wolfe JHN, Tyrrell MR *et al*: Graft stenosis; justification for 1-year surveillance. Br J Surg 77:1125–1128, 1990
12. Mills JL, Harris EJ, Taylor LM, Beckett WC, Porter JM: The importance of routine surveillance of distal bypass grafts with duplex scanning: A study of 379 reversed vein grafts. J Vasc Surg 12:379–389, 1990
13. Bandyk DF: Postoperative surveillance of femorodistal grafts: the application of echo-Doppler (duplex) ultrasonic scanning. *In* Reoperative Arterial Surgery, Bergan JJ, Yao JST (Eds). Orlando, London: Grune & Stratton, pp. 59–79, 1986

Vein Graft Surveillance by Duplex Scanning and Pressure Measurement

P. R. F. Bell and J. Brennan

Autologous veins have been known to develop stenoses since this was first shown by Szilagyi[1] in 1973 when they were thought to be a possible cause of graft failure. We now know that fibrous stenoses can occur in up to 30% of patients in the first year after surgery.[1-3]

In Leicester over a 7-year period from 1981 to 1988 31% of vein grafts occluded in the first year, which could have been due to stenoses leading to thrombosis of the graft. Although haemodynamically significant stenoses can cause clinical symptoms and do cause a fall in the ankle brachial pressure index (ABPI)[4,5] relatively few are said to be detected in this way and exercise testing only improves sensitivity but to a minor degree.[3,6,7] As a result of this poor sensitivity, more complex screening tests have been devised, including intravenous digital subtraction angiography (IVDSA) and duplex scanning.[7,8]

The discovery of such stenoses has led, in recent years, to their treatment by percutaneous angioplasty (PTA) or surgery because of the risk of occlusion although no randomized studies are available to indicate if this is necessary. However, this policy has been shown to improve graft patency by over 20%[8-10] after intervention by PTA or surgery. Duplex scanning is expensive and digital subtraction angiography (DSA) is invasive and expensive. As a result we have re-examined the reliability of ABPIs for the detection of stenoses and report our results in this chapter.

PATENTS AND METHODS

Since August 1988 all patients undergoing reconstructive surgery with autologous vein have been prospectively examined 4–6 weeks, 3, 6, 9 and 12 months post-operatively. During this time 50 grafts in 48 patients have been studied. Of these grafts 38 were *in situ* vein, 11 reversed and one arm vein. The distal anastomosis was to the above knee popliteal vein in three patients, the below knee popliteal in 16 and the crural vessels in 31. Surgery was undertaken for critical ischaemia in 33 patients, pain at rest in three, severe claudication in 13 and a popliteal aneurysm in one (Table 1). At each visit the patients were examined clinically and the ABPI measured before and after exercise which consisted of walking for 2 minutes on a treadmill with a 10% incline at either 1 or 2 miles per hour. After this had been done the entire graft was scanned with a 7.5 MHz duplex probe and areas of stenosis diagnosed by a characteristic increase in velocity and spectral broadening over a short segment (Fig. 1). The degree of narrowing was estimated using peak velocity criteria as described elsewhere.[3] The pressure measurements were recorded prior to the duplex examination.

Table 1. Prospective follow-up of 50 grafts in 48 patients

Type		*Distal anast*	
in situ	38	AK pop	3
reversed	11	BK pop	16
arm	1	crural	31

Indications	
critical ischaemia	33
rest pain	3
severe claudication	13
popliteal aneurysm	1

If there was clinical deterioration, a serial fall in resting ABPI, a positive exercise test, or a significant stenosis determined by duplex scanning, the patient was assessed by angiography. Initially we used a peak velocity ratio greater than 2 for duplex scanning but this has now been increased to greater than 4. In severe stenoses the peak velocity was not recordable due to the phenomena of aliasing. In this situation, of spectral broadening throughout, the pulse cycle was taken to indicate a severe stenosis. Frequently, although the velocity disturbance could be seen the actual stenosis was not visible on duplex.

Provided the stenosis was technically accessible (Fig. 2) PTA was used as a first line of treatment. This was performed at the same session as the arteriogram in order to minimize the number of interventions. Surgical repair was undertaken if the lesion

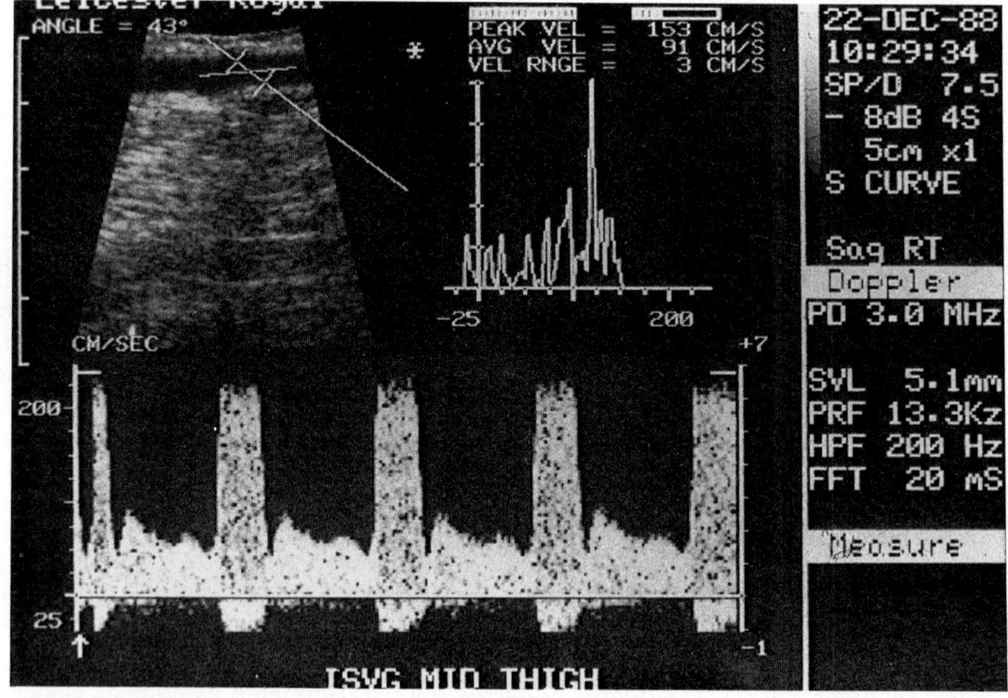

Fig. 1. Velocity increase and spectral broadening seen at a vein graft stenosis.

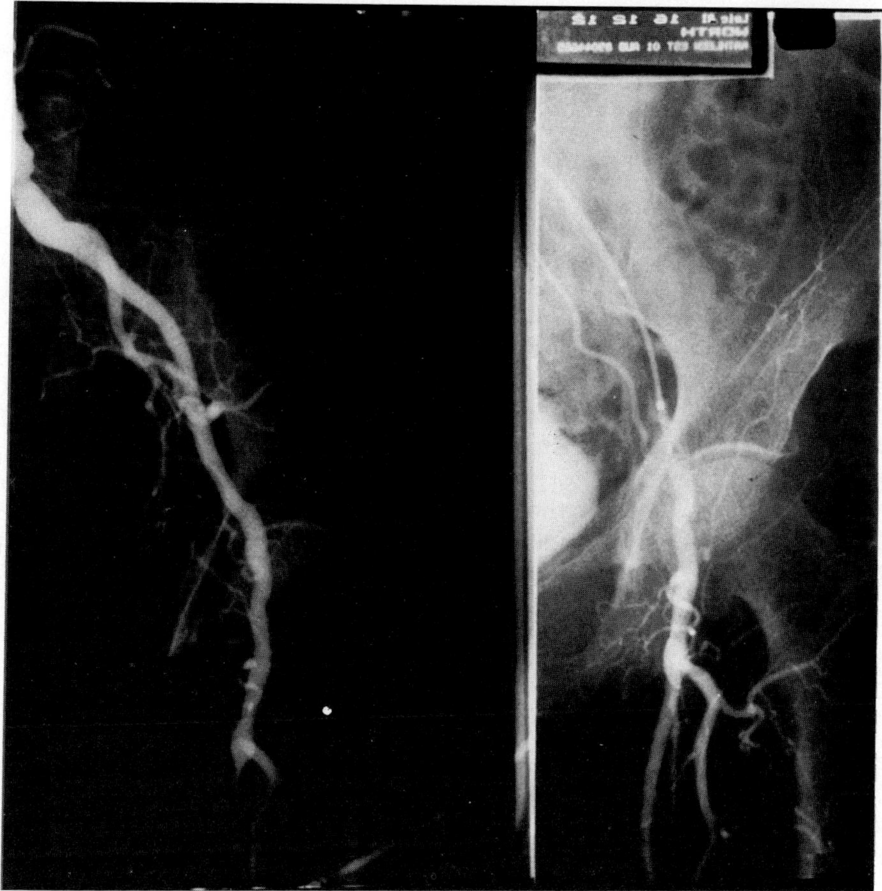

Fig. 2. (Left): A typical stenosis confirmed by angiography. **Fig. 3.** (Right): A vein graft stenosis successfully treated by PTA.

was unsuitable for PTA or after failed PTA. Following treatment graft follow-up was started again at 4–6 weeks, 3 months etc.

RESULTS

Duplex examination detected 25 stenoses in 24 (48%) grafts which was confirmed on subsequent arteriography. The lesions were scattered throughout the graft, seven being proximal, eight mid-graft and ten distal with 17 *in situ* and eight in reversed grafts (Table 2). The majority of the stenoses were discovered in the first 3 months (Table 3).

Clinical examination of these patients revealed only two with clinical deterioration (one with claudication and the other gangrene of one toe). Ankle pressure analysis successfully diagnosed stenoses in 18 of the grafts at risk. In nine of these there was a resting fall in ABPI and in a further nine a fall occurred after exercise. In the

Table 2. Duplex results of 25 stenoses in 24 (48%) grafts

Site		Grafts	
proximal	7	*in situ*	17
mid	8	reversed	8
distal	10		

remaining six, ABPI was normal but the patient was not able to walk because of healing foot lesions or a stroke in one of them (Table 4). Resting ABPI fell by a mean of 0.14 in nine patients and the median fall was 0.19 in those in whom it fell after exercise, with fall of greater than 0.1 in all 18 and 0.2 in six (Table 5). Twenty-three stenoses were subsequently treated, 20 by percutaneous angioplasty (Fig. 3) and three by surgery (one vein patch, one excision with primary anastomosis and one jump graft). Of those treated by PTA, one recurred after 3 months and was subsequently treated by vein patch, and this has been the only recurrence to date. Follow-up times vary from 3 to 18 months (mean 9.8). In the series as a whole no graft has thrombosed within the first year after the surveillance and treatment programme began compared with the 30% we used to lose before surveillance started.

DISCUSSION

This study in common with others, has shown quite clearly that there is a high rate of vein graft stenosis in the first year following surgery; thereafter there tends to be no further stenosis in the graft itself but run-off problems may occur in the vessels below the graft. Our finding that 48% of our grafts have such lesions is higher than in most other series which report an incidence of between 25 and 33%.[1–3,7] In some series, however, screening has not been uniform with only a proportion of grafts being assessed at varying intervals which may have given a falsely low incidence.[1–2] A significant number of our grafts have been to crural vessels rather than to popliteal arteries and we have used smaller veins as a consequence. It may be that this is the reason why we have had a higher stenosis rate than others.

The importance of vein graft surveillance has been documented by Grigg[7] and his colleagues who found that 19 stenoses in 75 grafts were present on follow-up and five of these developed symptoms which were treated successfully. Three occluded without warning. Moody[2] similarly detected 22 stenoses in 80 grafts, five of which subsequently occluded, compared with four occlusions in 58 grafts with no stenosis. These figures suggest that once a stenosis develops there is a sixfold

Table 3. Time to detection

Interval	No. detected
4–6 weeks	8
3 months	9
6 months	3
9 months	4
12 months	1

Table 4. Standard testing results

Duplex scanning 24 'at risk' grafts	
Clinical deterioration	2 / 24 (8%)
Fall in resting ABPI	9 ↘
Normal ABPI +ve walk test	9→24
Normal ABPI no walk test	6 ↗

chance that the graft will occlude but equally a certain significant number of stenoses do not progress to occlusion and the grafts can remain patent. Recently Moody and his colleagues did not observe any failures in the nonstenosed group of grafts.[8]

As a number of these stenoses appear to be benign it would be useful to try and pick out factors which demand treatment and not treat those that will not progress to occlusion. Unfortunately however, this information is not available and controlled studies have not been performed nor are they likely to be because of the high chance of occlusion.[2,7] Once a stenosis causes symptoms there is no doubt that it ought to be treated; however, whether an asymptomatic stenosis needs to be dealt with—and when—remains to be resolved. Important features of possible occlusion are stenoses which occur early (in the first 3 months) and those which occupy more than two-thirds of the vessel diameter. In our own series nonhaemodynamically significant lesions which were asymptomatic were relatively uncommon and were seen in only three of 24 grafts (12.8%), the remainder having ABPI changes at rest or after exercise. Although the trend has recently been towards examining patients by duplex imaging this is an expensive technique and not available to everybody. We examine our patients by ABPI testing which has previously been said to be too insensitive to detect such stenoses even though earlier papers did suggest that ABPI was useful. The main reason for the reported lack of sensitivity is probably that the fall in ABPI used (i.e. greater than 0.2)[2,3,8] is too high. In our own series, a fall of greater than 0.2 was only seen in six patients. Provided the test is carried out by an experienced technician and done carefully then a fall of greater than 0.1 is in our opinion, a more realistic sign of stenosis and needs further evaluation. In those patients who do not have a fall at rest, exercise testing has produced a fall of greater than 0.1 in nine further cases. Exercise testing has been rejected for screening purposes[3,6,8] by other authors as being of little use but we cannot agree with this point of view. In our experience only a moderate amount of exercise is required to produce an APBI fall of greater than 0.1 in a graft with a stenosis.

Although duplex scanning is a sensitive method for detecting stenoses, the grafts cannot be seen below the knee without difficulty. Assessment at this level is time consuming but the introduction of colour duplex may help[11] and a recently described technique to measure impedence may help. In a busy clinical practice, duplex

Table 5. AB/KA Brachial Pressure Indices

Resting ABPI fall (9 patients)		med 0.14 (range 0.11–0.3)
Postexercise fall (9 patients)		med 0.19 (range 0.13–0.4)
	fall >0.1 in all 18 >0.2 in 6 (33%)	

scanning is expensive and time consuming and the use of ABPI index is quicker and a more valuable screening test. Of the 26 patients who did not develop stenosed grafts five had a positive exercise test. Their ABPI has remained stable since that time and not progressed, which may indicate that distal disease is present in the draining artery rather than the graft.

Once a stenosis has been diagnosed and intervention decided upon, the choice lies between PTA and surgery. Initial reports have favoured surgery and stated that PTA does not produce durable results or a high recurrence rate.[5,7,12] In our experience we have found that PTA has been a very good way of treating such patients and 20 of our 23 grafts have had successful PTA. In three, PTA was thought not to be possible or failed and surgery was necessary. So far our follow-up has been for a mean of 8.4 months after PTA with a range of 3–18 months. Those grafts which had been subjected to PTA have remained patent and we feel that a high inflation pressure is the key to success. Upto 17 atmospheres have been used in our series and graft rupture has not been seen.[8] Deciding which stenoses to treat remains a problem and lesions which are causing two-thirds diameter reduction or which occur early are probably best treated, although we remain in ignorance of which ones to treat. Having said this and having treated most of our patients with the exception of three which were thought to be minimally stenosed, our graft patency of 100% at 1 year as opposed to 70% at 1 year prior to surveillance does tend to suggest that a policy of intervention is worthwhile.

In summary therefore our own policy is to follow all the patients at intervals of 4–6 weeks and 3, 6, 9 and 12 months with ankle brachial pressure testing at rest or after exercise. If there is a fall of more than 0.1 in APBI these patients are examined by duplex scanning and then by angiography. If a patient cannot walk then a duplex scan is used to look for a stenosis. With appropriate treatment PTA in particular can give excellent results with a 100% graft patency at 1 year.

REFERENCES

1. Szilagyi DE, Elliot JP, Hageman JH, Smith RF, Daall'olmo CA: Biologic fate of autogenous vein implants as arterial substitutes. Ann Surg 178:232–246, 1973
2. Moody P, de Cossart LM, Douglas HM, Harris PL: Asymptomatic strictures in femoro popliteal vein grafts. Eur J Vas Surg 3:389–392, 1989
3. Grigg MJ, Nicolaides AN, Wolfe JHN: Detection and grading of femorodistal vein graft stenoses: Duplex velocity measurements compared with angiography. J Vasc Surg 1:295–296, 1987
4. Berkowitz HD, Hobbs CL, Roberts B *et al*: Value of routine vascular laboratory studies to identify vein graft stenoses. Surgery 90:971–979, 1981
5. Cohen JR, Mannick JA, Couch NP, Whittemore AD: Recognition and management of impending vein graft failure. Arch Surg 121:758–759, 1986
6. Wolfe JHN, Lea Thomas M, Jamieson CW *et al*: Early diagnosis of femorodistal graft stenoses. Br J Surg 74:268–270, 1987
7. Grigg MJ, Nicolaides AN, Wolfe JHN: Femoro distal vein bypass graft stenoses. Br J Surg 75:737–740, 1988
8. Moody P, Gould DA, Harris PL: Vein graft surveillance improves patency in femoropopliteal bypass. Eur J Vasc Surg 4: 117–123, 1990
9. Bandyk DF, Kaerbrich HW, Steward GW, Towne JB: Durability of the *in situ* saphenous vein arterial bypass:a comparison of primary and secondary patency. J Vasc Surg 256–268, 1987

10. Bartlett ST, Kellwich LA, Fisher C, Ward RE: Duplex imaging of *in situ* saphenous vein bypass grafts and late failure reduction. Am J Surg 156:484–487, 1988
11. Polak JF, Donaldson MC, Dobkin GR, Mannick JA, O'Leary DH: Early detection of saphenous vein arterial bypass graft stenosis by color assisted duplex sonography:a prospective study. Am J Radiol 154:857–861, 1990
12. Thompson JF, McShane MD, Gazzard V, Clifford PC, Chant ADB: Limitations of percutaneous transluminal angioplasty in the treatment of femorodistal graft stenoses. Eur J Vasc Surg 3:209–211, 1989

The Use of Early Postoperative Digital Subtraction Angiography

B. C. Eikelboom, R. J. C. M. Donders, M. B. Baars and H. C. de Valois

Angiography is still the standard procedure for visualization of arteries before, during and after surgical reconstruction. Both the short- and the long-term outcome of the operation are to a certain extent determined by the technical perfection with which the operation has been performed. Poor technique leads to early occlusion, increased restenosis rates and maybe even to false aneurysm formation. Some form of quality control seems therefore warranted. Ideally, this is achieved intra-operatively, which allows instantaneous correction of imperfections. Intra-operative angiography, however, is cumbersome and has therefore never gained widespread acceptance. More sophisticated forms of ultrasound, such as duplex scanning, are usually not available during the operation and are often not feasible in the early postoperative period. Conventional intra-arterial angiography is invasive and is therefore rarely used routinely as a method for early postoperative assessment. Szilagyi is one of the very few who has reported on this application.[1] Intravenous digital subtraction angiography (IVDSA) has made it easier to perform angiography, pre- as well as postoperatively. The quality of the pictures that are obtained seems to vary among institutions to such a degree that it is not generally accepted as a worthwhile procedure. We perform around 90% of all carotid and abdominal aortic angiographic procedures as IVDSA, in addition to noninvasive techniques from the vascular laboratory. Only lower extremity reconstruction requires preoperative intra-arterial angiography in most cases, although femoropopliteal bypass is often performed on IVDSA alone. We published previously on routine application of IVDSA in the early postoperative period after almost all types of arterial reconstruction.[2] The following is an update of our experience with this procedure and reflects our current ideas about this application.

METHODS

Digital subtraction angiography was performed with a Philips DVI IV system with a 512×512 image matrix. The number of contrast injections varied from one to a maximum of five, each consisting of 40 ml contrast medium followed by 15 ml glucose. A short cannula, not longer than 5 cm, was inserted in a cubital vein. All investigations were done before discharge from the hospital. Contra-indications were renal failure, major cardiac insufficiency, patient refusal or a very poor general condition. In our previous report, DSA was performed on 678 of 892 operated cases, which is 76%. More recently, in the year 1989, this percentage was 87.

CAROTIDS

The carotids lend themselves very well to postoperative DSA evaluation. It is obvious that carotid endarterectomy should preferably be checked during the operation to obtain the best possible technical and clinical result. Postoperative DSA has revealed to us that, without intra-operative assessment, sufficient numbers of abnormalities are present to justify intra-operative assessment, which will inevitably lead to uncertainties about the need to re-open the vessel and will lead to a prolonged operation time. In 339 carotids, there were 224 (66%) without problems, 75 (22%) with stenosis less than 30%, 34 (10%) with stenosis greater than 30% and six (2%) occlusions. Postoperative DSA has served as a baseline for follow-up studies with duplex scanning.[3] Approximately half of the arteries with a significant stenosis at 1 year postoperatively already demonstrated this lesion on early postoperative IV DSA. In a prospective randomized patch-primary closure study, we showed that the number of residual lesions was similar in both groups, while the 1-year restenosis rate was significantly lower in the patched arteries.[4] After we had reached these conclusions, we stopped doing routine postoperative DSA and feel that it is justified only for specific clinical research studies but not for routine patient care.

FEMORODISTAL BYPASS PROCEDURES

The previous report on postoperative DSA consisted of 105 studies after 129 bypasses (81%). In 1989 we performed 35 femoropopliteal and 26 femorocrural bypasses. Postoperative DSA was performed in 54 cases, which is 90%. No abnormalities were seen in 37 cases, or 67%. One-third of the angiograms were abnormal. There were six occlusions and eight stenoses greater than 30% in the graft or at the anastomosis. Of special importance were four stenotic graft segments of several centimeters length. There were three kinks and one false aneurysm.

Graft failure in the first postoperative month is almost entirely due to technical problems and it is therefore obvious that early documentation of the status of the graft and its outflow is of great importance. It helps to find the reason for early failure and serves as a baseline for follow-up with noninvasive techniques or IVDSA. We have performed follow-up of grafts with DSA and duplex scanning and prefer the latter. Comparison between duplex scanning and DSA was made in 106 cases. Surgical revision for severe stenosis was done in 27 cases. In six of them there was disagreement between duplex and angiography. Of special importance were three cases of pseudoocclusion on angiography. Three other cases showed only minor lesions on angiography, while duplex scanning suggested a significant stenosis, which was confirmed during operation.

Early postoperative DSA has been replaced now by intra-operative intra-arterial DSA since a special operating room with dedicated radiology equipment and a radiolucent operating table has become available to us. It provides in an easy way real time subtraction fluoroscopy as well as instant review and hard copy documentation with excellent quality images.

ABDOMINAL AORTIC PROCEDURES

Reconstructions of the abdominal aorta for aneurysmal dilatation or occlusive disease are common procedures that have proven to be durable. Major late complications include anastomotic aneurysm formation and graft occlusion. Although these conditions are relatively rare, they represent such a significant morbidity and mortality that attempts to obtain early diagnosis are warranted. The true incidence of anastomotic aneurysms is hard to determine. Although an aneurysm in the groin may be felt as an enlarging pulsatile mass, the first signs of an intra-abdominal anastomotic aneurysm are often rupture or bleeding into the bowel, both conditions that may lead to a sudden death. The incidence of anastomotic aneurysms may for this reason be higher than reported in the literature.[5] Even less is known about the time interval between operation and anastomotic aneurysm formation as no prospective serial angiographic or ultrasound studies exist. In retrospect, most authors mention a period of 5 years, but reports have been published on 'early' diagnosis after 6 months. Among reasons for graft occlusion may be the presence of residual lesions left behind or new stenosis made at the time of operation. Data on these technical problems are scarce.

In 1989, we performed 126 primary operations for infrarenal abdominal aortic aneurysms. Re-operations and high abdominal or thoraco-abdominal aneurysms were not included in this series. Postoperative DSA was performed in 106 cases (84%). The series consists of 79 elective operations and 27 operations for ruptured aneurysms. In the elective cases, there were 48% tube grafts ($n=38$), while this was 74% for ruptured aneurysms. DSA results are given in Table 1. Completely normal angiograms were seen in 73% (58/79 cases) of elective operations, and only in 52% (14/27 cases) of ruptured aneurysms. Abnormalities were significantly more often present after ruptured aneurysm surgery. Roughly speaking, one out of every four elective and half of all urgent operations showed abnormalities. Several patients had more than one abnormality. Figure 1 shows a tube graft implantation for a ruptured aneurysm. There were a residual common iliac stenosis, a minor iliac aneurysm and a residual, unexpected high abdominal aneurysm, which later proved to be a thoraco-abdominal aneurysm. Remaining aneurysms, mainly in the iliac

Table 1. Postoperative IVDSA findings after aortic aneurysm surgery and aortic bifurcation bypass procedures

	Elective-AAA-rupture				*Bypass*
	tube	*bif.*	*tube*	*bif.*	*bif.*
Total number	38	41	20	7	36
Normal	27	30	10	4	32
Normal (%)	71	76	50	57	89
Residual aneurysm	7	2	9	2	0
Residual stenosis	3	2	4	0	0
Anastomotic aneurysm	2	1	0	1	0
Anastomotic stenosis	2	6	2	0	4

AAA = Abdominal aortic aneurysms.

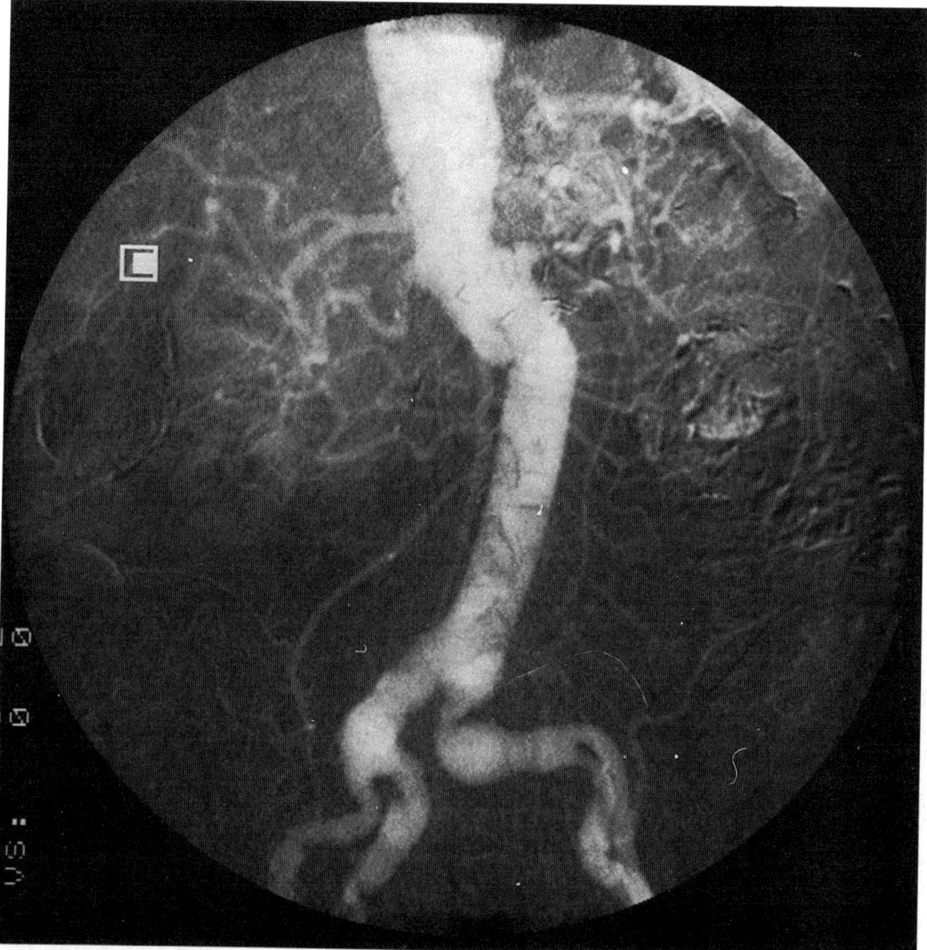

Fig. 1. Postoperative IVDSA after tube graft implantation for ruptured abdominal aortic aneurysm, showing residual common iliac stenosis, a minor common iliac dilatation and residual thoraco-abdominal aneurysm.

arteries, were the most common finding, which is no surprise when one takes into account that the majority of cases had tube graft implantations. The percentage of tube graft implantations has increased significantly during the last years, especially, but not only, for ruptured aneurysms. This procedure has the advantage of reducing the operating time and the amount of blood loss, but carries the risk of leaving iliac aneurysms behind. Especially in ruptured cases with a large haematoma, it is not always easy to judge the status of the iliac arteries. Moreover, it is not yet known which dilatations of the iliac arteries should be repaired.

We encountered one case of tube graft implantation with good backbleeding from the common iliac artery, an uneventful postoperative course and an unexpected external iliac occlusion on DSA, while the common and internal iliacs had remained patent. Although we noted 10 cases of anastomotic stenosis, this was never so severe that re-operation seemed indicated. Nevertheless, when graft occlusion would occur, this abnormality would be a probable explanation. The same holds true for residual stenoses in the iliac arteries. Obviously, this was mainly seen after tube graft implantation. There were four cases of anastomotic aneurysms. Three of these were unexpected and one patient was symptomatic and was re-operated.

Figure 2 shows a small aneurysm on the right side of the proximal anastomosis. It was confirmed on CT-scanning and treated conservatively. DSA some months later showed that it had thrombosed. To our knowledge, there are no reports in the literature on these very early anastomotic aneurysms and it has to be determined what their natural course will be. We have no firm criteria for re-intervention. Although this study shows that the anastomotic aneurysms are more often present than expected, the true number may be even higher. In a previous series, we encountered a patient with pain and a normal DSA, but an aneurysm on CT-scanning. Interestingly, all anastomotic aneurysms in this series as well as in the

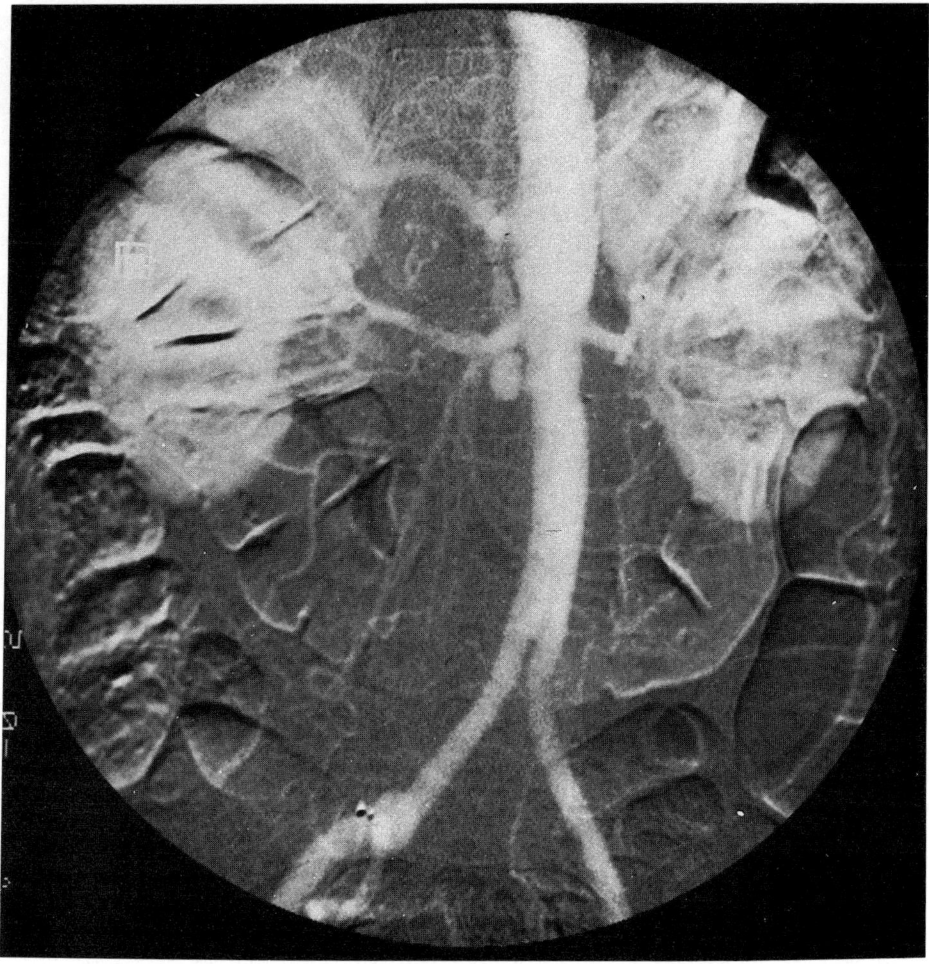

Fig. 2. Postoperative IVDSA after implantation of a bifurcation prosthesis for aneurysm. Small false aneurysm on the right side of the proximal anastomosis.

previous one, were in operations for aortic aneurysms and never for obstructive disease, which suggests that the quality of the vessel wall may be an important aetiological factor. Abdominal aortic bypass procedures in general showed less abnormalities than aneurysm operations. We performed 40 bypasses in 1989, of which 36 (90%) could be evaluated with DSA. There were 32 patients (89%) who had completely normal angiograms. No residual aneurysms or stenoses were seen, only four stenoses at, or near, the anastomotic sites. An example is given in Fig. 3. This patient was operated for a Leriche syndrome. The aorta was occluded just below the renal arteries. The infrarenal part was thrombectomized and the graft was implanted in an end-to-end fashion. Postoperatively, there were good femoral pulses, but in spite of this, the DSA showed a major stenosis. A similar case was encountered some years ago. The patient remained asymptomatic, no re-intervention was performed and DSA 1 year later showed marked improvement. This phenomenon may represent spontaneous lysis of residual thrombus.

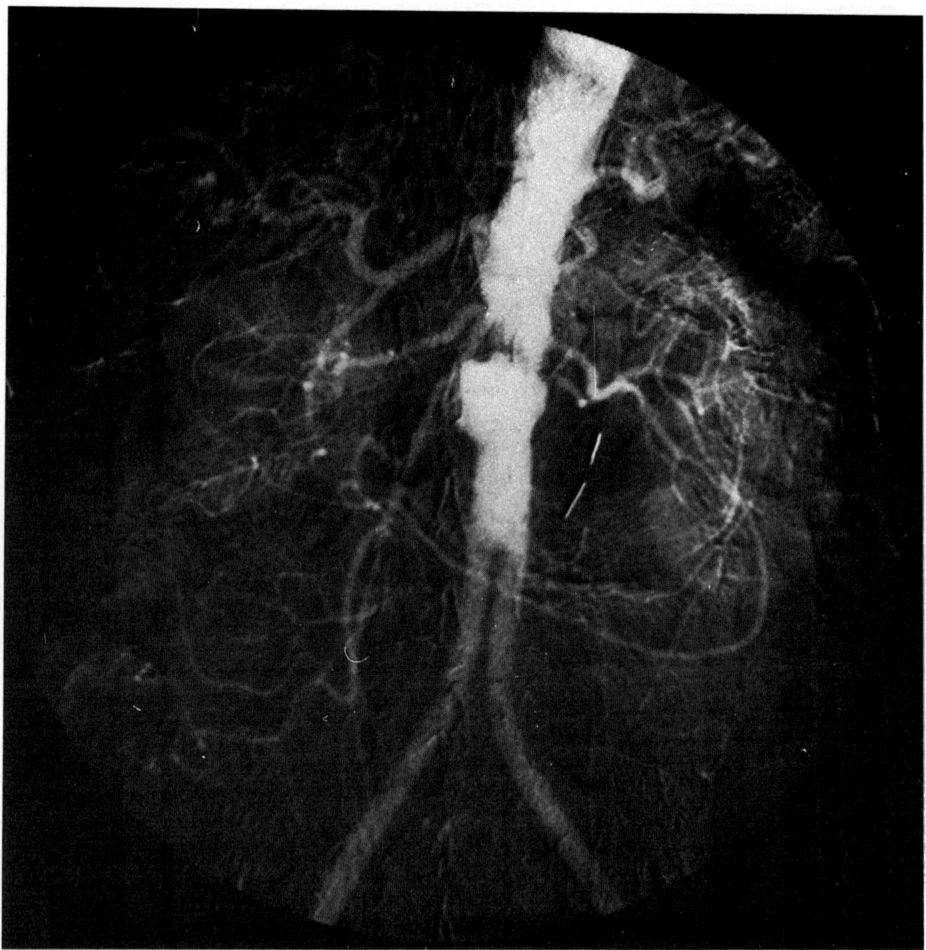

Fig. 3. Postoperative IVDSA after graft implantation for Leriche syndrome. Residual thrombus and major stenosis below the renal arteries.

CONCLUSION

There are few reports in the literature on early postoperative angiography. Intravenous DSA, in our hands, provides images of sufficient quality to detect abnormalities that would otherwise remain undetected. These are more frequently present than expected. It is not always easy to determine the clinical significance of these abnormalities. Only rarely was it felt necessary to perform re-operations based on the DSA findings. In many patients, however, it led to more scrutinized follow-up, which may not only be important for patient care but has certainly contributed to our knowledge about the behaviour of these unrepaired abnormalities. This was clearly seen in carotid endarterectomy, as mentioned above.

Postoperative DSA is not done any more on a routine basis after carotid endarterectomy or femorodistal bypass. In these cases we prefer now to do intra-operative intra-arterial DSA with dedicated equipment. Aortic reconstruction does not lend itself so well to intra-operative evaluation. This is most clearly seen in surgery for ruptured aortic aneurysms. It is here where postoperative IVDSA proved to have its greatest value. Our policy for ruptured aneurysms is to do as minimal repair as possible and we feel that this is an important reason for achieving good results. The price that one pays is the need to do some secondary operations for iliac aneurysms. Such an elective operation in a patient who has survived the operation for rupture is usually not too much of a problem. This study shows that anastomotic false aneurysms may occur early after aortic aneurysm surgery, and not, or less frequently, in aortic bypasses.

Aortic bypass operations showed few significant abnormalities, and it is questionable whether routine postoperative DSA in this area can be justified for other than scientific reasons. Postoperative DSA is certainly useful after special uncommon procedures where one may have doubts about the quality of the reconstruction. Actually, an important aspect of postoperative DSA is that all these angiograms are shown at the weekly vascular conference. It leads nearly always to fruitful discussions about the operative technique that has been used and serves as means of quality control as well as a means to educate the surgeons, residents and students.

REFERENCES

1. Szilagyi DE, Smith RF, Elliot JP *et al*: Anastomotic aneurysms after vascular reconstruction: problems of incidence, etiology, and treatment. Surgery 78:800–816, 1975
2. Teeuwen C, Eikelboom BC, Ludwig JW: Clinically unsuspected complications of arterial surgery shown by post-operative digital subtraction angiography. Br J Radiol 62:13–19, 1989
3. Sanders EACM, Hoeneveld B, Eikelboom BC *et al*: Residual lesions and early recurrent stenosis after carotid endarterectomy. J Vasc Surg 5:731–737, 1987
4. Eikelboom BC, Ackerstaff RGA, Ludwig JH *et al*: Benefits of carotid patching; a randomized study. J Vasc Surg 7:240–247, 1988
5. Sieswerda C, Skotnicki SH, Barentsz JO *et al*: Anastomotic aneurysms—an underdiagnosed complication after aorto-iliac reconstructions. Eur J Vasc Surg 3:2373–2238, 1989

Will Intra-arterial Ultrasound Catheters Improve Localization of Disease Treated by Endovascular Methods?

Hero van Urk and Elma J. Gussenhoven

Although intravascular catheter tip echography is nowadays being introduced as a new and exciting tool for diagnostic procedures in the field of cardial and vascular diseases, the development of such instruments has a history of 35 years, since the first application of intraluminal echography by Ciezynski[1] in 1956. With his single element (nonrotating) ultrasonic catheter he was able to obtain ultrasonic reflections of the inner walls of the right and left ventricle and pulmonary artery in dogs. He noted that the method was harmless to the animals' health and concluded that this procedure might open new possibilities for the diagnosis of heart failure in man.

In 1969 Bom and his co-workers started to develop a two-dimensional real-time intravascular ultrasonic imaging device, using a 32-element circular phased array with an outer diameter of 3.2 mm mounted at the tip of a 9 French catheter. This design operated at 5.6 MHz with a narrow beam and produced intraluminal images such as left ventricular cross-sections.[2]

Only during the last decade, as percutaneous interventional techniques such as percutaneous transluminal angioplasty (PTA) and laser-assisted PTA have been introduced, has the need arisen for these ultrasound devices. This has also led to the idea of combining cross-sectional real-time imaging in one catheter with laser or mechanical techniques, such as an atherectomy catheter. At present, most experience is based on intra-arterial echo catheters alone, used before and after recanalization procedures in peripheral or coronary arteries.[3]

We will describe our experience with the intravascular ultrasound catheter devised by Bom and associates at the Department of Biomedical Engineering of the Erasmus University in Rotterdam.[4–7]

METHODS

In vitro experiments were carried out using a 40 MHz single element rotating transducer mounted on the tip of an 8 French catheter (Fig. 1). Axial resolution of the system was 75 μm, with lateral resolution better than 200 μm at a depth of 1 mm. Cross-sectional images were obtained by catheter tip rotation. Data acquisition time for one complete image was 20 s. The resulting images were displayed on a monitor by means of a video-scanned memory of 512×512 pixels with 256 shapes of grey. Marker lines at 1 mm were displayed for calibration purposes.

Specimens of normal and diseased human arteries were either removed at surgery or at autopsy and stored at 20°C. For carrying out the *in vitro* experiments the

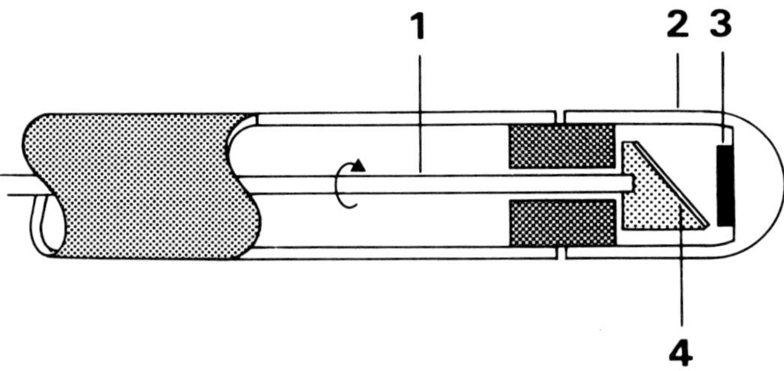

Fig. 1. Echo element (1); rotating mirror (2) and spark erosion electrode (3). Mechanically driven echo catheter tip with mirror (4).

specimens were thawed and embedded in a 1.2% solution of agar–agar. The arterial sections were positioned vertically in order to allow adequate access of the ultrasound catheter.

The lumen of the specimens was filled with purified water. After placing the catheter in the lumen of the specimen, ultrasonic cross-sections were obtained from proximal to distal with 1 mm intervals between each. After marking the cross-sectional sites with ink the specimens were fixed in 10% buffered formalin, decalcified and processed for routine paraffin embedding. Transverse sections of 5 μm were cut at 1 mm intervals. The sections were stained with a Verhoeff's elastin van Gieson and the haematoxylin azophloxine technique. Histologic characteristics were compared with the corresponding echo cross-section.

In vivo experience was obtained using a 32 MHz single element rotating transducer, mounted on the tip of a 5 French catheter (Fig. 2). Patients with long or short superficial

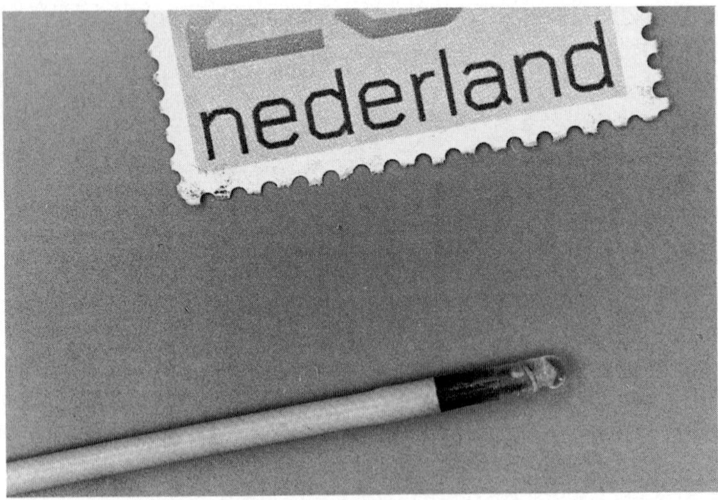

Fig. 2. Catheter tip with single element transducer for two-dimensional scanning compared in size with a regular postage stamp.

femoral artery (SFA) occlusions or severe stenoses were selected for a recanalization procedure consisting of a Nd:Yag laser-assisted balloon angioplasty or a thermoplaster-assisted balloon angioplasty.

Patients with an occlusion at the level of the orifice of the SFA were treated in the operating room through a surgical exploration of the common femoral artery. Patients with an open proximal SFA and occlusion in the midportion or at the level of Hunter's canal were explored percutaneously in the angiography suite.

IN VITRO RESULTS

Normal vessel wall

Several lessons learned in the past have to be learned again: many histological aspects of the normal arterial wall and of the atherosclerotic diseased vessel wall can be recognized, both histologically, and echographically. Basically, there are two types of arteries: the elastic type and the muscular type. Because the two types gradually merge into each other many mixed forms will be seen.

The elastic type is primarily confined to the aorta, pulmonary trunk, and the proximal segments of the brachiocephalic, carotid, subclavian and common iliac arteries. All other arteries, such as the femoral, renal and coronary arteries are of the muscular type. The main difference between the two types of arteries is found in the composition of the media: in the elastic artery the media consists of circularly arranged elastin fibres which have smooth muscle cells sandwiched in between (Fig. 3), resulting in an elastin-rich media in this type of artery. There may be a varying amount of intercellular connective tissue and mucopolysaccharide-rich ground substance.

Echographically an elastic artery was recognized by a media which was as echogenic as the adjacent intima and adventitia. The presence of circularly arranged elastin fibres in the media of an elastic artery resulted in a significant amount of acoustic backscatter with a power level comparable to that of the surrounding tissue.

On the other hand the media of a muscular type artery predominantly consists of circularly arranged smooth muscle cells (Fig. 3). Only a few elastin fibres may be present, particularly in the larger arteries, as well as some intercellular connective tissue.

Echographically these muscular type arteries are easily recognized as a typical three-layered vessel wall: an hypo-echoic media amidst the intima and adventitia which are both represented by bright echoes.

The gradual merging of an elastic artery into a muscular artery could be observed based on the echo characteristics of the media. Studies in proximal coronary artery specimens revealed that the media was of an elastic nature, whereas a few millimetres more distally the media became progressively more muscular.

ATHEROSCLEROTIC LESIONS

The early atherosclerotic lesions or fatty streaks are composed of agglomerates of foam cells containing lipids. The more advanced lesions, the atherosclerotic plaques,

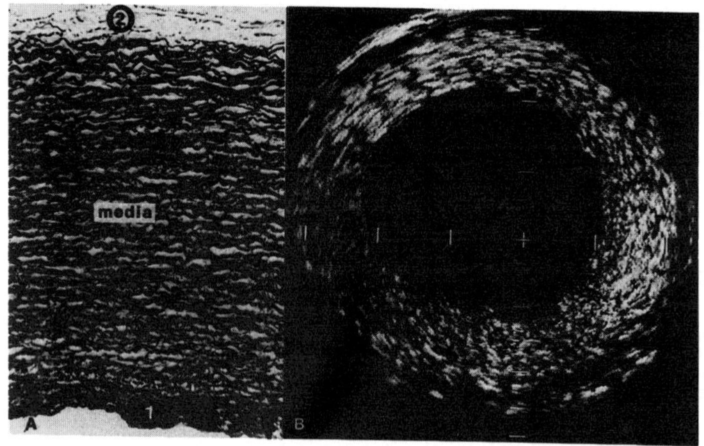

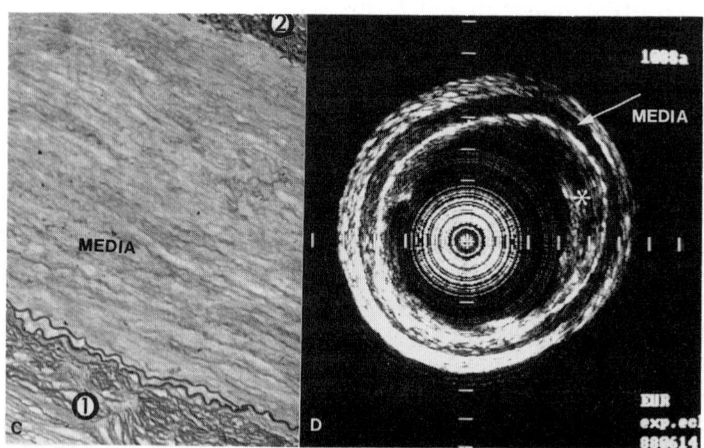

Fig. 3. Photomicrographs showing detailed characteristics of the media of an elastic artery (left panel) and a muscular artery (right panel) interposed between intima (1) and adventitia (2) together with the representative ultrasonic cross-sections. The media of an elastic artery is densely packed with elastin fibres (black stained) whereas the media of a muscular artery is mainly composed of smooth muscle cells. (Note that the presence of an echolucent media facilitates visualization of a superimposed lesion (asterisk)). Verhoeff van Gieson stain.

show extensive variability in composition. At one end of the spectrum the atherosclerotic plaque may be almost entirely composed of fibromuscular tissue i.e. connective tissue, smooth muscle cells and disorganized elastin fibres with an important collagenous component. At the other end of the spectrum, the plaque may consist of a large central atheroma with a scanty fibrous capsule composed of collagen-rich connective tissue. The classical atherosclerotic plaque is localized in the intima and is composed of a lake of fatty debris with cholesterol crystals, sometimes fibrin and calcium deposits, while the atheroma is surrounded by macrophages and lymphocytes and a fibromuscular layer. Towards the lumen the lesion is bordered by a fibrous tissue capsule covered by endothelium. Towards the media the border of the plaque may be easily recognizable by a still present internal elastic lamina, but may also be interrupted or fragmented or duplicated. In some instances the internal elastic lamina and the media may even totally disappear and the atherosclerotic lesion can reach as far as the adventitia. Such a lesion will evoke inflammatory infiltrate in the adventitia. When the fibrous capsule becomes extremely thin it may rupture and allow blood or blood components to enter the plaque leading to plaque haemorrhage.

A complication of ruptured or cracked plaque is thrombus formation on its surface. The thrombus is composed of a meshwork of strands of fibrin in which red cells, leukocytes and platelets are entrapped. If the thrombus does not dissolve it becomes organized by ingrowth of fibrovascular tissue.

Intravascular ultrasound could distinguish four basic types of plaque components, based on the echogenecity of the components of the atherosclerotic plaque.

1. *Hypo-echoic:* a reflection of a significant amount of lipid deposits.
2. *Soft echoes:* representing diffuse intimal thickening (intimal proliferation and atherosclerotic lesions consisting of fibromuscular tissue and diffusely dispersed lipids).
3. *Bright echoes:* representative for collagen-rich fibrous tissues.
4. *Bright echoes* with shadowing behind the lesion: representative for calcium deposits.

By systematically scanning the arterial segments with ultrasound going from proximal to distal at 1-mm intervals, the presence and extent of the lesions could be assessed correctly. The location and composition of atherosclerotic lesions showed marked variations, belying the general assumption that most of the atherosclerotic lesions are located at the dorsal side of the arteries (Fig. 4).

In the presence of calcification, problems were encountered in identifying echographically the internal elastic lamina, because of strong reflection and attenuation, thus obscuring the echoes of the structures behind the calcification i.e. internal elastic lamina. Both calcification and dense fibrous tissue containing a significant amount of collagen produce bright echoes. The typical presence of shadowing behind calcified structures allows a marked distinction between calcification and dense fibrous tissue (Fig. 5).

It must be stressed that in the *in vitro* experiments the lumen of the arteries was filled with purified water and not with blood.

IN VIVO RESULTS AND CLINICAL EXPERIENCE

The step from *in vitro* experiments with intravascular ultrasound in arterial specimens to the use of the ultrasound catheter in the clinical situation turned out to be a major one. Several animal experiments had been performed before the ultrasound catheter was introduced in the human situation. From these experiments on pigs and rabbits it had already become clear that the presence of blood and bloodflow was an important aspect that greatly influenced the interpretation of the ultrasound images.

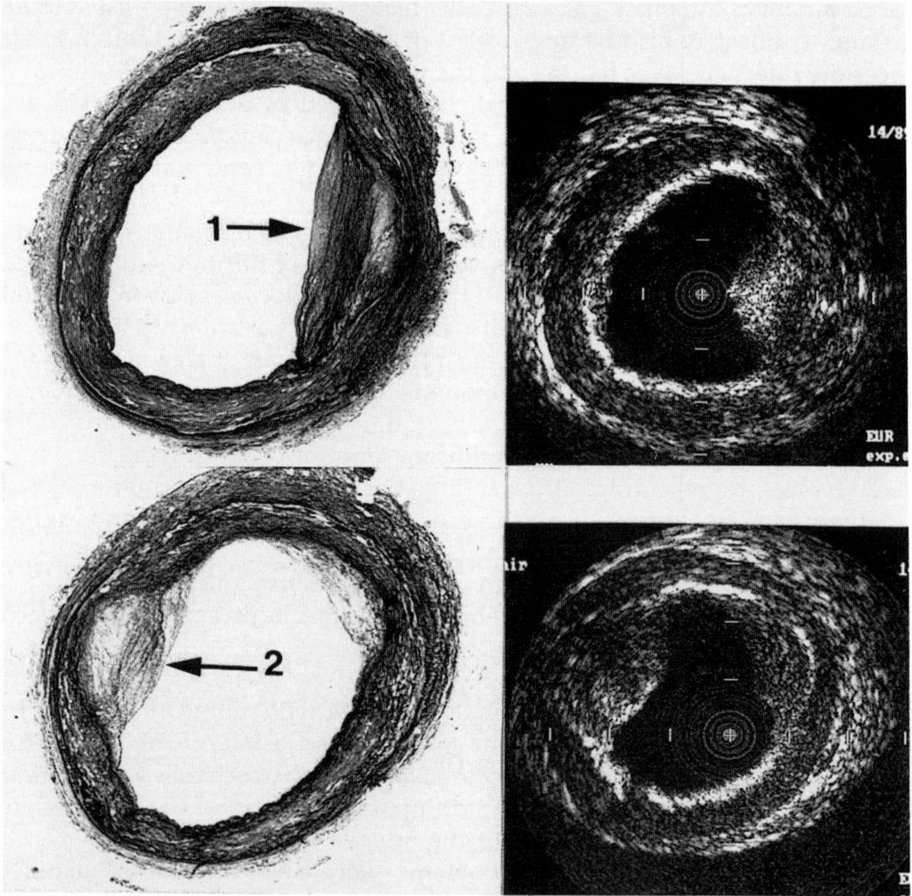

Fig. 4. Photomicrographs of histologic cross-sections obtained from the mesenteric superior artery together with the corresponding ultrasonic cross-sections. The media of this typical muscular artery mainly composed of smooth muscle cells, appears characteristically hypoechoic on ultrasound. Note that the eccentric atherosclerotic lesion barely visible at 9 o'clock (upper panel) is of marked larger size compared with the cross-section obtained 4 mm distally (lower panel). Both lesions (arrows 1 and 2) were of amorphous noncalcific tissue character containing fibromuscular tissue and lipid. Bright echoes of intima and adventitia circumscribing the hypoechoic media. Verhoeff van Gieson stain.

The different particles in blood, like red cells and leucocytes, produce a typical pattern of moving and constantly changing echoes, which can clearly be recognized. In animal experiments and in human arteries without stenotic atherosclerotic lesions a pulsatile flow pattern can be seen which does not interfere with the detection of the normal configuration of the vessel wall and its layers.

However, if bloodflow is reduced as a result of atherosclerotic stenoses, echogenecity of the erythrocytes increases and can obscure the outline of the lumen of the vessel. It also attenuates the resulting signal that is reflected by the various wall layers.

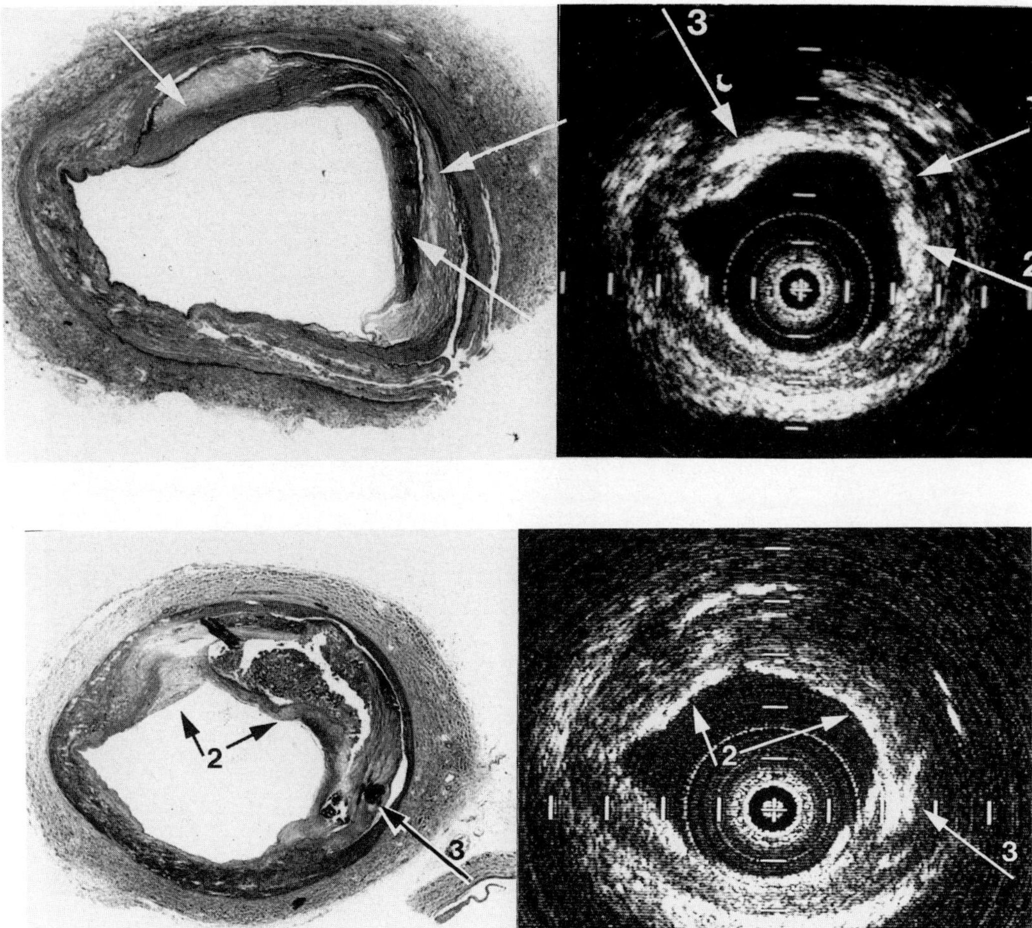

Fig. 5. Histologic cross-sections of a femoral artery showing a classical obstructive atherosclerotic lesion with corresponding ultrasonic cross-sections. Fatty debris appearing as hypo-echoic (arrow 1), collagen as bright echoes (arrow 2) and calcium as bright echoes with shadowing (arrow 3), are the major plaque constituents. Distribution of calcium within the lesion varies significantly (11 o'clock in upper panel, 4 o'clock in lower panel), Verhoeff van Gieson stain upper panel. Haematoxylin azophloxin stain lower panel.

Flushing of the interrogated artery with small amounts of saline solution through the introducer sheath immediately results in a clear outline of the lumen area and clearly allows identification of wall irregularities, obstructive lesions or plaque rupture (Fig. 6). The latter finding is especially interesting in case of balloon angioplasty interventions.

From angiographic control studies it has been known for a long time that balloon dilatation of atherosclerotic lesions frequently if not always results in longitudinal ruptures of the atheromatous plaque, sometimes leading to dissection of the vessel wall and not infrequently the cause of early (re)occlusion of the treated artery

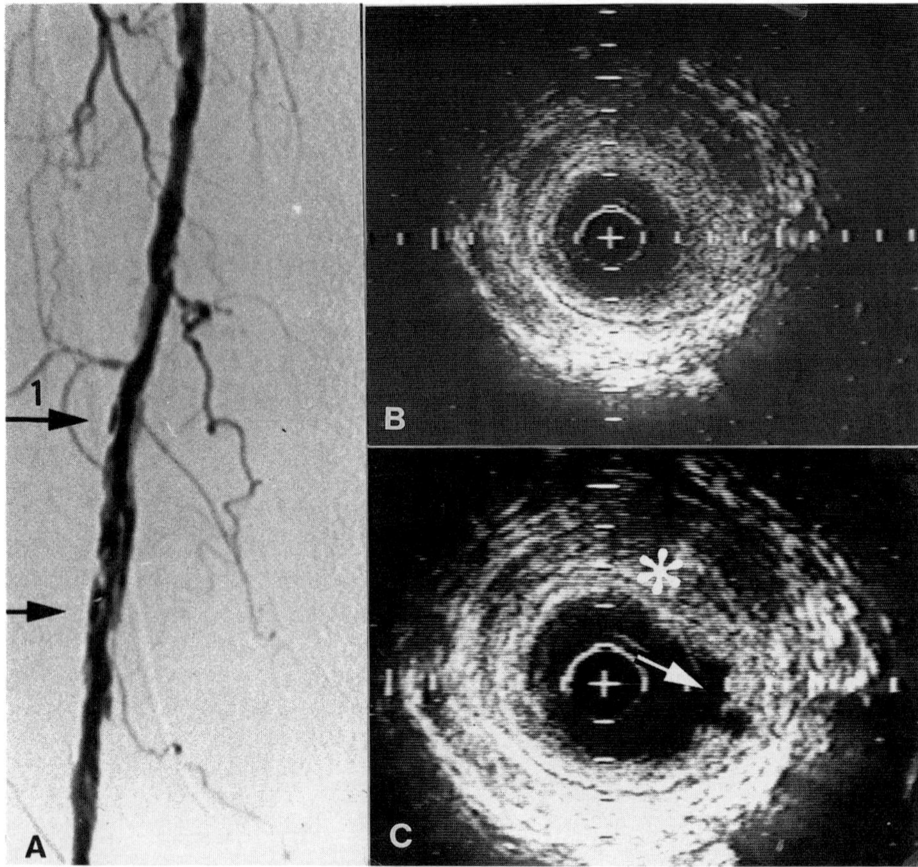

Fig. 6. Photographs of a superficial femoral artery angiogram (A) and intravascular ultrasound image following balloon angioplasty (B,C). Angiographically there was evidence of wall irregularities (arrows). Corresponding ultrasonic cross-sections obtained at level arrow 1 are indicative of a plaque rupture. Note that the echogenicity of blood hampers adequate visualization of the lesion (B). Injection of saline solves this problem (C). Note the plaque rupture at 4 o'clock. The hypo-echoic media is visible between 5 and 7 o'clock. The atherosclerotic lesion is still present between 11 and 5 o'clock (asterisk). Calibration 1 mm.

(Figs 6, 7). These longitudinal plaque ruptures are not always shown clearly on angiography, depending on the direction of the projection of the X-rays. Tangential projection may cause a somewhat irregular depiction of the lumen filled with contrast, but will not always show the real extent of the damage to the vessel wall (Fig. 8). This may result in an unclear situation for the interventionist: is the vessel lumen sufficiently enlarged and a sufficient blood flow produced to ensure the maintenance of a patent vessel, or will the free end of the ruptured plaque and the accompanying false lumen lead to early occlusion?

As intravascular ultrasound produces a cross-section of the total vessel wall throughout the entire length of the 'dissection', the beginning and end of the rupture

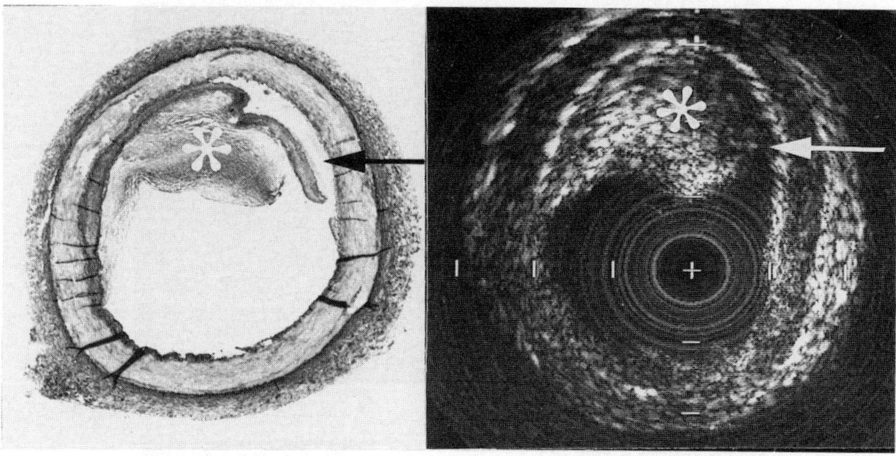

Fig. 7. Histologic and corresponding ultrasonic cross-sections obtained from the femoral artery after angioplasty. The artery presents an eccentric obstructive atherosclerotic lesion (asterisk) recognized as relative soft echoes. The corresponding histologic cross-section shows that the lesion mainly consists of connective tissue and fatty deposits. The dilatation procedure had resulted in a dissection (arrow). Verhoeff van Gieson stain.

together with the remaining vessel lumen can be localized and measured, and the policy for further intervention (or the decision to perform immediate bypass surgery) can be influenced by this new type of information, not available by angiography alone (Fig. 8). Another aspect of intravascular ultrasonic imaging is formed by the potential evaluation of vessel wall dynamics and compliance. As the real-time images can be stored with the use of a videorecorder, different sectors of the vessel wall can be evaluated and dynamic properties of normal vessel wall compared with parts of the same vessel with atherosclerotic changes or with other vessels and/or arterial substitutes like polytetrafluoroethylene (PTFE) or venous bypass materials.

Vessel wall dynamics also play a role in the process of balloon dilatation. From our experience so far, we conclude that the only sector of the arterial circumference that is actually being dilated or stretched by the force of the inflated balloon, is—in the case of an eccentric lesion—the relatively 'most normal' part of the vessel wall: the sector containing the atherosclerotic lesion stays virtually unchanged and will not be stretched. The marginal area between 'normal' and 'diseased' arterial wall appears to be the most vulnerable area for the origin of plaque ruptures or dissections (Fig. 6).[8] The site of a plaque rupture may well be the stimulus for a fibrocellular reaction leading to early restenosis. Identification and documentation of these sites may provide valuable information about the pathophysiology of the process of recurrent stenosis.

Another disadvantage of angiography is that it can only visualize the remaining vessel lumen at the site of a stenosis, or the distal vessels beyond a more proximal occlusion. The latter are only visualized in case of sufficient collateral blood supply to the distal tract of the occluded artery. Angiography can not distinguish between

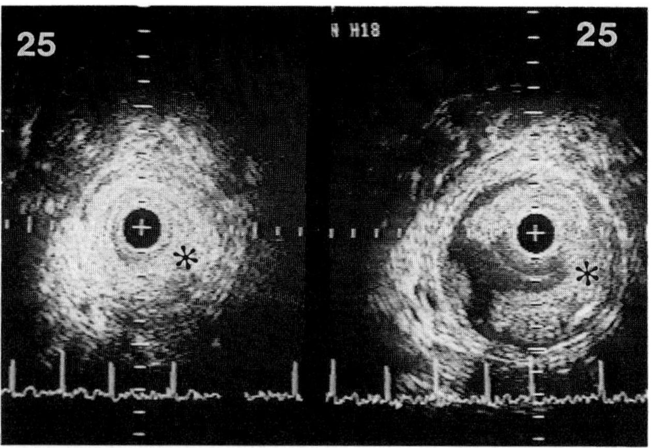

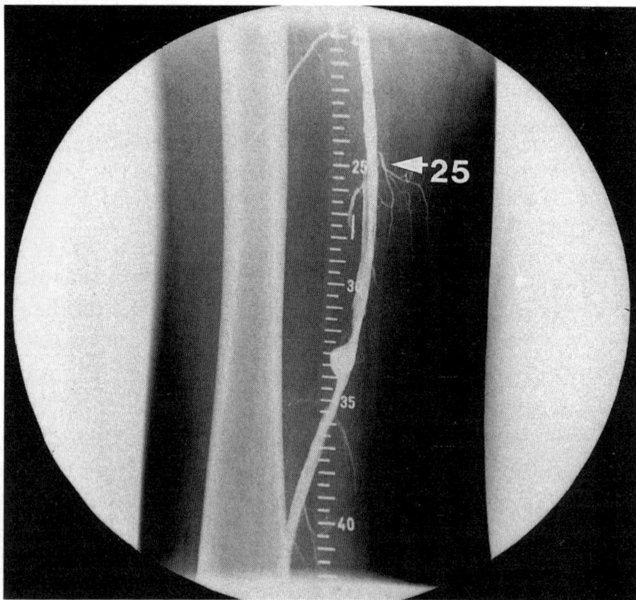

Fig. 8. Ultrasound cross-sections obtained before (left) and after (right) balloon angioplasty and angiogram. Note disagreement in the outcome of balloon angioplasty between angioplasty and intravascular ultrasound. Ultrasound cross-section corresponds with level 25 at angiography. A satisfactory result was suggestive from the angiogram. Echographically it was noted that the lesion was still present. The effect of angioplasty was increased arterial lumen with dissection of the lesion from the arterial wall. Calibration 1 mm.

a total occlusion of a long arterial segment and a short atherosclerotic occlusion with subsequent retrograde or antegrade thrombosis up to the level of the next major collateral branch.

Naturally, in cases of total occlusion, intravascular ultrasound can only be used after some recanalization procedure has been performed primarily. However, comparable to the mechanical recanalization that can frequently be obtained with the use of a relatively stiff laser-catheter—without the use of the laser energy—the ultrasound catheter can also be used as a mechanical means of producing a thin canal through an occluded vessel. In doing so, the ultrasound catheter has the advantage that it produces a simultaneous image of the kind of obstruction—atheroma or bloodclot—that is being passed through.

We have found that this phenomenon provides a safe passage through a recently thrombosed part of, for example, the superficial femoral artery resulting from a severe stenosis at the level of Hunter's canal.

The distinction between thrombus and fibromuscular atherosclerotic lesions or intimal hyperplasia can easily be made based on the ultrasonic appearance. Both thrombus and soft atherosclerotic lesions produce relatively soft echoes and therefore identification cannot be based on their ultrasonic appearance. However, in a relatively nondiseased arterial wall of a muscular artery, the media can easily be identified as an hypo-echoic circular structure with a diameter of approximately that of the normal vessel that is being interrogated, and a clockwise evenly distributed thickness. On the other hand a localized atheromatous lesion, even at a very early stage, invariably will be accompanied by a local diminishing or—in later stages—almost disappearance of the media; the thickness appears to be inversely related to the extent of atherosclerosis.[9] The lumen of the artery initially stays approximately the same as a result of this 'compensatory' process. This phenomenon was first described by Glagov *et al.*[10] in coronary arteries, but appears to occur also in peripheral arteries. The clinical relevance of this observation was not appreciated until we realized that it reliably served as a criterium for the presence of an atherosclerotic lesion.[10] We now use this phenomenon as an indicator for the arterial tract that is most critical for balloon dilatation.

LIMITATIONS OF ULTRASOUND

Identification of atherosclerotic lesions largely depends on identification of a highly reflective intima and a hypoechoic media. As a consequence, adequate discrimination of a lesion in a muscular artery is easily facilitated, but in an elastic artery the echo characteristics of the lesion are similar to the echo response generated by the intima and media, thus preventing distinction of the lesion.

The ultimate ultrasonic response is intimately dependent on the angle of insonification. Perpendicular insonification results in an optimal response. Only under these conditions is one able to make adequate distinction between the size and composition of the atheromatous lesion involved. This observation should be taken into account when *in vivo* application is considered.

CONCLUSIONS

Cross-sectional ultrasonic images appear to have a close relationship with histologic structures when a high frequency transducer is used in *in vitro* studies. A clear difference between elastic and muscular arteries was observed with ultrasound, which was caused by the presence or absence of elastin tissue in the media.

Comparison between ultrasonic images and corresponding histologic cross-sections showed that characteristics of the echo image of an atherosclerotic lesion relate to the histologic composition of the lesion.

In the clinical situation the effect of intervention techniques like laser ablation and balloon dilatation was studied. Thrombus formation and diffuse intimal thickening could be identified and discriminated, primarily based on the identification of a normal or thinned arterial media.

Calcified atherosclerotic lesions can easily be identified because of the shadowing that these lesions produce; no reliable ultrasonic information can be obtained of the arterial wall behind a calcified lesion.

Plaque rupture and dissection as well as vessel perforation can be seen on sonography with greater accuracy than on angiography. However, whether intravascular ultrasound imaging will improve our understanding of the pathophysiological processes that are involved with atherosclerotic disease and the treatment of such disease by endovascular methods is a question that cannot be answered at the current stage of clinical experience. Further studies will be necessary to elucidate the question put forward in the title of this chapter.

REFERENCES

1. Ciezynski T: Intracardiac method for the investigation of structure of the heart with the aid of ultrasonics. Arch Immun Ter Dosw 8:551–557, 1960
2. Bom N, Lancée CT, van Egmond FC: An ultrasonic intracardiac scanner. Ultrasonics 10:72–76, 1972; and US patent No. 1, 402, 192 filed 22 February 1973
3. Yock PG, Linker DT, White NW *et al*: Clinical applications of intravascular ultrasound imaging in atherectomy. Int J Cardiac Imag 4:117–125, 1989
4. Gussenhoven WJ, Bom N, van Egmond FC *et al*: A high frequency ultrasound catheter for intravascular imaging. Eur Heart J (abstr) 9:802, 1988
5. Gussenhoven WJ, Essed CE, van Egmond FC *et al*: Intravascular ultrasonic imaging: histologic and echographic correlation. Eur J Vasc Surg 3:571–576, 1989
6. Gussenhoven WJ, Essed CE, Lancée CT *et al*: Arterial wall characteristics determined by intravascular ultrasound imaging: an *in vitro* study. JACC 14:947–952, 1989
7. Gussenhoven WJ, Essed CE, Frietman P *et al*: Intravascular echographic assessment of vessel wall characteristics: a correlation with histology. Int J Card Imag 4:105–111, 1989
8. Essed CE, van den Brand M, Becker AE: Transluminal coronary angioplasty and early stenosis. Fibrocellular occlusion after wall laceration. Br Heart J 49:393–396, 1983
9. Gussenhoven WJ, Pijl P, Frietman P *et al*: Thinning of the media in atherosclerosis: an *in vitro/in vivo* intravascular echographic study. Circulation Suppl. III: 82, 1990
10. Glagov S, Weisenberg E, Zarins CK, Stankunavicius R, Kolettis GJ: Compensatory enlargement of human atherosclerotic coronary arteries. N Engl J Med 316: 1371–1375, 1987

Improvement of Distal Bypass Reconstructions by the Use of Intra-Operative Angioscopy

M. Loeprecht, K. D. Woelfle, U. Kugelmann and R. Jakob

The *in situ* vein technique for bypass offers advantages in femorotibial as well as in popliteopedal reconstructions, in terms of the vein utilization rate and the size of the vein relative to the recipient artery. For good results a reliable method of proof of complete valvulotomy is required which method should also demonstrate venous side branches, a potential source of arteriovenous fistula.

Completion intra-operative arteriography has been standard procedure and intra-operative ultrasound has also been used[1] and occasionally the ultrasound has been used in the form of duplex scanning.[2] Intra-operative angiography can demonstrate incomplete valve ablation, where the whole valve cusp is not divided but it is also possible for the contrast to lie over the thin venous valve and fail to demonstrate the problem. B-Mode ultrasound is capable of detecting arteriovenous fistulae and with duplex scanning, views of ablated venous valves are achieved but the resolution is rather poor on intra-operative scans.[2] Intra-operative detection of arteriovenous fistulae after *in situ* bypass has been achieved with the use of simple Doppler ultrasound with satisfactory results.[3] We looked for a method to achieve both assessment of complete valve ablation and to demonstrate the site of side branches. Experience with angioscopy is now well established[4,5] particularly with the larger endoscopes measuring some 5 mm diameter. Therefore when endoscopes of smaller diameter and longer length became available, these were obvious candidates to assess *in situ* bypass.

PATIENT SERIES AND METHODS OF ANGIOSCOPY

For veins of small diameter, flexible scopes with a diameter of 2.7 mm or less with a steerable tip became available and this enabled us to view every aspect of the luminal service. As a routine device we presently use a steerable scope of 2.2 mm diameter and a working length of 80 cm.

In contrast to the larger diameter endoscopes with an in-built channel for irrigation, some of the smaller diameter endoscopes require an additional special cannula, which we have constructed, which allows for irrigation. Ringers solution is used under pressure achieved by a pneumatic cuff of under 300 mmHg. A flow ranging from 0–400 ml/min can be achieved by control with a foot pedal. This method is easy to use and conserves volume of irrigated fluid.

After preparation of the proximal and distal portions of *in situ* vein before bypass, the angioscope and cannula are introduced from above and the valvulotome is introduced from below. Irrigation from above closes the valves and the valvulotome is observed as it cuts each valve closed by the irrigating pressure. The completeness of valve ablation is assured and where not performed adequately, is repeated. The main danger is of endothelial damage when the vein becomes too narrow to accommodate the scope. Another problem occurs when blood from side branches will not allow an adequate view. Occasionally kinking of a vein makes endoscopy more difficult. It is advisable to advance the instrument very gently under continuous irrigation down the central part of a vein to minimize the risk of damage to the endothelium.[6] Damage usually occurs when the endoscope is advanced without continuous visual control.

STERILIZATION OF THE ANGIOSCOPE

At the present time the cost of an angioscope is approximately £5000 but the tendency is for the price to fall as more angioscopes are being used. The nonsteerable scope is satisfactory for valve ablation if the vein does not have too many kinks. A 1-mm scope is now available[7] (Fig. 1). Such endoscopes of the diameter of less than 1 mm can be used for coronary vessels and also give a very adequate view of the inside of the vessel. These do not have a steerable tip and a balloon catheter is required to move the tip. This is used alongside the angioscope for attempted control. Ethyleneoxide is used for sterilization and it takes approximately 24 hours before an angioscope is returned for use in the sterile condition and so a number of scopes are required in the operating room complex so that one is always available. It is

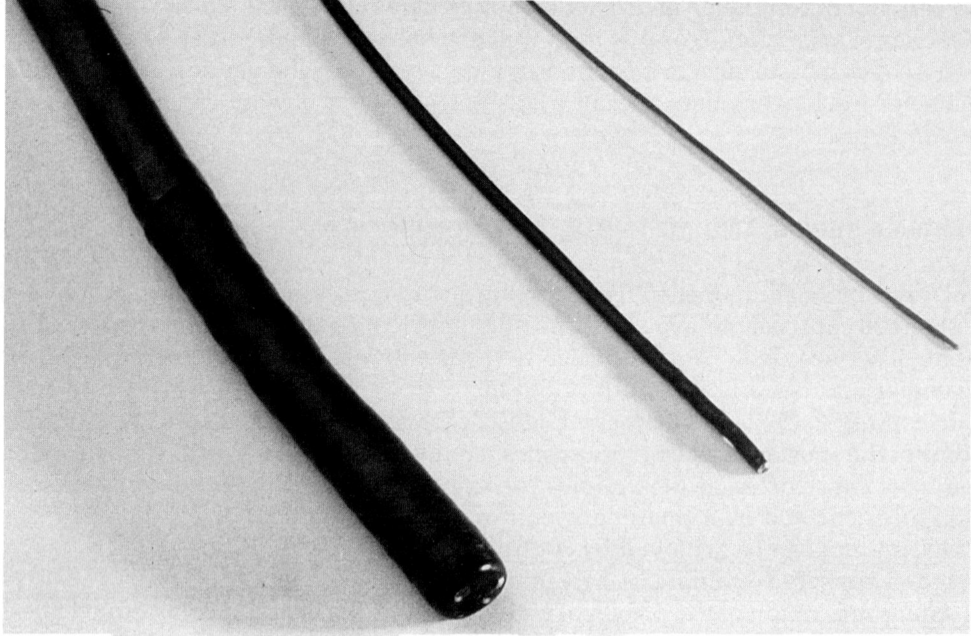

Fig. 1. New and smaller diameter endoscope (6 mm, 2.2 mm and 1.2 mm left to right).

important that the staff that are responsible for sterilization avoid kinking the scope. Otherwise the fibres will break and the optical system is ruined.

FINDINGS IN ENDOSCOPIC ABLATION

The completeness of valve ablation depends upon the technique used. Angiography identifies the cause of incomplete valve disruption, nondivided valves and also intravascular abnormalities such as thrombosis and double lumen.[8] Such abnormalities can also be detected using intra-operative angioscopy.[9] There is a learning curve for achieving completeness of valvulotomy using the angioscope and in Fig. 2 the scope demonstrates the division of a valve cusp by a valvulotome. The use of video is an excellent adjunct for teaching the system[10] and many centres have recommended the use of endoscopy routinely.[11] Intimal flaps, dissections and thrombi have been removed.[12]

IDENTIFICATION OF VENOUS SIDE BRANCHES

It is usual to have a continuous skin incision over the long saphenous vein to ligate every side branch. This may increase the time for healing and cause greater skin necrosis. Using angioscopy especially with the steerable tip, it is possible to identify the light shining at the level of a side branch and to make a smaller incision to find the branch demonstrated internally by the scope. By interrupting irrigation it is sometimes possible to see bleeding from a side branch to detect the tributary which cannot be visualized and many of the branches are identified by this method.

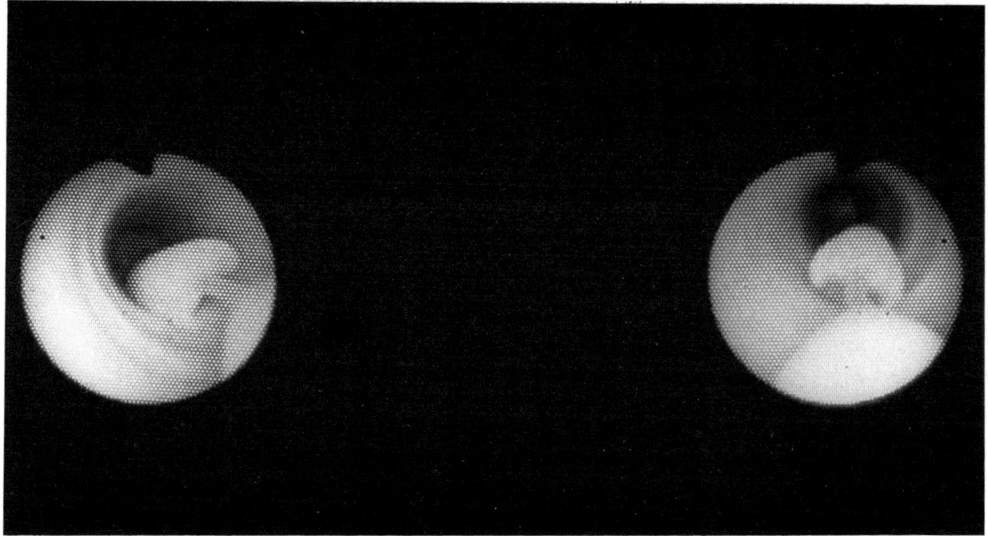

Fig. 2. Valvulotome seen cutting a venous cusp during *in situ* vein bypass.

ASSESSMENT OF DIFFERENT VALVULOTOMES WITH THE INTRA-OPERATIVE ANGIOSCOPE

In Germany, Hall type valvulotomes are widely used and these can be seen to produce a very satisfactory venous valve cusp division in our experience. However, without adequate intra-operative monitoring, it is possible for only one cusp to be disrupted or a side branch to be missed. The Mills hook provides satisfactory ablation, but there is the chance of leaving floating cusps which is less likely with the Hall or Leather valvulotomes. Another type of valvulotome is the bell shaped device introduced by Sandmann. Using this, we found disruption of valve cusps and incompetence, but occasionally larger cusp remnants floated in the lumen (Fig. 3). We do not know whether this leads to early failure but we prefer to abandon this device.

CLINICAL EVALUATION OF ANGIOSCOPY IN BELOW KNEE RECONSTRUCTIONS

In a prospective study including patients operated upon between October 1983 and October 1986, differences in early and intermediate graft failure were noted in 155 procedures checked by conventional angiography and 55 procedures assessed by endoscopy. The series was randomly allocated and there was a variety of procedures used, including differences of materials such as PTFE, composite grafts and vein grafts, but there is no difference in age, clinical stage or sex distribution in the series. The majority had primary procedures, but 31% had re-do operations.

The purpose of description of this series is to describe our early observations in 51 mixed graft failures, which occurred during the first 6 months after operation. Of the endoscopically examined patients, 12 failed (18.5%) against 39 (25%) of the conventional angiography group. The difference was not significant, but we did

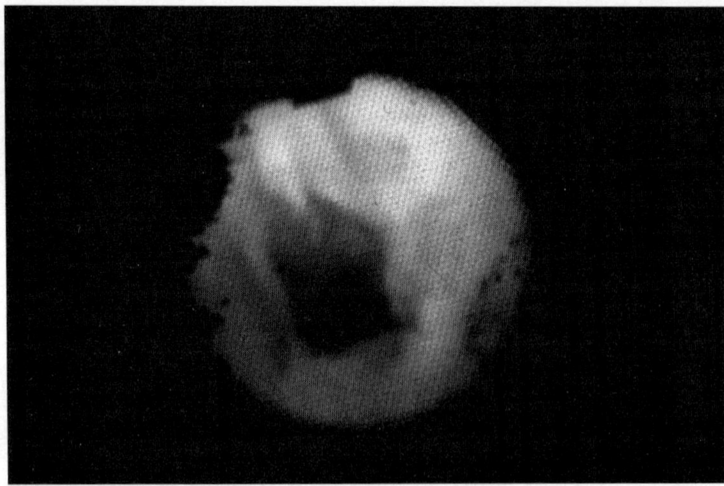

Fig. 3. Floating valve cusp after the Sandmann bell shaped valvulotome has been passed.

notice, as might be expected, that most early failures occurred when prosthetic bypass materials were used. Indeed of the 51 occlusions 21 occurred within the first 48 h and all of these were PTFE. It is interesting that the endoscope revealed thrombi on the internal wall of the prosthetic material and these could be removed by simple balloon thrombectomy. Our experience with the endoscope and completion angiography failed to leave any definite view as to which of these methods was more reliable—both had their value.

ANGIOSCOPY USED FOR *IN SITU* VEIN BYPASS

Our early results in a series of 17 patients were reported in 1988[13] in which a series of 17 patients had five valve remnents which caused a stenosis and three nondivided valve cusps despite what was considered to be a correct valvulotomy procedure. However, only in 14 of the 17 patients could we have visualized the distal anastomosis because the scopes used at the time were too big (2.7 mm). More reliable data on the usefulness of the method began with a prospective study which we began in March 1990. Using a smaller endoscope, by December 1989, we had experience of 30 patients assessed angioscopically and also by completion angiography and it is our intention to compare both methods of assessment at the end of the trial. So far, half of the bypass procedures have had *in situ* and half have had nonreversed procedures. The distal diameter of the vein ranged from 2.5 to 6.0 mm. The bypass length was as long as 63 cm in one case with an average of 44 cm for the series. The endoscope achieved optical visualization in 28 of the 30 patients but in the other two it was poor. The time required for the investigation was 5–10 min in 22 patients and less than 5 min in the other eight patients. The maximum fluid volume required was 750 ml (mean 290 ml). The full length of bypass was visualized in 27 patients and in two, three-quarters of the length was visualized using a 2.2 mm endoscope. Only in one patient were we completely unable to achieve an adequate vision. Valvulotomy was complete in 28 patients, incomplete in one and in the last, visualization was inadequate. We have discovered that angioscopy missed two problems demonstrated by arteriography. In one reversed saphenous vein, thrombus material accumulated above the distal anastomosis beyond a venous valve cusp resulting in a bypass stenosis, which was revised and valvulotomy performed. In the second patient, a side branch was missed which resulted in an arteriovenous fistula.

In conclusion, monitoring of valve ablation is essential after the *in situ* vein bypass procedure has been performed and our suspicion is that angioscopy could be developed to be the best method of the future. At present it is a very useful tool and instruments are getting better all the time, but there are similar improvements and developments in the digital subtraction systems for mobile intra-operative arteriography and we can expect further developments in these systems also.

REFERENCES

1. Bandyk DF, Schmitt DD, Seabrook GR, Adams MB, Towne JB: Monitoring functional patency of *in situ* saphenous vein bypasses: The impact of a surveillance protocol and elective revision. J Vasc Surg 2:286–296, 1989

2. Cullen PJ, Lehay AL, Ryan, SB *et al*: The influence of duplex scanning on early patency rates of *in situ* bypass to the tibial vessels. Ann Vasc Surg 1:340–346, 1986
3. Heather BP, Green IL, McCollum CN, Greenhalgh RM: Intraoperative detection of arterovenous fistulae after *in situ* vein bypass. *In* Diagnostic Techniques and Assessment Procedures in Vascular Surgery, Greenhalgh RM (Ed.). London and New York: Grune & Stratton, pp. 297–302, 1985
4. Vollmar JF, Storz LW: Vascular endoscopy: possibilities and limits of its clinical application. Surg Clin North Am 54:111–122, 1974
5. Vollmar JF, Loeprecht H, Hutschenreiter S: Advances in vascular endoscopy. Thorac Cardiovasc Surg 35:34–41, 1987
6. Matsumoto T, Koyanagi N, Hashizume M *et al*: Angioscopy and intimal response. *In* Angioscopy Vascular and Coronary Applications, White GH and White RA (Eds). Chicago, London, Boca Raton: Year Book Medical Publishers, 1989
7. Grundfest WS, Litvack F, Sherman T *et al*: Delineation of peripheral and coronary detail by intraoperative angioscopy. Ann Surg 202:394–400, 1985
8. Hackler MT, Bunt TJ: Negative impact of routine postreconstructive intraoperative angiography in lower extremity revascularization. Am Surg 49:15–17, 1983
9. Loeprecht H, Weber H, Monnig J: Vascular endoscopy. *In* Diagnostic Techniques and Assessment Procedures in Vascular Surgery, Greenhalgh RM (Ed.). London and New York: Grune & Stratton, pp. 303–317, 1985
10. Mehigan JT, Olcott C 4th: Video angioscopy as an alternative to intraoperative arteriography. Am J Surg 152:139–145, 1986
11. Miller A, Campbell D, Gibbons GW *et al*: Routine intraoperative angioscopy in lower extremity revascularization. Arch Surg 124:104–108, 1989
12. White GH, White RA, Kopchok GE *et al*: Endoscopic intravascular surgery removes intimal flaps, dissections and thrombus. J Vasc Surg 11:280–286, 1990
13. Woelfle KD, Loeprecht H, Weber H, Zinkl K: Intraoperative assessment of *in situ* saphenous vein bypass grafts by vascular endoscopy. Eur J Vasc Surg 2:257–262, 1988

The Management of Vein Bypass Strictures

P. L. Harris and A. P. Moody

In 1973 fibrous strictures were identified by Szilagyi in nearly 30% of femoropopliteal saphenous vein grafts.[1] He anticipated that such strictures might be an important cause of graft failure and advocated an aggressive policy of prophylactic surgical intervention. This proposition was based on data obtained from repeated postoperative angiography, this being the most effective means available for detecting strictures at the time. The importance of fibrous strictures has now been confirmed by others using intravenous digital subtraction angiography (IVDSA)[2,3] and duplex ultrasonic scanning.[3,4] The advent of these newer techniques has permitted repeated, detailed surveillance of vein grafts safely, and with a minimum of discomfort and inconvenience to the patient, and has made possible a thorough re-appraisal of the problem.

It has now been verified that strictures develop in 20–30% of all vein grafts during the first 6–9 months after operation and the incidence appears to be similar whether the vein is utilized *in situ* or reversed.[2] The majority are asymptomatic and undetectable by simple clinical examination.[4,5] The spur to treatment is therefore in most cases entirely preventive, based on the hypothesis that graft failure may thereby be averted.

Given its essentially prophylactic nature, the formulation of a rational policy for the management of vein graft strictures first requires a detailed knowledge of the natural history of these lesions, and specifically their effect on graft patency. Second, reliable information is required about the relative merits or otherwise of the treatment options available, and finally it must be demonstrated that the natural history of strictures can be modified beneficially to a worthwhile degree by the application of these techniques.

WHAT IS THE NATURAL HISTORY OF VEIN GRAFT STRICTURES?

A series of 80 femoropopliteal saphenous vein bypasses from Broadgreen Hospital, which included equal numbers of *in situ* and reversed grafts, were screened during the first year after operation using IVDSA. All of the grafts were clinically patent and the patients were free from ischaemic symptoms in their relevant limb. The overall incidence of fibrous strictures detected by this examination was 27.5%, with similar numbers in *in situ* and reversed grafts. In order to determine the natural history of these lesions, a policy of nonintervention was followed provided that the patients remained asymptomatic. At an average of 13 months after the initial examination all strictured and nonstrictured grafts were reassessed by IVDSA. Those patients who developed symptoms in the interval were re-Xrayed immediately and were subjected to remedial reintervention as appropriate. At the end of this study there were five occlusions of 22 grafts in the strictured group (22.7%) compared to only five of 58 (6.9%) in the nonstrictured group ($\chi^2=4.0$, $p<0.05$). Therefore the strictured grafts had threefold risk of occlusion compared to the nonstrictured grafts.

WHICH STRICTURES CARRY THE GREATEST RISK?

Not all strictured grafts progress to occlusion if left untreated. In the above study 77% of such grafts remained patent and their owners asymptomatic. Surprisingly some of these lesions appeared to be very tight and yet remained clinically silent, but there was a trend for the most tightly stenosed grafts and those with strictures which developed soon after operation to be associated with the highest risk of occlusion. Although insufficient numbers of strictures in each subgroup precluded statistically valid analysis, these observations formed the basis for the following criteria for elective intervention; 1) associated symptoms; 2) an area stenosis of greater than 50% as determined by duplex derived peak systolic velocity ratios (this is equivalent to a 70% diameter stenosis); 3) fall in ankle brachial pressure index of greater than 0.2 after exercise; 4) progression of a stricture on subsequent examinations and 5) the majority of strictures occurring within the first 6 weeks after operation (Table 1).

Although these criteria were to a certain extent originally derived empirically, subsequent experience has not led to any significant changes in policy, and it now seems clear that a selective approach to treatment is most appropriate.

WHAT ARE THE OPTIONS AVAILABLE FOR THE TREATMENT OF VEIN GRAFT STRICTURES

The options available for treatment of graft strictures are limited (Table 2). Surgical management comprises patch angioplasty, interposition grafting, or sequential ('jump') grafting (Fig. 1). Nonsurgical intervention comprises percutaneous transluminal angioplasty.

SURGICAL CORRECTION

Techniques for surgical management of strictures are well established and fundamental to vascular surgery in general. Patch angioplasty is best undertaken

Table 1. Criteria for treatment of vein graft strictures[4]

Area stenosis >50%
Symptomatic stricture
ABPI fall >0.2 on exercise
Stricture progression
Early lesions (<6 weeks)

Table 2. Options for treatment of vein graft strictures

Surgical
Patch angioplasty
Interposition graft
Sequential graft
Interventional radiology
Balloon and angioplasty

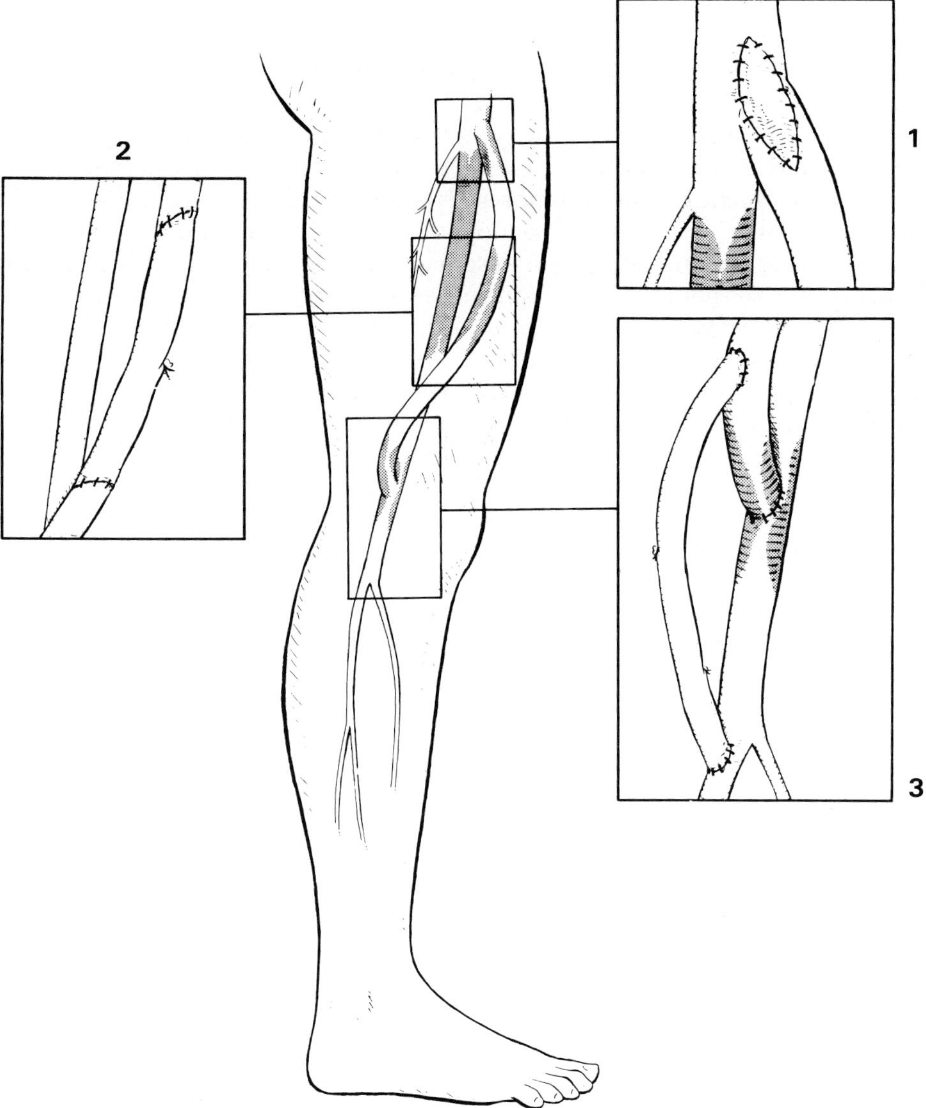

Fig. 1. Open surgical options for the treatment of vein graft strictures. 1. Vein patch angioplasty. 2. Interposition graft. 3. 'Jump' graft.

with an autologous vein patch. Interposition grafting involves the resection and replacement of the strictured section of graft. Again, the preferred conduit is a length of autologous vein. Sequential or 'jump' grafts are most appropriate for the bypass of strictures at the distal anastomosis, the proximal and distal end-to-side anastomoses being constructed by standard techniques. Alternative materials such as PTFE have been described[6] although numbers are small. The poorer results of prosthetic conduits in other situations compared with autologous vein might be expected to translate directly to graft revision and the use of such materials in this situation is rarely if ever justified.

PERCUTANEOUS TRANSLUMINAL ANGIOPLASTY (PTA)

Percutaneous transluminal angioplasty as first described by Dotter was improved by Gruntzig and Hopff in 1974[7] and popularized in Britain by Cumberland in 1981[8] as a means of correcting arterial stenoses. The basic technique now applied to graft strictures is similar and utilizes balloon dilatation, although the use of teflon 'nonballoon' catheters has also been described.[9] The technique for dilating fibrous strictures differs in that relatively high pressures of up to 24 atmospheres may be required. This is compared to a pressure of around 4 atmospheres necessary to treat atheromatous lesions in natural arteries. With such high pressures, it is clearly essential to employ catheters of appropriate specification and to choose very carefully the size of balloon to avoid overdistension and rupture of the graft.

Some vein graft strictures may not be accessible for PTA by standard arterial puncture, for example, those at or near the proximal anastomosis. Direct puncture of the graft has been shown to be a safe procedure[10] and the anatomical site of the stricture should not therefore necessarily preclude treatment by this method.

TREATMENT BY OPEN SURGERY AND PERCUTANEOUS BALLOON ANGIOPLASTY

The first attempts to treat vein graft strictures were by open surgical techniques, and very good results were then, and have continued to be, reported. Unfortunately, many series include only small numbers with limited duration of follow-up.[11,12] Patch angioplasty was used by Disselhoff *et al.*[13] in 12 strictures with good results, improving patency of femorodistal grafts from 63% to 79% at 2 years, and Bandyk *et al.*[14] describe secondary patency rates in grafts treated for strictures of 81% at 3 years compared with a primary patency of 86% for unstrictured grafts. In another large series, by Cohen *et al.*,[15] a mixture of open surgical techniques was used in 22 grafts with 100% initial patency, and a 5-year secondary patency rate of 82%. Surgery is, therefore, both reliable and durable (Table 3a).

Treatment by balloon angioplasty is more controversial. Advantages over surgery are obvious: a further anaesthetic and incision are avoided, and the entire procedure is less invasive. It is certainly more convenient than open surgery, but is it as effective? Doubts have been expressed particularly about durability of results obtained. Initial success rates appear high, but long-term follow-up is lacking in many

Table 3a. Summary of the reported results of surgical corrections of vein graft strictures

Ref.	*Treatment*	*No.*	*Occlusions*	*Follow-up (max. months)*
11	Vein patch	3	0	12
6	PTFE/vein patch	22	(76% patent at 5 years)	
12	Mixed	6	0	24
15	Vein patch	22	(82% patent at 5 years)	
13	Vein patch	12	(79% patent at 5 years)	
14	Vein patch	22	(81% patent at 4 years)	

reports, with patency rates at only 1 year (or less) often being quoted.[9,16,17] Most workers report graft occlusion rates on follow-up of between 10% and 20%[18,19] (Table 3b) and restenosis rates of 9% to 20%.[18,19] Restenosis after angioplasty appears to be a more common problem in coronary artery bypass grafts, with rates of 28% to 58%,[20–22] and in one series of shunts for vascular access, PTA was associated with a survival time for the conduit of only 4 months.[23] However, technical details such as inflation pressure and an assessment of the immediate success in dilating the strictures is omitted in many of these reports. Another criticism of many of these series is the failure to include any classification of strictures or to identify common factors which may affect the outcome of treatment. Germane to this are such factors as the site and length of the stricture and its severity in terms of reduction in cross-sectional area.

In order to assess the efficacy of balloon angioplasty further, a joint study has been undertaken between Broadgreen Hospital, Liverpool, and St Mary's Hospital, London (Table 4) (unpublished). The pooled data include 34 stenoses within 30 grafts, 21 *in situ*, nine reversed and one PTFE. Eighteen stenoses (53%) were related to the distal anastomosis, nine (26%) to the body of the graft and seven (21%) to the proximal anastomosis. Twenty-seven (79%) were less than 1 cm in length, two (6%) were between 1 and 2 cm, and four (12%) were greater than 2 cm. One graft developed extensive atheroma. All were treated by balloon angioplasty and 27 were successfully dilated without any residual stenosis. Three (9%) had a slight residual stenosis, and two (6%) had a marked residual stenosis. Two (6%) occluded immediately after the procedure. Of the original 30 grafts, 19 (63%) remain patent

Table 3b. Summary of the reported results of balloon angioplasty for vein graft strictures

Ref.	*Treatment*	*No.*	*Occlusions*	*Restenosis*	*Follow-up (max. months)*
16	Balloon	12	0	1	7
18	Balloon	27	4	5	24
9	Teflon	5	2	1	15
19	Balloon	6	0	3	26
15	Balloon	7	(43% patent at 5 years)		
17	Balloon	6	2	0	—
4	Balloon	8	2	0	18
Harris/Wolfe (unpublished)	Balloon	30	5	2	30

Table 4. Summary of a combined series of vein graft strictures (Broadgreen and St Mary's hospitals) treated by balloon angioplasty (unpublished)

Stricture length (cm)	*No.*	*Restenosis*	*Occlusions*	*Follow-up (max. months)*
<1	27	2	2	27
1–2	2	0	0	19
>2	4	—	3	12
Extensive atheroma	1	1	1	2

at an average follow-up of 22 months. Six (20%) occluded at an average of 12.6 months after dilatation. Two grafts restenosed at an average of 5 months and, together with the two stenoses which failed to dilate originally, underwent tertiary surgical intervention. Three of the four grafts with stenoses greater than 2 cm (Fig. 2) subsequently occluded, as did the graft with extensive atheroma, despite an apparently satisfactory initial result from balloon angioplasty. Of the 23 grafts with strictures of less than 1 cm in length which were successfully dilated (Fig. 3), only two occluded, at an average of 22.5 months and two restenosed. The secondary patency rate for these grafts was 86% at 22 months.

From these data it is apparent that strictures of less than 1 cm in length can usually be treated successfully by balloon angioplasty and the effect is durable up to 2 years. The results for longer strictures are, however, poor. These lesions are preferably treated surgically by excision and replacement or in the case of a distal lesion by means of a jump graft.

Compared with the results following attempted salvage of thrombosed vein grafts, the prophylactic treatment of strictures by either technique is greatly superior. Cohen and Mannick reported a secondary patency rate of only 19% in femoropopliteal grafts after surgical thrombectomy,[14] and Graor achieved only 20% patency at 12 months after thrombolysis.[24] On this basis alone, the case for elective urgent treatment of strictures is a cogent one.

TO WHAT EXTENT DOES THE TREATMENT OF VEIN GRAFT STRICTURES MODIFY THEIR NATURAL HISTORY?

In 1987 a prospective programme of postoperative vein graft surveillance and selective treatment of strictures was instituted at Broadgreen Hospital based upon principles derived from our previous studies as described above.

All patients undergoing femoropopliteal bypass using autologous vein had their grafts assessed postoperatively by clinical examination including measurement of ankle brachial pressure indices before and after exercise, by IVDSA, and by duplex scanning. The clinical assessment and scans were performed at 6 weeks, 3 months, 6 months, 9 months and 12 months from operation. IVDSA was performed at 3, 6 and 12 months.

In a 12-month period, 79 grafts were surveyed prospectively in this way, and 22 strictures were identified in 18 grafts, an incidence of (22.8%). Eight of the 18 strictured grafts fulfilled our criteria for elective secondary intervention and were treated

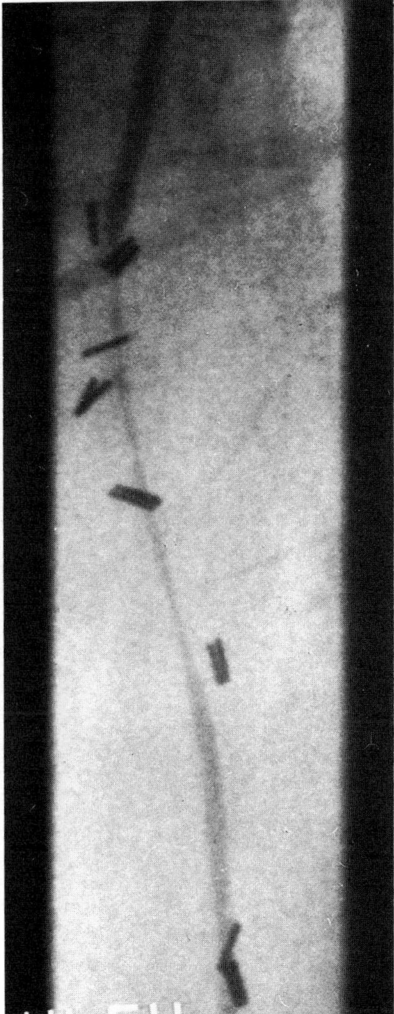

Fig. 2. Long segment stricture of the body of a vein graft. This graft occluded 4 weeks after balloon angioplasty.

accordingly. Figure 4 shows the secondary cumulative patency analysis of the 79 patients entered into this prospective screening and selective intervention programme and compares it with the primary cumulative patency curve of our previous series of 216 unscreened grafts. Although these two sets of data are not contemporaneous they are similar in all other respects and it would appear that a selective policy of prophylactic intervention has improved patency rates in the medium term by about 12%.

CONCLUSIONS

The case for vein graft screening during the first 6–9 months after operation has become compelling. But, since the majority of strictures do not progress inevitably

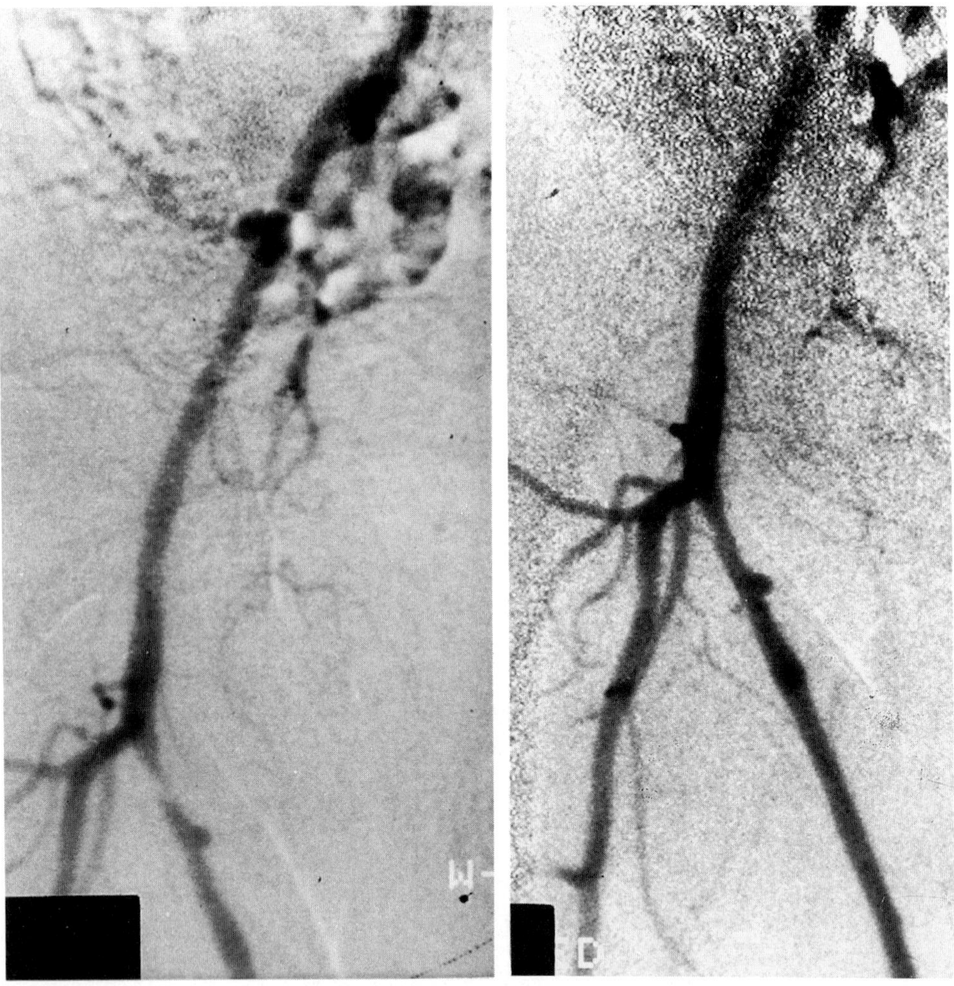

Fig. 3. Stricture of the proximal end of a femoropopliteal vein graft, a (left): before and b (right): 2 years after balloon angioplasty.

to graft occlusion, a selective policy of secondary intervention is appropriate, based upon the now well established principles that those associated with the greatest risk occur early and cause the greatest reduction in cross-sectional area. All such strictures should be regarded as surgical urgencies to be treated with minimal delay. It is also advised that strictures associated with symptoms and those with a clinically demonstrable haemodynamic effect warrant treatment.

Of the two principal methods available for treatment, open operation is almost universally applicable and gives excellent long-term results. Percutaneous balloon angioplasty is more convenient but is ineffective for lesions greater than 1 cm in length and is technically more complicated for strictures at or adjacent to the proximal anastomosis. The treatment of short strictures by PTA appears to be very effective

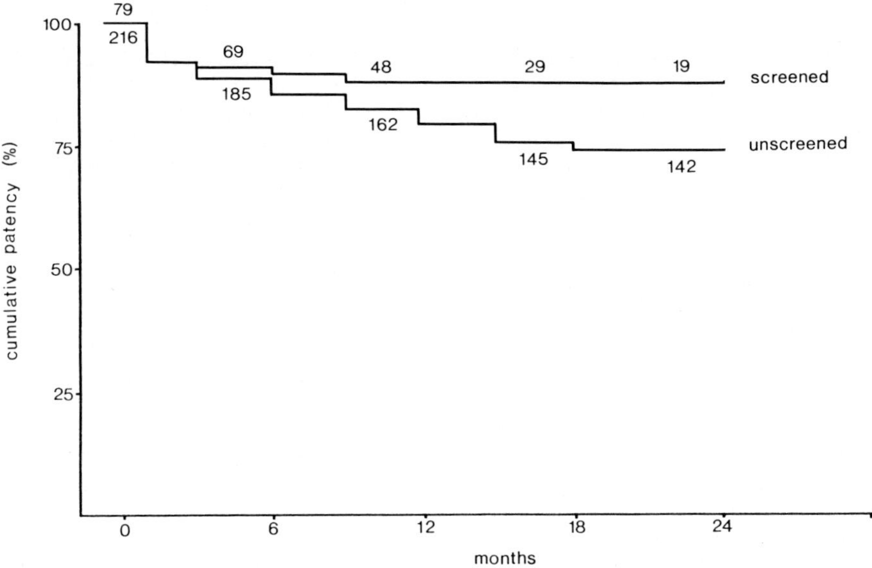

Fig. 4. Cumulative patency rates of 79 vein grafts screened and selectively treated for fibrous strictures (upper curve) compared to that of a previous series 216 untreated grafts ($p<0.002$, log rank test).

in the short term provided high dilatation pressures are used when necessary, but questions regarding the long-term efficacy of this technique remain pending the publication of larger series with adequate duration of follow-up.

REFERENCES

1. Szilagyi DE, Elliott JP, Hageman JH, Smith RF, Dallomolmo CA: Biologic fate of autologous vein implants as arterial substitutes. Ann Surg 178:232–246, 1973
2. Moody P, deCossart LM, Douglas HM, Harris PL: Asymptomatic strictures in femoropopliteal vein grafts. Eur J Vasc Surg 3:389–392, 1989
3. Grigg MJ, Nicolaides AN, Wolfe JHN: Femoro-distal vein bypass graft stenoses. Br J Surg 75:737–740, 1988
4. Moody AP, Gould DA, Harris PL: Vein graft surveillance improves patency in femoropopliteal bypass. Eur J Vasc Surg 4:117–121, 1990
5. Benveniste GL, Royle JP, Roberts AK *et al*: The detection of early femoro-distal vein graft stenosis by treadmill exercise testing. J Cardiovasc Surg (Torino) 29(6):723–726, 1988
6. Sladen JG, Gilmour JL: Vein graft stenosis: characteristics and effect of treatment. Am J Surg 141:549–553, 1981
7. Gruntzig A, Hopff H: Perkutane rekanalisation chronischer arterieller verschlusse mit einem neuen dilatationskatheter. Deutsch Medizine Wochenschrift 99:2502–2505, 1974
8. Cumberland DC: Percutaneous transluminal angioplasty: experience in balloon dilatation of peripheral, coronary and renal arteries. Br J Radiol 55:330–337, 1982
9. Sprayregen S, Veith FJ: Vein graft angioplasty with nonballoon catheters. Radiology 146:224–225, 1981
10. Zajko AB, McLean GK, Freiman DB *et al*: Percutaneous puncture of venous bypass grafts for transluminal angioplasty. Am J Rent 137:799–802, 1981

11. McNamara JJ, Darling RC, Linton RR: Segmental stenosis of saphenous vein autografts. N Engl J Med 277(6):290–292, 1967
12. Bandyk DF, Seabrook GR, Moldenhauer P *et al*: Haemodynamics of vein graft stenosis. J Vasc Surg 8:688–695, 1989
13. Disselhoff B, Buth J, Jakimowicz J: Early detection of stenosis of femoro-distal grafts. A surveillance study using colour duplex scanning. Eur J Vasc Surg 3:43–48, 1989
14. Bandyk DF, Cato RF, Towne JB: A low flow velocity predicts failure of femoropopliteal and femorotibial bypass grafts. Surgery 98(4):799–809, 1985
15. Cohen JR, Mannick JA, Couch NP, Whittemore AD: Recognition and management of impending vein graft failure. Arch Surg 121(7):758–759, 1986
16. Alpert JR, Ring EJ, Berkowitz *et al*: Treatment of vein graft stenosis by balloon catheter dilatation. J Am Med Ass 242(25):2769–2771, 1979
17. Sniderman KW, Kalman PG, Schewchun J, Goldberg RE: Lower extremity *in situ* saphenous vein grafts: angiographic interventions. Radiology 170(3):1023–1027, 1989
18. Berkowitz HD, Hobbs CL, Roberts B *et al*: Value of routine vascular laboratory studies to identify vein graft stenosis. Surgery 90(6):971–979, 1981
19. Greenspan B, Pillari G, Schulman ML *et al*: Percutaneous transluminal angioplasty of stenotic deep vein arterial bypass grafts. Arch Surg 120(4):492–495, 1985
20. Jones EL, Douglas JS, Gruntzig AR *et al*: Percutaneous saphenous vein angioplasty to avoid reoperative bypass. Ann Thorac Surg 36(4):389–395, 1983
21. Reeder GS, Bresnahan JF, Holmes DR *et al*: Angioplasty for aortocoronary bypass graft stenosis. Mayo Clin Proc 61(1):14–19, 1986
22. Marquis JF, Schwartz L, Brown R *et al*: Aldridge H, Henderson M. Percutaneous transluminal angioplasty of coronary saphenous vein bypass grafts. Can J Surg 28:335–337, 1985
23. Brooks JL, Sigley RD, May KJ, Mack RM: Transluminal angioplasty versus surgical repair for stenosis of haemodialysis grafts. Am J Surg 153:530–531, 1987
24. Graor RA, Risius B, Young JR *et al*: Thrombolysis of peripheral arterial bypass grafts: surgical thrombectomy compared with thrombolysis. J Vasc Surg 7:347–355, 1988

NEWER ENDOVASCULAR TECHNIQUES

The Impact of Nonoperative Therapy on the Clinical Management of Peripheral Arterial Disease

Frank J. Veith

Nonoperative therapy of arterial disease may be defined as including all conservative noninterventional treatments and those which are interventional but which do not require traditional open operation. The latter nonsurgical endovascular interventions include percutaneous transluminal balloon angioplasty (PTA) and techniques to ablate atherosclerotic plaque using a variety of laser energy systems or atherectomy devices. Although these endovascular interventions may be performed percutaneously, they can also be carried out via direct surgical access to an artery at a point remote from the site of proposed treatment. In general, most of the laser systems and some of the atherectomy devices have been used in combination with balloon angioplasty to enhance luminal restoration of the occluded or narrowed arterial segment being treated.

One purpose of the present article is to consider the impact of PTA and other newer endovascular techniques with laser or atherectomy devices on the treatment of lower limb ischaemia produced by aorto-iliac and infra-inguinal arteriosclerosis. A second purpose is to examine the role of conservative, noninterventional treatment, which in many instances amounts to nontreatment, in the management of this common disease entity.

To achieve these goals it is necessary to review briefly the natural history of the various clinical stages of lower limb ischaemia from arteriosclerosis as well as the current ability to deal with this process by open surgical operations, which include primarily bypass procedures. With these facts in mind we can evaluate the roles and potential impact of conservative noninterventional treatment and the nonoperative endovascular interventions in managing atherosclerotic lower limb ischaemia. To this end, the following questions must be addressed: How can these endovascular interventions better *or worsen* the natural history of the disease process? Should they justify a change in the indications for intervention? Can they replace or facilitate standard operative treatment? To answer these questions we need to know the relative safety and efficacy, both short-term and long-term, of standard operations, the newer endovascular treatments and conservative treatment for various stages of the disease process. In most instances precise data to answer these complex questions with certainty are not available. The following discussion will therefore largely be an expression of opinion based on reasonable extrapolations of what is currently known about an extraordinarily common and usually benign disease process and its response to standard operative treatment and PTA. It will also highlight gaps in knowledge that need to be filled to provide precise answers to the questions posed. Finally, it will address the issue of who, by virtue of their experience in dealing with this disease process, are best qualified to treat it and provide definitive answers to these questions.

NATURAL HISTORY, STAGING AND TREATMENT OF LOWER EXTREMITY ISCHAEMIA: ROLE OF CONSERVATIVE TREATMENT AND NONTREATMENT

Arteriosclerosis may involve the infrarenal aorta, the iliac arteries, the common femoral artery and its branches, the above knee and below knee popliteal artery, any of the infrapopliteal arteries including their terminal branches, or any combination of these arteries. This involvement generally begins early in adult life and progresses slowly to the point where a flow reducing stenosis or occlusion occurs in one or more of the arteries below the renal segment of the aorta. As the average age of our population increases, the number of individuals with this haemodynamically significant infrarenal arteriosclerosis also increases.

Obviously, this disease is associated in varying degrees with arteriosclerotic involvement elsewhere in the body, and this fact must constantly be considered when making therapeutic decisions in afflicted patients. It is this consideration which should guide the physician correctly to seek palliation rather than cure and to attempt a lesser intervention or operation that maintains function rather than one that will restore a normal circulation. The generalized and slowly progressive nature of the disease process and the imperfect results of all interventional treatments should also deter any who might be unwisely tempted to treat asymptomatic or minimally disabling arteriosclerotic occlusive lesions. In the management of the increasingly common entity of lower extremity arteriosclerosis, diagnostic and therapeutic restraint and the desire to minimize risks and avoid doing harm must be paramount principles if the disease is not producing major functional impairment or tissue necrosis. On the other hand, despite the advanced age and poor generalized condition of the afflicted population, aggressive intervention for both diagnosis and treatment is justified if limb loss is truly threatened by the disease process.

The reserve of the human arterial system is enormous. Haemodynamically significant stenosis or major artery occlusions can exist in the infrarenal arterial tree with no symptoms or with only minimal symptoms. This is particularly true if collateral pathways are normal or the patient's activity level is limited by coronary arteriosclerosis or other disease processes. Accordingly, the most common manifestation of a short segmental occlusion of the superficial femoral artery, the most common site of major arteriosclerotic involvement below the inguinal ligament, will be mild intermittent claudication. Similarly, this lesion will often be totally asymptomatic, and this is usually the case if only one or two tibial arteries are occluded without other significant lesions. Thus the usual patient who presents with severe disabling intermittent claudication or tissue necrosis has multiple sequential occlusions or so-called combined segment disease with haemodynamically significant lesions at the aorto-iliac level and the superficial femoropopliteal level, or either or both of these combined with severe infrapopliteal disease as well.

Staging

Patients with haemodynamically significant infrarenal arteriosclerosis may be classified into one of five stages depending on their clinical presentation as indicated in Table 1. Patients in Stage III and Stage IV are those with so-called *critical ischaemia*

Table 1. Staging of infrarenal arteriosclerosis with haemodynamically significant stenosis or occlusions

Stage	*Presentation*	*Invasive diagnostic and therapeutic intervention at present*
0	No signs or symptoms	Never justified
I	Intermittent claudication (>1 block) No physical changes	Usually unjustified
II	Severe claudication (<1/2 block) Dependent rubor Decreased temperature	Sometimes justified Not always necessary May remain stable
III	Rest pain Atrophy, cyanosis Dependent rubor	Usually indicated but may do well for long periods without revascularization
IV	Nonhealing ischaemic ulcer or gangrene	Usually indicated but not always

and whose limbs may be considered imminently threatened, although some patients with mild ischaemic rest pain may remain stable for many years and an occasional patient with a small patch of gangrene or an ischaemic ulcer will heal their lesion with conservative in-hospital treatment.[1] With the exception of these few patients, invasive diagnostic procedures such as angiography are usually justified for those with Stage III and IV disease, which is usually associated with disease and significant lesions at several levels.

Rest pain as an isolated symptom in patients with infra-inguinal arteriosclerosis can be difficult to evaluate unless it is accompanied by other findings. Many patients with significant arterial lesions have pain at rest from causes other than their arteriosclerosis, such as arthritis or neuritis. Such pain will not be relieved by even a successful revascularization. Significant ischaemic rest pain must be associated not only with decreased pulses but also with other objective manifestations of ischaemia such as atrophy, decreased skin temperature when compared to the other extremity, and rubor and relief of pain with dependency. In some patients with a complex aetiology to their rest pain, it may be necessary to perform a noninvasive laboratory and angiographic evaluation before the predominant cause of the symptom can be determined and appropriate treatment instituted. Every patient with pain at rest and decreased pulses is not a candidate for angiography and an arterial intervention. Some of these patients will be relieved by appropriate treatment for gout or osteoarthritis. Others can be well managed with simple analgesics and reassurance that their limb is not in jeopardy. Such reassurance generally suffices for patients with Stage I disease and those with Stage II disease who are elderly (>80 years) or at high risk because of intercurrent disease or atherosclerotic involvement of other organs such as the heart, the kidneys, or the brain.

This conservative approach to patients with Stage I involvement from lower extremity arteriosclerosis is widespread among surgeons, albeit not universally so.[2] Conservatism appears to be clearly justified by the numerous reports of the benignancy and slow progression of Stage I disease to more advanced stages.[3–5]

Without treatment, 10–15% of patients in Stage I will improve over 5 years, and 60–70% will not progress over the same period. The 10–15% who do worsen are, in our opinion, best treated with a primary nonoperative intervention or operation after their disease progresses. This conservative approach to Stage I disease is justified by the greater surgical difficulty encountered when a procedure for claudication fails in the early or remote postoperative period and the patient then has a threatened limb, a situation that we have observed all too frequently.

The fact that some patients in Stage II and a few in Stage III or Stage IV may remain stable and easily managed without operation for protracted periods of 1 or more years justifies a cautiously conservative noninterventional approach to selected patients in these stages.[1] This often requires hospitalization so that the patient and the progress of his ischaemia can be assessed. Moreover, this conservative approach is particularly indicated if the patient is elderly and a poor surgical risk from a systemic and a local point of view. An example of this would be an octogenarian with intractable congestive failure in whom a difficult distal small vessel bypass would be required to alleviate Stage III signs and symtoms. Close observation can and often should be the preferred management for such a patient for several months or even years; however, we would not hesitate to revascularize such a patient when his rest pain became intolerable or he developed a small progressive patch of gangrene.[6]

PRESENT STATUS OF SURGICAL TREATMENT FOR LOWER EXTREMITY ISCHAEMIA

Details of this are presented elsewhere in this volume and are beyond the scope of this article. However, several generalities concerning arterial surgery for lower limb ischaemia are relevant to the theme of this chapter and the questions already posed.

One such generality is that most patients who currently require treatment for severe limb threatening lower extremity ischaemia have a pattern of arterial disease that is amenable to some form of bypass operation. In the past many patients were thought to have arteries that were 'unsuitable for reconstruction' because of extensive, multilevel occlusive disease in the leg arteries. However, we and others have shown that, with appropriate commitment, high quality arteriography and use of technical innovations, very few patients with lower limb ischaemia cannot be revascularized successfully. In one study published in 1981, we found that only 6% of patients with threatened limbs had arteries unsuitable for a bypass operation.[6] With more recent technical improvements, particularly use of distal origin, short vein grafts and the ability to perform bypasses to arterial segments in the ankle region or foot, less than 1% of previously unoperated cases and less than 2% of all patients with limb threatening ischaemia are unsuitable for some operative attempt at limb salvage with more than an 80% chance of initial success.[7,8] On the other hand many of these very distal small artery limb salvage operations are difficult, time consuming and technically demanding. If the ischaemia is associated with extensive necrosis or infection in the foot, multiple debridements and protracted hospitalizations may be required. Nevertheless, these are usually successful and result in limb salvage and normal ambulation, a state often not achieved after major amputation.[6] For this reason most vascular surgeons currently believe that aggressive efforts at limb salvage are worthwhile. This is true even if the patient with a threatened limb has multiple risk factors which might appear to increase operative mortality and limit life expectancy. With improved anaesthetic management and perioperative intensive care, it has been possible to perform long complex operations on patients with severe coronary artery disease, recent congestive heart failure, diabetes and advanced age with an acceptably low 30-day operative mortality of 2–5%.[6,9,10]

A second generality is that all interventions that manipulate arteries including operations carry risks. In addition to the obvious risks of provoking a myocardial infarction or thrombosis or bleeding from instrumented arteries, surgical operations may be complicated by wound infection. When this involves an arterial suture line or graft it may be difficult to treat, result in further arterial occlusions and require complex revascularizations and protracted hospitalization. Moreover any reconstructive arterial procedure, even if initially successful, can be complicated by subsequent failure with thrombosis.[11] When this occurs immediately after operation, it may be due to an imperfect repair or the choice of the wrong procedure. Late failure, usually within 2–20 months of operation, may be produced by the healing process in the traumatized artery or the arterial graft. Such fibro-intimal hyperplasia can occur after any manipulation of a blood vessel. Its aetiology is poorly understood, but fortunately its occurrence is not universal. Late failure, after 2 years, is usually due to progression of arteriosclerosis.[11]

All these processes produce a substantial late failure rate for arterial reconstructions particularly those to the popliteal or infrapopliteal arteries. Because of this, most vascular surgeons generally have a conservative attitude regarding arterial interventions for anything less than critical Stage III or Stage IV ischaemia, and this is certainly true when an arterial reconstruction extending below the popliteal artery is required. This conservatism is further supported by the fact that failure of a primary arterial intervention is sometimes associated with ischaemia greater than that originally present, necessitating secondary interventions which are often rendered difficult by scarring, obliteration of previously patent arterial segments and sometimes infection. Nevertheless, when such difficult re-operative procedures are required, appropriate strategies and operative techniques have been developed so that they can be carried out effectively with resulting benefit to most patients.[11,12]

A third generality which is related to some of the foregoing points is that patients whose arteries are easy to operate upon, in terms of having relatively normal arteries proximal and distal to a single severe stenosis or occlusion, probably do not require any operation since they will have relatively nondisabling claudication. In contrast, patients who have Stage III or IV ischaemia which requires revascularization usually have arteries that are difficult to operate on by virtue of having diffuse disease often with calcification and thick diseased walls in even their patent arterial segments.

A fourth therapeutic generality is that the arterial intervention, when performed in these very ill, end stage disease patients with complex multilevel peripheral arteriosclerosis, should be the simplest procedure possible to salvage the patient's extremity or relieve the patient's most troublesome symptom. If the patient has Stage II or III ischaemia or trivial necrosis in the foot, correction of the most proximal haemodynamically significant lesion will generally suffice even if multiple distal occlusions remain. Only if extensive necrosis or infection are present in the distal limb is it usually necessary to restore straight line arterial flow to the foot to achieve healing.[6,13]

IMPACT OF NONOPERATIVE INTERVENTIONS ON PATIENTS PRESENTLY UNDERGOING OPERATION

To replace operation

In light of all the foregoing considerations, it is clear that we believe that patients who presently have valid indications for operative therapy, if they have one or more haemodynamically significant lesion suitable for treatment by PTA at this time, should have that technique used to treat that lesion. This applies to stenoses and short (<5 cm) occlusions of the common and external iliac arteries, the superficial femoral and popliteal arteries and tibial arteries.[6,14] Although the success rates of PTA for such lesions in mostly Stage III and IV ischaemia varies depending on the nature and location of the lesion, the criteria of success and the presence of associated lesions, it is high enough to warrant such treatment. The morbidity of the procedure is <8% and the mortality <1%.[15] More than 50% of the patients will derive benefit for at least 2 years, and when complications or early or late failure occur, they can be managed by operative intervention generally no more complex and risky than if the PTA had not been performed.[15] However, these good results in this group of patients with diffusely diseased arteries requires close collaboration and co-operation between the radiologist and the vascular surgeon.[15,16] The proportion of operative candidates who can be treated by PTA varies depending on the aggressiveness of the radiologist and how far from the ideal short, stenotic lesion he is willing to extend his or her attempts at PTA. Success rates vary inversely with the radiologist's boldness, and complication rates vary directly. We as surgeons remain enthusiastic about these extended indications for PTA in these patients because they usually apply to those who would be difficult, high risk operative candidates as well. Presently approximately one-third of our limb salvage operative candidates undergo PTA of one or more lesions. Some of these patients never require operation.

To facilitate operation

Approximately two-thirds of our patients undergoing PTA or one-quarter of all our limb salvage operative candidates require an operation after the PTA. Most of these operations are bypass procedures to overcome a lesion other than the one treated by PTA, and some may be required because a PTA fails or has a complication. PTA of significant iliac lesions are often performed proximal to a distal operative procedure originating from the common femoral artery. Complex aortofemorodistal operations are thereby avoided, and treatment simplified and rendered less risky in this group of patients with multiple systemic risk factors and complex multilevel disease. The enthusiasm that we and others had for this approach many years ago has now been verified by recent late observations showing durable long-term results.[6,17,18] More recently we have also used PTA to treat popliteal and tibial lesions distal to a bypass when the distal lesions were impairing healing of the foot.[14]

Another way that PTA can facilitate or improve operative treatment is to correct a haemodynamically significant lesion that develops in, proximal to or distal to a bypass graft without yet causing graft thrombosis. This condition which we have termed a 'failing graft' must be treated or the graft will thrombose (fail), and this treatment may be by operation or PTA.[19] We currently favour PTA for short inflow and outflow lesions and <1.5 cm stenoses in vein grafts. Although others have had poor results with PTA of vein graft stenoses, some of our patients have had arteriographically good results for 3–6 years.

Other new nonoperative interventions

To date most laser systems have facilitated balloon angioplasty by enabling passage of a guide wire through otherwise impassible occlusions, and atherectomy devices have restored luminal patency by excising plaque thereby removing lesions that might otherwise be treated by balloon angioplasty. Larger diameter laser systems which can ablate sufficient plaque to restore an adequate arterial lumen are just beginning clinical trials. All these methods are interesting and attractive because of their promise of effective treatment with a lower morbidity. All therefore deserve to be tried clinically. However, it is well known that all arterial trauma induces a healing response and that this may lead to fibrointimal hyperplasia. This in turn may not only overcome the benefit of the therapeutic intervention, it may also produce more extensive luminal obliteration than was present before the treatment and thereby worsen the patient. Poor 1-year patency results after hot-tipped laser assisted balloon angioplasty[20–22] and mixed anecdotal reports after various atherectomy device treatments underscore this potential risk. It is mandatory, therefore, that all clinical trials with newer endovascular interventions include late arteriographic follow-up extending for at least 2 years after the procedure. Until such observations are available to allow comparison of the newer method with operative treatment and standard PTA to treat various lesions in various stages of the disease, the exact role of these newer technologies in the management of lower limb ischaemia cannot be defined.

IMPACT OF NONOPERATIVE INTERVENTIONAL TREATMENTS ON THE THRESHOLD FOR THERAPY

Because PTA of ideal iliac and superficial femoral artery lesions is simple, reasonably safe and reasonably durable, it seems logical to extend the indications somewhat beyond those for operation. This is particularly true for short stenoses in otherwise undiseased arteries. Patients with such lesions and Stage I or Stage II disease certainly may be subjected to PTA. However, complications and failures can occur and patients should be informed of the risks and that the treatment is not intended to prevent disease progression, since it does not, but only to relieve the symptom. On this basis we have performed PTAs on a few patients who we would not have subjected to operation. However, the number of such individuals is small, comprising <1% of our treated patients. The philosophy underlying this therapeutic restraint is reinforced by recent data showing that conservative therapy for claudication may offer benefits equal to PTA after several years.[23] This underscores our belief that arteriosclerotic medical regimens to delay progression of arteriosclerosis may be more important than PTA for patients with Stage I disease. However, this remains unproven.

The relative simplicity of other newer endovascular treatments using laser and atherectomy devices with or without PTA has prompted many physicians and surgeons to recommend the extension of indications and the lowering of therapeutic thresholds for lower limb arteriosclerosis. Some surgeons, radiologists and particularly cardiologists new to the peripheral vascular field and armed with these new techniques and devices have used them routinely to treat Stage I and even Stage 0 disease detected incidentally during physical examination or coronary arteriography. Their rationale is that such treatment may prevent disease progression, an assumption for which there is not one shred of evidence. This practice is to be condemned at this time. The mid- and long-term safety and efficacy of these newer treatments remain totally unknown. Even if they are successful immediately, they can initiate a healing process in the artery which causes late failure or worse an acceleration of the occlusive process and ultimately net harm to the patient. Therapeutic thresholds should not be lowered until clinical trials demonstrating mid- and long-term safety and efficacy are available. Moreover these trials must include arteriographic follow-up at least 2 years after the intervention.

QUALIFICATIONS AND CREDENTIALS OF INDIVIDUALS WHO SHOULD TREAT PERIPHERAL VASCULAR DISEASE PATIENTS

The introduction of many new devices that can potentially treat peripheral atherosclerotic lesions has provoked much interest in the field of lower extremity ischaemia. However, the mere presence of a flow reducing lesion in the infrarenal arterial tree does not mean that it should be treated. Those who care for this disease entity should be familiar with the natural history of all stages of the disease. They should be aware of other manifestations of arteriosclerosis and other disease processes that are rampant in this patient population. Most importantly, they should be aware of the relative benignancy of the disease in most patients and how effective conservative treatment and nontreatment can be. Finally they should be aware of how difficult it can be to treat effectively some patients with true limb threatening ischaemia.

To determine qualifications and credential requirements for specialists who should treat lower limb ischaemia goes beyond the scope of this article. However, a few relevant points can be made. For years vascular surgeons have managed the vast majority of lower extremity circulatory problems. They have administered both operative and nonoperative treatment for these patients, and they are aware of the value of conservative treatment. Clearly vascular surgeons should be among those who continue to care for these patients in the future, and an article on guidelines for hospital privileges in this specialty has recently appeared.[24] One year of special training in this field is the fundamental requirement for credentials and hospital privileges in vascular surgery.

With the introduction of PTA, interventional radiologists have become involved in the management of patients with lower limb ischaemia. Generally these radiologists work in close collaboration with vascular surgeons. They provide the surgeon with high quality arteriograms, they collaborate in joint therapeutic decisions, and individuals from the two complementary specialties help to take care of each other's complications. Interventional radiologists, too, have 1 year of specialized training devoted in large part to the diagnosis and management of lower limb ischaemia. Clearly they, too, should continue their role in the management of these patients.

More recently cardiologists have professed an interest in these patients and they have begun to treat them interventionally.[25] Clearly cardiologists can contribute to improved care. They know about coronary artery disease and its management, and they may be able to bring special expertise in the use of the newer endovascular devices, some of which were specifically designed for use in the coronary arteries. However, if cardiologists wish to become involved in the care of peripheral vascular disease, they, too, should fulfill two requirements. First they should have 1 year of training during which they have broad exposure to peripheral vascular disease patients of all stages, including those that require all kinds of treatment—nontreatment, conservative, nonoperative interventional, operative and a combination of these modalities. Second, they should work together as part of a team which includes interventional radiologists, vascular surgeons and cardiologists. Only in that way will patients with lower extremity ischaemia get the safest, least meddlesome and most effective management.

SUMMARY

Nonoperative therapy includes conservative noninterventional and endovascular interventional modalities. The latter includes percutaneous transluminal angioplasty (PTA) and a variety of laser systems and atherectomy devices. This article considers the role and impact of all nonoperative treatments in the perspectives of the natural history of lower extremity arteriosclerosis and its current surgical (operative) treatment. Nonoperative treatments may replace and/or facilitate surgical treatment in operative candidates. Nonoperative methods may also justify treatment in patients who cannot or should not be subjected to operation. Facts and opinions relating to these uses of nonoperative treatments are presented. The issue of qualifications and credentials of individuals who should be treating patients with lower extremity ischaemia from peripheral arteriosclerosis is discussed.

REFERENCES

1. Rivers SP, Veith FJ, Ascer E, Gupta SK: Successful conservative therapy of severe limb threatening ischemia: The value of non-sympathectomy. Surgery 99:759–762, 1986
2. Donaldson MC, Mannick JA: Femoropopliteal bypass grafting for intermittent claudication. Is pessimism warranted? Arch Surg 15:724–727, 1980

3. Boyd AM: The natural course of arteriosclerosis of the lower extremities. Proc R Soc Med 55:591–593, 1962
4. Coran AG, Warren R: Arteriographic changes in femoropopliteal arteriosclerosis obliterans: A five year follow-up study. N Engl J Med 274:643–645, 1966
5. Imparato AM, Kim GE, Davidson T, Crowley JG: Intermittent claudication: Its natural course. Surgery 78:795–797, 1975
6. Veith FJ, Gupta SK, Samson RH *et al*: Progress in limb salvage by reconstructive arterial surgery combined with new or improved adjunctive procedures. Ann Surg 194:386–401, 1981.
7. Veith FJ, Ascer E, Gupta SK *et al*: Tibiotibial vein bypass grafts: A new operation for limb salvage. J Vasc Surg 2:552–557, 1985
8. Ascer E, Veith FJ, Gupta SK: Bypasses to plantar arteries and other tibial branches: An extended approach to limb salvage. J Vasc Surg 8:434–441, 1988
9. Rivers SP, Scher LA, Gupta SK, Veith FJ: Safety of peripheral vascular surgery after recent myocardial infarction. J Vasc Surg 11:70–76, 1990
10. Taylor LM, Edwards JM, Porter JM: Present status of reversed vein bypass: Five year results of a modern series. J Vasc Surg 11:207–215, 1990
11. Veith FJ, Gupta SK, Ascer E, Rivers SP, Wengerter K: Improved strategies for secondary operations on infrainguinal arteries. Ann Vasc Surg 3:85–93, 1990
12. Bartlett ST, Olinde AJ, Flinn WR *et al*: The reoperative potential of infrainguinal bypass: Long-term limb and patient survival. J Vasc Surg 5:170–179, 1987
13. Veith FJ, Gupta SK, Daly V: Femoropopliteal bypass to the isolated popliteal segment: Is polytetrafluoroethylene graft acceptable? Surgery 89:296–303, 1981
14. Bakal CW, Sprayregen S, Scheinbaum K, Cynamon J, Veith FJ: Percutaneous transluminal angioplasty of the infrapopliteal arteries: Results in 53 patients. Am J Roentgen 154:171–174, 1990
15. Samson RH, Sprayregen S, Veith FJ *et al*: Management of angioplasty complication, unsuccessful procedures and early and late failures. Ann Surg 199:234–240, 1984
16. Franco CD, Goldsmith J, Veith FJ *et al*: Management of arterial injuries produced by percutaneous femoral procedures. J Cardiovasc Surg 30:7, 1989
17. Alpert JR, Ring EJ, Freiman DB *et al*: Balloon dilatation of iliac stenosis with distal arterial surgery. Arch Surg 115:715–717, 1980
18. Brewster DC, Cambria RP, Darling RC *et al*: Long-term results of combined iliac balloon angioplasty and distal surgical revascularization. Ann Surg 210:324–330, 1989
19. Veith FJ, Weiser RK, Gupta SK *et al*: Diagnosis and management of failing lower extremity arterial reconstructions. J Cardiovasc Surg 25:381–384, 1984
20. Wright JG, Belkin M, Greenfield AJ *et al*: Laser angioplasty for limb salvage: Observations on early results. J Vasc Surg 10:29–38, 1989
21. Perler BA, Osterman FA, White RI, Williams GM: percutaneous laser probe femoropopliteal angioplasty: A preliminary experience. J Vasc Surg 10:351–357, 1989
22. Harrington ME, Schwartz ME, Sandborn T *et al*: Expanded indications for laser assisted balloon angioplasty in peripheral artery disease. J Vasc Surg, 1990 (in press)
23. Van Rij AM, Packer SGK, Morrison ND: Angioplasty for claudicants with femoropopliteal disease. J Cardiovasc Surg 30:88, 1989
24. Moore WS, Treiman RL, Hertzer NR, Veith FJ *et al*: Guidelines for hospital privileges in vascular surgery. J Vasc Surg 10:678–682, 1989
25. De Maria AN: Peripheral vascular disease and the cardiovascular specialist. J Am Col Cardiol 12:869–870, 1988

Angioplasty Using the Pulsed Dye Laser

R. F. M. Wood, D. C. Mitchell and A. Murray

Laser ablation of atheroma offers a potentially less invasive means of achieving revascularization of the ischaemic limb than reconstructive surgery. The procedure has the advantage over percutaneous transluminal angioplasty (PTA) of debulking plaque and recanalizing long occlusive lesions through which a guidewire cannot be negotiated.

A variety of intravascular devices are now available and it is possible to produce a profile of the ideal device and to measure the performance of any system against this standard.

PROFILE OF THE IDEAL INTRAVASCULAR DEVICE

1. Capable of percutaneous insertion.
2. Able to recanalize total occlusions, by removal of atheroma.
3. Low rate of vessel perforation.
4. Minimal risk of producing embolic fragments.
5. Capable of being imaged and guided within the artery.
6. Producing a satisfactory channel without the need for adjunctive balloon dilatation.
7. Leaving a vessel wall surface which produces a low thrombotic and intimal hyperplastic response.
8. Able to ablate calcified disease.

It is clear that none of the available systems meet all these requirements. In this chapter we will examine the performance of the pulsed dye laser against this exacting specification.

THE PULSED DYE LASER

The wavelength of light transmitted by a pulsed dye laser is controlled by the colour of dye pumped through the laser head (Fig. 1). Theoretically it is possible to produce light output at any wavelength within the visible spectrum. In practice the selection of wavelengths depends upon finding dyes which will remain sufficiently stable within the operating system. The coumarin group of dyes produce wavelength outputs at the blue/green end of the visible spectrum and are particularly suitable for use in treating atherosclerotic plaque.

The work of Prince *et al.*[1] has demonstrated that there is an approximately twofold increase in the absorption of light by atheroma compared with normal arterial

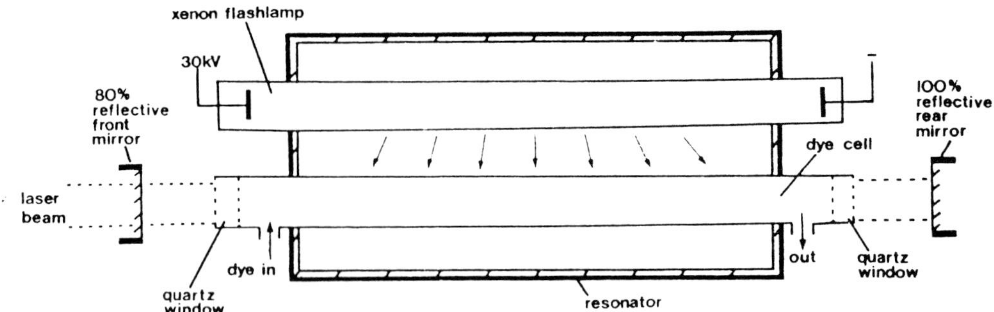

Fig. 1. The flashlamp-pumped dye laser. Cooled coumarin dye at either 480 nm or 504 nm is circulated through the resonator. Laser light is fully reflected from the rear mirror and emerges through the 80% reflecting front mirror to be focused onto the end of the quartz delivery fibre.

wall at wavelengths from 420 to 530 nm (Fig. 2). This wavelength difference can be exploited to produce preferential ablation of atheroma. The work of Murray *et al.*[2] has shown that at a wavelength of 480 nm the same output energy will produce deeper craters in atheroma than in normal arterial wall (Fig. 3). In addition *in vitro* experiments have demonstrated that the pulsed dye laser has the capacity to cause disruption of calcified plaque.[3–5]

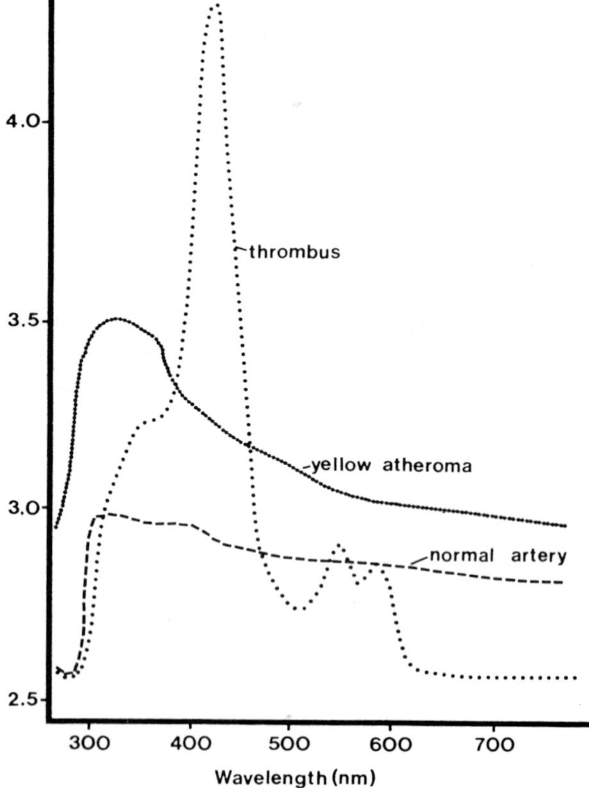

Fig. 2. The absorbtion spectrum of thrombus, normal arterial wall and atheroma (Prince *et al.*, 1986)[1].

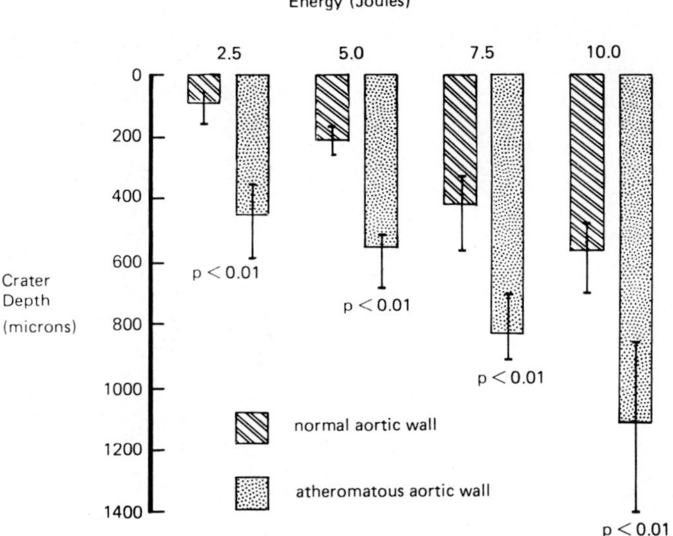

Fig. 3. Crater depth related to energy applied (median and range) in normal and atheromatous aortic specimens produced by firing a 600 μm 'bare' fibre at four different energy levels. (Statistics: Mann-Whitney U-test.)

THE ADVANTAGES OF PULSED ENERGY

The ability to deliver energy in short pulses has two advantages. First it enables very high peak powers to be produced. As currently tuned, the MDL-1P pulsed dye laser (Candela Laser Corp, Wayland, MA) produces a 1 μs pulse ten times per second. The peak power is of the order of 10^5 Watts. The delivery of energy in pulses to the target tissue allows any heat generated to dissipate before the next pulse arrives. The time that it takes for the temperature of a heated volume of given radius to fall exponentially can be calculated mathematically and is known as the 'thermal relaxation time'. Using energy delivered through a 600 μm ball-tipped fibre, the approximate thermal relaxation time of arterial wall is of the order of 100 ms.

Studies *in vitro* have shown that the pulsed dye laser causes minimal thermal injury to nonablated tissue. The craters produced in arteries by firing at right angles to the surface are smooth walled (Fig. 4) and transmission electron microscopy confirms that there is preservation of cellular architecture. In comparison if ablation is carried out with a continuous laser at a similar wavelength (Argon laser, 504 nm) there is marked charring and vacuolation of adjacent normal structures in the vessel wall.

DELIVERY DEVICES

The majority of intravascular devices have been designed to be inserted over a guidewire. The standard probes for the 'hot tip' argon laser have an eccentric channel in the tip which allows the assembly to be advanced over an 0.38 guidewire. The use of a guidewire undoubtedly adds safety to the procedure by reducing the risk of perforation. However, although it is possible to pass guidewires through tight

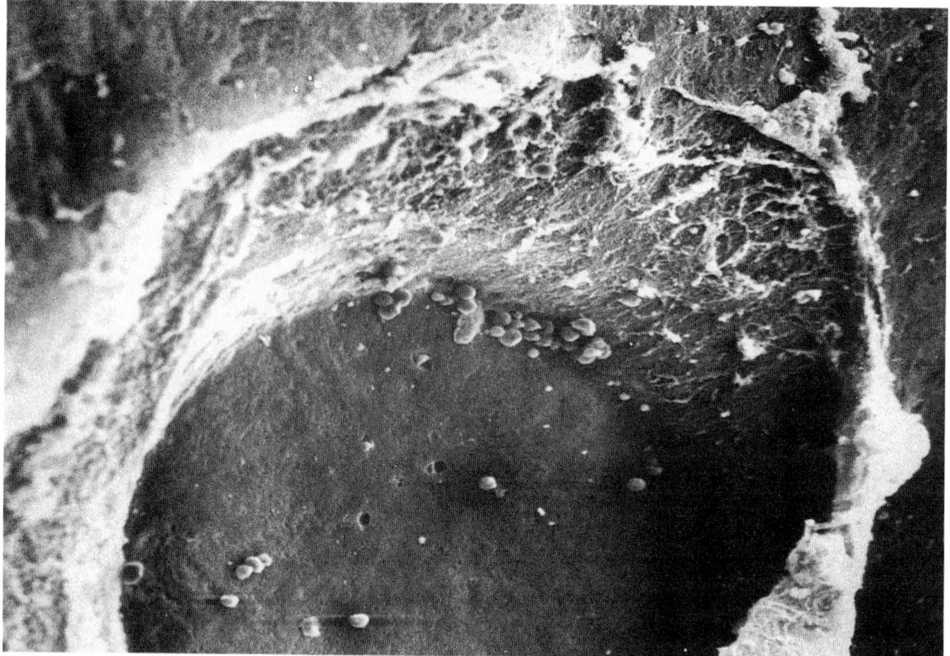

Fig. 4. Scanning electron micrograph of the crater produced in an atheromatous specimen using the pulsed-dye laser.

stenoses and short segment occlusions it is much more difficult to tackle long superficial femoral artery occlusions. In working towards a clinical programme for angioplasty with the pulsed-dye laser we felt that the system should aim to recanalize lesions which would otherwise require surgical treatment.

Bench testing with bare 600 μm and 400 μm fibres demonstrated that it was possible to achieve recanalization of totally occluded arterial segments. Unfortunately our pilot clinical studies with bare fibres were disappointing. It proved extremely difficult to devise a reliable means of keeping the end of the fibre in the correct alignment. When advancing through an occluded lesion the fibre tended to become embedded in the plaque and readily deviated through the vessel wall. The high peak power produced by the pulsed-dye laser precludes attaching an atraumatic tip to the fibre, such as the industrial sapphires which have been used with the Nd:YAG laser.[6,7]

The solution devised was to spin the fibre while heating the tip in an oxyacetylene flame. This produced a molten ball of silica. Ball tips up to 4 mm in diameter can be created on 600 μm diameter fibres, although a considerable amount of skill is required to achieve consistent results. In bench testing these ball-tipped fibres (Dunn Labs, St Bartholomew's Hospital) transmitted pulsed laser energy without being damaged and were capable of recanalizing occluded cadaveric femoral arteries through which a guidewire would not pass.

Following these experiments a clinical programme of laser angioplasty was developed in patients facing amputation, who were not suitable for bypass surgery or PTA. Initial success allowed us to broaden our treatment group to include patients with arterial occlusions which would require bypass, but were not suitable for PTA.[8]

The ball-tipped fibre was used alone initially. This necessitated recrossing the occlusion with a guidewire to augment the lasered channel by balloon angioplasty—a situation which can give rise to arterial dissection. To avoid this problem we have backloaded the sterile ball-ended fibre into a balloon angioplasty catheter—creating a combined laser and dilatation device (Fig. 5). The low profile of the uninflated balloon allows it to follow the ball tip easily as the occlusion is recanalized. The lasered channel can then be dilated as the device is withdrawn.

To date, we have treated 74 limbs in 68 patients with a mean age of 70 years. In 55% of limbs there was evidence of critical limb ischaemia,[9] the limbs in the remaining patients having severe claudication.

Preoperative assessment involved arteriography or intra-arterial DSA, with doppler pressure measurements and duplex scanning to characterize plaque morphology. There was a defined protocol for postoperative follow-up. Patients were rescanned and exercised prior to discharge home. They were then seen at 2 weeks, 1, 2, 3, 6, 9 and 12 months and then at half-yearly intervals. At each visit Doppler pressure testing was carried out at rest and after exercise. Duplex scans were carried out at 1, 3, 6 and 12 months and annually thereafter. Arteriography was not used routinely. During duplex scanning evidence of restenosis was sought. This was achieved by examination of waveform, peak velocity measurement and imaging of luminal narrowing. Restenosis was defined as a fall of the ankle brachial indices (ABI) to within 0.15 of the preoperative value, return of original symptoms, or further symptoms requiring retreatment.

Technical success is defined as successful crossing of the lesion and balloon dilatation when required. This was achieved in 56 limbs (76%). Clinical success is defined as abolition of rest pain, healing of gangrene or ulcer, improvement in claudication and a rise in the ABI of 0.15. Where obvious clinical benefit is obtained without significant change in the ABI (e.g. abolition of rest pain) this is allowed to override the ABI requirement. Clinical success was achieved in 46 of the 74 limbs (62%). The ABI rose from a mean preoperative value of 0.51 to 0.83 postoperatively $p<0.0001$ (Student's paired *t*-test).

We have identified a subgroup of patients with marked discrete arterial calcification in whom there was a significantly reduced rate of technical success. These were cases where the calcified lesions occupied a significant proportion of the vessel diameter rather than the scattered 'speckled' calcification which was a common finding in many patients in the series.

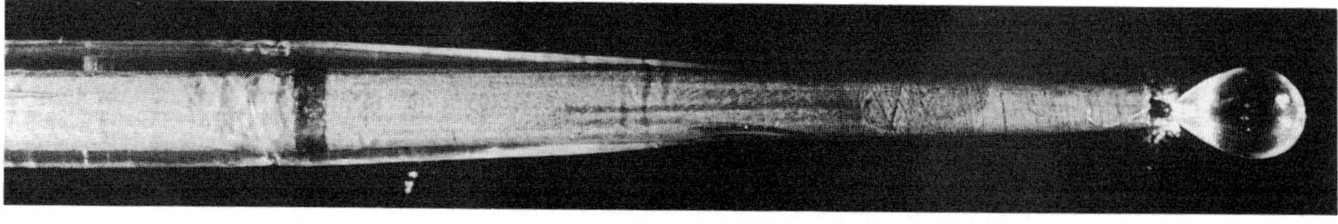

Fig. 5. The combined laser and balloon dilatation device, showing the ball end fibre backloaded into a standard angioplasty catheter.

Overall the cumulative patency for technically successful cases was 66.7% at 6 months and 49.2% at 12 months. Six-month cumulative patencies were 80% in calcified and 64% in noncalcified cases (p=NS log-rank test) (Fig. 6). Patency was adversely affected by lack of run-off vessels, being 62% at 6 months and 40.5% at 12 months in those with less than two patent tibial vessels. Similar figures for those with two or more patent tibial vessels were 70.4% and 55.4%, but these differences failed to reach statistical significance (Fig. 7).

During follow-up of between 1 and 22 months, a total of 22 limbs have re-occluded. A total of 21 further procedures have been carried out in 12 limbs. Only six limbs have come to major amputation; for unsalvagable ischaemia in five and as a life-saving procedure to eliminate a septicaemic focus in one. In three cases, bypass grafting was not feasible following failed laser assisted angioplasty.

A total of six patients are known to have died. There were two deaths within 30 days of surgery. One death followed myocardial infarction 10 days after successful

Table 1. Results of laser assisted angioplasty

	Occlusion length (cm ± SD)	*Technical success n (%)*	*Clinical success n (%)*
Non calcified $n=52$	21.4 ± 13.5	45 (87)*	36 (69)**
Calcified $n=22$	20.1 ± 14.1	11 (50)*	9 (41)**
Total $n=74$	21.0 ± 13.5	56 (76)	46 (62)

*$p<0.001$, **$p<0.05$, χ^2 test.

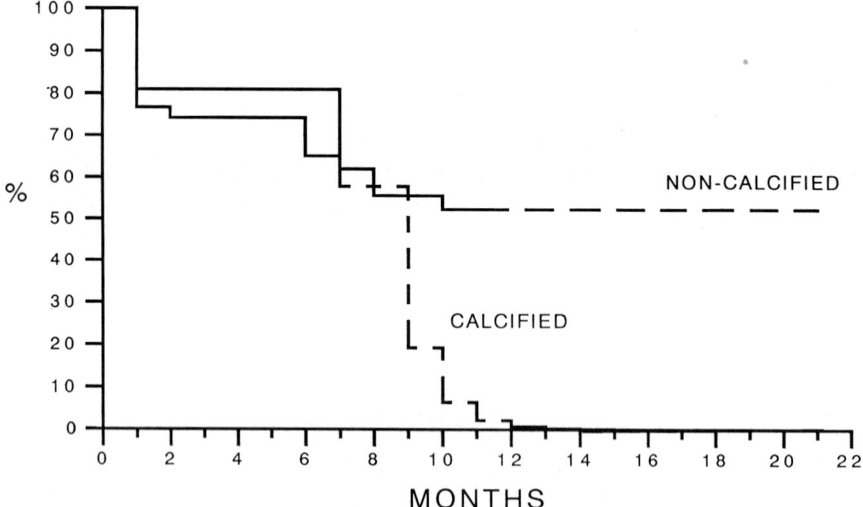

Fig. 6. Laser assisted angioplasty. Patency by lesion morphology. Arterial patency on follow-up in calcified and non-calcified cases; p=NS (log-rank test).

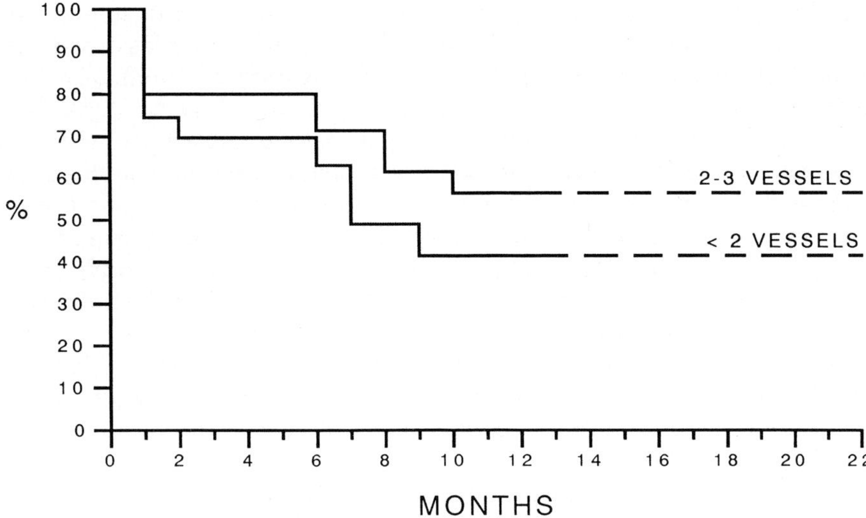

Fig. 7. Laser assisted angioplasty. Patency by run-off. The effect of run-off on cumulative long-term patency following laser angioplasty; $p = \mathrm{NS}$ (log-rank test).

aortobifemoral grafting and laser angioplasty in a 71-year-old man. The other early death was in a male respiratory cripple of 74 who died of respiratory failure despite a successful procedure carried out percutaneously under local anaesthesia. The remaining deaths were all due to myocardial infarction and illustrate the severity of disease seen in many of the patients in our practice.

SUMMARY

This series demonstrates that recanalization of long arterial occlusions is feasible in patients with advanced vascular disease. Occlusion length is not a determinant of immediate outcome, though occlusion morphology has a significant effect on the initial technical success of the procedure.

The restenosis figures are broadly similar to those seen when PTA is applied to shorter occlusions of the lower limb arteries, but the two groups are not comparable. The rates are not as good as the patency data for grafting with vein or PTFE above the knee, but approach those of below knee synthetic grafts, especially if antiplatelet agents are not given. It is in the patient with distal disease requiring below knee prosthetic grafting that laser assisted angioplasty may have most to offer. However, until a randomized prospective trial of laser angioplasty against grafting is undertaken it will not be possible to reach a firm conclusion about the relative merits of each approach.

CONCLUSIONS

Laser angioplasty is in its infancy at present, but holds the promise of a less invasive approach to severe peripheral vascular disease. Restenosis is a problem common to all intraluminal interventions in arteries below the inguinal ligament. Greater understanding of the events which lead to intimal hyperplasia will permit modification of this response and enhance the results of minimally invasive techniques.

The ability of the pulsed dye laser to cross lesions of great length, which would not be suitable for PTA, allows the clinician to extend the application of this approach to patients with severe disease. Although success rates are lower than those seen after grafting, the use of the laser does not prejudice the results of surgery where it is subsequently required. The pulsed dye laser has a role to play in the treatment of peripheral vascular disease in the young patient in whom it is desirable to avoid grafting, and in the frail elderly patient with critical limb ischaemia for whom life expectancy is short. For this latter group, the relative lack of durability of intraluminal recanalization procedures may not be an important factor, whereas the avoidance of major surgery and a prolonged hospital stay will have a profound effect on the quality of life that remains.

Reviewing laser angioplasty with the pulsed dye laser against the exacting specification given at the beginning of this chapter it will be seen that the procedure still has some way to go to become an established part of the treatment of peripheral vascular disease. On the positive side, the device undoubtedly ablates atheroma, is capable of recanalizing long occlusions and can be inserted percutaneously. Distal embolization has not proved a problem and there is at least the potential of treating calcified disease. The surface created after lasing is smooth but whether it is of low thrombogenicity is a subject of on-going study. The pulsed dye laser is extremely effective in vapourizing thrombus. In many long occlusions there may be several centimetres of thrombus lying above a short segment of occlusive atheroma. In this situation laser treatment will frequently produce a lumen proximal to the atheroma which does not require dilatation. However, bench experiments indicate that with the energy levels currently delivered, the volume of atheroma ablated is relatively small. Further research on delivery devices and laser output will be required to produce a channel which does not require adjunctive balloon dilatation. With ball-tipped fibres the perforation rate has been low although dissection remains a significant problem. Improvements require an effective imaging and guidance system to keep the device in the line of the true lumen of the vessel. Ultrasound would appear to hold out the best prospect for noninvasive guidance. In-line ultrasound probes are already available but at this stage they can only image the vessel around the tip and not forward from it.

In the medium term trials of laser assisted angioplasty combined with agents capable of modifying the cellular proliferation leading to restenosis will determine the place of this promising technique in the therapeutic armamentarium.

REFERENCES

1. Prince MR, Deutsch TF, Mathews-Roth MM *et al*: Preferential light absorption in atheromas *in vitro*: implications for laser angioplasty. J Clin Invest 78:295–302, 1986
2. Murray A, Crocker PR, Wood RFM: The pulsed dye laser and atherosclerotic vascular disease. Br J Surg 75:349–351, 1988

REFERENCES

3. Prince MR, LaMuraglia GM, Teng P, Deutsch TF, Anderson RR: Preferential ablation of calcified arterial plaque with laser-induced plasmas. IEEE J Quantum Electron QE-23(10):1783–1786, 1987
4. Prince MR, Anderson RR, Deutsch TF, LaMuraglia GM: Pulsed laser ablation of calcified plaque. Society of Photo-optical Instrumentation Engineers 906:305–309, 1988
5. Murray A, Basu R, Wells C, Wood RFM: Defining parameters for peripheral laser angioplasty. Eur J Vasc Surg 3:31–36, 1989
6. Ashley S, Brooks SG, Gehani AA, Kester RC, Rees MR: Thermal and optical behaviour of sapphire fibretips for laser angioplasty. Society of Photo-optical Instrumentation Engineers 1201:137–144, 1990
7. Kvasnicka J, Stanek F, Boudik F *et al*: Percutaneous peripheral laser angioplasty with a pulsed Nd:Yag laser and sapphire tips. Society of Photo-optical Instrumentation Engineers 1201:211–218, 1990
8. Murray A, Wood RFM, Mitchell DC *et al*: Peripheral laser angioplasty with the pulsed dye laser and ball-tipped optical fibres. Lancet ii:1471–1474, 1989
9. Dormandy J (Ed.): European Consensus on Critical Limb Ischaemia. Berlin: Springer-Verlag, 1989

Cw-Nd: YAG vs Excimer Laser for Peripheral Angioplasty: Comparison with Conventional Balloon Angioplasty

Johannes Lammer, Ernst Pilger, Günther E. Klein, Fritz Flückiger and Klaus Hausegger

The first experimental work and clinical feasibility studies of laser-assisted angioplasty were done with continuous wave (cw) lasers, such as Argon or Nd:YAG lasers.[1–9] Scepticism was caused by the thermal side-effects due to heat accumulation in subsurface tissue layers, which caused a large zone of thermal necrosis.[10–12] This led to a search for laser systems, which caused less, or ideally no, thermal damage. Grundfest *et al.*, have shown that excimer lasers can ablate plaque tissue by nanosecond pulses.[13,14] These short pulses did not cause heat accumulation or thermal damage. Daikuzono and Joffe[15] have developed sapphire contact probes which in combination with cw-lasers permit ablation of large tissue volumes.[16–18] Direct laser–tissue interaction through the sapphire lens markedly reduced heat accumulation as observed with the hot tip system.[12] Despite these major developments for laser-assisted balloon angioplasty the question whether laser angioplasty enables better results than conventional balloon angioplasty remains unanswered.

METHODS AND MATERIALS

Our cw-Nd:YAG laser (Surgical Laser Technologies, USA) operating at 1064 nm has been in use since 1986. The laser beam was conducted through a 600 micron (μm) glass fibre. A 2.2 or 3.0 mm sapphire lens, with a 60–80% transmission rate for laser light, was attached to the tip of the fibre. The highest energy density was in the centre of the sapphire probe; this avoided peripheral thermal damage. The Nd:YAG laser was applied in 1-s pulses with a power of 10–15 Watts.

Our pulsed XeCl excimer laser (Technolas, Germany) operating at 308 nm has been in use since 1989. The laser beam was conducted through a multifibre catheter 2.2 mm in diameter containing up to 30 fibres 100 μm in diameter. The maximum energy output of the laser was 300 mJ/pulse. The maximum energy at the tip of the catheter was 30–40 mJ/pulse. The pulse width was 115 ns, the repetition rate 20 Hz.

For conventional recanalization and balloon angioplasty various steerable guidewires (Terumo, Magnum-Schneider, Lunderquist) were used. After successful recanalization by means of a guidewire, balloon dilatation of the stenosis was performed (Fig. 1). All recanalization procedures were done percutaneously under local anaesthesia. Initially a 7 French catheter introducer sheath was inserted in antegrade fashion. Both laser catheter systems were used in contact with the occluding plaque tissue.

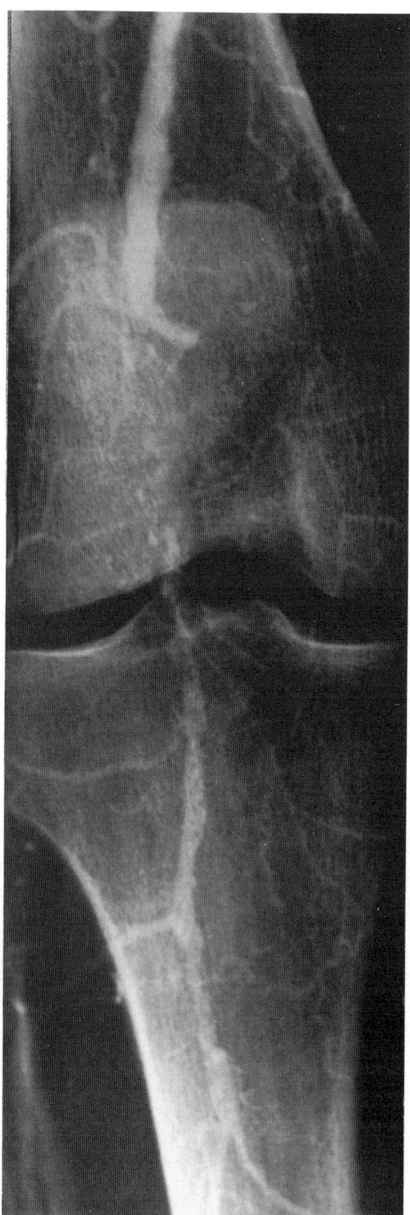

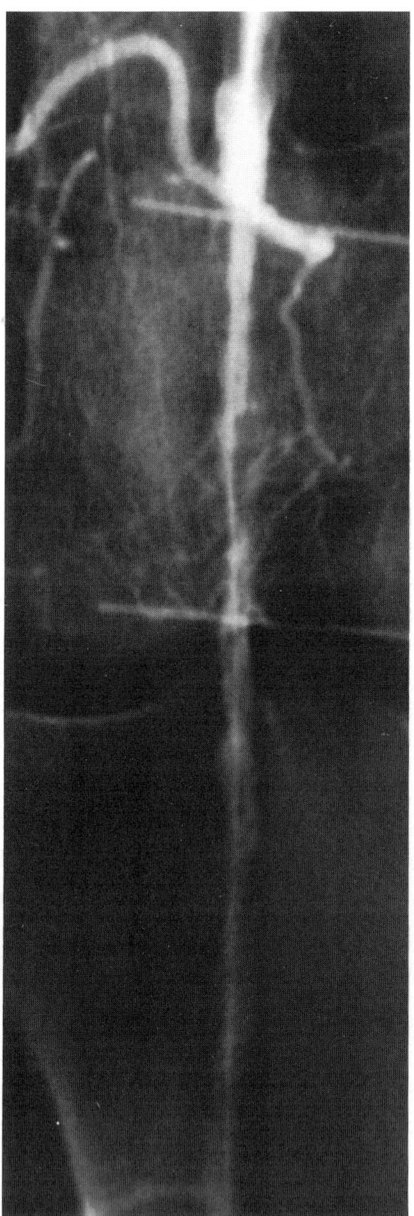

Fig. 1. Conventional recanalization of a calcified popliteal artery occlusion causing limiting claudication (walking distance 100 m). a (left): Angiogram demonstrating the popliteal artery occlusion. b (right): Angiogram after guidewire recanalization.

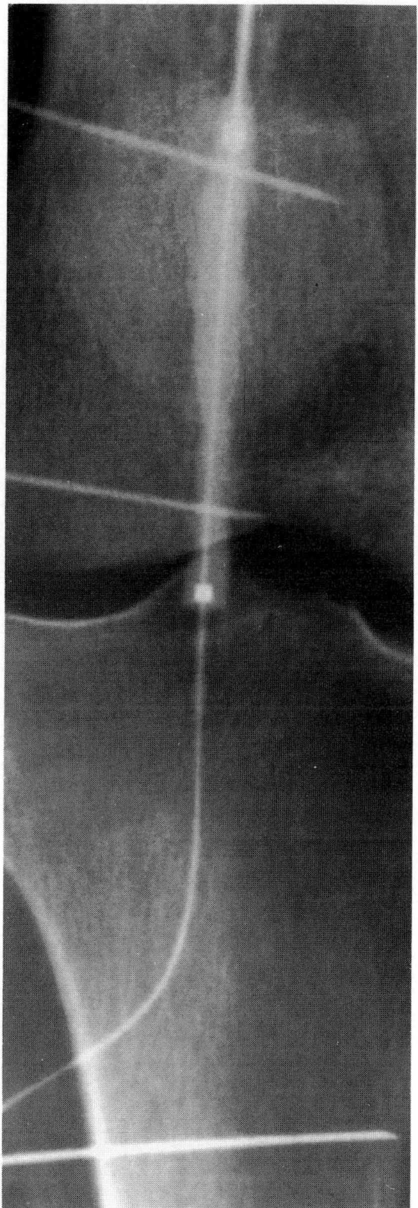

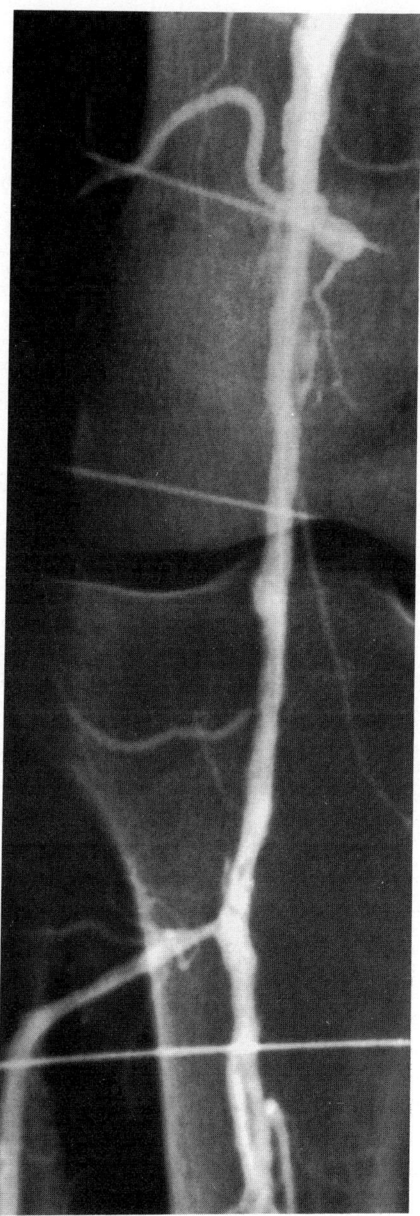

Fig. 1. c (left): Balloon angioplasty of the recanalized artery. d (right): Angiogram after PTA.

After successful recanalization, balloon dilatation was performed with a 5–7 mm angioplasty balloon (Figs 2, 3).

Patients were anticoagulated during the procedure by means of 5000 U heparin intra-arterially and by means of intravenous heparin (1000 U/h) after a successful procedure. After discharge from the hospital the patients were continued on platelet inhibition therapy (acetylsalicylic acid 330 mg/day, dipyridamole 75 mg/day) or

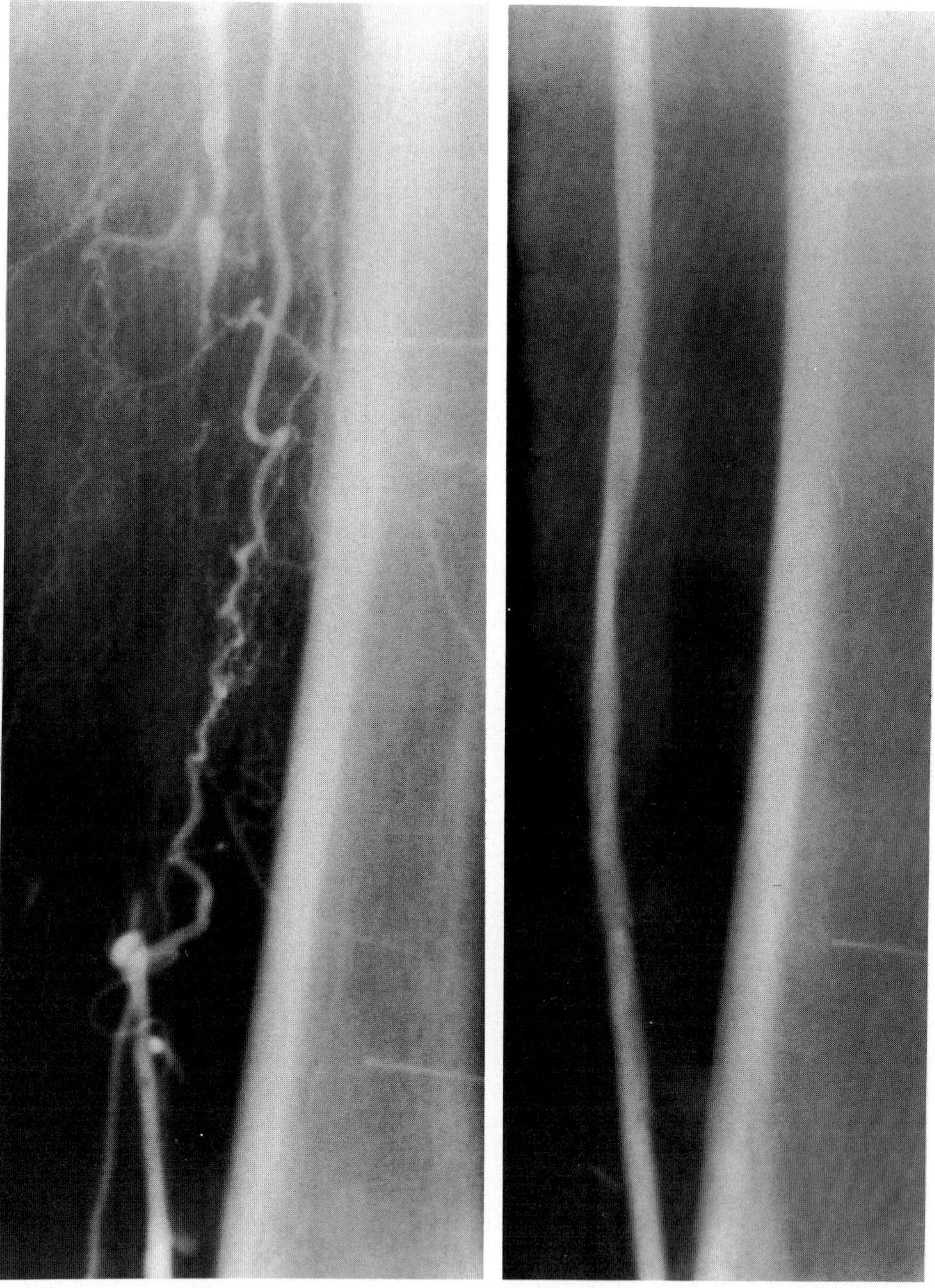

Fig. 2. Excimer laser-assisted balloon angioplasty of a superficial femoral artery occlusion causing severe claudication (walking distance less than 50 m). a (left): Angiogram demonstrating the superficial femoral artery occlusion. b (right): Angiogram after laser-assisted balloon angioplasty.

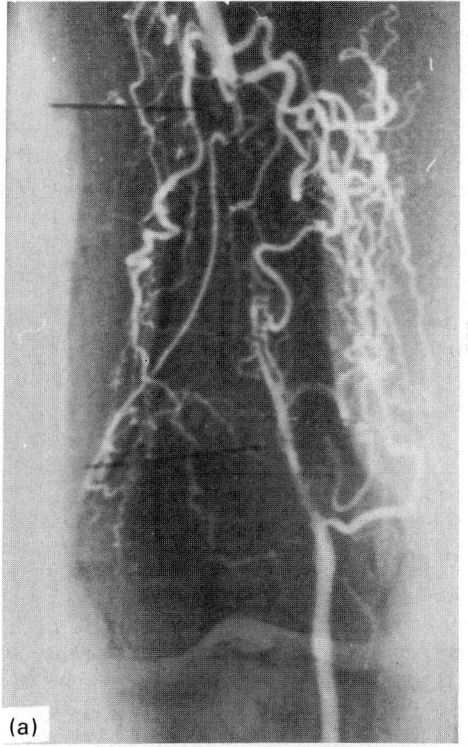

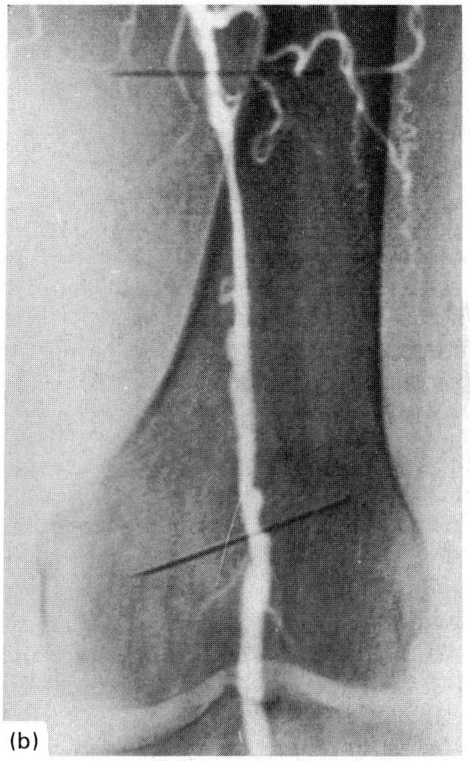

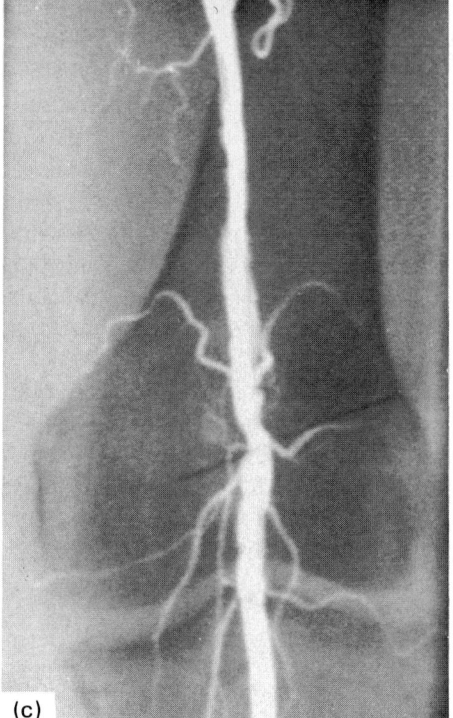

Fig. 3. Cw-Nd:YAG laser-assisted balloon angioplasty of a popliteal artery occlusion causing claudication (walking distance 200 m). a (top left): DSA before treatment. b (top right): DSA after laser recanalization alone. c (lower left): DSA after additional balloon angioplasty.

anticoagulated. Control studies were performed by Doppler ultrasound and digital subtraction angiography (DSA).

In order to compare the results of excimer laser-assisted angioplasty, Nd:YAG laser-assisted angioplasty and conventional angioplasty, a prospective randomized trial was initiated. The patients were stratified into three treatment groups (excimer-laser, Nd:YAG laser, conventional percutaneous transluminal angioplasty (PTA)), two groups of occlusion length (1–7 cm, 8–20 cm) and two groups of peripheral outflow (2–3 patent tibial arteries, 0–1 patent tibial artery). The criteria for inclusion were femoropopliteal artery occlusions causing limiting claudication (Fontaine Stage IIb), rest pain (Fontaine Stage III), or gangrene (Fontaine Stage IV). Excluded were patients with additional iliac artery obstructions, fresh thrombotic or embolic occlusions and diabetic patients.

RESULTS

Over 21 months 130 patients were included in this study; 37 were treated with the excimer laser, 49 patients with the cw-Nd:YAG laser and 44 patients by a conventional guidewire-balloon technique. The initial recanalization was successful in 26 of 37 patients with the excimer laser (70%); 39 of 49 patients with the Nd:YAG laser (80%); and 33 of 44 patients with conventional PTA (75%). In the group of short occlusions (1–7 cm in length) the initial recanalization rate was 79% for the excimer laser, 83% for the Nd:YAG laser and 85% for the guidewire. In the group of the long occlusions (8–20 cm in length) the highest recanalization rate was achieved by the Nd:YAG laser (76%), followed by the excimer laser (67%), and the conventional guidewire-balloon technique (61%). In 29 patients severe calcifications at the obstruction site were present. These calcifications reduced the initial recanalization rate in all three groups of treatment. The highest recanalization rate was achieved by a conventional PTA (60%), followed by the excimer laser (57%) and the cw-Nd:YAG laser (50%).

Complications were observed in 37 of 130 patients. Peripheral emboli to the tibial arteries were observed in four patients in each of the laser groups and in five patients after conventional PTA. A spasm of the popliteal artery was observed twice after excimer laser angioplasty and once after Nd:YAG and conventional angioplasty, respectively. Dissections or perforations of the arterial wall were observed in six patients after excimer laser angioplasty, in seven patients after Nd:YAG laser angioplasty and in seven patients after conventional PTA.

The long-term patency rate were calculated by life-table analysis. The patency rates in patients treated by excimer laser-assisted angioplasty were 70% after 2 weeks, 35% and 35% after 6 and 12 months, respectively. The patency rates after cw-Nd:YAG laser-assisted angioplasty was 80% after 2 weeks, 62% and 52% after 6 and 12 months, respectively. After conventional balloon angioplasty the 2-week patency rate was 75%, after 6 and 12 months it was 63% and 53%, respectively.

DISCUSSION

It has been shown by experimental work that the nature of laser–tissue interaction depends on whether continuous or pulsed lasers are used.[20] Tissue ablation by continuous wave lasers is caused by photothermal vapourization. Tissue ablation by pulsed lasers in the nanosecond range is caused not only by the photothermal effect but also by the photo-acoustic effect due to plasma formation. The photothermal effect alone can ablate fibrofatty plaque tissue, but cannot ablate the calcium within the plaques. In contrast the photo-acoustic effect can shatter calcified plaques into small particles, but has less effect on elastic soft tissue. Interestingly, in clinical practice excimer laser angioplasty did not show a higher recanalization rate in calcified obstructions than the cw-Nd:YAG laser.[17–19] This is probably due to the fact that the energy, which can be transmitted through 100 μm glass fibres, is too low for a sufficient ablation of calcified plaques.

Experimental studies have shown that thermal side-effects to the arterial wall caused by continuous wave lasers can cause arterial spasm. In our study, continuous wave lasers did not show a higher spasm rate than the other two recanalization methods. This was probably due to the fact that the sapphire contact probe in combination with the cw-Nd:YAG laser focuses the light to the centre of the artery. Thus the thermal damage to the outer vessel layers is minimized.

The overall results after recanalization of femoropopliteal artery occlusions revealed no difference between laser-assisted balloon angioplasty and a conventional guidewire-balloon technique.[17–19,21–24] In the group of the long occlusions (8–20 cm in length) Nd:YAG laser angioplasty revealed the highest recanalization rate. This could be explained by the fact that the continuous wave Nd:YAG laser in combination with the sapphire contact probe helps sufficiently to ablate plaques in those arterial segments which are completely obstructed. Therefore continuous wave laser-assisted balloon angioplasty seems to be beneficial in long femoropopliteal artery occlusions. The long-term patency rates were not improved by laser-assisted plaque ablation. The excimer laser which probably causes only minimal ablation due to the low energy has shown the poorest long-term results.

In conclusion, laser-assisted balloon angioplasty is helpful for recanalization of long femoropopliteal artery occlusions. The cw-Nd:YAG laser in combination with a sapphire contact probe has shown to be most effective. Nevertheless, none of the laser systems is ideal, because no system creates a channel large enough for sufficient antegrade flow. Subsequent balloon angioplasty thus is required after thermal or nonthermal laser recanalization. Therefore the long-term results are currently not improved by laser-assisted balloon angioplasty.

REFERENCES

1. Lee G, Ikeda RM, Kozina J, Mason DT: Laser dissolution of coronary atherosclerotic obstruction. Am Heart J 102:1074–1075, 1981
2 Choy DSJ, Sterzer SH, Rotterdam HZ, Sharrock N, Kaminow IP: Transluminal laser catheter angioplasty. Am J Cardiol 50:1206–1208, 1982
3 Abela GS, Norman S, Cohen D *et al.*: Effects of carbon dioxide, Nd:YAG, and Argon laser radiation on coronary atheromatous plaques. Am J Cardiol 50:1199–1205, 1982
4 Lee G, Ikeda RM, Herman I *et al.*: The qualitative effects of laser irradiation on human arteriosclerotic disease. Am Heart J 105:885–889, 1983
5 Lee G, Ikeda RM, Stobbe D *et al.*: Effects of laser irradiation on human thrombus: Demonstration of a linear dissolution-dose relation between clot length and energy density. Am J Cardiol 52:876–887, 1983

6. Geschwind H, Boussignac G, Teisseire B *et al*: Percutaneous transluminal laser angioplasty in man (letter). Lancet i:844, 1984
7. Ginsburg R, Kim DS, Guthaner D, Toth J, Mitchell RS: Salvage of an ischemic limb by laser angioplasty: Description of a new technique. Clin Cardiol 7: 54–58, 1984
8. Choy DSJ, Sterzer SH, Myler RK, Marco J, Fournial G: Human coronary laser recanalization. Clin Cardiol 7:377–381, 1984
9. Lammer J, Ascher PW, Choy DSJ: Transfemorale Katheter-Laser-Thrombendarterektomie (TEA) der Arteria carotis. Dtsch Med Wschr 11:607–610, 1986
10. Lee G, Ikeda RM, Chan ML: Dissolution of human atheriosclerotic disease by fiberoptic laser heated metal cautery cap. Am Heart J 107:777–778, 1984
11. Sanborn TA, Haudenschild CC, Faxon DP, Ryan TJ: Experimental angioplasty: Circumferential distribution of laser thermal energy with a laser probe. J Am Coll Cardiol 5:934–938, 1985
12. Lammer J, Kleinert R, Pilger E, Schmidt-Kloiber H, Reichel E: Contact probes for intravascular recanalization. Experimental evaluation. Invest Radiol 24:190–195, 1989
13. Grundfest W, Litvak F, Forrester J: Pulsed ultraviolet lasers provide precise control of atheroma ablation (abstr.). Circulation 70 (Suppl II):35, 1984
14. Grundfest W, Litvak F, Forrester J: Laser injury of human atherosclerotic plaque without adjacent tissue injury. J Am Coll Cardiol 5:929–933, 1985
15. Daikuzono N, Joffe SN: An artificial sapphire probe for contact photocoagulation and tissue vaporization. Med Instrument 19:173–178, 1985
16. Lammer J, Pilger E, Kleinert R, Ascher PW: Laserangioplastie peripherer arterieller Verschlüsse. Experimentelle und klinische Ergebnisse. Fortschr Röntgenstr 147:1–5, 1987
17. Lammer J, Karnel F: Percutaneous transluminal laser angioplasty with contact probes. Radiology 168:733–737, 1988
18. Lammer J, Pilger E, Karnel F *et al*: Austrian multicenter trial for laser angioplasty: 3-year results of a prospective clinical study. Radiology 1991 (in press)
19. Litvak F, Grundfest WS, Adler L, Hickey AE, Segalowitz J *et al*: Percutaneous excimer laser and excimer laser assisted angioplasty of the lower extremities: results of initial clinical trial. Radiology 172:331–335, 1989
20. Cragg AH, Gardiner GA, Smith TP: Vascular applications of laser. Radiology 172:925–935, 1989
21. Johnston KW, Lae M, Hogg-Johnston SA *et al*: Five-year results of a prospective study of percutaneous transluminal angioplasty. Ann Surg 206:403–413, 1987
22. Murray RR, Hewes RC, White RI *et al*: Long-segment femoropopliteal stenoses: is angioplasty a boom or a bust? Radiology 162:473–476, 1987
23. Zeitler E: Percutaneous dilatation and recanalization of iliac and femoral arteries. Cardiovasc Intervent Radiol 3:207–212, 1980
24. Krepel VM, van Andel GJ, von Erp WFM, Breslau PJ: Percutaneous transluminal angioplasty of the femoropopliteal artery: initial and long-term results. Radiology 156:325–328, 1985

ATHERECTOMY DEVICES

Peripheral Arterial Atherectomy with the TEC and Simpson Atherocath Devices

R. L. McCann, G. E. Newman and M. H. Sketch Jr

Percutaneous treatment of atherosclerotic obstructive disease was introduced by Dotter and Judkins in 1964.[1] The technique of co-axial percutaneous transluminal dilatation was limited in that lumen size could not be increased beyond the size of the puncture one was willing to make at the entry site. In 1974, Grüntzig[2] introduced the dual lumen catheter incorporating an inflatable balloon on the tip for the treatment of peripheral vascular obstructive disease. This allowed creation of virtually any size lumen while maintaining a puncture site size compatible with haemostasis and an acceptable rate of entry site complications. The mechanism by which this dilatation occurs is now recognized in most cases to be mechanical fracture of the atherosclerotic plaque and stretching of the underlying media. The atherosclerotic material is not changed in any significant way and remains in the vessel wall. While percutaneous dilatation has achieved a significant and permanent role in the treatment of peripheral vascular obstructive disease, there remains considerable room for improvement. Failure to maintain an adequate dilatation occurs in between 30 and 50% of cases, depending upon the site of the lesion, lesion length, length of follow-up observation, and sensitivity of the method used to determine recurrence.[3] An intrinsically attractive hypothesis is that if significant volumes of the atherosclerotic material itself are physically removed from the vessel wall that tendency to recurrence of obstruction might be diminished. Several approaches are currently undergoing exploration and have yielded promising initial results. We have focused on techniques by which miniature cutting devices have been mounted upon angiographic catheters with the intention of performing an 'intraluminal endarterectomy' as a means of removing atherosclerotic plaque from obstructing lesions in the peripheral circulation. In this area technological advances continue to be achieved at a rapid rate but their application to man must be scrutinized carefully and the results compared both with traditional transluminal angioplasty and conventional surgical reconstructions before the role of these new technologies can be determined in the armamentarium of the treatment of peripheral vascular disease.

Patient selection

Proper patient selection is a critical feature of the application of this new technology to the patient with peripheral vascular obstructive disease. This became abundantly evident early in the development of these new catheters. It is vitally important to be fully cognizant of the natural history of peripheral vascular obstructive disease and, in particular, to be able to distinguish a threatened from a nonthreatened limb so that patients with a benign condition are not subjected to excessive risk and that the full spectrum of surgical and percutaneous treatment is available so that the most appropriate treatment can be offered to each patient based upon the severity of his symptoms and anatomy of his disease. In this regard, we advocate that patients be evaluated in an environment which includes not only those involved in developing these new interventional technologies but also those experienced in the management and natural history of patients with peripheral vascular disease. Using this team approach obviates the 'turf' battles which have emerged in some centres much to the detriment of patient care and vascular science.[4]

THE SIMPSON ATHEROCATH

The Simpson atherocath (Devices for Vascular Intervention, Redwood City, Calif.) was the first atherectomy catheter released for general use in the USA. The system (Fig. 1) consists of a multilumen catheter which is usually passed through a conventional indwelling arterial sheath. The 7, 9 and 11 French systems are available. At the end of the catheter is a fixed floppy spring tip. This is similar to a guidewire but is fixed in position. Proximal to the tip is a cylindrical metallic housing. This housing has a longitudinal opening on one side referred to as the window. On the cylinder opposite the window is mounted a balloon which is similar to an angioplasty balloon but it is intended that inflation pressures will not exceed 35 psi. This balloon is used to firmly press the window on the reciprocal surface into the vessel wall so that the plaque protrudes through the window into the housing cavity. A

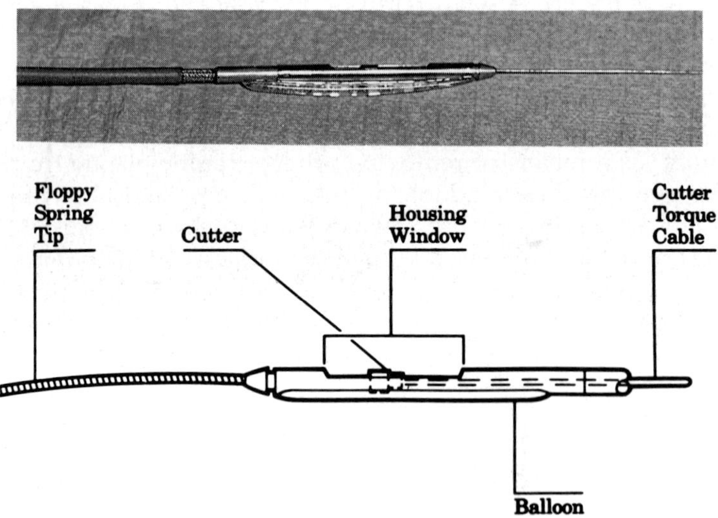

Fig. 1. A (Upper): Photograph of the Simpson atherocath tip. B (Lower): Diagrammatic representation of the photograph. This illustrates the housing window located on the reciprocal surface of the low pressure balloon. It also shows the floppy spring tip and the rotational cutting blade attached to the torque cable.

cylindrical blade is mounted on the end of a torque wire. A battery-powered motor at the hub of the catheter is activated, rotating the torque wire and attached cutter at 2000 rpm. The cutter is advanced through the housing while being rotated and the trapped protruding plaque in the housing window is shaved off (Fig. 2). The fragment is compressed into the receptacle tip where it is later retrieved after the catheter has been removed from the patient. The specimen can be submitted for histological examination and considerable information regarding plaque morphology has been obtained in this manner.[5]

PROCEDURE

The procedure is performed utilizing sedation and local anaesthesia. It must be performed where adequate fluoroscopic facilities are available and this usually is an angiographic or catheterization suite. After diagnostic angiography, an arterial sheath is inserted either antegrade or retrograde, depending upon the target vessel. The appropriately sized catheter is advanced under fluoroscopic control until the housing is located at the site of the lesion. The balloon is inflated to less than 2 atmospheres, pushing the housing window up against the vessel wall. The motor is actuated and the cutter is advanced, shaving the atheroma and collecting the specimen in the tip. The catheter may then be rotated 90 degrees and the procedure repeated a number of times before removing the catheter to empty the tip receptacle.

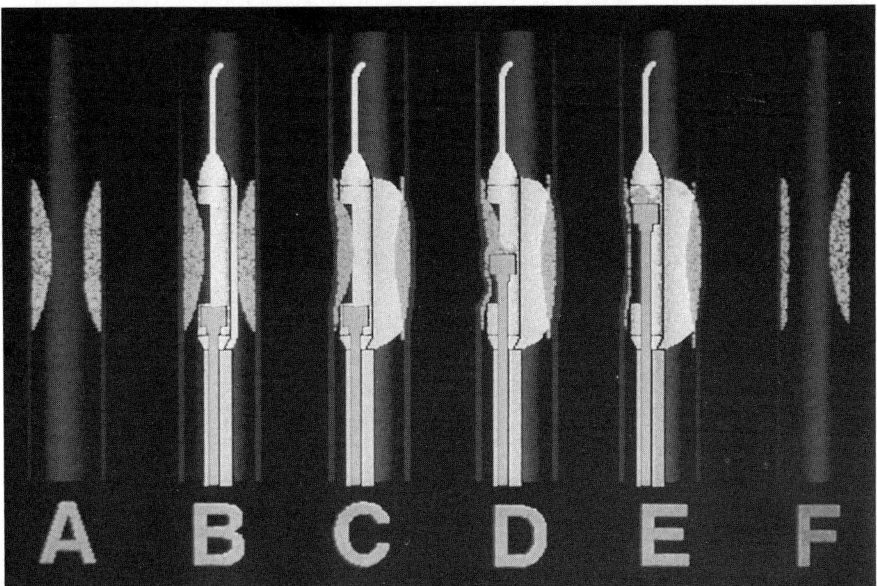

Fig. 2. Diagrammatic illustration of the Simpson atherocath mechanism of lumen enlargement. A stenosis is represented at A. B shows the catheter in position with the window adjacent to the protruding plaque. In C, the balloon is inflated and the plaque firmly pushed into the window. In D, the cutter is being advanced and at E, the specimen is shaved and compressed into the receptical tip.

As shown in Fig. 3, a relatively large volume of tissue can be removed. Figure 4 shows the typical histologic appearance of the atheromatous material retrieved. This appearance is quite similar to an endarterectomy specimen as it includes areas of smooth muscle cell proliferation, plaque neovascularization, and lipid accumulation.[5]

UTILITY

The Simpson atherocath has been used for both peripheral and coronary lesions. The system is best suited to treatment of eccentric stenoses. While total occlusions, especially when short, have been treated successfully, they require creation of a channel sufficient for passing the catheter. This has been achieved by passage of a coaxial dilating catheter or the use of small coronary-type balloon angioplasty catheters. Once an adequate channel has been achieved, the atherocath is then passed and the vessel is atherectomized. Similarly, the most favourable lesions are those that are relatively short. A typical example is shown in Fig. 5. An eccentric stenosis is present in the external iliac artery (single arrow) and after treatment (double arrow), a significant increase in luminal area is achieved.

The housing at the tip of the catheter is rigid and thus the axial vessels are more favourable rather than visceral vessels that require acute angulation of the catheter. We have found that the ideal lesion then is in a relatively large axial vessel such as the common iliac or femoral, and the lesion is eccentric and stenotic rather than occlusive. Most tibial vessels are too small for even the smallest catheter and the largest catheter seldom will be satisfactory to achieve an adequate lumen in the aorta.

Because multiple passes are required, the procedure often takes two to three times the amount of time of a conventional balloon angioplasty and the catheters are considerably more expensive. It is not yet clear whether the long-term results will justify this increased cost.

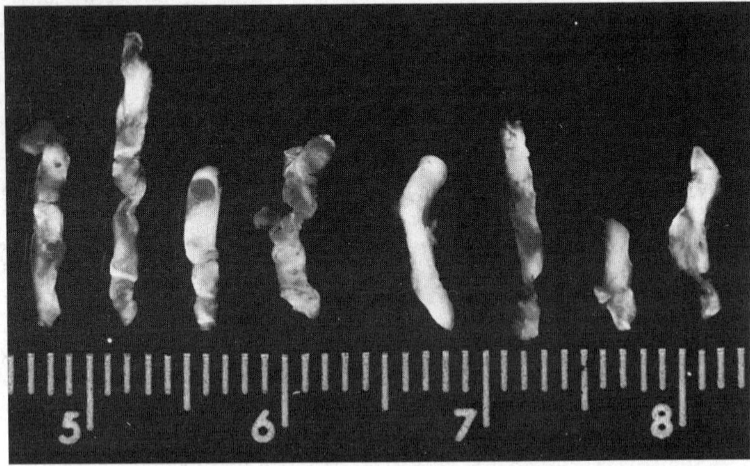

Fig. 3. A number of plaque shavings can be removed from each lesion. These typically measure 1 × 8–12 mm.

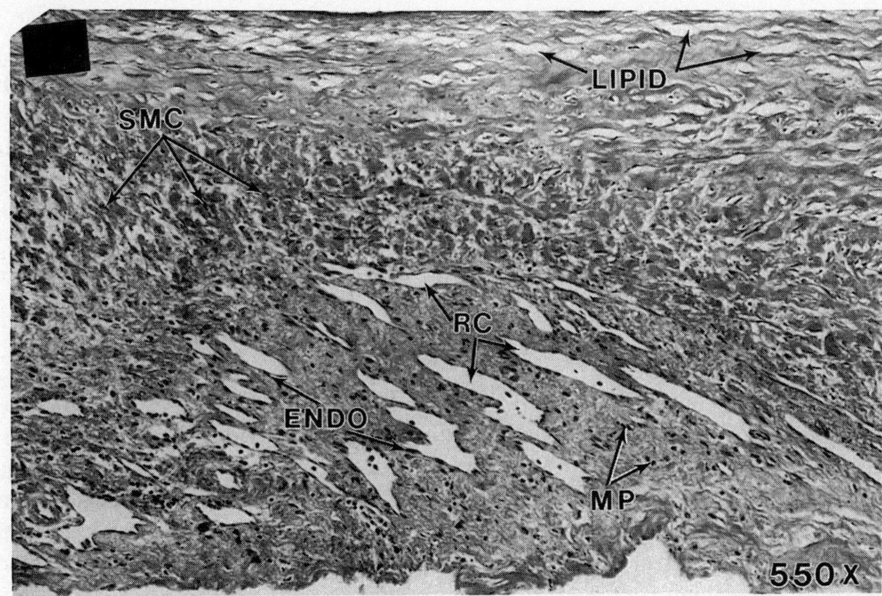

Fig. 4. Histologic examination highlights the presence of modified smooth muscle cells (SMC), macrophages (MP), and marked neovascularization (Neo). These small vessels are lined with endothelial cells (Endo). There is also moderate extracellular lipid (Lipid). From Barbano EF, Newman GE, McCann RL *et al*: Atherosclerosis 78:187, 1989 with permission.

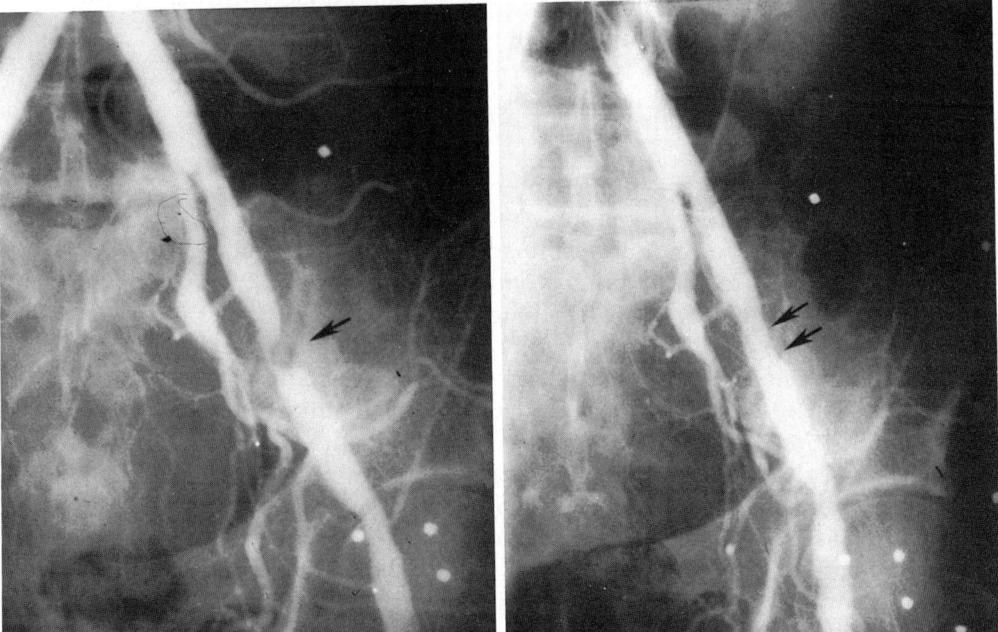

Fig. 5. A (Left): An eccentric severe stenosis of the mid-external iliac artery before treatment (single arrow). B (Right): After treatment (double arrow), the lumen is significantly enlarged.

SAFETY

Because the catheter cutting device is contained within the housing and cuts from the side rather than the tip, very few perforations occur.[6–8] Local dissection has occurred but is less frequent than with balloon angioplasty.[8] Because of the large size of the sheath, haematoma and groin complication at the puncture site have been relatively frequent.[7] Distal embolization and local spasm have also been reported but are unusual. Emergency bypass surgery has been required in less than 2% of patients.[9]

LONG-TERM FOLLOW-UP

Initial success has been achieved in 85–95% of lesions attempted.[6–8] Clinical and angiographic follow-up at up to 1 year have demonstrated recurrent stenoses and occlusions to occur. Longer lesions, initial incomplete atherectomy (i.e. 30% or greater residual stenosis), and occlusions have yielded significantly greater recurrence rates than simple lesions, particularly eccentric stenoses. For occlusions, recurrence rates of up to 50% have been reported.[10] Unfortunately, no randomized comparison has been performed between Simpson atherectomy and traditional balloon angioplasty. Because of the realization that residual stenosis yields significantly poor results, it is becoming increasingly popular to combine atherectomy and balloon dilatation when the former does not result in complete resolution of the lesion. This combination has further confused the issue of comparison with simple balloon angioplasty.

THE TRANSLUMINAL EXTRACTION CATHETER (TEC)

The transluminal extraction catheter (Interventional Technologies, Inc., San Diego, Calif.) was designed to overcome some of the disadvantages of other atherectomy devices. In contrast to the Simpson atherocath, this catheter travels over a conventional guidewire and thus is potentially directly applicable to any lesion that can be crossed by a guidewire. The catheter design incorporates a guidewire based motor-driven, rotating flexible torque tube ending in a conical head containing two rotating, short, stainless steel cutting blades. The blades first shred and then extract atherosclerotic plaque material. The catheter is depicted diagrammatically in Fig. 6. The blades rotate at a speed of 750 rpm. The fragments cut from the plaque are extracted through the central lumen by application of a continuous vacuum. The material is collected in a vessel at the hub of the catheter (Fig. 7). Figure 7 also shows the hand gun assembly which houses the motor and trigger with sites for attachment of a remote battery-power source and the vacuum bottle for retrieval of the excised material. The trigger activates both the cutting blade rotation and the vacuum system. On the top of the gun assembly is a lever which controls the relative position of the cutting blades with respect to the lumen of the catheter. The TEC system is inserted through a 9 French arterial sheath and tracks over a 0.014 guidewire. The 5, 7 and 9 French sizes are available.

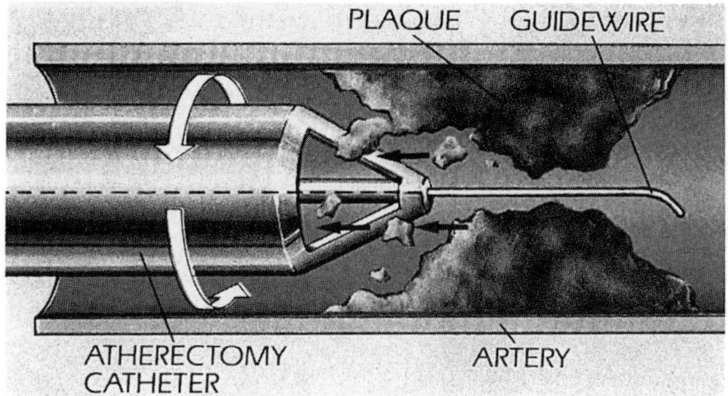

Fig. 6. Diagrammatic representation of the TEC catheter. The catheter travels over a guidewire. The rotating conical, sharp, stainless steel blades shave small fragments of the atheroma which are then aspirated through the central lumen.

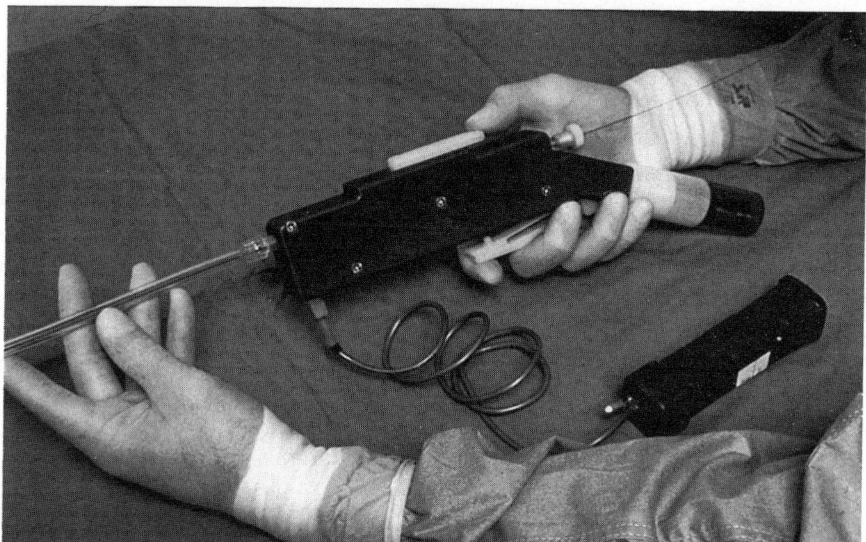

Fig. 7. Photograph of the hub of the transluminal extraction catheter system. The hand gun houses a trigger which activates the cutting blade rotation and simultaneously the vacuum system which provides 29 cm of water suction. The slide on the top controls the relative position of the cutting blades with respect to the lumen of the catheter.

PROCEDURE

This procedure also must be performed where adequate fluoroscopic facilities are available. An arterial sheath is inserted antegrade or retrograde depending upon the target vessel. The steerable guidewire is positioned across the lesion and the TEC catheter is advanced to a position just proximal to the lesion. The trigger is activated, initiating both rotation and suction, and then the rotating catheter tip is advanced through the lesion. Simultaneous with advancement of the tip is infusion of a saline solution which is aspirated through the central lumen and which serves to collect the debris excised by the sharp cutting blades as they are advanced.

As opposed to the atherocath, this system is directly applicable to total occlusions. Virtually any lesion which can be crossed by the guidewire can theoretically be treated with the TEC device. However, our experience has suggested again that the most favourable lesions are short and discrete. This catheter will not make as large a lumen as the atherocath and thus is less suitable for the larger vessels such as the iliac. The maximum size of the largest catheter will provide only a 3 mm lumen. On the other hand, the smaller size has been more useful for treating lesions in distal vessels such as smaller popliteal and tibial arteries. Figure 8 shows a typical distal superficial femoral artery occlusion. Following treatment with the TEC device, an adequate lumen has been restored in this vessel.

The debris retrieved consists primarily of small fragments of atheromatous material (Fig. 9). Plaque fragments ranging in size from 0.1 to 2.8 mm are retrieved. When examined histologically, these fragments consist of a mixture of collagen, elastic tissue, and modified smooth muscle cells. Cholesterol deposits are also recognized.

CLINICAL RESULTS

Primary success has been achieved in 95% of patients and 97% of lesions attempted.[11] Success is defined as 50% or less residual diameter stenosis by quantitative digital angiography. Eleven of 67 lesions in our initial study were total occlusions. The majority of the lesions treated (51) have been in the superficial femoral. Two technical failures occurred, both due to dissection. One required bypass surgery 10 days later. Mean luminal diameter narrowing has been reduced from 82 to 22% visually, and from 73 to 33% by quantitative digital angiography. Lumen diameter has been increased and average 1–2.5 mm. In our patients treated, the mean lesion length was 17 mm, ranging from 2 to 90. Follow-up angiography 6 months after the procedure has been performed in 22 of 28 eligible patients (79%). Restenosis was found in seven of 22 or 32% of patients. Restenosis is defined as greater than

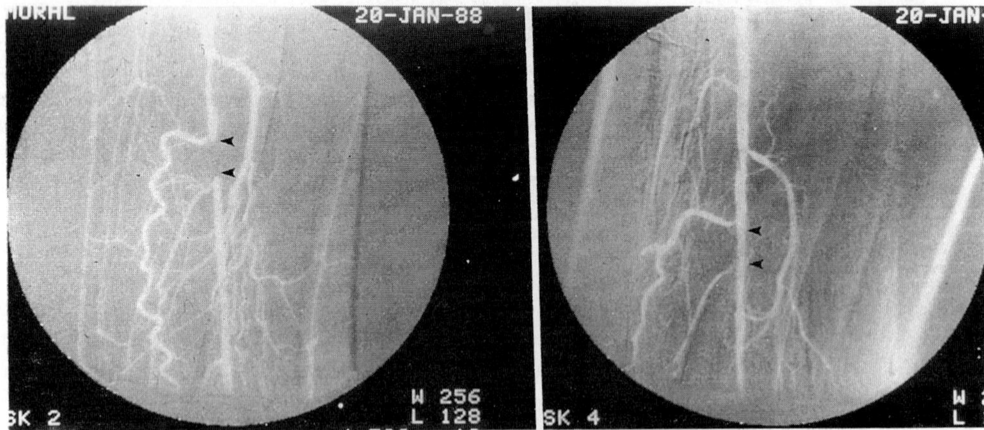

Fig. 8. On the left is a short segmental superficial femoral artery occlusion before treatment. Following transluminal extraction catheter atherectomy, the lumen is restored.

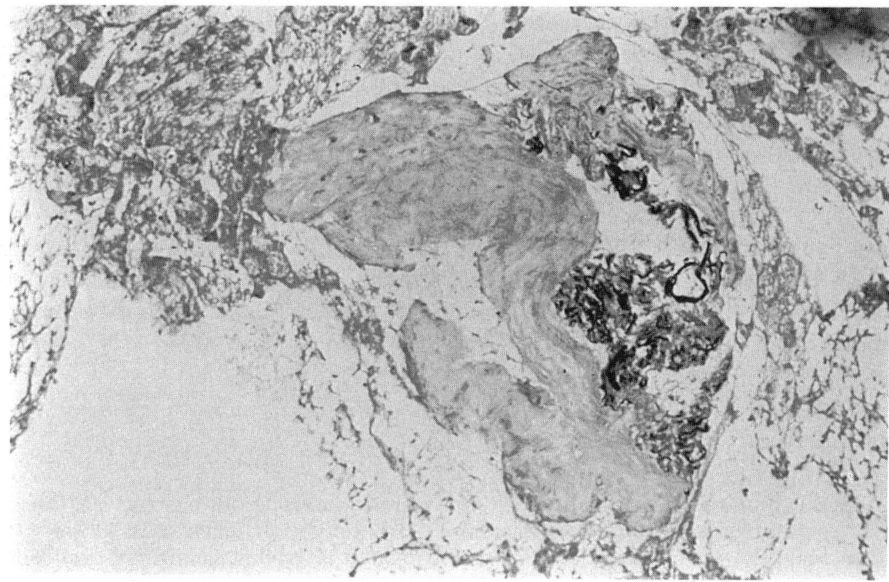

Fig. 9. Small 1–2 mm fragments of atheromatous tissue are retrieved. These fragments consist of smooth muscle cells and extracellular lipid.

60% luminal diameter narrowing by quantitative digital angiography at the site of the treated lesion. Factors associated with the reduced probability of recurrent stenosis included if the target lesion was not the site of a previous PTA, only five of 20 or 17% of the lesions had restenosis. If a target lesion had a good distal run-off, only 15% recurred. If the residual stenosis following the procedure was less than 30%, only one of 12 or 8% restenosed.

COMPLICATIONS

Major complications have been limited to the puncture site. Up to 8% of the patients have significant haematoma and/or false aneurysms. Distal embolization, acute occlusion due to spasm or dissection, and thrombosis at the treatment site are rare. Despite the small size of the fragments excised with the TEC system, distal embolization of this material has not been recognized. Larger plaque fragments have been dislodged and embolized distally and one of our patients required tibial bypass for treatment of this.

The TEC procedure also requires additional angiographic time and expense compared to balloon angioplasty. Long-term results are also complicated by the concurrent use of balloon angioplasty which has been applied when stenoses could not be reduced to less than 30%.

SUMMARY AND CONCLUSIONS

Both the Simpson atherocath and the TEC device are useful for treatment of patients with peripheral vascular obstructive disease. Both devices, however, have best success in treating short, uncomplicated lesions and thus are most useful for treating patients with claudication rather than those with threatened limb. Neither device has demonstrated any significant success in treating patients with long superficial femoral artery occlusions or the severely diseased superficial femoral artery with multiple lesions in series. Thus, it is not expected that application of this technology in its present form will improve limb salvage in patients with severe obstructive disease. The catheters are useful in treating patients who present with lifestyle-limiting claudication and, because they have been shown to be safe in this population, we feel it is reasonable to offer patients, whose lifestyles are significantly altered by inability to walk, a treatment that has reasonable chance of improvement with a demonstrably small risk.

REFERENCES

1. Dotter CT, Judkins MP: Transluminal treatment of arteriosclerotic obstruction. Description of a new technique and a preliminary report of its application. Circulation 30:654–670, 1964
2. Grüntzig A, Hopff H: Percutaneous recanalization after chronic arterial occlusion with a new dilator-catheter (modification of the Dotter technique) (Author's transl.) Dtsch Med Wochenschr 99:2502–2510, 2511, 1974
3. Johnston KW, Rae M, Hogg-Johnston SA *et al*: Five year results of a prospective study of percutaneous transluminal angioplasty. Ann Surg 206:403–413, 1987
4. Zarins CK: The vascular war of 1988: The enemy is met. JAMA 261:416–417, 1989
5. Barbano EF, Newman GE, McCann RL *et al*: Correlation of clinical history with quantitative histology of lower extremity atheroma biopsies obtained with the Simpson atherectomy catheter. Atherosclerosis 78:183–196, 1989
6. Newman GE, Miner DG, Sussman SK *et al*: Peripheral artery atherectomy: Description of technique and report of initial results. Radiology 169:677–680, 1988
7. Simpson JB, Selmon MR, Robertson GC *et al*: Transluminal atherectomy for occlusive peripheral vascular disease. Am J Cardiol 61:96G–101G, 1988
8. Graor RA, Whitlow PL: Transluminal atherectomy for occlusive peripheral vascular disease. J Am Coll Cardiol 15:1551–1558, 1990
9. Hinohara T, Selmon MR, Robertson GC, Braden L, Simpson JS: Directional atherectomy. New approaches for treatment of obstructive coronary and peripheral vascular disease. Circulation (Suppl IV) 81:IV79–IV87, 1990
10. von-Poinitz A, Nerlich A, Berger H, Hofling B: Percutaneous peripheral atherectomy: angiographic and clinical follow-up of 60 patients. J Am Coll Cardiol 15:682–688, 1990
11. Sketch ME, Jr, Newman GE, McCann RL *et al*: Transluminal extraction-endarterectomy in peripheral vascular disease: Late clinical and angiographic follow-up. Circulation (Suppl II) 80:II305, 1989

The Rotablator Atherectomy Device for Peripheral Arterial Disease

Samuel S. Ahn

In the emerging field of endovascular surgery, transluminal balloon angioplasty has become an established effective alternative and adjunct to peripheral arterial reconstruction in selective cases.[1] Laser assisted balloon angioplasty and mechanical atherectomy are currently being developed as alternative methods to recanalize occluded arteries. Several atherectomy catheters are now approved for clinical use and these include the Simpson athrocath, the Kinsey atherectomy catheter, the transluminal extraction catheter, and the Auth rotablator. This chapter will describe the Auth rotablator atherectomy device for peripheral arterial occlusive disease.

DESCRIPTION OF THE DEVICE

Figures 1 and 2 show the atherectomy device. This device is a high speed rotary atherectomy catheter designed to remove atherosclerotic plaques directly and transluminally. A high speed rotary burr tracks along a central coaxial guidewire and selectively grinds hard calcified arteries into a liquid colloidal suspension. Figure 1 shows the diamond coated metal burr welded to a flexible drive shaft that rotates and tracks along a central coaxial guidewire. The burr is available in various sizes and is selected to match the luminal diameter of the artery. The diamond chips measure up to 120 micron (μm) in diameter and are embedded in the brass burr. The drive shaft is encased within a protective plastic sheath to form a system capable of delivering a flexible catheter. The drive shaft is connected to a turbine that is housed in a plastic casing and driven by compressed air (Fig. 2). The turbine rotates the drive shaft at 100 000 to 200 000 rpm. A fibre optic light probe measures the number of revolutions per min displayed on a control panel. The rotational speed is controlled by the air pressure within the system and this pressure in turn is

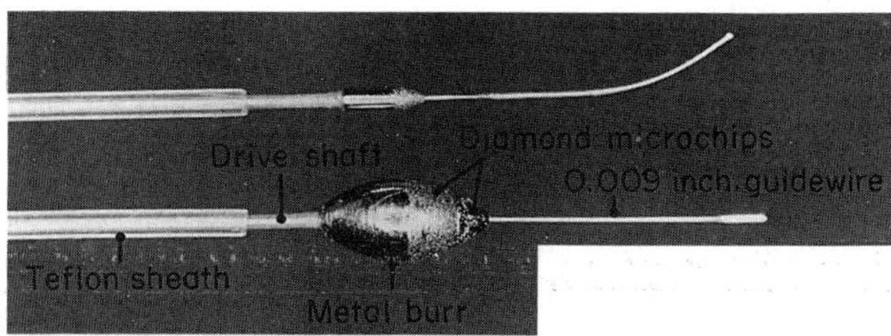

Fig. 1. Atherectomy burr and guidewire. Burrs of 1.25 (upper) and 4.5 mm (lower) in diameter, respectively, are shown. Note the micro diamond chips embedded in distal half of the burr. Also note the coaxial spring tip (top) and semirigid (bottom) guidewires.

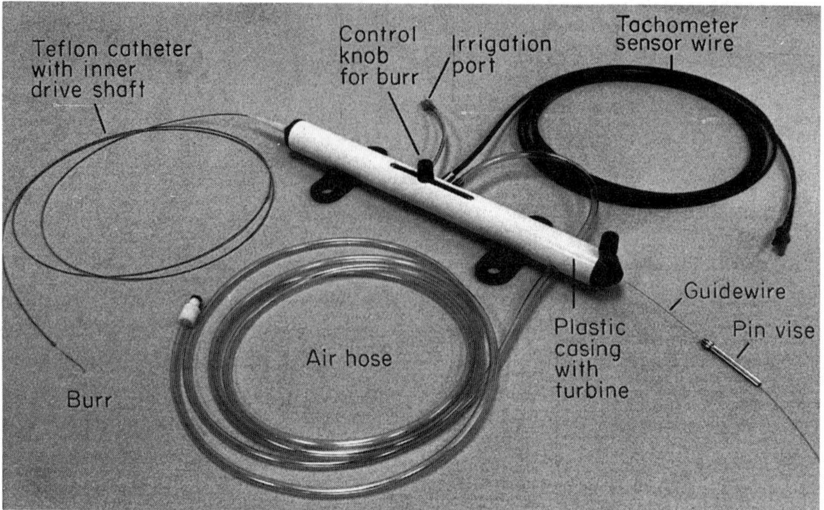

Fig. 2. Atherectomy catheter system. See text for details.

controlled by a separate foot pedal. The turbine also pumps sterile saline irrigation solution into the plastic sheath to lubricate and cool the rotating drive shaft and burr. A control knob on top of the plastic casing allows the operator to advance the burr over the guidewire. The entire system is disposable.

This athrectomy device preferentially attacks hard calcified atheroma because of its selective differential cutting of hard rather than soft tissue. As shown in Fig. 3, soft elastic tissue is deflected away by the rotating diamond chips. However, hard rigid tissue is fixed, and thus cannot move out of the way and accordingly gets chipped off as micro particles.

PRECLINICAL STUDIES

The safety and efficacy of this device was tested extensively prior to initiation of clinical trials. The device was first tested in harvested *ex situ* cadaver arteries.[2] The overall efficacy of the device in harvested superficial femoral artery, popliteal artery and tibial arteries was 25 of 30 or 83%. The success rate in stenotic arteries was 17 of 17 or 100% but for total occluded arteries was only 8 of 13 or 62%. The main limiting factor was the inability of the guidewire to cross totally occluded lesions. The next studies were performed in fresh whole human cadavers.[2] Similar to the *ex situ* harvested arteries, atherectomy was highly successful in stenotic arteries (19 of 20 or 95%) but less successful in totally occluded arteries (10 of 18 or 56%). In both the *ex situ* and whole cadaver studies the atherectomy device was equally effective in the popliteal and tibial arteries as well as the superficial femoral artery.

Histologic specimens of successfully treated arteries revealed a smooth, highly polished luminal surface (Fig. 4). The elastin of the external media and adventitia tissue were intact. We observed no intimal dissections. Scanning electron microscopy (SEM) confirmed a smooth polished surface with intact side branches[3] (Fig. 5).

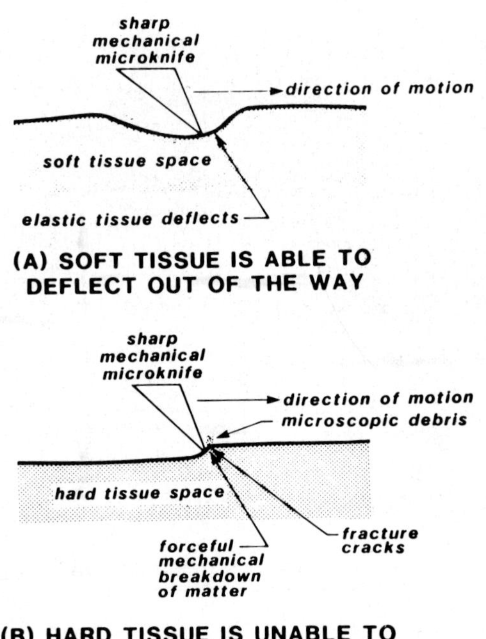

Fig. 3. Differential cutting: its application in soft and hard tissue.

However, higher magnification views of the atherectomized surfaces revealed endothelial peeling and denuded lumen as well as etchings of the diamond chips within the smooth muscle layers[3] (Figs 6 and 7).

The particles resulting from the atherectomy procedure were analysed by Coulter counter and were noted to be mostly 2–10 μm in size[2] (Fig. 8). However, some of the particles resulting from the atherectomy procedure particularly with the larger burrs, were 15–20 μm which are larger than red blood cells. Subsequent studies in which the particles were labelled with technetium^{99} and injected into the common femoral artery of a dog revealed no apparent thromboembolic complications from these particles. In fact, most of the particles passed through the capillary circulation of the lower extremity and were taken up in the lung, liver and spleen, the reticulo-endothelial system[2] (Fig. 9).

After these feasibility, efficacy and safety studies, clinical trials were initiated in the peripheral arteries.

CLINICAL STUDIES

Technique of the procedure

Atherectomy can be performed percutaneous or openly. The open technique is preferred since the percutaneous technique limits the burr size to 3.0 mm diameter.

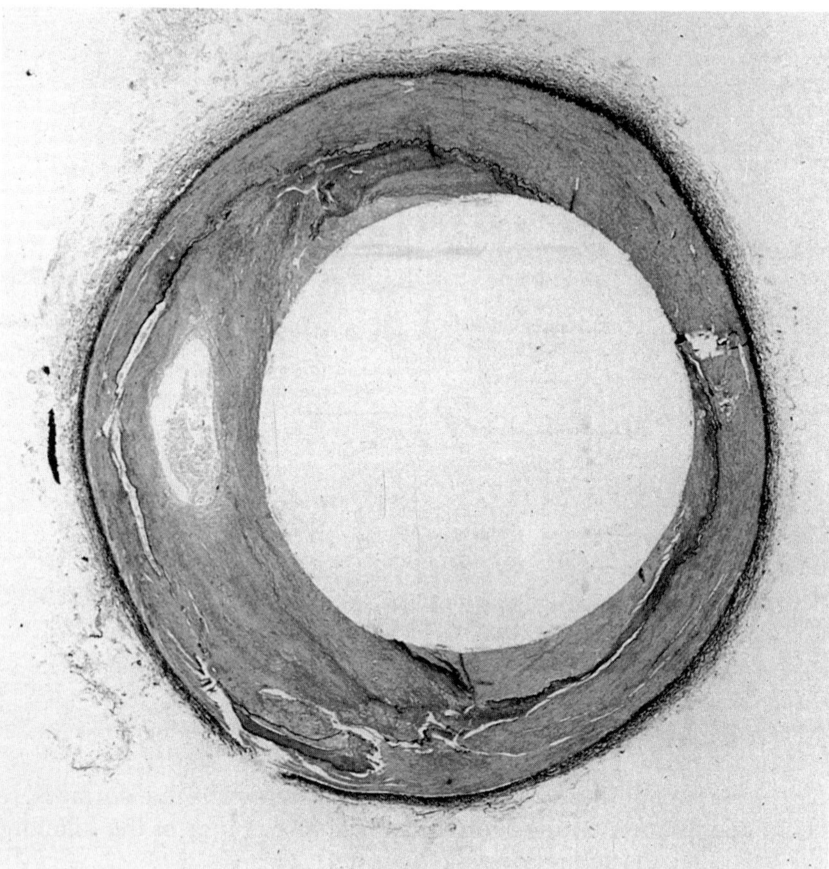

Fig. 4. Photomicrograph of successfully atherectomized artery seen in cross-section. Note the smooth highly polished intraluminal surface (Verhoeff-van Gieson Stain; ×40).

The artery proximal to the atherectomy site is dissected and exposed. An introducer sheath ranging from 9 to 14 French (depending on the size of the artery) is inserted into the artery using the Seldinger technique or through a transverse arteriotomy. This sheath prevents repeated trauma to the artery by multiple passages of the instrument. It also prevents back bleeding and minimizes the blood loss. A vascular endoscope is passed through the sheath and the lesion is documented. Then under direct angioscopic and fluoroscopic guidance a 0.014 high torque floppy atraumatic guidewire is passed through the stenotic lesion. With the guidewire in place the vascular endoscope is removed in exchange for a 4 French guide catheter. The atraumatic guidewire is removed and is replaced by a stiffer 0.009 diameter athrectomy guide wire that comes with the system. This atherectomy guidewire is stiffer and rigid enough to support the rotating burr.

The burr and drive shaft are fed over the guidewire and positioned just proximal to the obstructive lesion. Initially a burr size approximately half the diameter of the native artery is used. The atherectomy turbine is connected to pressurized

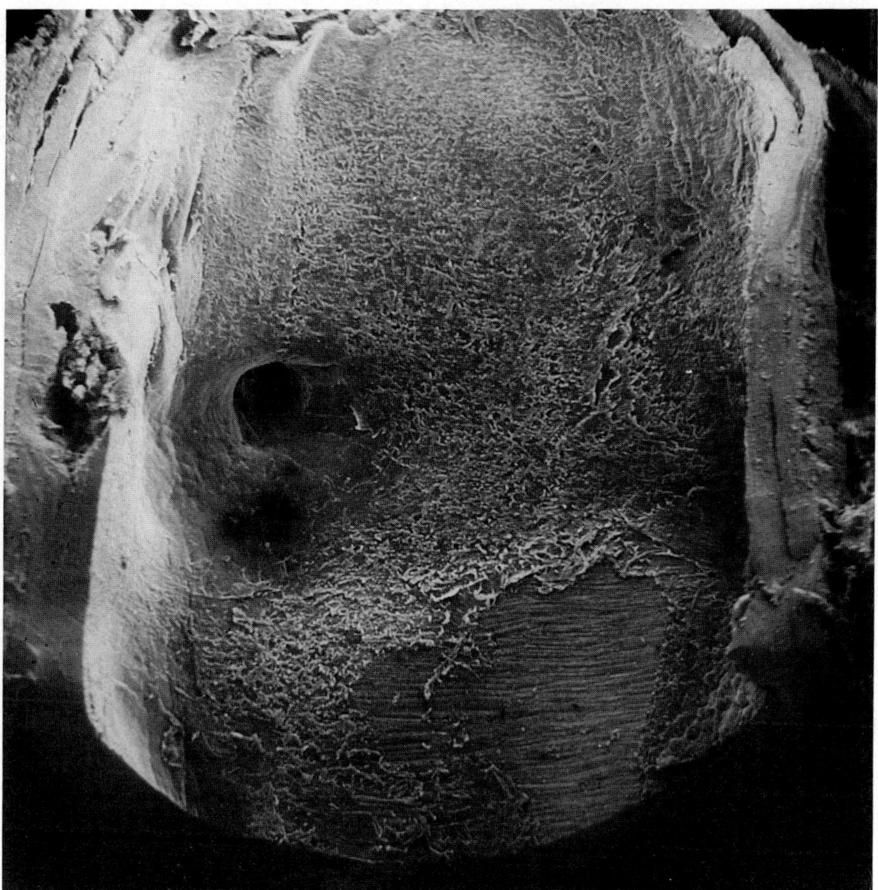

Fig. 5. Scanning electron microscopy (SEM) of sizeable section of a successfully rotary atherectomized popliteal artery (× 40). Note the smooth contoured luminal surface and the intact patent geniculate branch orifice.

nitrogen set at 40–45 psi. Normal saline solution mixed with dextran and papaverine is connected to the irrigation port. Atherectomy is started by pressing the foot pedal and slowing advancing the burr using the control knob. The rotational speed is kept at 100 000–175 000 rpm. Care must be taken not to advance the burr too rapidly which will slow the speed below 100 000 rpm which will cause the burr to snag and stall the device. The burr should not be kept in one spot too long which could lead to overheating of the atherectomized area. Ideally a vibratory action should be used to manipulate the control knob to create a fine darting in and out motion of the burr.

After the burr traverses the obstructive lesion an interval angiogram is performed. If this is satisfactory then a larger sized burr is selected and used to complete the atherectomy. The residual luminal stenosis should be less than 20%, and achievement of this result generally requires the passage of two or three incrementally larger burrs. After the final atherectomy completion angiography and vascular endoscopy are performed.

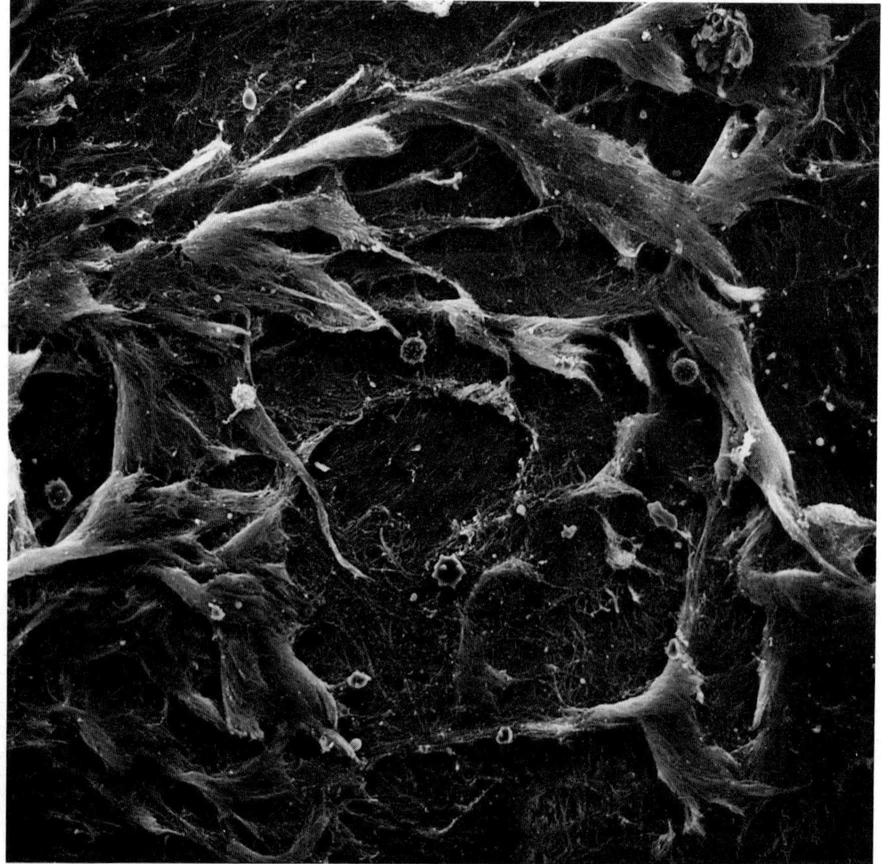

Fig. 6. Higher magnification of SEM seen in Fig. 5 ($\times 600$). Note the endothelial peeling and smooth intact muscle layer underneath.

Postoperatively the patient should be maintained on anticoagulation therapy for 48 hours. The patient should be discharged on long-term antiplatelet agents. Standard vascular reconstructive procedures can be performed simultaneously with the atherectomy procedure. Such strategies using combined vascular reconstruction and atherectomy have been previously described.[4]

Clinical results

The UCLA series currently includes 40 arteries, in 24 patients, including the superficial femoral, popliteal and tibial arteries.[5] The overall initial success rate was of 22 of 24 cases (92%), and 38 of 40 arteries (95%). Mechanical problems caused two early technical failures. Four early thromboses occurred in patients who subsequently proved to have a hypercoagulable state. Follow-up of 1–22 months (average 9 months), revealed seven late failures (29%). Two-year follow-up revealed only a 25% primary patency rate. Further analysis revealed that the longer lesions

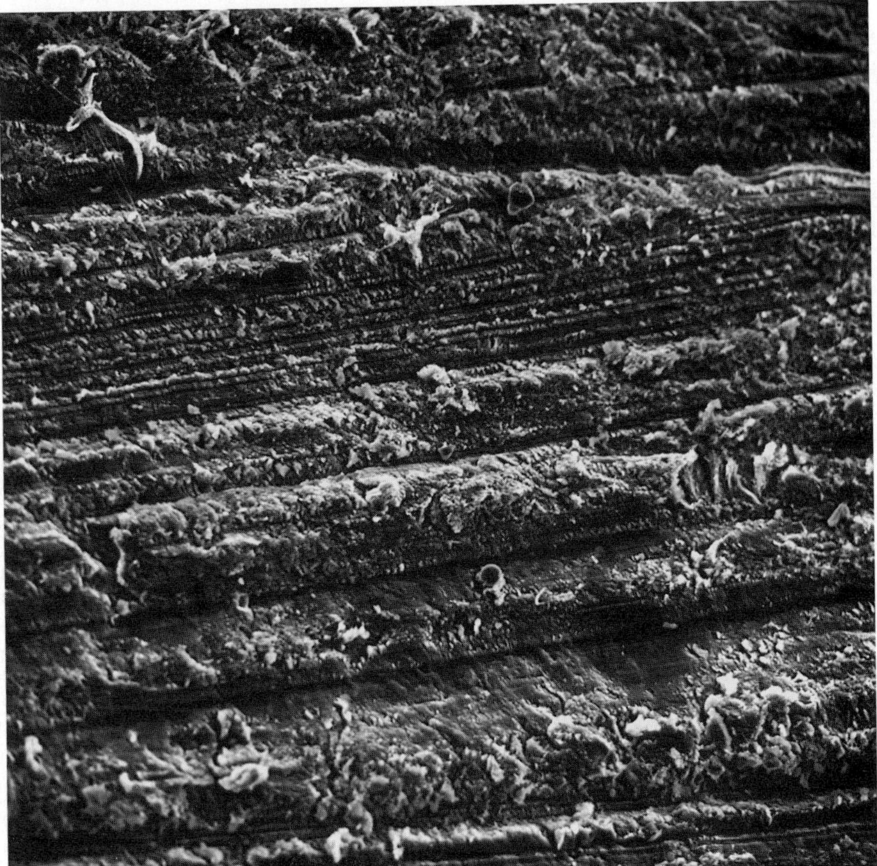

Fig. 7. Higher magnification of SEM seen in Fig. 5 (×600). Note the etching of diamond bits of burr within media smooth muscle.

had worse early and late failures. Curiously the best results occurred in the tibial arteries and the worse results in the superficial femoral arteries. The reason for this probably reflects the length of lesion treated. The tibial lesions tended to be short, while the superficial femoral artery lesions tended to be greater than 10 cm and up to 40 cm in length.

John Mehigan has recently reported the Stanford series which includes 42 patients, 21 treated openly and 21 treated percutaneously.[6] This series includes superficial femoral and popliteal artery stenosis. The angiographic success rate was 81%. However, in hospital, clinical success was only 52% and 6-month clinical follow-up showed a 43% success rate.

Complications and limitations

Misplacement of the guidewire in a subintimal plane is a potentially common complication. This complication can be avoided by the use of good fluoroscopic and

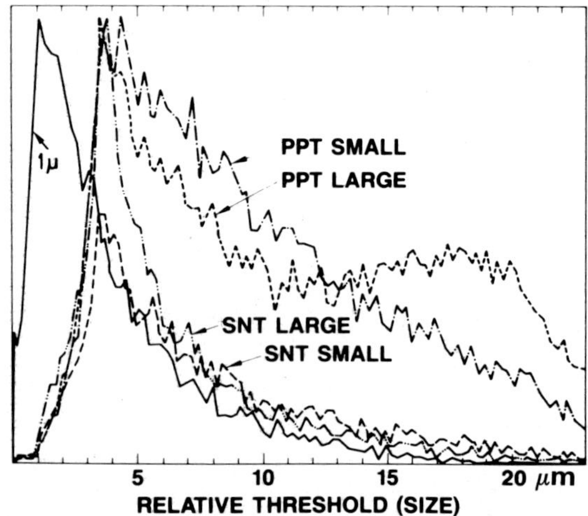

Fig. 8. Coulter counter analysis of atherectomized particles. Vertical axis is the distribution of particles. Horizontal axis is the relative threshold in size of the particles. PPT small = precipitate of particles generated by 2.5 mm burr; PPT large = precipitate of particles generated by 4.5 mm burr; FNT small = supernatant of centrifuged colloidal suspension generated by 2.5 mm burr; SNT large = supernatant of centrifuged colloidal suspension generated by 4.5 mm burr. Note that particles are generally smaller than 10 µm.

angioscopic equipment and the initial use of an atraumatic, high torque, floppy guidewire to cross the stenotic lesion. Burr entanglement can occur if the burr is advanced too rapidly or if an oversized burr is chosen for the initial treatment. A few cases of thromboembolic problems have been noted. Most were microscopic and clinically insignificant. However, one patient in the UCLA series developed diffuse microemboli in the presence of a hypercoagulable state and ultimately lost a limb.[5] Microscopic haematuria has occurred in approximately 10% of the patients and occurs when the larger size burrs, 4 mm or greater are used. However, this complication has had a clinically benign course and has resolved within 12 hours in the UCLA and Stanford series.[5,6] Other complications include groin haematoma and wound infections. Only two perforations have been noted in the Stanford series and none in the UCLA series.

The Auth rotablator has several limitations. The same differential cutting that allows the rotablator to preferentially attack hard calcified plaques also prevents its efficacy in treating chronic thrombus which is often rubbery in character.[7] These rubbery lesions preferentially deflect away from the rotating burr leading to suboptimal recanalization. The multiple burr requirements and exchanges slow down the procedure. The clinical results also suggests that long lesions have suboptimal long-term results and thus the atherectomy device appears better suited for short lesions.

Although the particle problems have been minimal so far, a large particle burden resulting from treatment of a long occluded lesion could potentially lead to problems which have not yet been clearly identified. These problems could include diffuse intravascular coagulopathy and limb loss. The device should not be used for carotid or vertebral arterial lesions since the microemboli could lead to focal neurological deficits and even frank global cerebral dysfunction.

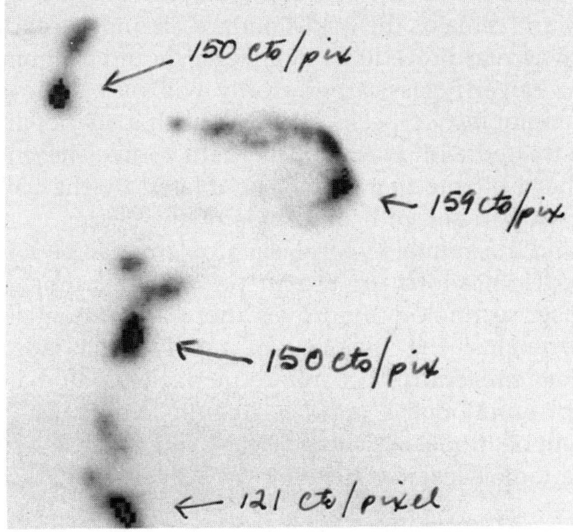

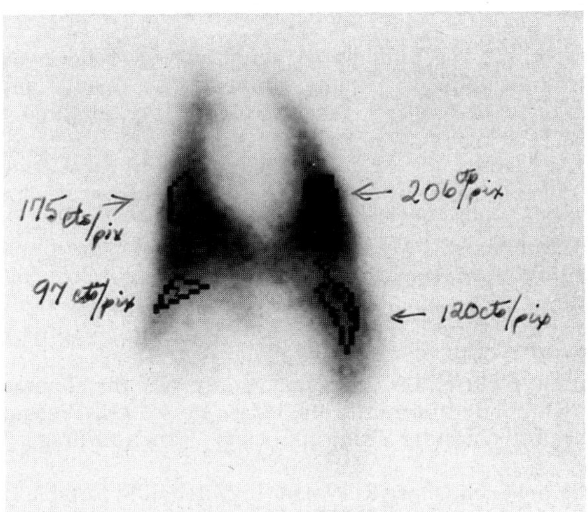

Fig. 9. Radionuclide scan of dog injected with technetium^{99m}-labelled atherectomized particles. Note that most particles past through the leg and accumulate in the lung, liver and spleen, the reticulo-endothelial system.

CONCLUDING REMARKS

Despite actual removal, debulking, and polishing of the stenotic plaque, arterial trauma invariably occurs as demonstrated by our histological studies. This arterial trauma almost certainly induces intimal hyperplasia which clearly causes intermediate and late failures in many of these patients. Thus the restenosis rate following rotary atherectomy has not improved significantly over balloon angioplasty. Our results suggest that, like other atherectomy and laser assisted balloon angioplasty catheters, balloon angioplasty still remains the gold standard among the endovascular devices. Furthermore, endovascular procedures in general should be limited to short lesions of less than 10 cm. Nevertheless, atherectomy will play an important role as an adjunct to balloon angioplasty. Specifically, lesions that are not amenable to balloon angioplasty can be treated with mechanical atherectomy. These lesions include the severely calcified hard plaque that cannot be dilated by the balloon catheter and ulcerated lesions that present with thromboembolic events.

If the restenosis and the intimal hyperplasia problems can be solved, the rotablator will have expanded indications for use in peripheral arterial occlusive disease. Furthermore, as laser technology improves there is a potential for laser assisted atherectomy to recanalize the majority of totally occluded arteries. Thus as endovascular surgery procedures become refined, the combination of the various devices used in a multimodality approach could eventually become the major therapeutic treatment of arterial occlusive disease. However, the restenosis problem, particularly for the longer lesions, needs to be solved first.

REFERENCES

1. Deutsch LS: Chapter 21. Techniques of percutaneous balloon angioplasty including aortoiliac and femoropopliteal systems: Indications, results and complications. *In* Endovascular Surgery, Moore WS, Ahn SS (Eds). Philadelphia and London: W. B. Saunders, pp. 163–208, 1989
2. Ahn SS, Auth DA, Marcus DR, Moore WS: Removal of focal atheromatous lesions by angioscopically guided high speed rotary atherectomy preliminary experimental observations. J Vasc Surg 7:292–300, 1988
3. Ahn SS, Arca MJ, Marcus DR, Moore WS: Histologic and morphologic effects of rotary atherectomy on human cadaver arteries. Ann Vasc Surg 4:563–569, 1990
4. Ahn SS, Moore WS: Lesions amenable to mechanical atherectomy: Clinical strategies. *In* Endovascular Surgery, Moore WS, Ahn SS (Eds). Philadelphia and London: W. B. Saunders, pp. 299–309, 1989
5. Ahn SS, Yeatman LR, Deutsch LS, Auth DC, Moore WS: Intraoperative peripheral rotary atherectomy: Early and late clinical results. J Vasc Surg 1991. Presented at the 6th annual meeting of the Western Vascular Surgical Society, Rancho Mirage, California, USA, Jan 13–16, 1991
6. Jennings LJ, Mehigan JT, Ginsberg R, Wexler L, Mitchell S: Rotablator atherectomy: Early experience and six month follow-up. J Vasc Surg 1991. Presented at the 6th annual meeting of the Western Vascular Surgical Society, Rancho Mirage, California, USA, Jan 13–16, 1991
7. Ahn SS: The rotablator—high speed rotary atherectomy: Indications, techniques, results, and complications. *In* Endovascular Surgery, Moore WS, Ahn SS (Eds). Philadelphia and London: W. B. Saunders, pp. 327–335, 1989

Peripheral Vascular Experience with the Trac-Wright Atherectomy Device

Stanley O. Snyder Jr, Jock R. Wheeler, Roger T. Gregory, Robert G. Gayle and F. Noel Parent

The Trac-Wright® system (formerly Kensey atherectomy catheter) (Fig. 1) is a recanalization/atherectomy device utilizing a rotating cam tip driven by an internal torsion wire to traverse occlusive arterial lesions. The cam tip, rotating at speeds of up to 100 000 rpm, is designed to use the concept of viscoelasticity to permit deformation of the normal arterial wall without significant energy absorption or tissue damage while selectively pulverizing the firm atherosclerotic lesions within the arterial lumen. The coaxial system permits constant radiographic contrast infusion to cool the tip and allow fluoroscopic visualization and control of the catheter progress.

NORFOLK EXPERIENCE

Patients and methods

During the period from 4 December 1986 to 31 July 1990, 41 patients underwent 46 procedures (five bilateral) to attempt recanalization of atherosclerotic superficial femoral artery (SFA) lesions; 28 were complete occlusions and 18 were high grade stenoses. Lesion length ranged from 2 to 20 cm with a mean of 7.15 cm. Patient age ranged from 44 to 83 years with a mean of 68 years. There were 24 procedures in males and 22 in females with claudication the indication in 31, tissue loss in 11 and rest pain in four.

All procedures were done in the operating room under spinal anaesthesia using a groin incision to expose the femoral vessels. Seldinger techniques were used to insert a 9 French introducer into the femoral artery with angiography and fluoroscopic monitoring to define the lesion site and visualize catheter progress (Fig. 2). A Hexabrix solution (60 ml Hexabrix contrast, 40 000 units urokinase, 140 ml dextran, and 1000 units heparin) was injected at 30 ml/min as the catheter cam tip was advanced through the lesion rotating at 60 000–90 000 rpm. Early in the series, catheter manipulation persisted until the lesion was successfully traversed or until vessel perforation was encountered. In the latter half of the series, continued inability to traverse the lesion was also considered an end point. Successful catheter passage was followed by attempted balloon angioplasty while vessel perforation or inability to traverse the lesion was followed by standard femoropopliteal bypass procedures. Five patients required intraoperative balloon angioplasty procedure of the ipsilateral iliac vessel prior to the atherectomy procedure distally.

All patients were given aspirin (5 grains) the night prior to surgery, and were fully anticoagulated with heparin (100 units/kg) intraoperatively. Following completion of

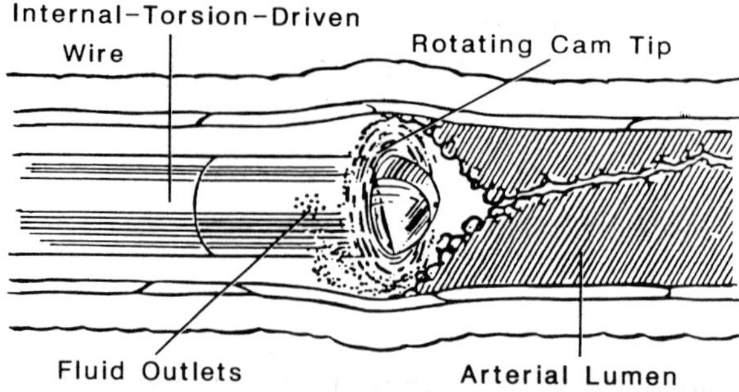

Fig. 1. Trac-Wright catheter.

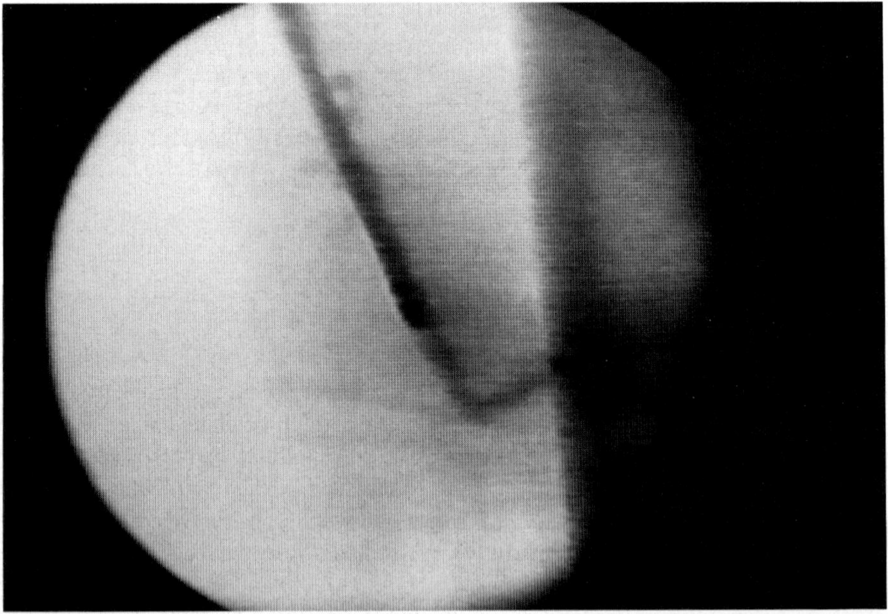

Fig. 2. Fluoroscopic view of Trac-Wright catheter.

successful cases, the heparin was only partially reversed with protamine and a low dose heparin drip (400 units/h) was maintained for 48 h. Patients were discharged on low dose aspirin therapy (1.5 grains daily) and all had ankle brachial indices (ABIs) measured preoperatively, 24 h postoperatively, and on routine postoperative office visits.

Results

Immediate technical success was achieved in 31 of 46 (67%) with balloon dilatation accomplished in 27 of these procedures. Initial clinical evaluation (palpation of popliteal pulses, evaluation of pedal doppler signals, and evaluation of ankle brachial indices) revealed immediate haemodynamic failure (ABI increase <0.15 above pre-operative levels) despite successful catheter passage in four patients (two had successful balloon passage, two did not) producing an overall initial haemodynamic (clinical) success rate of 59% (27/46).

Fourteen immediate technical failures and one of the four immediate haemodynamic failures underwent standard revascularization procedures (Table 1) utilizing the spinal anaesthesia employed for the initial atherectomy attempt. One immediate technical failure (perforation) had a balloon dilatation procedure after a guidewire successfully traversed the lesion despite the perforation. The remaining three demonstrating technical success but immediate haemodynamic failure required: 1) a femoropopliteal *in situ* bypass (at 2 months); 2) conversion of an ischaemic below knee amputation to the above knee level (3 days); 3) continued observation with stable claudication and ABIs initially unchanged from preoperative levels.

COMPLICATIONS

Vessel perforation (Fig. 3) occurred in 11 limbs (eight SFA, three popliteals) and was the most frequent complication. The perforation rate of the initial series was high (7/19) as only technical success or perforation were regarded as end points to the procedure and the operators persisted until one or the other was achieved. Several factors, including operator learning curve, manufacturer rotating cam tip modifications, and attempts at passage through long complete occlusions contributed to the high perforation rate. In phase two, after modification of the catheter tip and acceptance of inability to traverse the lesion as an end point, the perforation rate (4/27) was significantly lower. Perforation, however, did *not* lead to significant haemorrhage in any patients and required suture closure in only one patient in whom the perforation site was exposed at the same operative procedure to facilitate the distal anastomosis of an above knee bypass graft.

Three groin incisional haematomas occurred (one requiring re-exploration and drainage) and one patient developed a draining groin lymphocele requiring operative closure. There were no documented cases of clinically significant distal embolization, but a single patient developed an acute popliteal occlusion secondary to a flap created by plaque dissection.

FOLLOW-UP DATA

Follow-up ranges from 2 weeks to 37 months with life table analysis for *all* patients (Fig. 4) yielding a cumulative primary patency of 37.5% (SE±7.7) at 1 year and

Table 1. Procedures required at time of immediate technical failure

Location	*Procedure*	*No.*
Femoropopliteal	AK Gore-Tex	6
Femoropopliteal	BK Vein	8
Femoroposterotibial	Vein	1

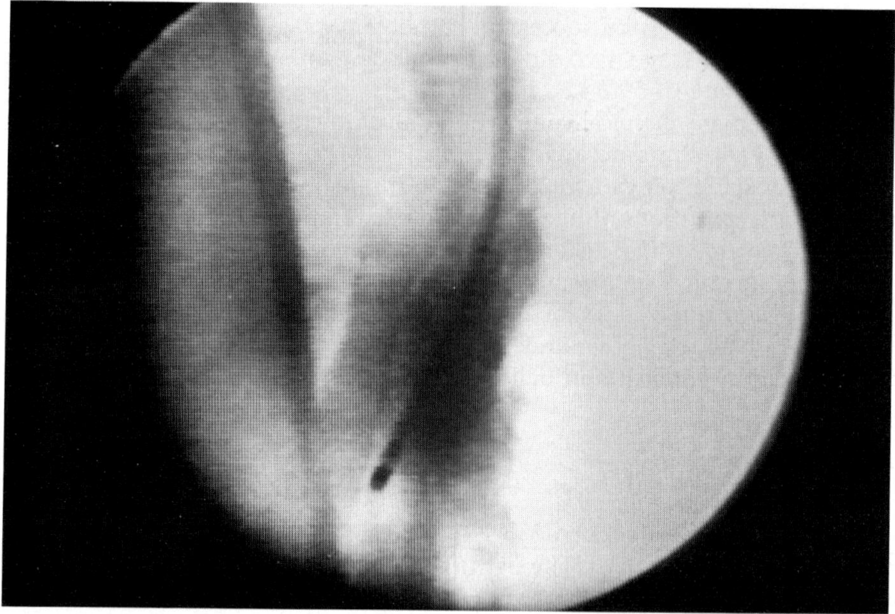

Fig. 3. SFA perforation with Trac-Wright catheter.

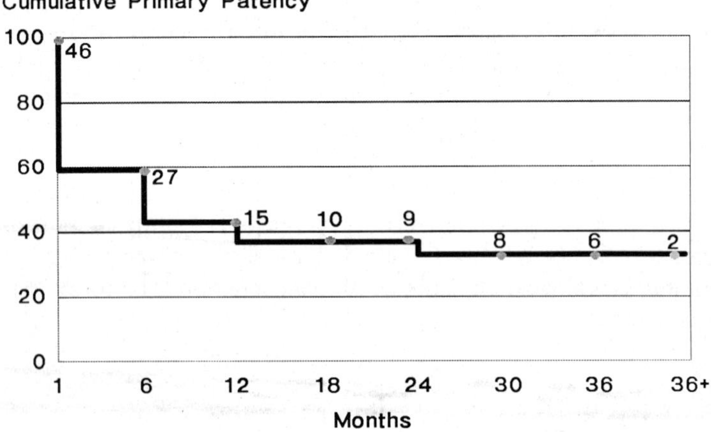

Fig. 4. Life table analysis for all procedures.

33.3% (SE±9.1%) at 2 years. Analysis of 'adjusted' life tables (Fig. 5), i.e. follow-up of only patients with initial haemodynamic success (27/46), as is often reported for endovascular procedures, reveals a continued haemodynamic success rate of 63.9% (SE±9.9%) at 1 year and 57% (SE±12.5%) at 2 years.

Continued haemodynamic success (ABI >0.15 above preoperative ABI level) was required to categorize a vessel as having maintained primary patency. Ankle brachial index measurements are often inaccurate or incorrect and angiographic follow-up is desirable but the invasiveness of angiography hinders follow-up of endovascular

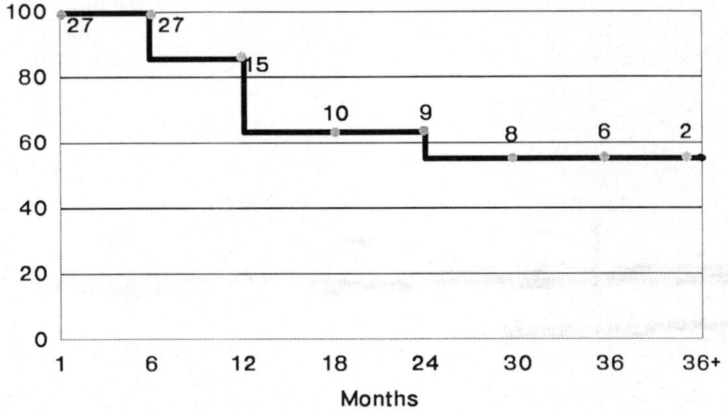

Fig. 5. Life table analysis for patients with initial clinical success.

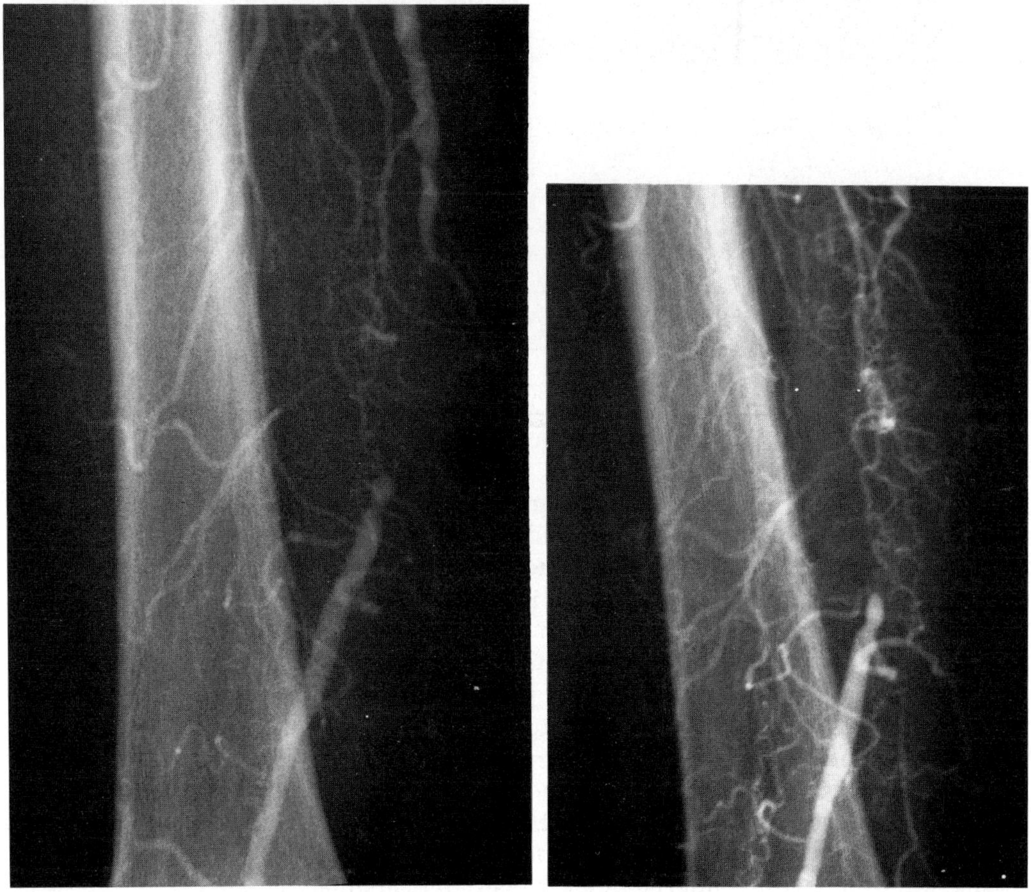

Fig. 6. Case 1. a (Left): Preoperative angiogram ABI 0.73. b (right): Follow-up angiogram ABI 0.85 despite re-occlusion.

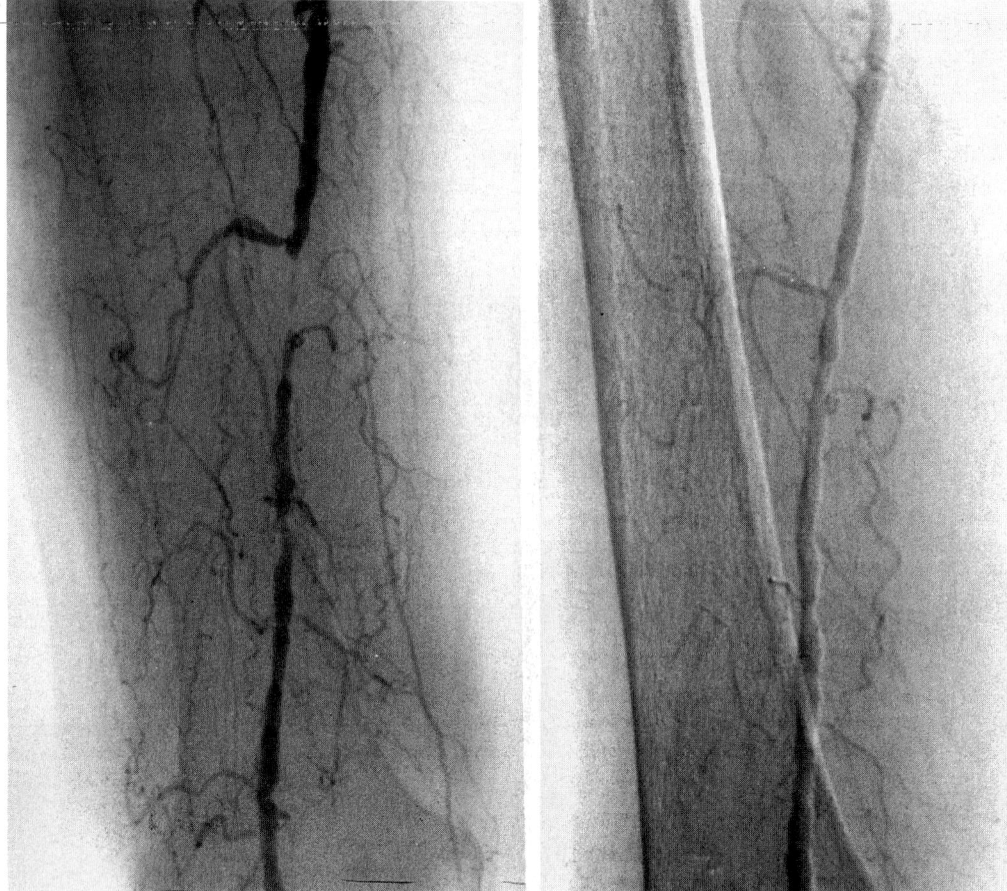

Fig. 7. Case 2. a (Left): Preoperative angiogram ABI 0.37. b (Right): Postoperative angiogram ABI of 0.52 but SFA segment remains patent.

interventional procedures. In Case 1 (Fig. 6) the ABI remains stable despite complete occlusion of the region of atherectomized superficial femoral artery seen on a follow-up angiographic study. Conversely, Case 2 (Fig. 7) is recorded as haemodynamically failing despite the follow-up angiographic evidence of wide patency of the superficial femoral artery segment in question. In addition, ankle brachial indices have been condemned as inaccurate secondary to calcification of vessels and difficulty in reproducing pressure measurements, particularly in patients with tibial disease and/or limited distal run-off.[1] This problem is more significant in endovascular follow-up than in bypass procedure follow-up where a palpable graft and/or intragraft duplex velocity studies can help define patency and haemodynamics.

There have been nine haemodynamic failures from the original 27 haemodynamic success procedures. Four have undergone bypass operations (two femoropopliteal, two femorotibial), one underwent laser assisted balloon angioplasty and four have been observed nonoperatively (two of which have haemodynamic failure but patent atherectomy segments). One patient with initial technical success but initially

Table 2. Results and follow-up for all procedures

	Procedures	*Initial technical success*	*Technical success haemo failure*	*Initial haemo success*	*Late haemo failure during F/U**	*Cont'd haemo success*
Occlusion	28	17	3	14	3	11
Stenosis	18	14	1	13	6	7
Total	46	31	4	27	9	18
Claudicants	31	21	1	20	8	12
Salvage	15	10	3	7	1	6
Total	46	31	4	27	9	18

*ABI<0.15 of preoperative levels.

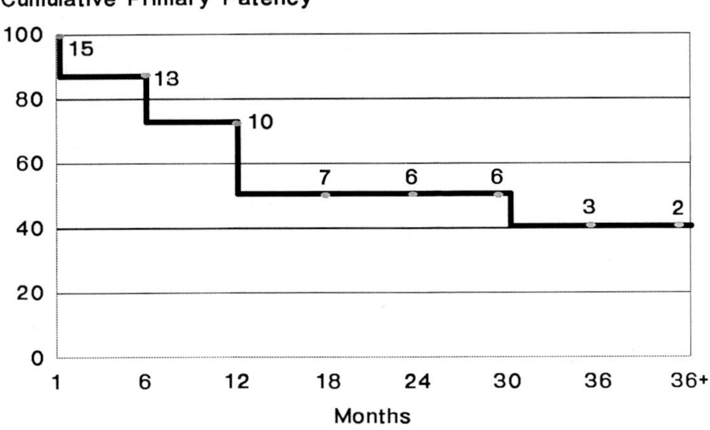

Fig. 8. Life table analysis for bypass procedures done at the time of immediate technical failure.

designated as an immediate haemodynamic failure has remained stable clinically and at 19 months follow-up has an ABI 0.19>than preoperative level. The 18 patients (Table 2) with continued haemodynamic success to the point of follow-up represent 11 cases done for occlusion (14/28 initial haemodynamic success) and seven cases done for stenosis (13/18 initial haemodynamic success).

Alternate procedure follow-up

Fifteen patients (Fig. 8) had bypass procedures done at the initial failed atherectomy operative procedure and eight of these have subsequently failed yielding a 24-month cumulative primary patency of 51%. Limb loss occurred in three patients (two limb salvage, one claudication), all of which were initial technical failures. The two limb salvage patients had required femoral to tibial graft procedures (occluded and required below knee amputation at 2 months, 7 months) and the claudicant developed a Charcot foot at 5 months, requiring below knee amputation despite

Table 3. Technical success in multiple US sites

Centres participating	*Main physician(s)*	*Patients*	*Limbs*	*Lesions*
Sentara Norfolk Norfolk, VA	Drs Snyder & Wheeler	31	34	37
Western Medical Anaheim, CA	Dr Matthews	11	15	25
Methodist Lubbock, TX	Dr Overlie	18	20	21
Humana Cypress Pompano Beach, FL	Dr Avila	16	17	22
Heart Institute of Nevada Las Vegas, NV	Dr Siragusa	17	17	19
Palm Beach Gardens Palm Beach Gardens, FL	Dr Wilbur	11	14	15
St Lukes Episcopal Houston, TX	Dr Krajcer	9	15	18
Total		113	132	157

Table 4. European technical success and perforation rates

Physician	*Technical success rate*	*Immediate clinical success rate (%)*	*Perforation (P) or dissection (D) rate*
Lundquist	50%(3/6)	50	D 1/6
Snyder & Wheeler	65%(24/37)	59	P 9/37
Siragusa	67%(10/15)	67	P 4/15
Schmitt	81%(25/31)	61	P 3/31
Ulrich	63%(10/16)	50	P 6/16
Zeitler	89%(24/27)	89	P 1/27
Mahler	96%(24/25)	80	P 0%
Rousseau	92%(24/26)	92	P/D 5/26
Dyet	86%(12/14)	79	0%
Desbrosses	76%(35/46)	76	P 4/46

a patent above knee femoropopliteal graft with ankle pressure indices of 1.0 and strongly palpable pedal pulses. One patient underwent thrombectomy, four had successful revision/extension procedures and one has been followed nonoperatively. Two patients (four procedures) died during the follow-up period.

FOLLOW-UP OTHER CENTRES

A compiled series of 157 cases in 113 patients from seven US centres (Table 3) yielded initial technical success in 117 cases (75%). This represented technical success in 34/42 (80%) of stenotic lesions and 83/115 (71%) of occlusions. European technical success rates (Table 4) have been similar to US reports but perforation rates have been variable from 0% (Mahler) to 37% (Ulrich) (Technical data: Dow Corning Wright). Published long-term follow-up has been limited until recently but Dr P. Overlie (personal communication) reports initial clinical success in 17/20 patients. Four patients were lost to follow-up but six of 11 cases followed for 1 year remain patent. Excellent follow-up results were recently published by Debrosses *et al.*[2] with initial clinical success in 40/46 cases. Venous angiographic studies were obtained at 48 h, 6 months and 1 year with confirmed patency of the treated artery in 35/46 (76%) procedures at 48 h. Life table analysis was not available for this group but 14 of 20 patients followed for at least 12 months remain patent.

Research

In an effort to quantitate and characterize the particles generated by Trac-Wright® catheter passage, we conducted an *in vivo* research protocol[3] to study distal effluent

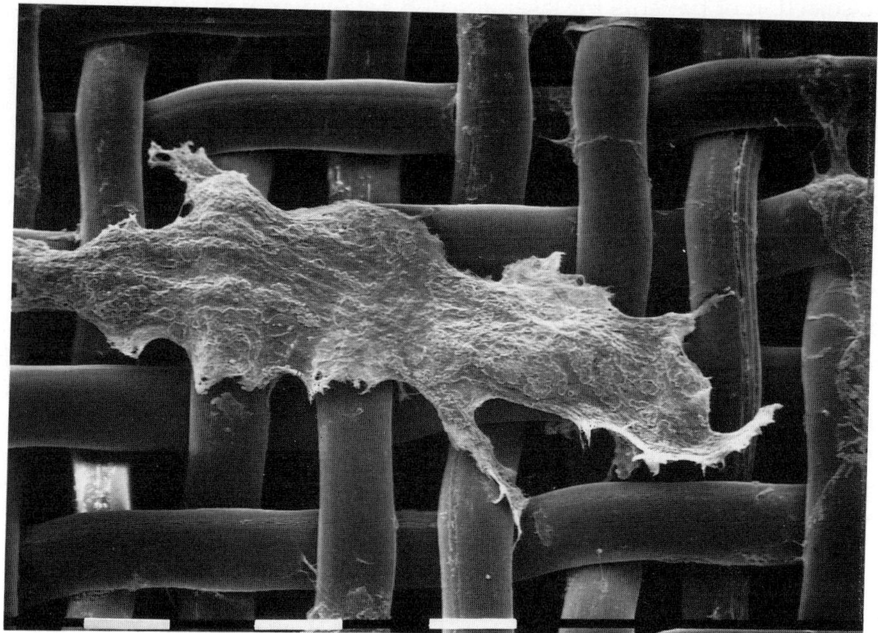

Fig. 9. Effluent particle SEM 74 m filter × 110. Bar division 0.1 mm at bottom.

Table 5. Trac-Wright catheter effluent analysis

Filter pore size (μm)	*Total no. of particles*	*Volume (μm³)*	*Area (μm²)*	*Longest dimension (μm)*
1000	20	– [c]	923008	1525
500	131	31636450	174573	748
74	5974	120502	28035	253
12	109347	7521	915	43
5	788782	3108	156	18

particle size and volume following Trac-Wright catheter passage through occluded superficial femoral arteries. A Javid shunt was inserted into the popliteal artery to collect the distal effluent during catheter passage. Scanning electron microphotographs (Fig. 9) demonstrated varied atheromatous particles, and analysis with Coulter counter and Particle Data Elzone 180 XY techniques after glutaraldehyde fixation indicated that both micro and macro particles (Table 5) are generated by Trac-Wright catheter passage through obstructed arteries. The effluent was serially filtered through 1000, 500, 74, 12, and 5 mm membranes and particles were measured for particle volume, area and longest dimension. The average longest dimension ranged from 18 to 1525 mm but only 0.7% of the particles generated had an average longest dimension greater than 43 mm. This was in marked contrast to a previous *in vitro* study in which passage of an 8 French Trac-Wright catheter through the relatively nondiseased portion of a superficial femoral artery in an above knee amputation specimen did not produce significant distal particle embolization.

We have previously studied (unpublished data) the role of plaque morphology in the selection of patients for laser assisted balloon angioplasty procedures. High resolution duplex scanning techniques in 19 cases categorized plaques (Type I–IV) based upon the ratio of echolucency to echogenicity within the arterial lesion. Laser tip passage was successful in 10 of 12 extremities with soft (Type I) lesions but was accomplished in only three of seven hard (Type IV) lesions. Preoperative plaque morphology assessment may become essential for endovascular procedures. Desbrosses *et al.*[2] experienced all four perforations from their series in heavily calcified lesions and subsequently considered these lesions to be formal contra-indications for use of the Trac-Wright catheter.

At present the catheter is commercially available only in the 8 French catheter size which creates a 2.4–2.8 mm lumen. A 5 French system for tibial and distal popliteal lesions is being clinically investigated. A 10 French size to create a larger lumen (3.3 mm) in superficial femoral artery lesions and possibly obviate the need for balloon angioplasty will undergo animal testing in the near future. Although perforation has *not* been a clinical problem it often precludes successful recanalization and extensive engineering research is underway to convert the Trac-Wright system to an over-a-guidewire exchange catheter system.

COMMENTS

The issue of atherectomy vs simple recanalization has not yet been totally defined. By definition, atherectomy would imply the physical removal of atheromata. The Simpson catheter mechanically removes atheromatous material from the arterial lumen utilizing a cutting edge and collection chamber.[4] The Trac-Wright system (Fig. 10) appears to simply recanalize a patent channel through which adjunctive balloon angioplasty may or may not be utilized. However, as previously described, effluent studies have generated significant numbers and volume of particles in the distal effluent. In effect, the rotating cam tip has 'atherectomized' the arterial segment through which the catheter was passed with variable amounts of atheromatous material being embolized distally. Ahn *et al.*[5] in experimental canine work with the rotoblator demonstrated similar distal embolization of large numbers of minute

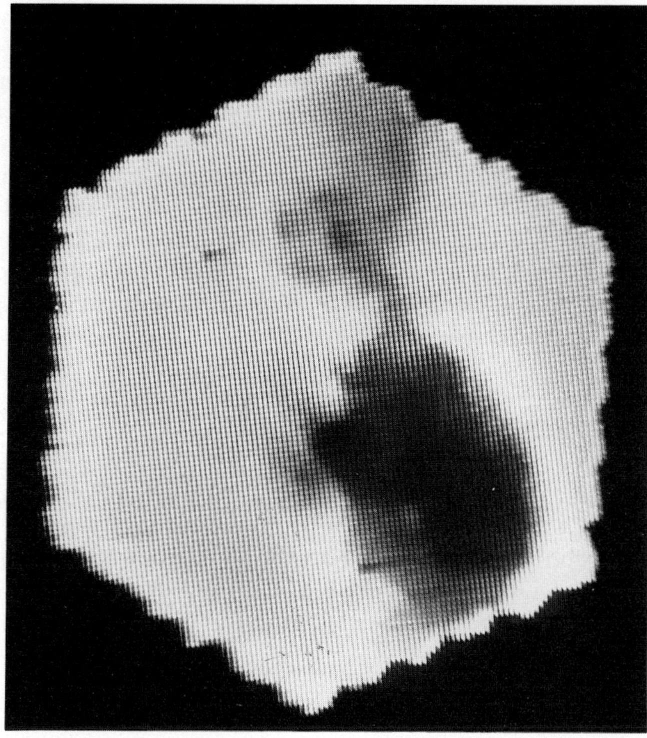

Fig. 10. Angioscopic visualization after Trac-Wright Catheter procedure.

particles. Isotope tagging of these particles revealed evidence of phagocytic removal of these particles into the reticuloendothelial system and in effect, a 'physiologic' atherectomy could be postulated.

SUMMARY

The Trac-Wright recanalization system has successfully recanalized (and/or atherectomized) total occlusions with approximately a 70% initial technical success rate in multiple US and European sites. In several series, the Trac-Wright recanalization system was utilized only after attempted passage of conventional guidewires had failed. The durability of the Trac-Wright recanalization system and other endovascular procedures remains an unanswered question. Our numbers of cases available for long-term follow-up are small and the standard error rates therefore high. Nevertheless, in patients with initial haemodynamic success, the life table analysis at 2 years reveals an acceptable cumulative primary patency rate of 57%. The potential for plaque morphology assessment in determining appropriate candidates for endovascular procedures may prove to be extremely beneficial. In addition, continued research to understand and manipulate the healing response in the recanalized artery may ultimately improve long-term patency rates with these procedures.

Patient follow-up to 37 months must be considered 'preliminary' in a surgical specialty where 5- and 10-year results are the accepted norm. Early results are clear that this technology in its present state cannot compare with the long-term patency of the gold standard of autogenous femoropopliteal bypass procedures. The questions to be answered of this technology, however, involve continued evaluation of the various endovascular devices results, taking into consideration their relative 'noninvasiveness' and lack of morbidity compared with traditional procedures as well as assessment of the future potential of these devices. It is our opinion that appropriately trained vascular surgeons are best suited to provide the operative skills, informed preoperative and postoperative evaluation, and diligent patient follow-up that will help answer these questions.

ACKNOWLEDGEMENTS

Gayle Adcock PhD, Ashwin Trivedi MD, James Chappell, and Steve Roth, Department of Physiology, Eastern Virginia Medical School, provided the photograph and preliminary data for the effluent particle study table. Richard L. Feinberg MD, assisted with statistical preparation of life tables. We are especially grateful to Martha Wimett for her assistance in the preparation of the manuscript.

REFERENCES

1. Samson RH, Sprayregen S, Veith FJ *et al*: Inadequacy of the noninvasive hemodynamic evaluation of percutaneous transluminal angioplasty. Am J Surg 147:212–215, 1984
2. Desbrosses D, Petit H, Torres E *et al*: Percutaneous atherectomy with the Kensey catheter: Early and midterm results in femoropopliteal occlusions suitable for conventional angioplasty. Ann Vasc Surg 4:550–552, 1990
3. Chappell JE, Adcock GD, Trivedi AN *et al*: The Kensey catheter: Characterization of effluent particle number, size, and morphology following catheterization of human superficial femoral arteries. Vasc Surg 1990 (submitted)
4. Simpson JB, Selmon MR, Robertson GC *et al*: Transluminal atherectomy for occlusive peripheral vascular disease. Am J Cardiol 61:96–101, 1988
5. Ahn SS, Auth D, Marcus DR, Moore WS: Removal of focal atheromatous lesions by angioscopically guided high-speed rotary atherectomy. J Vasc Surg 7:292–300, 1988

Current Experience with the Intravascular Balloon Expandable Stent in the Peripheral Circulation

Julio C. Palmaz

The notion of repairing a vessel with a prosthetic tube can be found as early as 1894 in early attempts to restore patency with surgically implanted glass or metal tubes.[1] However, the original idea of placing a prosthetic tube through a fluoroscopically guided catheter must be attributed to Charles Dotter. His simple experiment in dogs consisted of placing coil spring tubes in hind leg arteries that remained patent over 30 months.[2] The significance of Dotter's contribution must be found in the fact that in the late 1960s percutaneous angioplasty was at its very beginning and its limitations were not as yet defined. A dozen years later, the experience accumulated in percutaneous angioplasty clearly indicated the limitations imposed by elastic recoil and dissection (Fig. 1). Published work on intravascular stenting at this time specifically addressed these problems.[3–7]

Although the basic principle of placing an intravascular device through a remote access site is quite simple, the present status of knowledge of biocompatibility, rheology, biomaterials corrosion and fatigue resistance, prosthetic surface thrombogenesis, and management of coagulation and platelet function, makes the task of bringing a new device to clinical application a rather complex one. Setting aside all government-monitored regulatory matters regarding intravascular devices, the ethical issues related to the clinical application of intravascular implants dictate the need for thorough compliance with rigorous steps toward this end. These steps must include studies on long-term fatigue failure, local rheological phenomena, prosthetic–host interphase, long-term patency in animals, models of atherosclerotic and fibrous stenoses, acute and delayed effects of low flow states, altered coagulation and platelet function, and physical alterations of the prosthetic surface.[8]

Preclinical investigation of the balloon expandable intraluminal stent (Fig. 2) supported clinical studies that were instituted as multicentre trials monitored by a sponsor (Johnson and Johnson Interventional Systems) and the US Food and Drug Administration. These study protocols were designed in an attempt to address the main limitations of balloon angioplasty. The following is a brief description of the current status of these trials.

STENTING OF THE ILIAC ARTERIES

During the past 3 years significant experience was obtained from a multicentre trial of iliac artery stenting. The materials and methods used have already been described in detail.[3] The main indication for the procedure was ineffective balloon angioplasty as defined by a lumen reduction of 30% or more of the diameter achieved by maximum balloon inflation and/or the persistence of a mean pressure gradient of

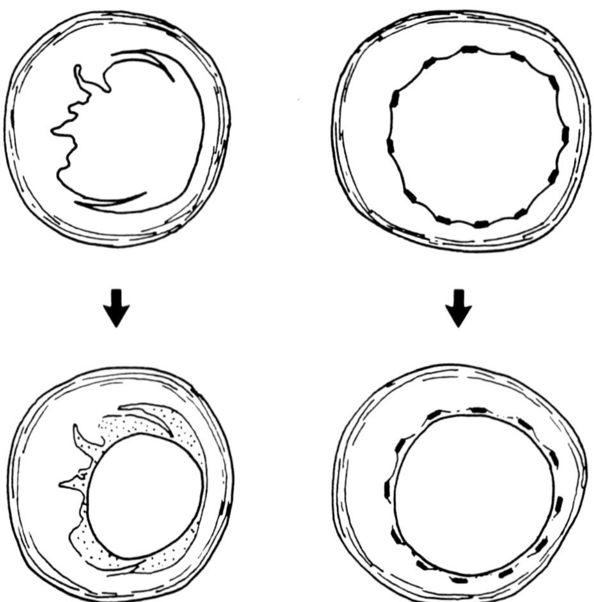

Fig. 1. Surface irregularities following balloon angioplasty lead to restenosis by thrombus deposition and late myointimal hyperplasia (left). Placement of a stent following angioplasty provides a smooth, cylindrical lumen that limits the amount of thrombus deposition and ultimately provides a wider lumen (right).

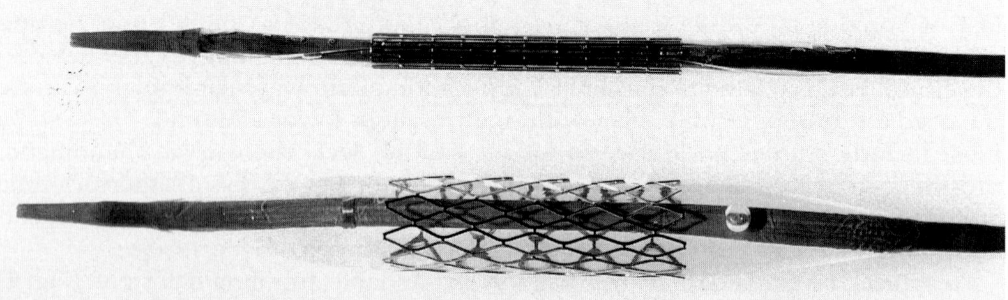

Fig. 2. Balloon expandable intraluminal stent (Johnson and Johnson Interventional Systems).

at least 5 mm mercury following the injection of vasodilators (Fig. 3). Additional indications were recurrent stenoses from previous balloon angioplasty, total iliac occlusion, and ulcerated plaque.

At the writing of this chapter, 294 consecutive patients with complete procedure and follow-up data were recruited. The mean age of this group of patients was 62.5 ± 10 years and was composed of 77.4% and 22.6% females. Atherosclerosis-risk profile in this patient population included 50% with coronary artery disease, 16% with cerebral vascular disease and 22% with diabetes mellitus (Fig. 4). Poor run-off vessels were present in 44.6% of the patients. Using a four-stage classification of peripheral vascular disease (Stage 1: asymptomatic, Stage 2: moderate claudication or claudication of more than 50 m, Stage 3: severe claudication or claudication of less

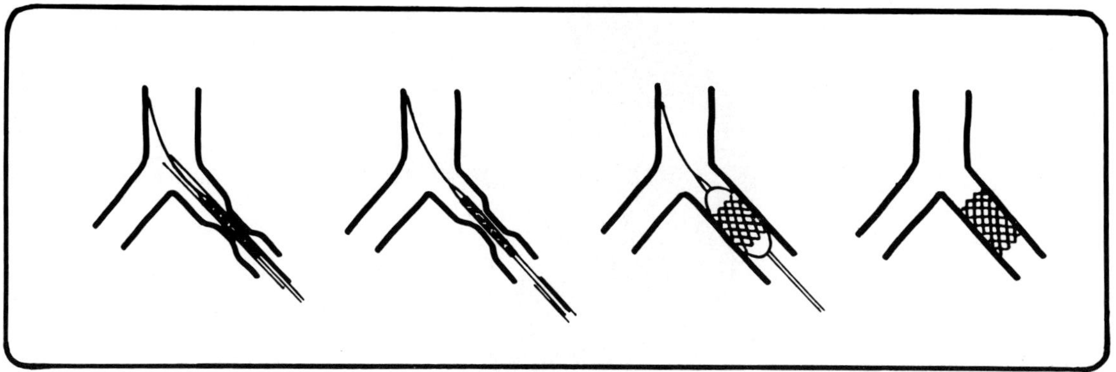

Fig. 3. Schematic representation of stenting of iliac artery stenosis.

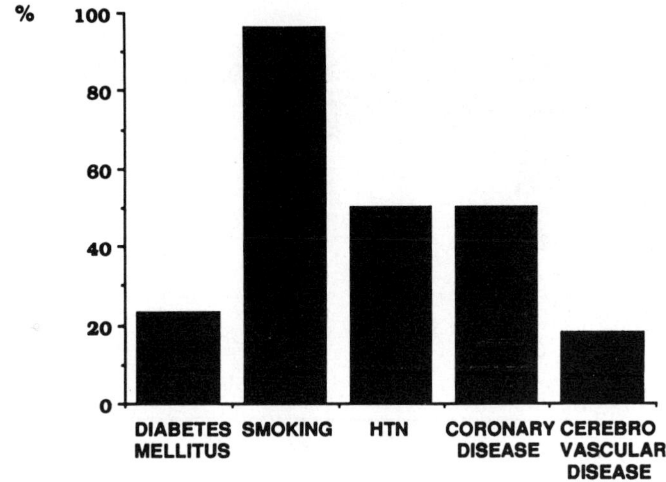

Fig. 4. Risk profile of the patient population with iliac artery disease.

than 50 m, and Stage 4: limb-at-risk of amputation as defined by the presence of rest pain, nonhealing ulcer, or gangrene), 44% of the patients had moderate intermittent claudication, 29% had severe intermittent claudication, and 27% had a limb at risk of amputation (Fig. 5).

The average iliac artery stenosis was 82.5 ± 15% and the average lesion length was 2.9 ± 2.6 cm. These lesions were unilateral in 257 patients and bilateral in 38. They were located in the common iliac artery in 71.7%, in the external iliac artery in 18.1% and in both in 10.2% of the patients. An average of 1.7 ± 1 stent per patients were placed, with 57% of the patients receiving one stent, 30% two stents, 5% three stents, 4% four stents, 2% five stents, 1% six stents, and 1% seven stents (Fig. 6). Transluminal pressure gradient across the lesions treated decreased from an average of 38.5 ± 24 ml of mercury to 1.5 ± 3 ml of mercury following stenting.

Clinical follow-up was carried out to an average of 10.7 ± 8.4 months (maximum 39 months) showing cumulative clinical success (success was defined as an increase

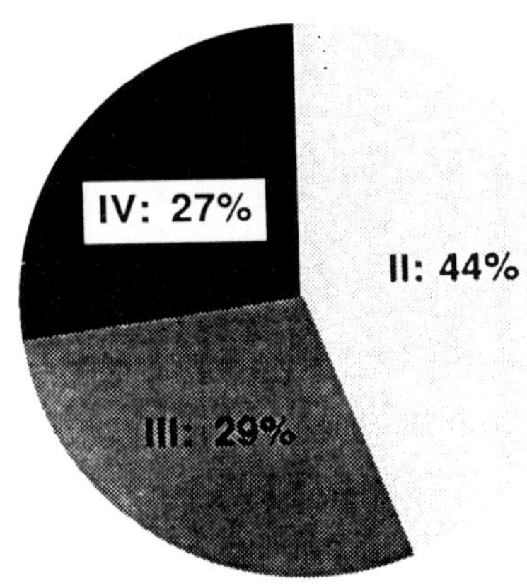

Fig. 5. Distribution of ischaemic staging in patients with iliac artery disease.

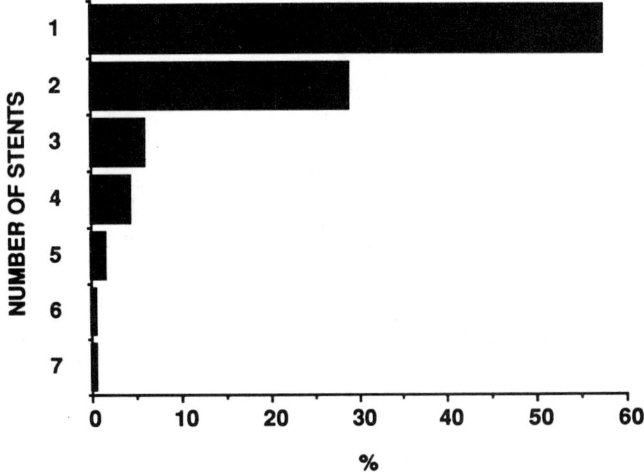

Fig. 6. Distribution of the number of stents employed per patient in the iliac stent trial.

of at least one clinical stage following treatment) of 78% at 20 months and 68% at 36 months (Fig. 7).

Using the generalized Wilcoxon test to compare product limit curves of clinical success between diabetics and nondiabetics, a significant difference was observed (Fig. 8). All other paired comparisons among risk factors and symptoms, yielded no significant differences. Comparison between clinical success of patients with stents in the common iliac artery as opposed to those with stents in the external iliac artery approached significance.

As part of the study protocol, the patients were offered an arteriogram 6-months after implant. Angiography was obtained in 48.1% of the patients at an average of 8.4±5.1 months following stenting. If patency was defined as a minimal luminal diameter equal or larger than 50% of the immediate poststenting diameter, patency was obtained in 94.2% of the patients. If the criterion for patency was set at 30% minimal luminal diameter, then patency was present in 85.6% of the

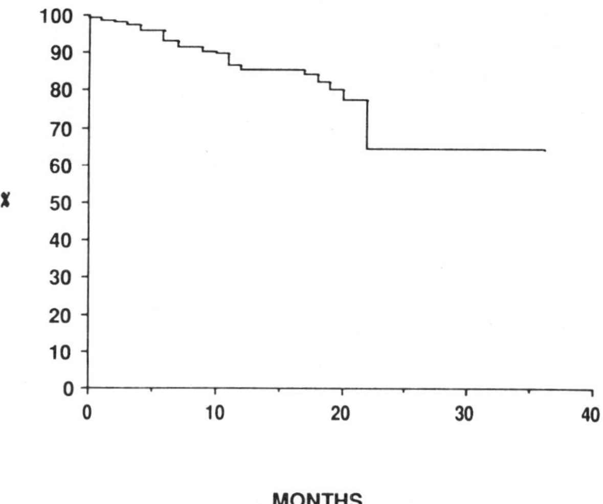

Fig. 7. Product-limit curve of clinical success in patients receiving iliac artery stenting. (SEM = < 10% for all points.)

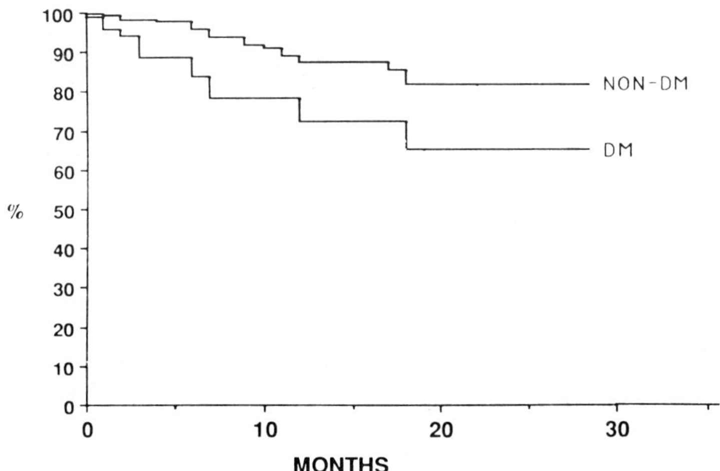

Fig. 8. Product-limit curves of clinical success following iliac artery stenting in patients with and without diabetes mellitus. The curves are significantly different by the generalized Wilcoxon test ($p = 0.006$) (SEM = < 10% for all points).

patients. The overall intimal thickness calculated as (stent diameter–stent lumen/2) was 0.65 mm.

Complications

Overall procedure complications occurred in 13.2% of the patients. In 10.2% of the patients, the complications were procedure related as follows:

six groin haematomas,
five distal embolizations,
three groin pseudo-aneurysms,
one groin AV fistula,
two puncture-site thromboses,
two puncture-site lacerations,
four angiographic extravasations or clinical evidence of bleeding at the angioplasty site,
two missed targets,
one subintimal dissection,
two contrast-induced renal failures,
one surgical arteriotomy bleed,
one arterial graft thrombosis.

In 3% of the patients, complications were directly related to a stent, including five stent thromboses, one dissection starting at the distal end of the stent, and three pseudo-aneurysms at the level of the stent. In all of these three cases, the pseudo-aneurysm occurred after stenting completely occluded iliac arteries recanalized by hot tip laser procedures.

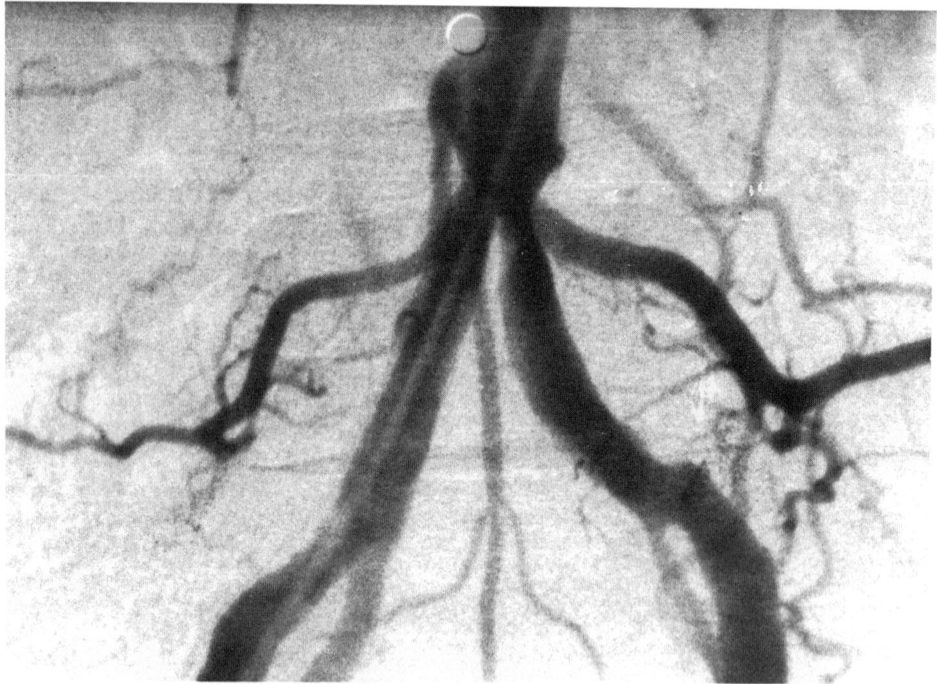

Fig. 9. Abdominal aortic bifurcation of a 64-year-old male with recurrent left lower extremity intermittent claudication following bilateral iliac artery balloon angioplasty 12 months prior to this procedure. The distal aortic diameter was 10.5 mm after correction for magnification. Intraluminal mean pressure gradients were 18 mm of mercury across the right common iliac artery stenosis and 11 mm across the left.

Amputation rate was 0.7% (two patients). One above the knee amputation occurred in a patient following stenting, and another patient had below the knee amputation 4 months following stenting. The 30-day mortality in the overall trial was 1.7%, or five patients. Two deaths were directly related to the stent procedure including one anaphylactic reaction to contrast injection, and one fatal episode of sepsis following an infected groin haematoma. Mortality rate beyond 30 days was 3.4%, or 10 patients. None of these deaths were related to the stent procedure.

Comment

Although longer follow-up is needed to definitely establish the safety and efficacy of iliac artery stenting, the experience accumulated by the co-operative trial suggests that the procedure is most useful in complete iliac occlusions,[10] long irregular stenoses, ulcerated plaques, and postangioplasty dissections.[11] Stents were also found useful in the treatment of distal aortic stenosis involving the origin of common iliac arteries (Figs 9–12).

Balloon angioplasty should always be tried prior to stent placement with the possible exception of ulcerated plaques. One purpose of preliminary angioplasty with the same balloon diameter as the one used to deploy the stent, is to test the

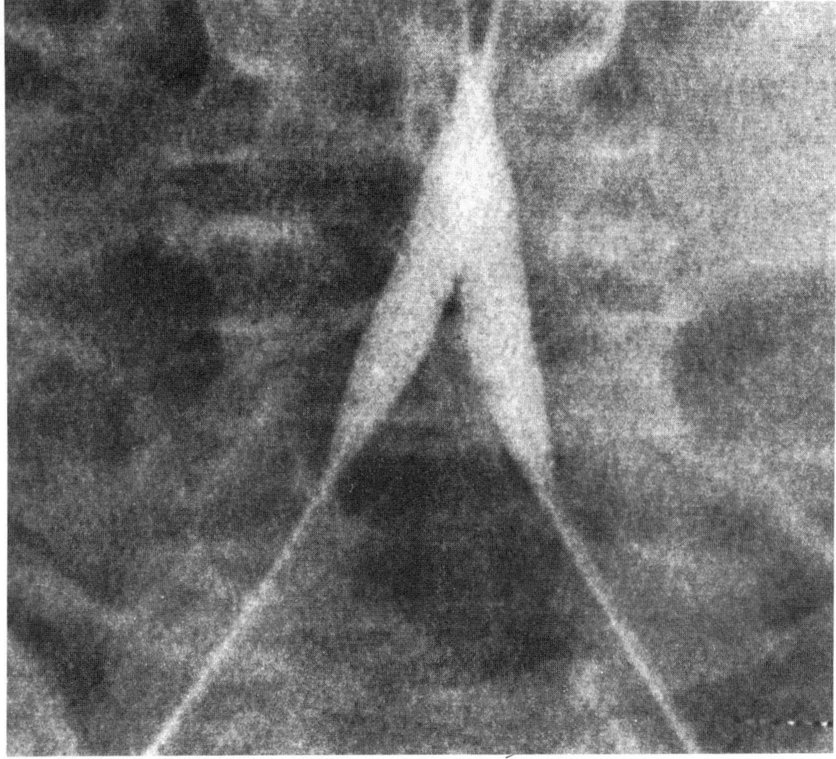

Fig. 10. Bilateral 'kissing' balloon angioplasty with 8 mm balloons.

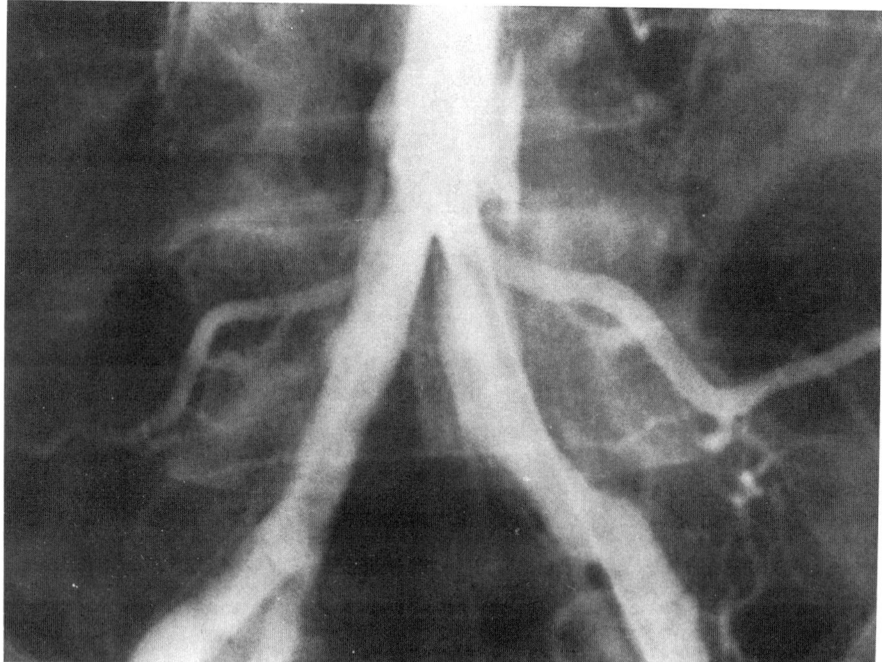

Fig. 11. Postangioplasty aortogram demonstrating subintimal dissection in the left distal aortic wall and persistence of the left proximal iliac stenosis.

distensibility of the arterial segment by monitoring pain sensation. An additional purpose is the prevention of stenting of those lesions that respond well to angioplasty. Localized short concentric stenoses of the iliac arteries are often treated adequately by balloon angioplasty alone. Caution should be exercised in placing stents after recanalization of long-term occlusion of the iliac arteries with atherectomy or laser since bleeding from a veiled perforation of the artery after this procedure may be intensified following stenting. In conclusion, the procedure is relatively safe in experienced hands. A high angiographic patency rate may be expected at 1 year, with moderate clinical success rate at 2 and 3 years following the procedure.

CLINICAL WORK IN PROGRESS WITH BALLOON EXPANDABLE INTRALUMINAL STENT

Renal artery stenting

In the USA, a multicentre trial of renal artery stenting approved by the Food and Drug Administration is currently underway.[12] Renal stents are mainly used in ostial atherosclerotic renal artery stenosis after failure of percutaneous renal balloon angioplasty (Figs 13–16). The experience accumulated is too small and the follow-up too short to draw any definitive conclusions. However, encouraging preliminary results and refinement in the materials and methods warrant the continuation of

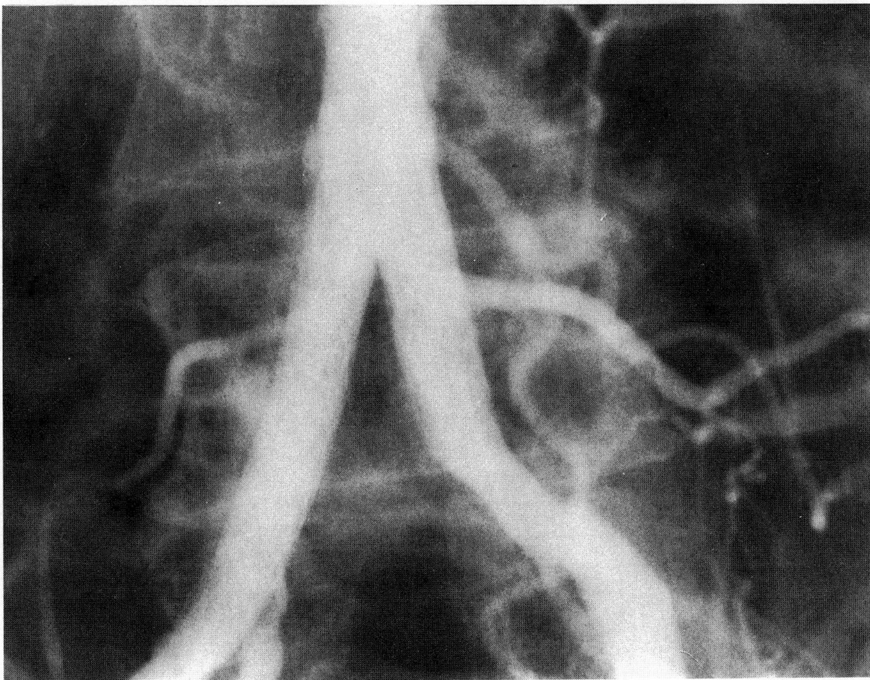

Fig. 12. Two stents placed in the right common iliac artery and one in the left provided restoration of the lumen of the aorto-iliac junction. The pressure gradients were reduced to zero bilaterally.

the trial. To date, a total of 28 patients with ostial renal artery atherosclerotic stenoses have received intrarenal stents. The average age of these patients is 66±8.8 years (48–80). This population includes 30 males and 15 females with renovascular hypertension of 10.1±10.3 years. The indications for stenting were previous percutaneous transluminal renal angioplasty with transient benefit in eight patients and technical failure following percutaneous transluminal renal angioplasty in 20 patients. The risk was marked by diabetes mellitus in 33%, renal insufficiency in 50%, smoking in 76%, coronary disease, peripheral vascular or cerebrovascular disease in 96%, and high blood pressure in 100% of the patients. The average renal artery stenosis prior to treatment was 75±16%. Following preliminary percutaneous transluminal renal angioplasty, the residual stenosis amounted to 46±18%. Following renal artery stent placement the residual stenosis was 9.8±12%.

The average clinical follow-up was 6.5±5.8 months (1–25). Clinical success was defined as the cure or improvement of hypertension and the persistence of success was evaluated by survival statistics. The cumulative success rate was 64.3% at 1 month, and 64% at 6 months. The 14 patients with renal failure as defined by serum creatinine equal or larger than 1.5 ml/dl had an average creatinine prior to stenting of 2.5±1.4 ml/dl. After stent, the average creatinine remained essentially unchanged. In five patients, the creatinine decreased, in three patients it did not change, and in six patients there was a slight increase.

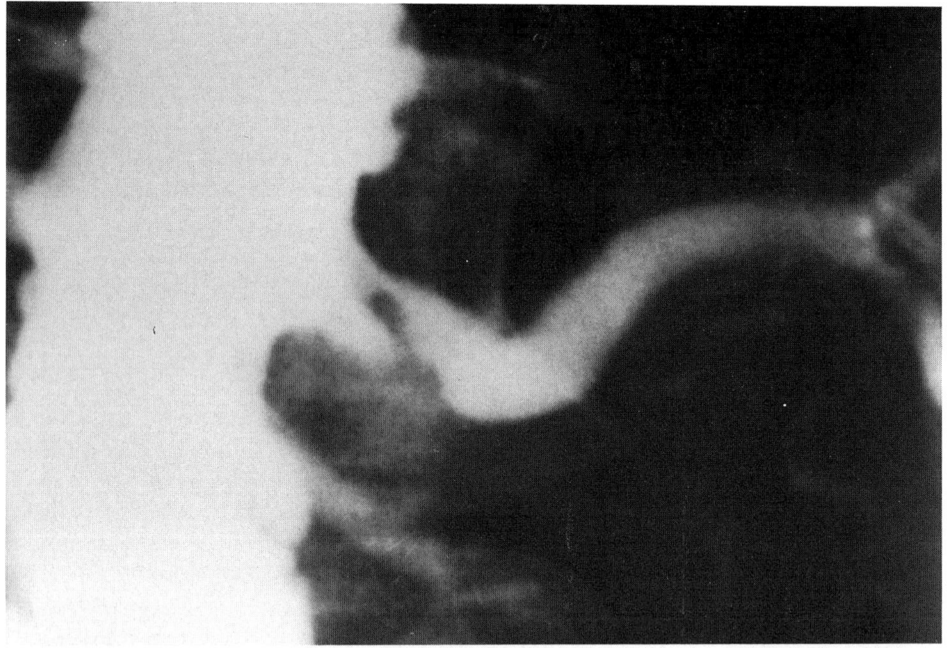

Fig. 13. Left proximal renal artery stenosis caused by an ulcerated atherosclerotic plaque in a 58-year-old man with hypertension and renal failure.

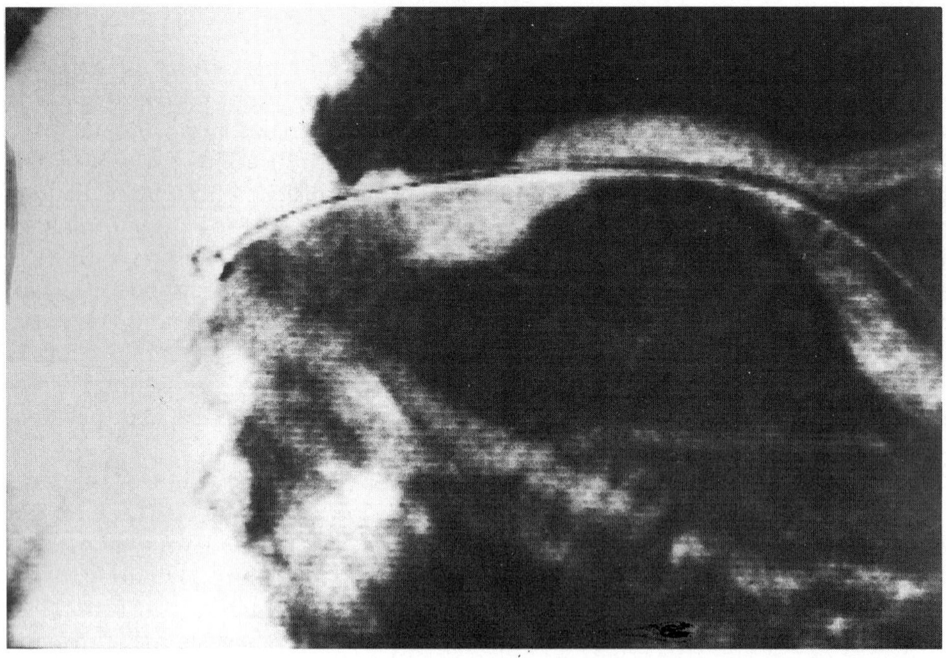

Fig. 14. Following percutaneous angioplasty a persistent filling defect is present.

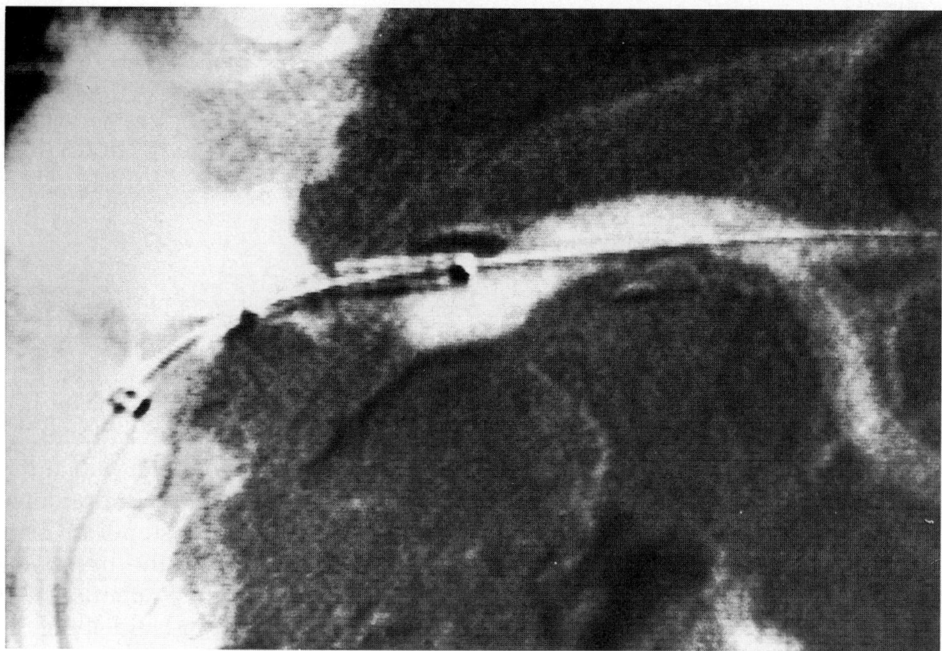

Fig. 15. A balloon-expandable stent mounted on a 5 French, 7 mm balloon is placed across the stenosis.

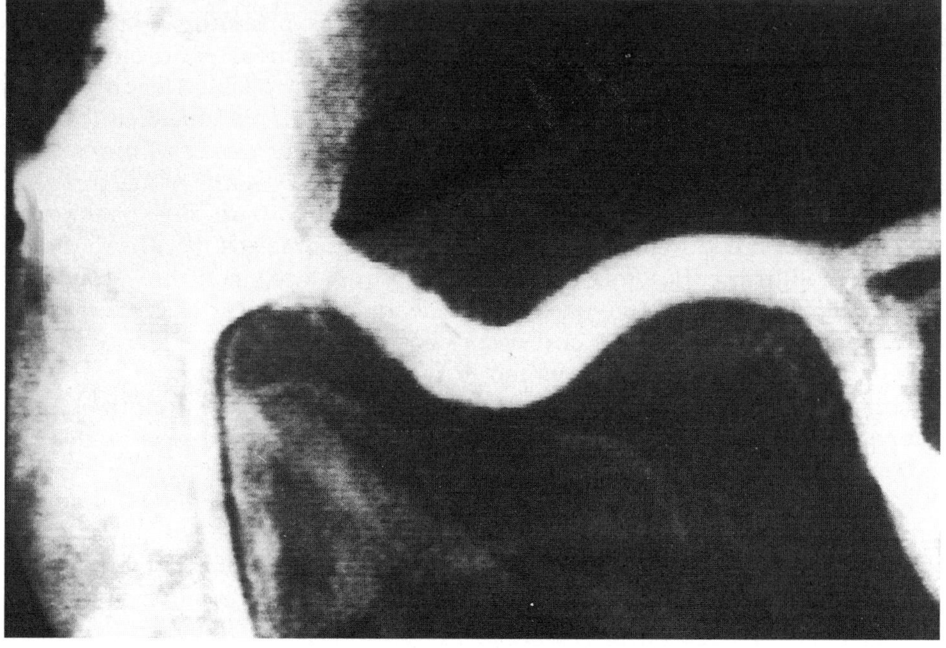

Fig. 16. Aortogram following stent deployment in the proximal renal artery.

Procedure complications amounted to 18% including two contrast-induced renal failures, one renal artery branch thrombosis with segmental infarct following guidewire injury, one transient sepsis, and one iliac dissection treated by iliac artery stent placement. Follow-up angiography was obtained in 18 patients at a mean of 7.5 ± 4.4 months. Restenosis ($\geq 50\%$ loss of lumen) occurred in seven patients (39%).

Transjugular intrahepatic portocaval shunt

A percutaneous transjugular intrahepatic portocaval stented shunt (TIPSS) is created by means of a combined jugular and transhepatic approach. The transhepatic portal vein access allows placement of a stone retrieval basket that serves as a target to direct the jugular needle tip. A long transeptal needle is introduced through the internal jugular vein sheath protected by an 8 French tapered Teflon catheter. The tissue tract is usually established between the proximal middle hepatic vein and the portal vein bifurcation or the proximal right or left portal branches. In the hepatic tissue tract joining the portal and hepatic veins, balloon-expandable stents are placed through 10 French sheaths in the jugular vein (Fig. 17). Most of the preliminary clinical experience has been accumulated at the University of Freibourg, West Germany, with additional centres contributing to this series from Heidelberg, and Miami.[13] Of 23 patients in whom the procedure was attempted, 18 had successful placement. No adverse effects were found among those in whom the shunt could not be established. The mean age of these patients was 61 years (34–84). Portal hypertension was due to alcoholic liver cirrhosis in 13 patients and postnecrotic cirrhosis in five. The metabolic Child's stage was C in nine patients, B in six patients, and A in three patients. Thirty-day mortality of this procedure was 11% (two patients). One death was due to adult respiratory distress syndrome 3 weeks poststent placement, and the other was related to uncontrollable bleeding through the liver capsule at the puncture access site. Following stent placement all 18 patients had an open shunt. The main portal-pressure prior to shunt was 28 ± 7 mm mercury. Following shunt placement the main portal-pressure was 15 ± 4 mm of mercury. Mean clinical follow-up was 11 months (2–27). At the latest follow-up—five patients have died. The causes of death include hepatocellular carcinoma at 4 months, perforated ulcer at 8 months, septicaemia at 13 months, shunt occlusion and oesophageal bleeding at 18 months, and one unexplained death in an 84-year-old patient. Except for the single stent thrombosis and oesophageal bleeding, no evidence of shunt failure or recurrent bleeding was noted in the surviving patients.

Percutaneous transjugular intrahepatic portocaval shunts were performed mostly in patients with poor metabolic status and recent history of life-threatening variceal bleeding. The procedure is still technically complicated and lengthy, but with increasing experience the technique is undergoing refinement. One such improvement is the avoidance of transhepatic portal vein catheterization for localization. At present, the portal vein bifurcation is localized by ultrasound preventing significant risk of peritoneal bleeding and allowing for shorter procedure time. Additional improvement was achieved by decreasing the needle size from 18 to 21 gauge and adding a tapered tip mandril (Richter GM, Heidelberg, Germany).

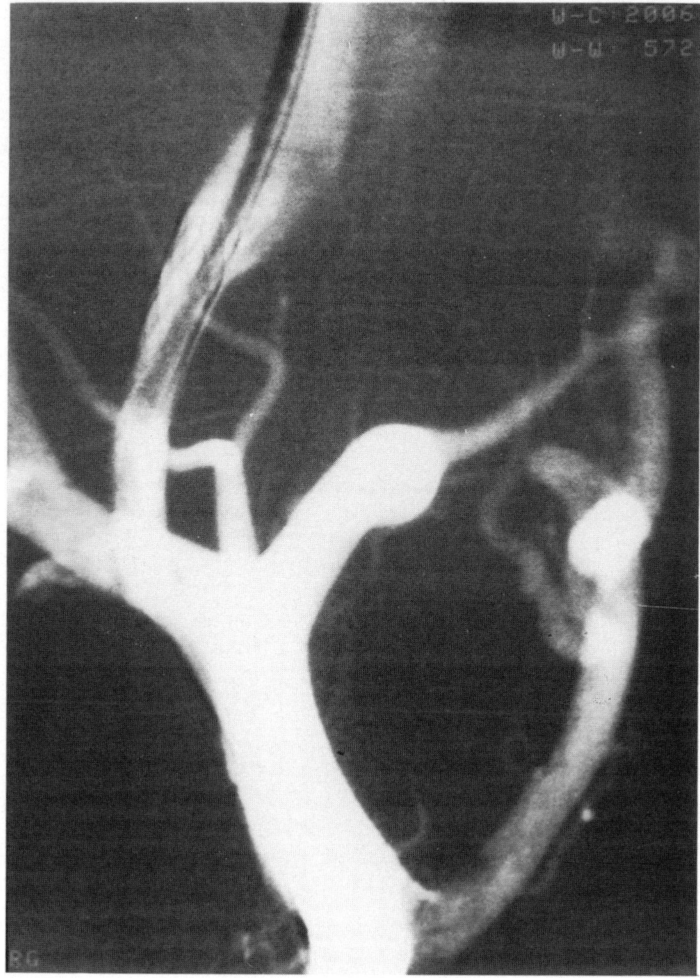

Fig. 17. Injection of contrast in the portal vein following transjugular intrahepatic portocaval stent shunt (TIPSS).

REFERENCES

1. Abbe R: The surgery of the hand. Transactions of the New York Academy of Medicine X:639–662, 1894
2. Dotter CT: Transluminally-placed coilspring endarterial tube grafts. Long-term patency in canine popliteal artery. Invest Radiol 4:329–332, 1969
3. Dotter CT, Bushmann RW, McKinney MR, Rosch J: Transluminally expandable nitinol coil stent grafting. Preliminary Report. Radiology 147:259–260, 1983
4. Cragg A, Lund G, Rysary J *et al*: Nonsurgical placement of arterial endoprostheses: A new technique using nitinol wire. Radiology 147:261–263, 1983
5. Maas D, Zollikofer Ch L, Largiarder F, Senning A: Radiological follow-up of transluminally inserted vascular endoprosthesis: An experimental study using expanding spirals. Radiology 152:659–663, 1984
6. Palmaz JC, Sibbitt RR, Reuter SR, Tio FO, Rice WJ: Expandable intraluminal graft: A preliminary study. Radiology 156:73–77, 1985

7. Wright KC, Wallace S, Charsangavej C, Carvasco H, Giantures C: Percutaneous endovascular stents: An experimental study. Radiology 156:69–72, 1985
8. Palmaz JC: Balloon-expandable intravascular stent. Am J Roent 180:1263–1269, 1988
9. Palmaz JC, Richter GM, Noeldge G *et al*: Intraluminal stents in atherosclerotic iliac artery stenosis: Preliminary report of a multicenter study. Radiology 168:727–731, 1988
10. Rees CR, Palmaz JC, Garcia O *et al*: Angioplasty and stenting of completely occluded iliac arteries. Radiology 172:953–959, 1989
11. Palmaz JC, Garcia O, Schatz RA *et al*: Balloon expandable intraluminal stenting of iliac arteries: The first 171 procedures. Radiology 174:969–975, 1990
12. Rees CR, Palmaz JC, Becker GJ *et al*: Restenosis of the renal artery after angioplasty: Treatment with the Palmaz balloon-expandable stent. Chicago: Radiological Society of North America, 1989
13. Richter GM, Noeldge G, Palmaz JC *et al*: Transjugular intrahepatic portocaval stent shunt: Preliminary clinical results. Radiology 174:1027–1030, 1990

The Medtronic-Wiktor Stent: A New Balloon Expandable, Flexible, Tantalum Stent

Bruce J. Brener, Victor Parsonnet, David E. Eisenbud, Frances L. Cross, Michael Trent, Kevin Lopyan, Michelle Ferrara-Ryan and Alex Villanueva

In 1985 a patient of ours underwent a thoracotomy to remove an aneurysm caused by dissection of the thoracic aorta. During his period of recuperation this patient, an engineer, began to think of ways to cure a dissection without surgery. He envisioned an intra-aortic mechanical stent to be inserted percutaneously that would close the intimal tear and push the dissected intima and media back to the adventitia, obliterating the dissected lumen and establishing flow through the true lumen.

This projected use of a stent co-ordinated with a worldwide interest in mechanical support of arterial lesions subjected to balloon angioplasty. Early abrupt failure and restenosis occurs in about 2% and 30% respectively after coronary angioplasty. These events have spurred the development of mechanical devices to prevent elastic recoil and stabilize dissection of the vessel after dilatation.

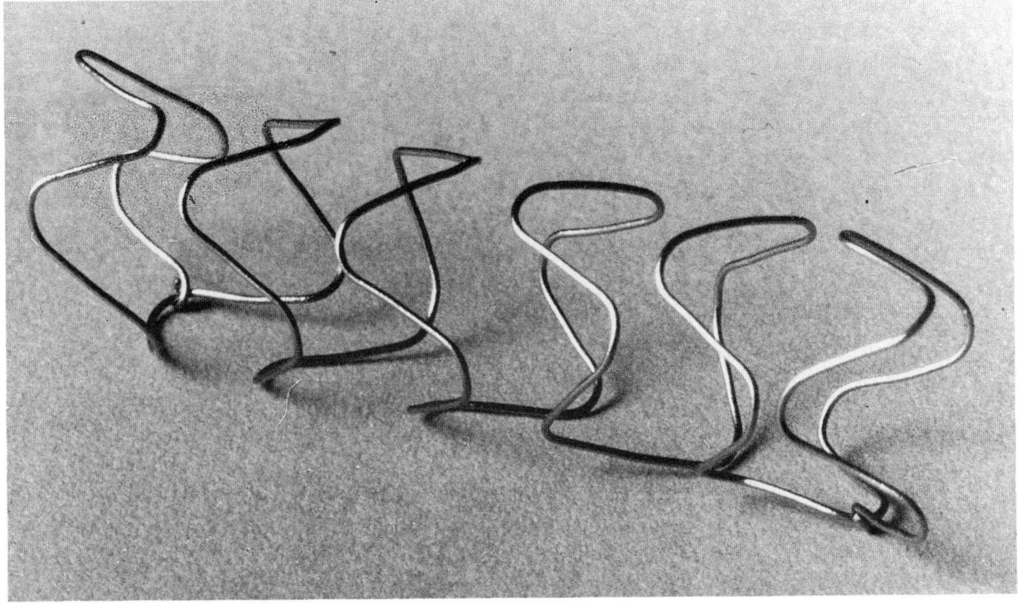

Fig. 1. The expanded stent has a coiled helial configuration with a secondary sinusoidal curve.

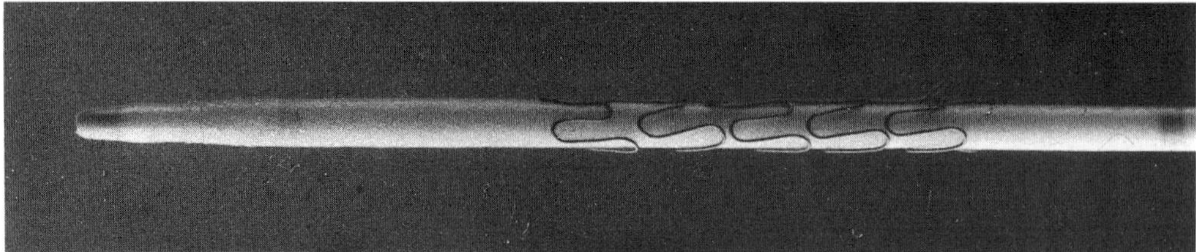

Fig. 2a. The stent is tightly crimped on a balloon catheter.

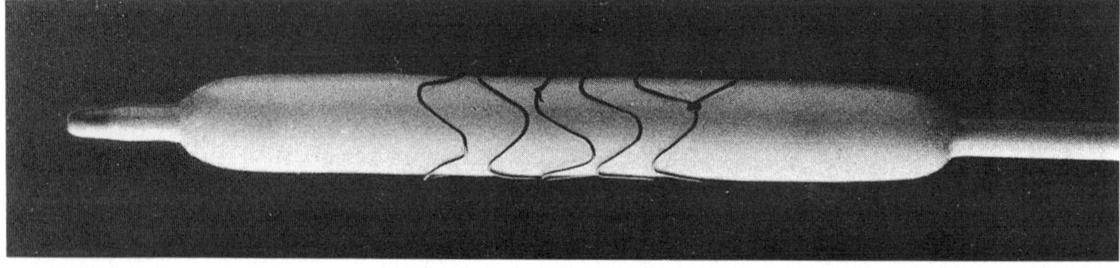

Fig. 2b. Balloon expansion partially straightens the sinusoidal wave, allowing the stent to expand to the diameter of the vessel.

Our experience with stenting has embraced several designs, each improving the previous model. Major considerations of all stents continue to include biocompatibility, ease of delivery, ability to expand from a contracted state, radiographic visibility, and suppression or induction of intimal hyperplasia.

After successful testing of a polyester mesh stent in animals,[1] a stainless steel and finally a tantalum stent evolved. This stent has the following characteristics. It is a continuously coiled flexible wire with a helical configuration and secondary sinusoidal wave and can be cut to any length. It is tightly crimped on an angioplasty catheter, and expanded by a balloon (Figs 1 and 2). It was hoped that it might be used to re-attach torn intima and media following balloon angioplasty, support an aortic dissection, hold open venous and arteriovenous strictures, and perhaps support a dilated prostatic urethra or trachea. The stent has been tested and studied in animals in three centres in the USA and accepted for clinical trial in Europe. Human trials for use in the coronary arteries have begun in the USA.

STENT CHARACTERISTICS

Stents are made from tantalum wire and meets the ASTM requirements for mechanical properties (tensile strength, elongation), chemical analysis, determination of contaminants, and purity of the base metal (minimum 99.70% Ta). Tantalum is nonmagnetic, highly visible under fluoroscopy, inert to body fluids and tissues, and corrosion resistant. Wire sizes are 0.005 and 0.010 inches in diameter and 17 mm and 2 or 3 cm in length. The ends are polished and tied back to the main stent body.

The percentage of open spaces of the stent ranges from 87% (4 mm–0.010 inch stent) to 95% (5 mm–0.005 inch stent). Radial strength has been shown to adequately resist spasm. Fine element analysis by computer modelling predicts that the device will not fail from stress-cycling in an arterial environment.

ANIMAL STUDIES

At least eight animal studies employing the Medtronic-Wiktor stent have been carried out. Seven of these tested the biocompatibility of the stent in arteries and one tested the reaction of veins to stent placement. After extensive bench-top design work, our first animal study of intravascular stents demonstrated the feasibility of inserting a polyester mesh stent into 13 dogs using a percutaneous technique.[1] The stents were well tolerated and had mild thrombogenicity that decreased as they were incorporated into the vessel wall. Neo-intimal thickness at 6 months was minimal. The self-expanding nature of this design made positioning the stent imprecise, and the material was difficult to visualize fluoroscopically. Concern over the strength of the material led to the use of metal wires.

The second study employed the current helical configuration with sinusoidal waves constructed from a single strand of 0.011 inch stainless steel wire. Twelve stents were placed in the thoracic aorta of 12 dogs through laparotomy and catheterization of the abdominal aorta using the Seldinger approach. Stents ranging from 10 to 35 cm in length were placed on commercially available balloon catheters. The balloon catheters with the stents crimped in place were directed into the aortic arch and

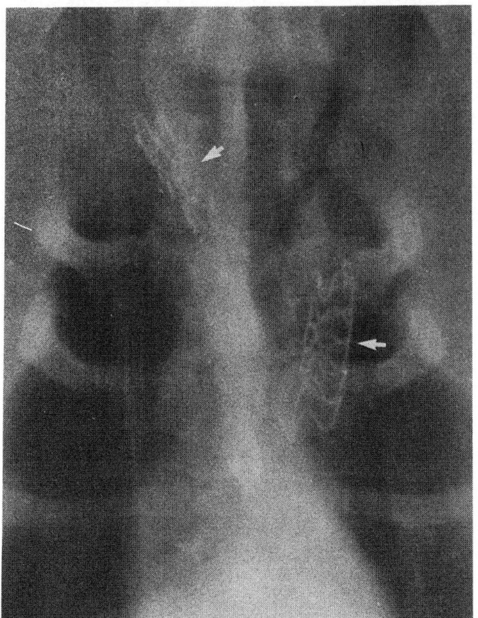

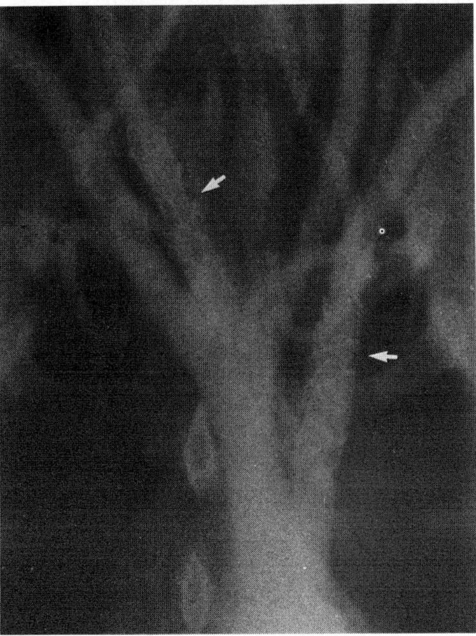

Fig. 3. Plain and contrast radiographs 3 months after implantation in mid-sized arteries demonstrate fully expanded stents with no migration, distortion or stenosis (0.010 inch wire).

descending thoracic aorta and the stents were deposited. Radiographic, gross visual, light microscopic and electron microscopic evaluations were performed after 6 weeks of implantation. The aorta and side branches traversed by the stents remained patent. The stents were incorporated into the aortic wall and covered by a thin neo-intimal layer.[2]

Sixty-nine tantalum stents were then placed in mid-sized arteries of 29 dogs.[3] These arteries included the brachiocephalic, subclavian, carotid and iliac arteries (Fig. 3). These stents were 0.005 and 0.010 inches in thickness and 1.5–3.7 cm in length, and were expanded in vessels 4–12 mm in diameter. Plain and contrast radiography and gross, light and electron microscopic studies were performed at 2 and 6 weeks, and 3, 6, and 12 months.

The tantalum stent was more readily visible than stainless steel during fluoroscopy. All vessels and side branches remained patent. No stent migration was observed. Changes in stent configuration were noted in eight of 69 instances. Two 0.005 inch stents in the carotid arteries were partly crushed by neck movement; two 0.005 inch stents dilated to 7 mm became elongated. The 0.005 inch stent may be too flexible when expanded in larger arteries and when exposed to twisting motions. Four 0.010 inch stents became deformed: two were incompletely dilated at the orifice of the conical-shaped brachiocephalic artery; the portion of stent not anchored at the orifice became stretched out into the aortic lumen. Two other stents became slightly deformed for no apparent reason.

At 2 weeks the stents and the vessels were covered by a thin layer of organized thrombus. At 6 weeks (Fig. 4) the lumen was covered by a confluent monolayer of cells which contained Factor VIII, confirming its endothelial structure. Under this layer was a neo-intima consisting of myofibroblasts in a sparse collagen network. Neovascularity was seen between the struts. At 3 months the vascularity was gone and the fibrous tissue was more atrophic. The neo-intima contained even fewer cells at 6 and 12 months (Fig. 4). Endothelium was again demonstrated. Neo-intimal thickness was less than 150 μm when 0.005 inch wire was used and less than 250 μm when the 0.010 inch wire was employed (Table 1). This measurement includes the thickness of the wire stents.

During the initial phases of this study stent misplacement occurred. The stent was easily retrieved with a biopsy forcep 2. The loose end of the stent was grasped and the stent was easily elongated and removed.

These stents have been employed in small arteries of dogs. Seventeen 0.005 inch stents 15 mm in length were placed in the coronary arteries and six in the renal artery

Table 1. Neo-intimal thickness after implantation of Medtronic-Wiktor stents in mid-size canine arteries

	0.005 inch Wire		*0.010 inch Wire*	
	No. of Arteries	*Mean (μm)*	*No. of Arteries*	*Mean (μm)*
2 weeks	4	129 ± 22	6	144 ± 14
6 weeks	4	149 ± 41	8	230 ± 105
3 months	6	97 ± 17	7	144 ± 26
6 months	13	129 ± 44	8	203 ± 43
12 months	4	149 ± 22	7	246 ± 27

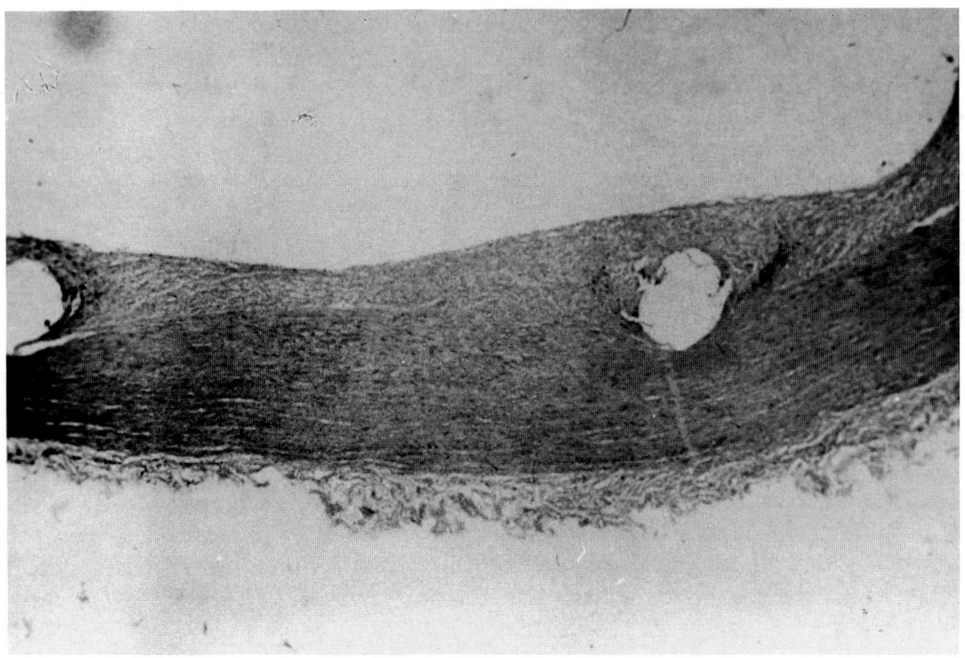

Fig. 4a. Microscopic study at 6 weeks demonstrates relatively thin neo-intima covered by endothelium. (Hematoxilin and eosin, ×3)

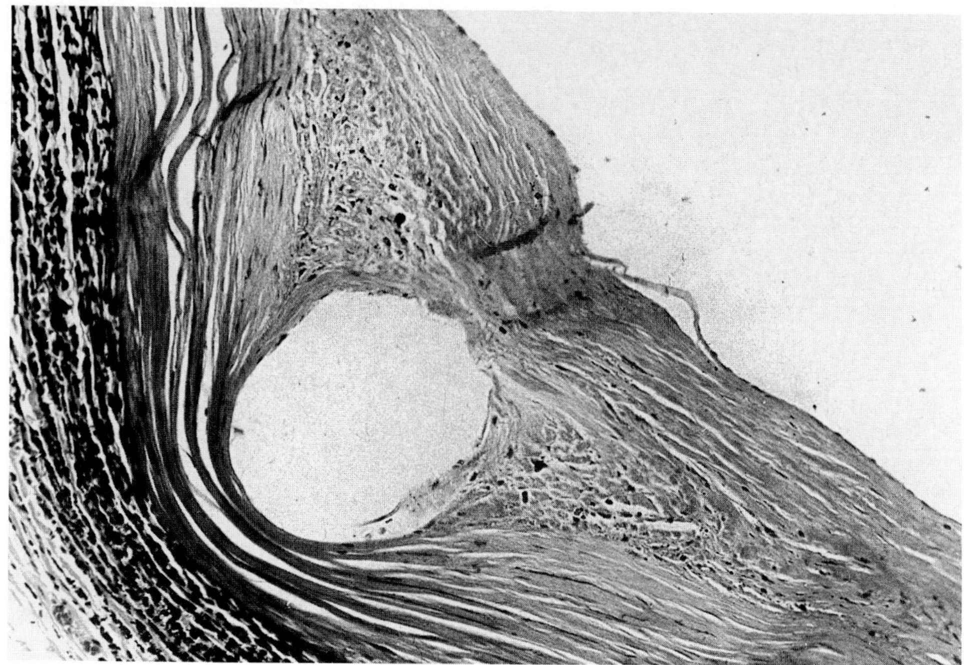

Fig. 4b. Microscopic study at 6 months shows mature fibrous neo-intima. (Trichrome, ×15)

of 17 dogs. Angiographic patency was confirmed in all instances at 2, 6, and 12 weeks, and at 6 months in the coronary arteries.[4]

Two studies have been carried out in pigs. White and colleagues[5] placed 0.005 inch stents in 19 coronary and 32 iliac arteries of 25 Yucatan miniswine who received atherogenic diets. Arterial diameter ranged from 2 to 4 mm. Angiographic patency was maintained in all arteries up to 32 weeks. Neo-intimal thickness went from 209 to 239 to 95 μm in 19 iliac arteries at 2, 6, and 24 weeks respectively. In 10 coronary arteries the neo-intimal thickness varied from 312, to 272, to 192 μm at 2, 6, and 24 weeks respectively (C. J. White, personal communication). This model is a rather severe test of the stent since balloon expansion alone in arteries of swine fed an atherogenic diet commonly results in stenosis.

Van der Giessen *et al.*[6,7] introduced 10 stents into 3 and 3.5 mm coronary arteries in pigs. Angiography at 4 weeks demonstrated patency and minimal decrease in mean luminal diameter (2.6 to 2.4 mm). The median neo-intimal thickness was 140 μm.

Stents have been tested in the venous circulation of dogs.[8] Thirty-six 0.010 inch stents were placed via the external jugular vein in the iliac veins and superior vena cavae of 12 dogs. Plain and contrast radiographs and light and electron microscopic studies were carried out at explant at 2 days, 2 and 6 weeks, and 6 months. All vessels

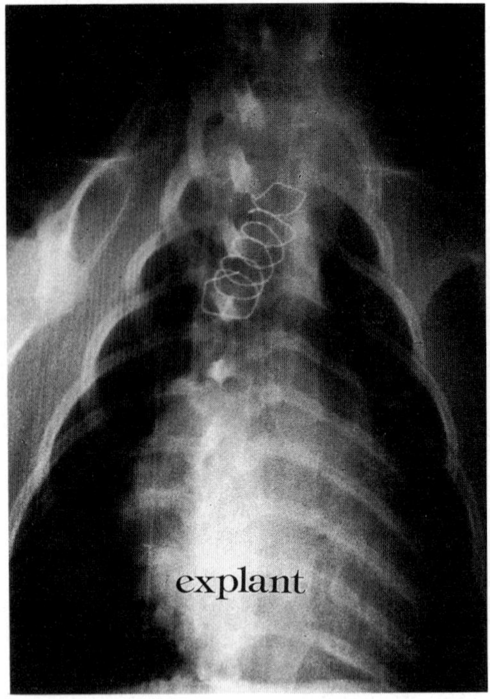

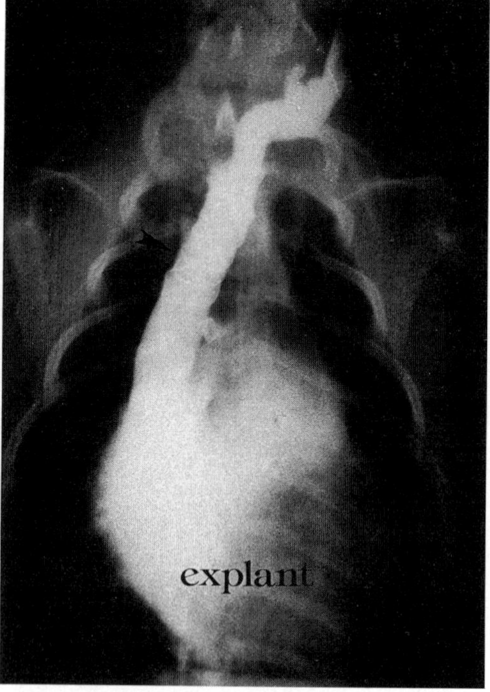

Fig. 5a/b. Plain and contrast radiograph of stents in the canine superior vena cava explanted at 6 weeks.

Table 2. Neo-intimal thickness after implantation of 0.010 inch Medtronic-Wiktor stents in canine veins

	No. of veins	*Mean (μm)*
2 days	9	78 ± 54
2 weeks	8	142 ± 62
6 weeks	9	210 ± 141
6 months	9	226 ± 111

and side branches were patent (Fig. 5). The metal was incorporated into the wall and covered with a thin neo-intima that was bounded on the luminal surface by endothelial cells. The thickness of the intima was varied from 78 ± 54 μm at 2 days to 226 ± 111 μm at 6 months (Table 2). There were two instances of stent migration from the superior vena cava due to improper sizing. Three stents in peripheral veins were deformed; two of the three vessels were stenotic but not occluded.

The Wiktor stent was originally designed to seal the intimal tear of an acute aortic dissection and to pin back the dissected intima. This use was tested in a dog model using the preparation of Blanton *et al.*[9] The thoracic aorta was opened transversely,

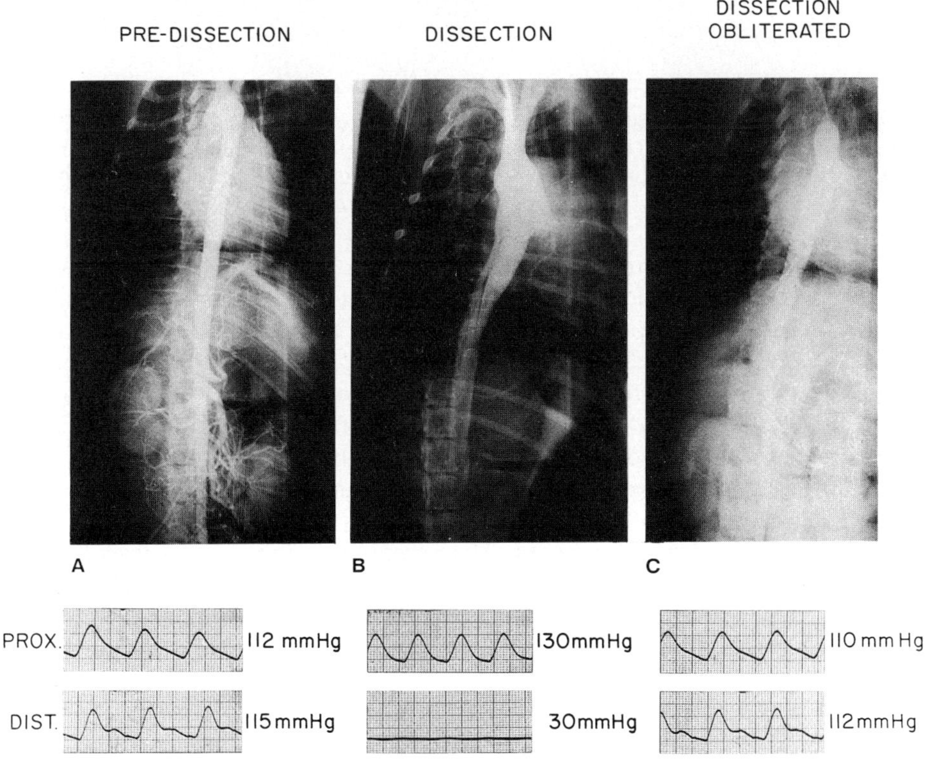

Fig. 6. Preoperative angiograms and pressure measurements (A) are compared with effect of experimental dissection demonstrated in (B). Dissection is obliterated and normal pressure is restored by insertion of a stent in the descending aorta (C). Reprinted with permission of the Journal of Vascular Surgery 11:707–717, 1990.

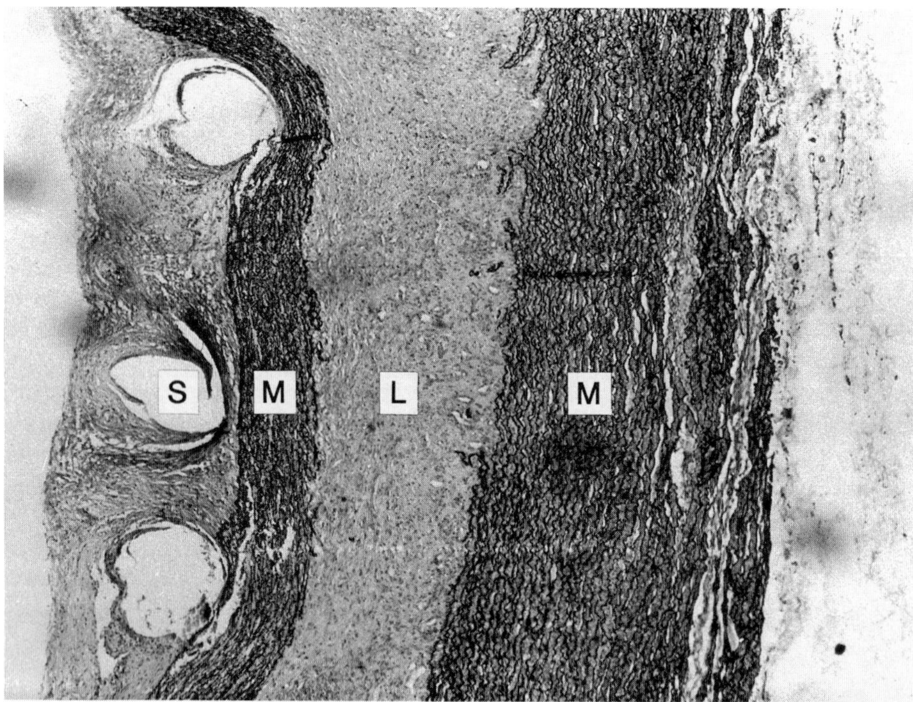

Fig. 7. Aortic photomicrograph 6 weeks after dissection has been obliterated. Portion of stent (S) shows the dissected lumen (L) between two layers of media (M) is obliterated and replaced with fibrous tissue (van Gieson elastic stain; ×80). Reprinted with permission of the Journal of Vascular Surgery 11:707–717, 1990

the media split with a spatula, the inner lining attached to the opposite wall with a suture and the arteriotomy closed. This uniformly created a dissection to the coeliac axis. In 12 dogs this acute dissection was treated with the immediate insertion of a balloon expandable stent which sealed the intimal tear and pinned back the dissected intima from the origin of the dissection to the diaphragm.[2] Ten of the 12 dogs lived to 6 weeks at which time angiography and autopsies were performed (Fig. 6). The dissection was obliterated as seen on angiography and light and electron microscopy (Fig. 7).

An additional 12 animals were allowed to survive after creation of the experimental dissection. Three dogs died within a week from rupture of the false lumen. In one animal a spontaneous cure occurred. The remaining eight dogs received a stent. In all cases the stent obliterated the false lumen both angiographically and on light microscopy.[2] Current experiments with chronic dissections revealed the need for a balloon mounted on a narrow catheter that can expand to a large diameter. Although aortic dissection is a rare disease, we feel that these experiments demonstrate the possibility of a percutaneous emergency treatment of this lethal entity. Certainly dissections in small vessels caused by angioplasty can be controlled.

HUMAN EXPERIENCE

Early reports on the use of the Medtronic-Wiktor stents in the human coronary circulation recently have been released. A multicentre co-operative study in Europe has begun using the stent in patients who have had recurrent coronary stenosis following a previous angioplasty.[10] Angiograms in 24 patients revealed four instances of acute thrombosis after redilatation and stent placement. The authors speculated that an increase in anticoagulation using aspirin, dextran, and heparin may prevent this complication.

Angiographic analysis of the stented vessels showed a significant increase in luminal cross-sectional area following angioplasty.[11] The intimal cross-sectional area increased from 0.7 mm^2 to 2.4 mm^2 after angioplasty and to 4.5 mm^2 ($p=0.001$) after stent placement. Long-term follow-up was not available.

SUMMARY

The Medtronic-Wiktor stent displays many of the desirable characteristics of an intraluminal device. It is highly visible, balloon expandable, longitudinally flexible, occupies less than 5–10% of the surface area of the vessel, can be cut to any length, shortens very little upon expansion, and can be easily removed. Animal studies have demonstrated its compatibility in arteries and veins of dogs and pigs. All vessels remained patent and neo-intimal reaction was minimal and not progressive. Initial clinical results are promising.

REFERENCES

1. Eisenbud DE, Parsonnet V, Wiktor D, Ferrara-Ryan M, Villanueva A: A polyester intravascular stent for maintaining luminal patency. Texas Heart Inst J 15:12–16, 1988
2. Trent MS, Parsonnet V, Shoenfeld R *et al*: A balloon expandable intravascular stent for obliterating experimental aortic dissection. J Vasc Surg 11:707–717, 1990
3. Cross FL, Parsonnet V, Chokshi S *et al*: *In vivo* evaluation of a new, flexible, balloon expandable tantalum stent in canines. Presented at the International Congress III, Lasers, Stents and Interventions in Vascular Disease Meeting, Phoenix, Arizona, February 1990
4 White CJ, Ramee SR, Mesa JE *et al*: Angiographic patency of a balloon expandable tantalum coil stent in coronary and renal artery of dogs. Circulation 82 (Suppl III):655, 1990
5. White CJ, Ramee SR, Banks AK *et al*: Angiographic patency of a tantalum coil stent. J Am Coll Cardiol 15:118A, 1990
6. Van der Giessen WJ, Straus BH, van Beusekom HMM *et al*: Neointimal hyperplasia within three different stents after implantation in normal coronary arteries of pigs. Circulation 82 (Suppl III):315, 1990
7. Van der Geissen WJ, Serruys PW, van Woerkens LJ *et al*: Arterial stenting with self-expandable and balloon-expandable endoprosthesis. Int J Cardiac Imaging 5:163–171, 1990
8. Lopyan KS, Cross FL, Shoenfeld R *et al*: Use of Medtronic-Wiktor stent in the venous system (Abstract) Radiology (Suppl) 177:151, 1990
9. Blanton FS Jr, Muller WH Jr, Warren WD: Experimental production of dissecting aneurysms of the aorta. Surgery 45:81–90, 1959
10. Bertrand M, Kober G, Scheerder Y, Uebis R, Wiegand V: Initial multi-center human clinical experience with the Medtronic-Wiktor coronary stent. Circulation 82 (Suppl III):655, 1990
11. Serruys W, Bertrand M, Kober G *et al*: Morphological change of coronary stenosis stented with the Medtronic Wiktor Stent. Circulation 82 (Suppl III):658, 1990

LONG-TERM RESULTS OF ARTERIAL RECONSTRUCTION

Long-term Functional Results Following Carotid Endarterectomy

Jesse E. Thompson and C. M. Talkington

Carotid endarterectomy is the most frequently performed peripheral vascular operation in the USA. That it can be performed with acceptably low operative mortality and morbidity has been amply demonstrated. In a recent survey of 15 960 carotid endarterectomies performed for all indications, Hertzer found the overall average operative mortality to be 1.4% and the perioperative stroke rate to be 2.2%.[1] In a number of individual series operative mortality was under 1% and perioperative stroke less than 2%.

The goals of carotid endarterectomy are to relieve transient ischaemic symptoms, improve neurologic function and prevent the occurrence of strokes in patients with extracranial cerebrovascular occlusive disease, thereby improving the quality of life and hopefully lengthening survival. To date it has not been possible to document any significant increase in survival of these patients by means of carotid endarterectomy because of the high incidence of concomitant coronary artery disease. The only demonstrated increase in survival in patients having carotid endarterectomy has been in those who have also had myocardial revascularization by means of coronary artery bypass grafting.[2]

It is the purpose of this chapter to review the long-term results of carotid endarterectomy as regards the incidence of transient ischaemic attacks (TIAs) and strokes in both symptomatic and asymptomatic patients using our personal experiences as well as selective ones taken from the older and the recent literature. Carotid restenosis will not be discussed as this matter is covered elsewhere in this book. Emphasis will be placed on the results in patients with preoperative classifications of transient ischaemia and asymptomatic stenoses.

FRANK STROKES

The functional results of any method of treatment for frank strokes are difficult to assess since the clinical course is so variable and the natural history of improvement so well known. A patient who survives an initial stroke usually improves, at least for a time and to some degree. Conversely, as the years pass, patients with cerebrovascular insufficiency who were previously normal or improved postoperatively, in some instances may deteriorate and worsen functionally.

Evaluation of the efficacy of carotid surgery for frank strokes is also hampered by the lack of adequate control studies. In our personal series of operated patients, among 201 hospital survivors followed up to 13 years, 26% were normal, 53% improved, 11% the same, 4% worse and 5% improved and then worsened either at follow-up or at the time of death. Thus 80% were normal or improved following operation.[3] It is generally estimated that unoperated patients with prior strokes suffer subsequent strokes at the rate of 10% per year.

TRANSIENT CEREBRAL ISCHAEMIA

Patients with transient cerebral ischaemia (TIAs) are ideal candidates for surgical therapy since disabling symptoms can be relieved and frank strokes prevented. In our own series of 289 hospital survivors followed up to 13 years after carotid endarterectomy, 77.2% were normal, 16.6% improved, 0.7% the same, 3.8% worse, and 1.7% improved and then worsened either at follow-up or at the time of death. Thus, 93.8% were normal or improved during long-term follow-up. The long-term stroke rate following operation was 5.4% or 1.6% per year.[3] It is generally accepted that 35 to 40% of untreated patients with TIAs go on to suffer frank strokes if followed up to 5 years or more, or at an annual stroke rate of 6–10% per year.[4]

Table 1 displays results in several of the older series of patients with TIAs subjected to endarterectomy, testifying to the beneficial effects of operation in reducing the occurrence of TIAs and lowering significantly the incidence of subsequent strokes. The incidence of long-term stroke following endarterectomy is thus about one-seventh of that to be expected in untreated patients with TIAs.

In an important recent (1989) study, Callow and Mackey[8] have reported the long-term results of endarterectomy in 404 symptomatic patients followed up to 12 years, averaging 56 months. Operative mortality was 0.7% and perioperative stroke morbidity was 2.7%. The annual stroke incidence, including perioperative strokes, was 2.1%. The life table stroke free rate at 5 years was 89.3% and at 12 years was 80.8%. In another study from the Cleveland Clinic the life table stroke free rate for TIA patients was 89.3% at 5 years and 76.1% at 10 years.[9] Stewart *et al.*,[10] reporting on 100 TIA patients followed for a mean of 5.5 years, gave an annual stroke incidence of 2% and a 5-year life table stroke free rate of 90%.

From all the available data, it appears that carotid endarterectomy is effective in the treatment of transient ischaemic attacks, by abolishing the vast majority of ischaemic episodes and reducing significantly the expected occurrence of strokes had these patients not been operated upon.

Table 1. Results of carotid endarterectomy for transient cerebral ischaemia — older data

Ref.	*Normal or improved long-term (%)*	*Long-term strokes (%)*	*Length of follow-up (years)*	*Stroke rate per year (%)*
5	89	5	1–11	NA
3	93	5.4	1–13	1.6
6	94	5.7	1–10	NA
7	88	10.6	5 (all patients)	2.1

ASYMPTOMATIC STENOSES

There is still controversy regarding the advisability of performing endarterectomy on patients with asymptomatic carotid stenoses as a method of preventing strokes. A great body of data has accumulated over the years and two randomized trials are under way at the present time.

It is clear that these patients, properly chosen, can be operated upon safely with low morbidity and mortality. In our own series,[11] in 167 cases operative mortality was 0, and the incidence of permanent strokes related to the operation was 1.2%. In a survey of the recent literature, in 2183 cases operated upon, operative mortality averaged 0.7% and the incidence of permanent operation related strokes was 1.25%.[12]

A number of long-term follow-up studies on asymptomatic patients subjected to prophylactic carotid endarterectomy are now available for review. In our personal experience,[11] among 132 operated patients followed up to 15 years (average 55 months) TIAs occurred in 4.5% and strokes, fatal and nonfatal, occurred in 4.6%, while 90.9% remained asymptomatic. This is an incidence of stroke of 1% per year. By contrast in 138 comparable control patients not operated upon and followed for 16 years (average 55 months) 26.8% developed TIAs, 17.4% sustained strokes, and only 55.8% remained asymptomatic.

In a recent survey of the literature the annual stroke rate among operated patients with severe degrees of stenosis (usually 70% or greater) followed for long periods of time ranged from 0 to 2%, with an average rate of 1.2% per year[12] Table 2. By contrast, the long-term stroke incidence per year in patients with comparable severe degrees of stenosis not treated by operation ranged from 2.6% to 9.5% with an average rate of 5.27% per year.[12] The rate of 1.2% among operated patients represents a 77% reduction in the rate of stroke to be expected had these patients not been treated by carotid endarterectomy.[12]

Callow and Mackey,[8] in their recent long-term study of 179 asymptomatic patients subjected to carotid endarterectomy and followed up to 12 years (average 56 months), reported operative mortality of 0.56%, perioperative stroke rate of 1.1%, and long-term stroke incidence of 1.4% per year, results similar to those quoted above.

Table 2. Long-term follow-up stroke incidence per year in patients with asymptomatic carotid stenosis treated by carotid endarterectomy

Ref.	*Criteria for operation: Degree of stenosis (%)*	*Stroke rate per year (%)*
13	Severe	1.2
11	>50	1
14	>50	1.6
15	>80	2
16	>50	1
1	>70	1.4
17	>75	0
		Av. – 1.2

CONCLUSION

Carotid endarterectomy is an effective procedure for stroke prevention on the basis of 30 years of careful observation and experience. When critical selection of patients for operation is made according to proper indications, when angiography is performed by skilful persons, and when appropriate surgical therapy is carried out by well-trained experienced operators, the operative mortality and morbidity rates are low and acceptable, the immediate results are excellent, and long-term results are quite favourable when compared with the natural history of the untreated patient. Carotid endarterectomy is an established, worthwhile procedure.

REFERENCES

1. Hertzer NR: Presidential address: Carotid endarterectomy—a crisis in confidence. J Vasc Surg 7:611–619, 1988
2. Hertzer NR, Loop FD, Taylor PC, Beven EG: Combined myocardial revascularization and carotid endarterectomy. Operative and late results in 331 patients. J Thorac Cardiovasc Surg 85:577–589, 1983
3. Thompson JE, Austin DJ, Patman RD: Carotid endarterectomy for cerebrovascular insufficiency: Long-term results in 592 patients followed up to thirteen years. Ann Surg 172:663–679, 1970
4. Millikan CH: Treatment of occlusive cerebrovascular disease. *In* Cerebrovascular Survey Report, McDowell F, Caplan LR (Eds). Bethesda, Maryland: National Institute of Neurological Disorders and Strokes, pp. 149–187, 1985
5. DeBakey ME, Crawford ES, Cooley DA *et al*: Cerebral arterial insufficiency: one to 11-year results following arterial reconstructive operation. Ann Surg 161:921–945, 1965
6. Wylie EJ, Ehrenfeld WK: Extracranial Occlusive Cerebrovascular Disease, Philadelphia: W. B. Saunders, 1970
7. DeWeese JA, Rob CG, Satran R *et al*: Results of carotid endarterectomies for transient ischemic attacks—five years later. Ann Surg 178:258–264, 1973
8. Callow AD, Mackey WC: Long-term follow-up of surgically managed carotid bifurcation athersclerosis. Ann Surg 210:308–316, 1989
9. Hertzer NR, Aronson R: Cumulative stroke and survival 10 years after carotid endarterectomy. J Vasc Surg 2:661–668, 1985
10. Stewart G, Ross-Russell RW, Browse NL: The long-term results of carotid endarterectomy for transient ischemic attacks. J Vasc Surg 4:600–605, 1986
11. Thompson JE, Patman RD, Talkington CM: Asymptomatic carotid bruits—long-term outcome of patients having endarterectomy compared to unoperated controls. Ann Surg 188:308–316, 1978
12. Thompson JE: Carotid endarterectomy for asymptomatic carotid stenosis: an update. J Vasc Surg (in press)
13. Javid H, Ostermiller WE, Hengesh JW *et al*: Carotid endarterectomy for asymptomatic patients. Arch Surg 102:389–391, 1971
14. Moore DJ, Miles RD, Gooley NA, Sumner DS: Noninvasive assessment of stroke risk in asymptomatic and nonhemispheric patients with suspected carotid disease. Five-year follow-up of 294 unoperated and 81 operated patients. Ann Surg 202:491–504, 1985
15. Moneta GL, Taylor DC, Nicholls SC *et al*: Operative versus nonoperative management of asymptomatic high-grade internal carotid artery stenosis: Improved results with endarterectomy. Stroke 18:1005–1010, 1987
16. Rosenthal D, Rudderman R, Borreo E *et al*: Carotid endarterectomy to correct asymptomatic carotid stenosis: Ten years later. J Vasc Surg 6:226–230, 1987
17. Caracci BF, Zukowski AJ, Hurley JJ *et al*: Asymptomatic severe carotid stenosis. J Vasc Surg 9:361–366, 1989

Late Failure After Carotid Endarterectomy

Thomas S. Riles

Late failure after carotid endarterectomy may be defined in several ways. Postoperative neurologic symptoms from carotid bifurcation disease clearly constitute a failure, since the primary goal of the operation was to prevent strokes and transient ischaemic attacks. Failure of the operation, however, cannot only be defined in terms of recurrent symptoms. Asymptomatic patients with residual or recurrent carotid bifurcation lesions may also be considered failures. Most patients consent to carotid surgery with the view that if the operation is not performed, they face a 20–30% risk of stroke during their remaining year. If, after the operation has been successfully performed, the patient is found to have a high grade stenosis at the site of the surgery, an occlusion of the carotid artery, an aneurysm or intraluminal thrombus, the risk of stroke continues to exist. For these individuals the operation has failed in its goal of improving their prospects for good health in the future.

The first step in managing late failure of carotid endarterectomy is prevention. In general, lesions found after surgery are due to either a technical failure of the operation or a proliferation of hyperplasia or new plaque at the site of the endarterectomy. At the time that a surgeon is asked to evaluate a patient with a postoperative lesion, it is often difficult to differentiate between technical failures and recurrent pathology. In many cases, there is a combination of both. A clamp injury, for example, may initiate a host response which, years later, results in a recurrent stenosis. In as much as there is very little one can do to prevent the progression of myo-intimal hyperplasia and atherosclerotic degeneration in the postoperative patient, it is very important to avoid technical mishaps which may precipitate recurrent disease in future years.

TECHNICAL PROBLEMS RELATED TO LATE FAILURES

Most of our knowledge of technical failures of carotid endarterectomy come from the analysis of patients with perioperative stroke.[1] In these patients, the failures are usually sufficiently severe that, within minutes to hours, thrombus forms and cerebral ischaemia results from either embolization of thrombus or flow reduction due to occlusion of the internal carotid artery. It is likely that only a fraction of patients with technical problems will develop early postoperative symptoms. When oculoplethysmography (OPG) first became available, we studied 200 consecutive patients several hours after surgery. If the OPG test was abnormal, an angiogram was performed. Two patients had asymptomatic thrombosis of the carotid artery within hours after surgery. Several others were found to have flow restrictive stenosis without symptoms. Had the postoperative studies not been performed, these patients would have been considered surgical successes. Also, had the problems not been

Table 1. Technical problems which may result in late failure after carotid endarterectomy

Incomplete removal of the plaque
Ledge at the proximal or distal end of the endarterectomy
Kinking of the internal carotid after endarterectomy
Irregular or rough surface at site of the endarterectomy
Shunt or clamp injury
Stenosis from closure of arteriotomy
Aneurysm from expressive patch closure

recognized until several years later, the failures would have been attributed to recurrent disease rather than a residual of the first operation.

In some instances the technical problem is less severe and not recognized even with early postoperative testing. Over time, the host may respond to the technical defect with smooth muscle cell proliferation or thrombus formation. With the proliferative response, a lesion becomes recognizable in follow-up.[2] Unless neurologic symptoms develop, these late lesions may never be appreciated unless a follow-up study of the carotid artery is performed.

Surgeons experienced with carotid endarterectomy are familiar with the technical problems which may lead to failure, early and late.[3,4] A list of these mechanisms of failure is given in Table 1. A variety of surgical approaches have been devised for their prevention. Although it is beyond the scope of this chapter, several of these mechanisms and techniques for prevention should be mentioned.

Incomplete removal of plaque is a sure means of postoperative failure. This is rarely a problem if adequate dissection of the carotid artery is performed. Mobilization of the hypoglossal nerve is usually necessary to reach a soft portion of the internal carotid artery distal to the plaque. If the complete plaque cannot be removed, or if a ledge exists at the ends of the endarterectomy, tacking sutures may be used to bring the endarterectomized adventitia up to the intima. Using the adventitia to cover the edge of the plaque. A smooth arterial wall is left which hopefully will result in laminar flow rather than turbulence at this point.

Surgeons are increasingly aware of the problem of kinking after removal of the plaque in a tortuous or redundant carotid artery.[5] Postoperative ultrasounds show that severe kinks may result in a stenosis and turbulence. Many believe that the turbulence from a kink may lead to myo-intimal hyperplasia.[2] There are several technical solutions to kinking. These include re-implantation of the internal carotid to a more proximal position on the common carotid artery, resection of a piece of the internal carotid or common carotid artery and plicating the internal carotid artery by sewing a pleat in the endarterectomized portion of the vessel.

Rough adventitial surfaces after endarterectomy are seldom a problem with a primary endarterectomy. If difficulty is encountered finding a suitable plane, or if there is calcification of the adventitial layer, one may use an interposition graft as an alternative to endarterectomy.

With regard to clamp injuries, problems may result from improper design or improper use. Vascular clamps and shunt clamps used on the carotid artery should be designed to require two to three ratchets to approximate the jaws. This design permits gentle occlusion of the vessel and allows for various thicknesses of the artery. Misuse of any clamp or shunt may result in arterial injury. Restenoses at the sites of previous clamp placement suggest that the proliferative response may have resulted from a clamp injury.

Perhaps no facet of carotid surgery is as controversial as the choice of closure of the arteriotomy. Many series have shown excellent results with primary closure of the artery.[6,7] Several recent studies, however, suggest that, in some hands, results are superior with patch closure. Eikelboom and associates randomized primary vs patch closure.[8] They found not only a lower incidence of perioperative complications, but also demonstrated a lower incidence of restenosis (4% vs 21%) in the patched group. Fode and associates reported on a multicentre series of carotid endarterectomies.[9] The stroke and death rate was 6.6% for the patients who had primary closure and 2.3% for those closed with a vein patch. The incidence was 7%, with a fabric patch closure.

Lord and associates have performed a randomized study of 140 carotid endarterectomies, comparing primary closure to vein patch closure and polytetrafluoroethylene patch closure.[3] They found that neurologic complications were more frequent in the nonpatched group, but the differences between groups were not statistically significant. Follow-up intravenous digital angiograms showed a residual stenosis of 30–50% in 18% of the nonpatched group, whereas none of the patch closures showed residual stenosis ($p > 0.01$). Although others feel the patch is unnecessary or should be reserved only for selected cases,[10] we continue to favour vein patch closure for most all carotid operations.

Although patching the carotid artery may reduce the risk of recurrent or residual stenosis, the patch may itself result in late failure of the operation. One of the problems of patching is the formation of aneurysmal dilatation of the artery in follow-up. Although the incidence is low, the aneurysm may lead to neurologic symptoms as laminated thrombus forms on the inner surface. The problem may be more severe with vein patches than synthetic patches. In the study by Lord and associates, the arteries with vein patch closure frequently had larger luminal diameters than those closed with fabric patches.[3] Although the late follow-up data from that study is not yet available, the authors suggest that leaving a large lumen will accelerate the formation of aneurysms in years to come.

HOST FACTORS RELATED TO LATE FAILURE AFTER CAROTID ENDARTERECTOMY

A variety of host factors have been examined with regard to recurrent disease after endarterectomy. Eikelboom and associates noted that recurrent stenosis was more common among women than men.[8] A similar observation was reported by Das and associates, although it was not statistically significant.[11]

Clagett and co-workers found that patients operated on young in life were more prone to late failure.[12] In their study the mean age at time of the initial surgery was 54.6 years for patients who developed recurrent disease compared with a mean age of 61.3 years for their entire series. This relationship has also been noted by others.[11,13]

Clagett and associates found the continuation of smoking to be a particularly significant factor for recurrent disease.[12] This was also noted by Eikelboom.[8]

Hyperlipidaemia and hypertension have also been cited as causes for late failure after carotid endarterectomy.[14–16] The significance of these factors has been a matter of debate.[12]

THE ROLE OF ROUTINE SURVEILLANCE AFTER CAROTID ENDARTERECTOMY

Routine evaluation of postoperative carotid endarterectomy patients has become increasingly common over the past decade. The introduction of digital subtraction, intravenous angiography, oculoplethysmography and carotid ultrasonography has provided a means of examining the patient repeatedly in follow-up without the risk of intra-arterial angiography. Using these techniques, the incidence of restenosis has been reported to be as low as 0% and as high as 29%.[3,6–8, 17–20] The vast range is attributed to a number of factors including the method of surveillance, the definition of significant stenosis, the length of follow-up and the surgical technique used for the initial operation (patch or primary closure). Controversy continues regarding the significance of these findings, and in particular whether or not asymptomatic late failures of endarterectomy represent a risk of stroke to the patient. In a recent multicentre study by Rosenthal and associates, postoperative ultrasound examinations were performed on 717 patients with a mean follow-up time of 37.8 months after surgery.[4] Significant stenosis (>50% diameter reduction) was identified in only 3.3% of the patients. Most of these patients were asymptomatic. Only 0.5% of the patients in the study had asymptomatic restenosis.

On the basis of studies such as these, some have concluded that the yield of useful information is so low that the cost of frequent follow-up evaluation of the endarterectomy patient is not warranted. This is especially so if one is of the opinion that re-operation should be reserved for the symptomatic lesions.

We have found annual follow-up examination with duplex scan to provide useful information. First, it has enabled us to recognize early failures which has led to improvements in the operative technique. Secondly, as years progress, the risk of a late failure due to restenosis or aneurysm of a patch increases. Most of our reoperations for carotid endarterectomy failure are performed between the fifth and tenth postoperative years. If surveillance is not initiated during the first year after surgery, it is unlikely that the patients will have follow-up studies in subsequent years.

MANAGEMENT OF LATE FAILURES AFTER CAROTID ENDARTERECTOMY

Most surgeons would agree that re-operation is indicated for patients with symptomatic late failures. A more controversial issue is what to do for a patient who is found to have an asymptomatic lesion in the carotid artery or routine follow-up. Some pathologic studies of recurrent carotid lesions have shown that restenosis during the first 2 years is frequently due to myointimal hyperplasia.[12,13,17] Late lesions, however, are often atherosclerotic or due to thrombus formation on the inner

Table 2. Management of late failure after carotid endarterectomy

Residual stenosis Early myo-intimal hyperplasia	Patch angioplasty
Early myo-intimal hyperplasia Late atherosclerotic restenosis	Redo endarterectomy and patch angioplasty
Late atherosclerotic restenosis Aneurysmal dilatation	Interposition graft

surface of an aneurysm. Because these later lesions carry all of the potential for an embolic stroke as primary lesions, we have generally advised asymptomatic patients to have a re-operation if there is >80% recurrent stenosis, intraluminal thrombus formation or aneurysmal dilatation of the patch. In our experience with re-operation for these lesions, we have had no perioperative strokes or deaths.[13]

Finally, if it is decided that re-operation is necessary for a late failure after carotid surgery, the choices of procedure include a simple patch angioplasty, redo endarterectomy with patch angioplasty or an interposition graft to entirely replace the segment of recurrent disease. Patch angioplasty may be suitable for early lesions such as a surgically created stenosis, or for a smooth myo-intimal hyperplastic lesions.[21]

Redo endarterectomy has been successfully used for the early and late recurrent lesions. In a recent review of our experience with redo endarterectomy for recurrent stenosis, however, we found a high incidence of tertiary restenosis and occlusion.[13] Among the 29 patients who had re-operation, there was a 21% incidence of late failure which was a ten-fold increase when compared to late failure after primary carotid endarterectomy. In light of this, we now favour interposition grafts, either with vein or synthetic prosthesis for the management of most recurrent stenosis. Patients with aneurysmal formation should be repaired by an interposition graft, since the adventitial layer is unsuitable for endarterectomy[21] (Table 2).

In summary, late failure may be due to technical failures at the time of the first endarterectomy, the development of new host lesions, or a combination of both. Although the incidence of symptomatic failures after carotid surgery is low, we feel the same criteria one uses for primary lesions of the carotid bifurcation should be used for secondary lesions. The goals remain the same—the reduction in the patient's risk for future stroke. The choice of operation for secondary lesion depends upon the pathology. Except for early stenosis which can be managed by patch angioplasty, interposition grafting may be preferable to redo endarterectomy for most late lesions.

REFERENCES

1. Imparato AM, Ramirez A, Riles TS, Mintzer R: Cerebral protection in carotid surgery. Arch Surg 117:1073–1078, 1982
2. Imparato AM, Baumann G, Riles TS: Arterial wall response to hemodynamic stress and its evolution. *In* Occlusive Disease of the Lower Limbs in Young Patients, Vol 15, Fiorani P, Pistolese GR, Spartera C (Eds). New York: Raven Press, 1984
3. Lord RS, Raj TB, Stary DL, Nash Pa, Graham AR: Comparison of saphenous vein patch, polytetrafluoroethylene patch and direct arteriotomy closure after carotid endarterectomy. Part I. Perioperative results. J Vasc Surg 9:521–529, 1989

4. Rosenthal D, Archie JP Jr, Garcia-Rinaldi R *et al*: Carotid patch angioplasty: Immediate and long-term results. J Vasc Surg 12:326–333, 1990
5. Poindexter JM, Patel KR, Clauss RH: Management of kinked extracranial cerebral arteries. J Vasc Surg 6:127–133, 1987
6. Nicholls SC, Phillips DJ, Bergelin RO *et al*: Carotid endarterectomy-relationship of outcome to early restenosis. J Vasc Surg 2:375–381, 1985
7. O'Donnell T, Callow AD, Scott G *et al*: Ultrasound characteristics of recurrent carotid disease: hypothesis explaining the low incidence of symptomatic recurrence. J Vasc Surg 2:26–41, 1985
8. Eikelboom BC, Ackerstaff RGA, Hoeneveld H *et al*: Benefits of carotid patching: a randomized study. J Vasc Surg 7:240–247, 1988
9. Fode NC, Sundt TN Jr, Robertson JT, Peerless SJ, Schields CV: Multicentre retrospective review of results and complications of carotid endarterectomy in 1981. Stroke 17:370–376, 1986
10. Clagett GP, Patterson CB, Fisher DF Jr *et al*: Vein patch versus primary closure for carotid endarterectomy. J Vasc Surg 9:213–223, 1989
11. Das MB, Hertzer NR, Ratliff NB, O'Hara PJ, Beven EG: Recurrent carotid stenosis. A five year series of 65 reoperations. Ann Surg 202:28–35, 1985
12. Clagett GP, Rich NM, McDonald PT *et al*: Etiologic factors for recurrent carotid artery stenosis. Surgery 93: 313–318, 1983
13. Gagne P, Riles TS, Imparato AM *et al*: Redo endarterectomy for recurrent carotid stenosis. Eur J Vasc Surg 5:1991
14. Cantelmo NL, Cutler BS, Wheeler HB, Herrmann JB, Cardullo PA: Noninvasive detection of carotid stenosis following endarterectomy. Arch Surg 116:1005–1008, 1981
15. Cossman D, Callow AD, Stein A, Matsumoto G: Early restenosis after carotid endarterectomy. Arch Surg 113:275–278, 1978
16. Hertzer NR, Martinez BD, Benjamin SP, Beven EG: Recurrent stenosis after carotid endarterectomy. Surg Gynacol Obstet 149:360–364, 1979
17. Sundt TM Jr, Houser IW, Fode NC, Whisnant JP: Correlation of postoperative and two-year followup angiography with neurological function in 99 carotid endarterectomies in 86 consecutive patients. Ann Surg 203:90–100, 1986
18. Deriu GP, Ballotta E, Bonavin L *et al*: The rationale for patch-graft angioplasty after carotid endarterectomy. Early and long-term followup. Stroke 15:972–979, 1984
19. Ouriel K, Green RM: Clinical and technical factors influencing recurrent carotid artery stenosis and occlusion after endarterectomy. J Vasc Surg 5:702–706, 1987
20. Katz MM, Jones GT, Degenhardt J *et al*: The use of patch angioplasty to alter the incidence of carotid restenosis following thromboendarterectomy. J Cardiovasc Surg 28:2–8, 1987
21. Piepgras DG, Sundt TM, Marsh NR, Mussman LA, Fode NC: Recurrent carotid stenosis: Results and complications of 57 operations. Ann Surg 203:205–213, 1986

Carotid Restenosis

Alan C. Meek, Rachel Cuming and Roger M. Greenhalgh

Before noninvasive methods of carotid assessment were developed, restenosis after endarterectomy was seen most often in patients with recurrent symptoms. In view of the morbidity associated with angiography, asymptomatic patients were seldom studied and recurrent stenosis was identified only in patients who developed symptoms or had an audible carotid bruit; based on these criteria, very low rates of restenosis were quoted in reviews of carotid endarterectomy.[1]

Following improvements in noninvasive carotid assessment to determine restenosis, it became both practical and ethical to re-examine large numbers of asymptomatic patients following surgery.[2] This showed that restenosis occurs in significant numbers of asymptomatic patients following endarterectomy, with the reported incidence ranging from 6 to 22%.[3,4] In contrast, recurrent symptoms of cerebrovascular insufficiency associated restenosis is seen in approximately 2% of patients following carotid surgery.[5]

More recently the incidence of restenosis has been studied in several centres to examine the effects of patch closure of the endarterectomy segment. Most studies suggest that patch closure improves long-term patency with saphenous vein repair, however, those patients undergoing vein rather than prosthetic patch repair had a higher incidence of late aneurysmal dilatation.[6] Although venous patches had a lower risk of early postoperative thrombosis compared to prosthetic material, concern has been shown for the small but appreciable risk of venous patch blow-out.[7]

The significance of restenosis following carotid endarterectomy has been examined in series investigating the incidence of recurrent symptoms of cerebrovascular insufficiency and comparing those patients with restenosis with others where the endarterectomy segment remains widely patent. As yet there is no evidence to suggest that asymptomatic restenosis requires further surgery and re-operation or myo-intimectomy should be reserved for symptomatic patients.[8,9]

Histologically, carotid restenosis may be due to recurrent atheroma or intimal hyperplasia but the pathogenesis of either process remains obscure.[10] Technical factors may be responsible in some cases and clamp damage, intimal flaps and failure to remove the distal tongue of plaque have all been implicated.[11–13]

The macroscopic and histological differentiation between intimal hyperplasia and recurrent atheroma has been described in detail.[14,15] In the postoperative period and up to 24 months after surgery the lesion is smooth, fibrous and without ulceration. It has been suggested that the earlier lesion of intimal hyperplasia is a precursor of later recurrent atheroma. However, there is no histological similarity between the fibrous stroma of hyperplasia which under microscopy appears as a structure of spindle shaped nucleated cells in a fibromyxomatous matrix and the ulcerating, neovascularized, lipid lesions characteristic of recurrent atheroma.[16] The difficulties of studying the artery at the transitional stage, which may well link the two seemingly separate pathological appearances, have yet to be overcome.

NONINVASIVE ASSESSMENT OF CAROTID STENOSIS

Noninvasive assessment of the carotid arteries has changed the practice of vascular surgery for extracranial disease both in the identification of bifurcation atheroma and postoperative follow-up. Carotid stenosis, originally measured indirectly by Doppler sonography[17] and Oculoplethysmography[18] has been superseded by the combination of real-time B-mode imaging of the arterial wall and flow assessment with Doppler spectral analysis which together produce duplex ultrasound. This is now regarded as the optimal imaging technique for the carotid artery in the noninvasive laboratory.[19] A modern duplex scanner with the option of colour flow imaging has now become essential equipment in the vascular laboratory.

Patients and methods

At Charing Cross Hospital 178 carotid endarterectomies were performed, between 1984 and 1990, in 173 patients, five requiring bilateral operation. There were 119 men and 54 women with mean age at operation of 64.4 years (39–83 years) and 68.5 years (46–80 years) respectively.

Eighty-six patients required carotid surgery for transient cerebral ischaemia (48%) and 37 for amaurosis fugax (21%). Thirty-nine patients (22%) had suffered either an established or transient stroke and in 14 patients (8%) urgent endarterectomy was performed for either crescendo TIA or stroke in evolution. Only two patients underwent endarterectomy for asymptomatic internal carotid artery stenosis as a prophylactic measure, prior to coronary artery bypass grafting and abdominal aortic aneurysm repair.

All surgical procedures were carried out under general anaesthesia with endotracheal intubation and assisted ventilation. Continuous central venous and arterial pressures were monitored and blood pressure was maintained at normal levels during the operative and postoperative period. In patients with an internal carotid stump pressure of less than 50 mm Hg or a nonpulsatile waveform, an intraluminal Javid shunt was placed to maintain cerebral perfusion. This was required in 89 cases (50%). Endarterectomy was performed through a longitudinal arteriotomy and direct arterial repair performed in the majority. In 46 cases (26%) the origin of the internal carotid artery was thought to be sufficiently narrow to require vein (7%) or Dacron patch angioplasty (19%).

All patients underwent postoperative duplex scanning within 24 h of surgery to exclude asymptomatic thrombosis. Subsequently they were re-examined at 3 days and at 3-monthly intervals up to 1 year and annually thereafter. At each visit patients were evaluated for cerebrovascular symptoms and the degree of restenosis recorded as a reduction in the luminal diameter. The common carotid was measured at the proximal extent of the endarterectomy and at the level of the bifurcation, while the internal was assessed at the level of the bulb and then more distally but still within the operated segment. From 1984 to 1988 noninvasive assessment was performed with a Sonicaid Vasoview imaging system fitted with a 7.5 MHz duplex probe and from 1988 to 1990 with an Acuson 128 colour coded duplex using a 5 MHz probe.

Low grade restenosis in the carotid arteries was identified at 25–49% luminal narrowing, moderate stenosis at 50–74%, severe at 75–99% or complete occlusion.

RESULTS

Of 173 patients in this series, 17 patients (10%) died during the follow-up period of mean 35.3 months which extended from 1 to 6 years. Initial mortality was 1.8% at 30 days, 4.5% at 1 year with an overall mortality of 4.4% per year over 5 years. Only two deaths followed stroke, 15 patients died from myocardial ischaemia and survival, calculated by life table analysis, was 95% at 1 year, 90% at 3 years and 78% at 5 years. Overall stroke rate in this group of operated patients was 3.5% at 30 days, and 4.2% at one year giving an overall stroke rate over 5 years of 1.3% per annum.

RESTENOSIS

Out of the total of 178 endarterectomies 54 arteries (30%) were identified to have either minor degrees of restenosis (25–49%) or more severe luminal narrowing. The appearance of minor restenosis was seen as frequently in the common as in the internal carotid artery. The majority of these lesions were identified within the first year of surgery (Fig. 1). More significant stenosis of greater than 50% was seen in 16 cases (9%); however, this was seen more frequently in the internal than the common carotid (Fig. 2) and again most of these lesions were seen within 12 months of operation. Two patients were found to have early postoperative occlusion and one further patient occluded at 3 years.

In the 12 patients who underwent saphenous vein patch repair one suffered early stenosis but there was no further incidence of restenosis in the remainder throughout the rest of the study. Two patients with Dacron patches were found to have greater than 50% restenosis (6%) and this compared favourably with 14 restenoses (10.5%)

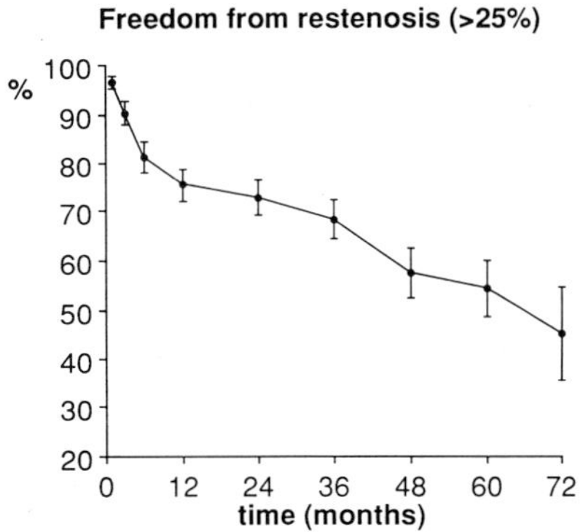

Fig. 1. Life table analysis of all patients developing any degree of restenosis greater than 25%. The majority occur in the first year after operation. These lesions were identified in both the common and internal carotid arteries.

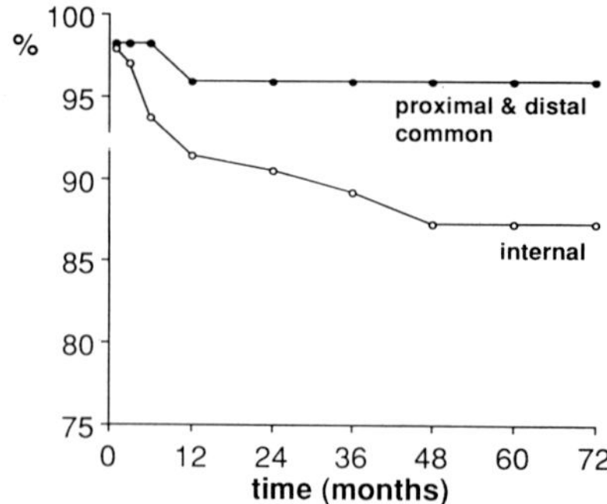

Fig. 2. Restenosis of greater than 50% is most often seen in the internal carotid artery ($0.05>p>0.02$).

in the 132 arteries which were closed by direct suture (Fig. 3). There was no difference in mortality comparing patients who developed restenosis of greater than 50% (11%) and those where the artery remained widely patent (9.5%). Only two patients suffered stroke during long-term follow-up at 18 months and 4 years and both of these had developed restenosis of greater than 25%.

There was no difference in rates of restenosis with respect to age or presenting symptomatology and similarly the incidence of restenosis was no higher in patients who suffered from diabetes, hypertension or had a history of ischaemic heart disease. There was a trend suggesting that former or current smokers had a higher incidence of restenosis when compared to nonsmokers (Fig. 4) but this failed to reach statistical significance ($p=0.059$). Restenosis was more common in female patients at 12.9% (7/54) compared to 7.3% (9/124) in males but this was again insignificant. Of the five patients who required bilateral carotid endarterectomy, none developed restenosis at follow-up.

DISCUSSION

The incidence of recurrent stenosis following carotid endarterectomy in this series is similar to other reports of noninvasive assessment.[20–22] The overall rate of

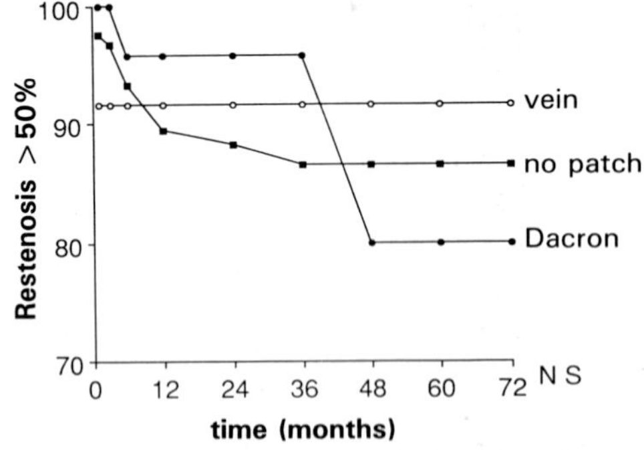

Fig. 3. Life table analysis showing the influence of patch repair. There was no significant difference between direct closure and patch angioplasty using either vein or prosthetic.

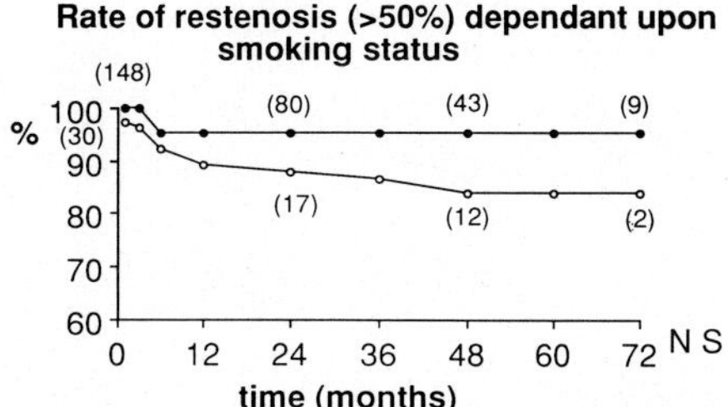

Fig. 4. Trend suggests that smokers have an increased risk of developing recurrent carotid stenosis (○ former/current smokers; ● nonsmokers).

restenosis of greater than 50% was 9%; however, minor degrees of restenosis was more frequent and 30% of patients were found to have luminal narrowing of greater than 25%. The low incidence of recurrent cerebrovascular symptoms (1.1%) during long-term follow-up suggests the efficacy of carotid surgery in the prevention of thromboembolic events.

The suggested management of those patients who develop restenosis following carotid surgery would seem to be conservative. The low incidence of symptomatic recurrence demonstrated in this and other series would suggest that asymptomatic patients should not undergo re-operation.[4] Although a proportion of asymptomatic patients with primary atheromatous lesions of the carotid arteries may develop neurological symptoms which require surgical intervention, this has not been found in patients with asymptomatic carotid restenosis.[23] Re-operative treatment is certainly more difficult and although it may be possible to identify an endarterectomy plane between the vessel wall and the restenotic lesion in cases of recurrent atheroma this is not found with intimal hyperplasia.[9] These procedures are technically exacting and in these circumstances patch angioplasty or interposition vein graft are most often required.

With the advantages of modern vascular imaging, we have been able to identify minor degrees of restenosis in 30% of cases after endarterectomy and these probably represent intimal hyperplasia seen in both the common and internal carotid arteries. The appearance of these lesions, most commonly within the first year of surgery, would be in keeping with current concepts of intimal hyperplasia which may yet be found to be the result of the healing response to the trauma of surgical endarterectomy. An appearance often seen on the earliest postoperative duplex studies is the step down from the full thickness of the common carotid artery to the thinner endarterectomy segment (Fig. 5). This irregularity will cause considerable disturbance to laminar flow and may accentuate the process of platelet aggregation already established by the collagen and smooth muscle in the exposed media of the arterial wall. The later result is seen in an image of the same artery at 3 months where the step defect has been replaced by homogeneous material which has eliminated the irregularity in the luminal surface (Fig. 6). However, in the first few days after surgery it is possible that the step defect has already been obliterated by fresh thrombus which has such similar ultrasonic density to blood that it is almost impossible to detect by noninvasive methods. The acoustic character of this tissue seen at 3 months is similar to the appearances of those early restenoses which are

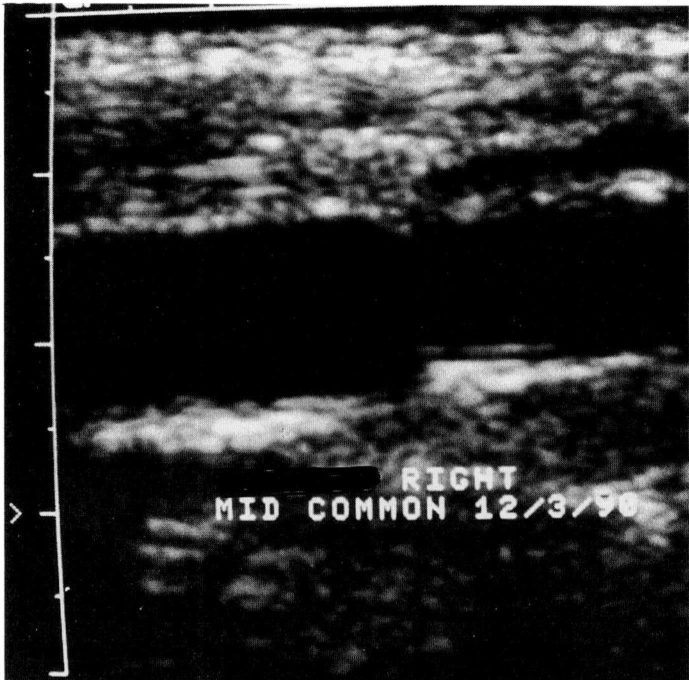

Fig. 5. Step down appearance on duplex scanning in the common carotid artery immediately after endarterectomy.

caused by intimal hyperplasia and we presume that this remodelling of the arterial wall will continue until the luminal surface is sufficiently smooth to allow laminar flow. What regulates normal healing and what constitutes the overexuberant response to arterial trauma has yet to be defined but the frequent identification of minor degrees of restenosis in the common carotid artery may reflect this phenomenon. A similar degree of intimal thickening in the internal carotid may well occur but because of its smaller diameter this will result in greater degrees of narrowing and hence the suggestion from our data that moderate and severe stenoses are seen most often at that site.

Duplex ultrasound can be used to monitor the appearance seen after patch repair of the arteriotomy. In transverse section, the initial postoperative appearance shows the artery to be widely patent but after 3 months the lumen is considerably reduced presumably by intimal hyperplasia (Fig. 7). The widening of the artery due to the increase in circumference depends on the width of the patch and excessive widening may promote intraluminal thrombus similar to that found in arterial aneurysms. Whether or not the degree of thrombus formation is related to the development of intimal hyperplasia remains unknown but the role of platelets and their associated growth factors have been suggested as one of the influences in arterial repair and the formation of arterial restenosis. It has been suggested that a policy of selective patching be adopted in patients with small carotid arteries, in women and in those at risk of restenosis. While this would seem appropriate, excessive widening should

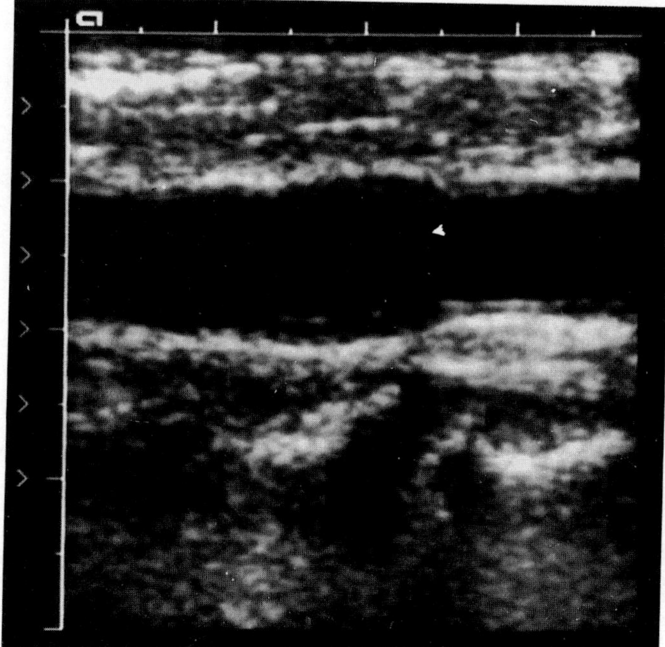

Fig. 6. Three months after surgery the angle between the full thickness of the arterial wall and the endarterectomy segment has been replaced by homogeneous low density material.

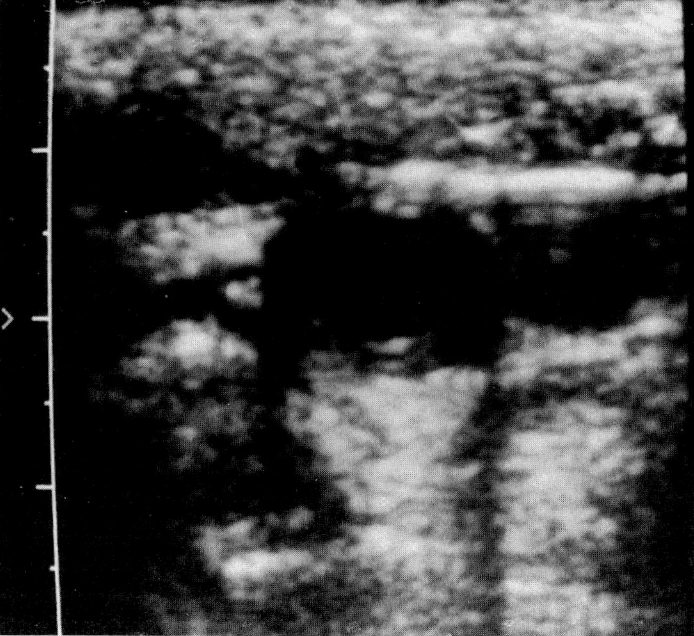

Fig. 7. Transverse section of a common carotid artery following patch angioplasty. Early postoperative appearance shows the artery to be widely patent but at 3 months considerable intimal thickening has occurred.

be avoided and carotid patching should attempt to reconstruct the normal configuration of the artery.

Despite these duplex appearances few patients develop recurrent cerebrovascular insufficiency and most restenoses identified in the first 12 months after surgery mature without evidence of further progression. This study has suggested that certain factors predispose to carotid restenosis. Women have been found more susceptible to restenosis and this has been noted previously. Whether or not this reflects the smaller size of the female carotid artery or there are other systemic factors is unknown.

REFERENCES

1. Thompson JE, Austin DJ, Patman RD: Carotid endarterectomy for cerebrovascular insufficiency—long term results in 592 patients followed up to 13 years. Ann Surg 172:663–679, 1970
2. Roederer GO, Langlois Y, Chan ATW *et al*: Post-endarterectomy carotid ultrasonic duplex scanning concordance with contrast angiography. Ultrasound Med Biol 9:73–78, 1983
3. Pierce GE, Iliopoulos JI, Holcomb MA *et al*: Incidence of recurrent stenosis after carotid endarterectomy determined by digital subtraction angiography. Am J Surg 148:848–853, 1984
4. Nicholls SC, Phillips DJ, Bergelin RO, Beach KW, Primozich JF: Carotid endarterectomy, relationship of outcome to early restenosis. J Vasc Surg 2:375–381, 1985
5. Hertzer NR, Martinez BD, Beven EG: Recurrent stenosis after carotid endarterectomy. Surg Gynaecol Obstet 149:360–364, 1979
6. Lord RSA, Baratha Raj T, Stary DL *et al*: Comparison of saphenous vein patch, polytetrafluoroethylene patch, and direct arteriotomy closure after carotid endarterectomy. Part 1. Perioperative results. J Vasc Surg 9:521–529, 1989
7. Eikelboom BC, Ackerstaff RGA, Hoeneveld H *et al*: Benefits of carotid patching: a randomised study. J Vasc Surg 7:240–247, 1988
8. Healy DA, Zierler RE, Nicholls SC *et al*: Long-term follow-up and clinical outcome of carotid restenosis. J Vasc Surg 10:622–629, 1989
9. Bartlett FF, Rapp JH, Goldstone J, Ehrenfeld WK, Stoney RJ: Recurrent carotid stenosis: Operative strategy and late results. J Vasc Surg 5:452–456, 1987
10. French BN, Rewcastle NB: Recurrent stenosis at the site of carotid endarterectomy. Stroke 8:597–605, 1977
11. DePalma RG, Chidi CC, Sternfeld WC, Doletsky S: Pathogenesis and prevention of trauma provoked atheromas. Surgery 82:429–437, 1977
12. Edwards WS, Wilson TAS, Bennett A: The long term effectiveness of carotid endarterectomy in prevention of strokes. Ann Surg 168:765–770, 1968
13. Javid H, Ostermiller WE, Hengesh JW *et al*: Natural history of carotid bifurcation atheroma. Surgery 67:80–86, 1970
14. Stoney RJ, String ST: Recurrent carotid stenosis. Surgery 80:705–710, 1976
15. Cossman D, Callow AD, Stein A, Matsumoto G: Early restenosis after carotid endarterectomy. Arch Surg 113:275–278, 1978
16. Callow AD: Recurrent stenosis after carotid endarterectomy. Arch Surg 117:1082–1085, 1982
17. Muller HR: The diagnosis of internal carotid artery occlusion by directional doppler sonography of the ophthalmic artery. Neurology 22:816–823, 1972
18. Kartchner MM, McRae LP, Morrison FD: Noninvasive detection and evaluation of carotid occlusive disease. Arch Surg 106:528–535, 1973
19. Strandness DE: Echo-Doppler (duplex) ultrasonic scanning. J Vasc Surg 2:341–344, 1985
20. Colgan MP, Kingston V, Shanik G: Stenosis following carotid endarterectomy. Arch Surg 119:1033–1035, 1984

21. Glover JL, Bendick PJ, Dilley RS *et al*: Restenosis following carotid endarterectomy. Arch Surg 120:78–684, 1985
22. Ackroyd N, Lane R, Appelberg M: Carotid endarterectomy. J Surg 27:418–425, 1986
23. Aldoori MI, Baird RN: Prospective assessment of carotid endarterectomy by clinical and ultrasonic methods. Br J Surg 74:926–929, 1987

Late Complications Following Graft Replacement of the Thoraco-abdominal Aorta

Larry H. Hollier, William M. Moore Jr and C. Daniel Procter Sr

Thoraco-abdominal aortic aneurysm repair is being done with increasing frequency in multiple centres in the USA, Europe, and Australia. Techniques have become relatively standardized and results have improved greatly over the past 15 years (Tables 1 and 2).[1–4] The risks of postoperative complications are well documented and methods have been described to minimize their occurrence.[3,4]

However, late complications associated with thoraco-abdominal aneurysm repair are infrequently discussed. In this chapter we attempt to detail the late complications we have seen in patients who had previously undergone thoraco-abdominal aortic graft replacement. We have included complications we have seen following operations we have done for aneurysmal disease, as well as those we have managed following operations done by others, and we have also included complications of any thoraco-abdominal graft, including those whose initial operations were not done for aneurysmal disease (e.g. supracoeliac co-arctation, infection, etc.).

Late complications we have seen following thoraco-abdominal graft replacement include development of secondary aneurysms, pseudo-aneurysms, graft infection, graft–pulmonary fistula, aortogastric fistula, and delayed-onset paraplegia, chylous leak, and delayed retroperitoneal haematoma.

SECONDARY ANEURYSM

In our experience, 21% of our patients had multiple aneurysms, of which 89% were managed by staged repair. Of the 130 patients who underwent thoraco-abdominal aortic graft replacement for aneurysmal disease, seven patients have developed a second aneurysm and undergone successful secondary aneurysm repair.

Approximately 20–40% of patients undergoing thoraco-abdominal aneurysm repair will have aneurysms separated by an intervening segment of relatively normal aorta or will develop a second aortic aneurysm at a later time; these patients will frequently undergo staged repair, wherein only one aneurysm is repaired at the initial operation

Table 1. Results of thoraco-abdominal aortic aneurysm repair

	Patients	*Mortality*	*Paraparesis*	*Paraplegia*
Intercostal re-implantation	66	5 (7.6%)	1 (1.5%)	2 (3.0%)
Intercostal re-implantation and CSF drainage	64	6 (9.4%)	3 (4.7%)	0
Total	130	11 (8.5%)	4 (3.1%)	2 (1.5%)

The initial group was repaired using routine attempts to re-implant intercostal arteries (it is incidentally noted that the two patients who developed paraplegia had not had intercostals re-implanted for technical reasons). The second group had intercostal re-implantation and cerebrospinal fluid drainage.

Table 2. Incidence of neurologic injury in relation to the extent of aneurysmal aorta replaced, using Crawford's classification of thoraco-abdominal aortic aneurysms

Aneurysm Type	*I*	*II*	*III*	*IV*	*Total*
No. of patients	26	22	32	50	130
Paraparesis	1	1	2	0	4 (3.1%)
Paraplegia	1	1	0	0	2 (1.5%)
Total neurologic deficit	2 (7.7%)	2 (9.9%)	2 (6.3%)	0	6 (4.6%)
	*8.3% (I + II)				
	*7.5% (I + II + III)				

* Combined neurologic deficit.

and the other repaired at a subsequent procedure. This has appeared, in our experience, to decrease the overall risk to the patient compared with repairing both aneurysms at one time.[5] Other patients, however, present with one aneurysm and undergo repair, only to develop another aneurysm at a later time. Crawford *et al.*[2] noted that 265 of 605 patients (44%) in their series underwent staged repair. In a similar report, Gloviczki *et al.*[5] noted that 201 (3.4%) of 5 837 aortic aneurysm operations were for multiple aortic aneurysms. Moreover, in 55 (54%) of those patients, multiple aortic aneurysms were present at the time of the initial aortic aneurysm repair.

We recently repaired a 7-cm type III thoraco-abdominal aortic aneurysm, replacing the distal one-third of the thoracic aorta and all of the abdominal aorta in a 66-year-old man; the proximal thoracic aorta was mildly ectatic but had no specific aneurysm. The patient made an uneventful recovery and was discharged on the eighth postoperative day. He was seen in clinic 4 days later and was doing well except for complaints of moderate back pain which was thought to be secondary to the thoracic aspect of the incision and the transection of the 7th and 8th ribs. Two days later, however, he complained of severe worsening of his back pain and was instructed to return for evaluation. Thirty minutes after walking into the emergency room he became paraplegic and mildly hypotensive. Computed tomographic scan and angiogram disclosed a large 9 cm thoracic aortic aneurysm above the previous graft (Fig. 1). At operation, the previous suture line was intact; the proximal aorta, however, had become aneurysmal and had ruptured posteriorly at the origin of several pairs of intercostal arteries. The aneurysm was successfully repaired but the patient has persistent paraplegia.

PSEUDO-ANEURYSMS

Thus far we have not seen any disruption or pseudo-aneurysm of a graft-to-aorta anastomosis in any of our patients who had repair of a thoraco-abdominal aneurysm. However, we have seen fairly prominent dilatation of the aortic cuff anastomosed to the aorta in two patients. One patient had a type II thoraco-abdominal aortic aneurysm graft repair that included re-implantation of an aortic cuff with several pairs of intercostal arteries. Routine follow-up after 1 year disclosed prominence of this area of the aortic cuff (Fig. 2); the patient remained asymptomatic and no interventions were undertaken.

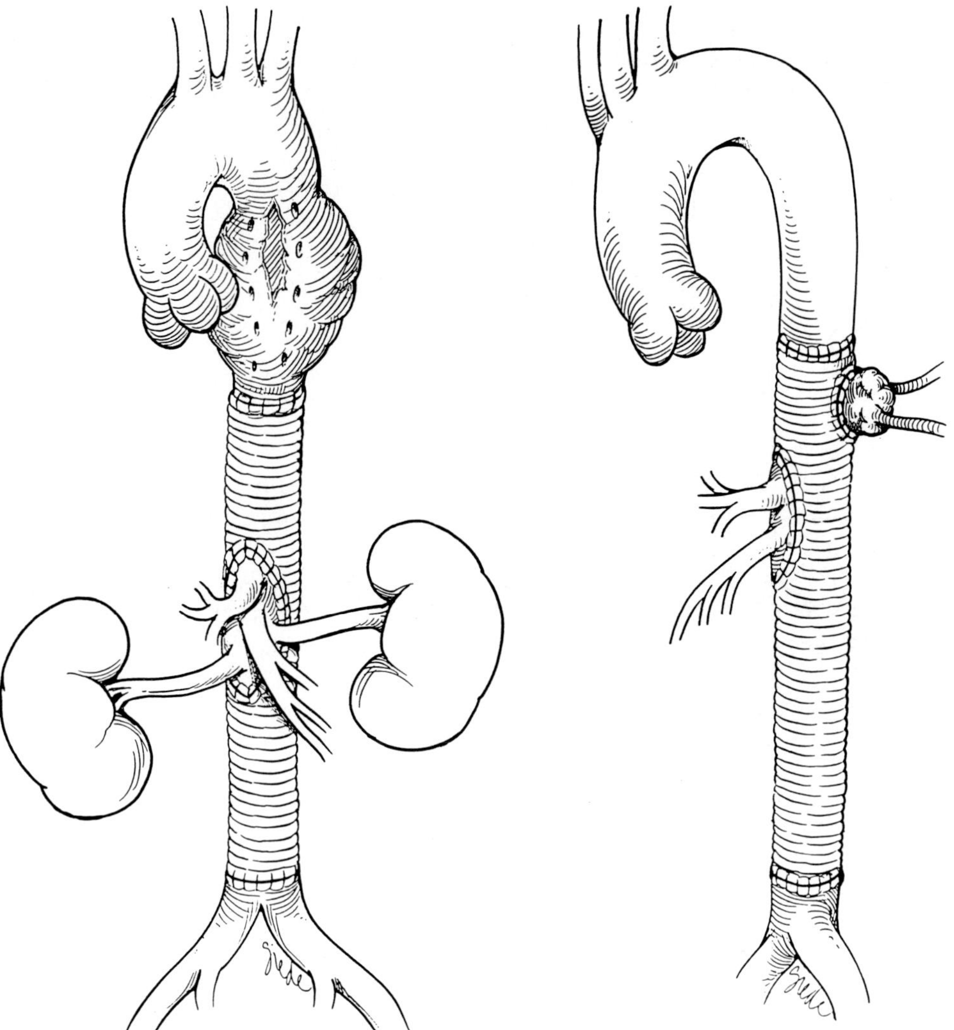

Fig. 1. Illustration of new aortic aneurysm in the proximal thoracic aorta that developed 2 weeks after repair of a large type III thoraco-abdominal aortic aneurysm. Note the site of rupture in the area of the origin of the intercostal arteries.

Fig. 2. Illustration of pseudo-aneurysmal dilatation of aortic cuff at site of re-implantation of several pairs of intercostal arteries.

A second patient developed aneurysmal expansion of the aortic cuff that included the origin of the coeliac, superior mesenteric, and right renal arteries (Fig. 3). Because of advanced age, renal dysfunction and a generally frail condition, no attempt was made to repair this area. The aneurysmal site has undergone only minimal further expansion with time and she remains asymptomatic now 5½ years after the original thoraco-abdominal aortic aneurysm repair.

Although cases may arise where these areas of cuff re-implantation associated with thoraco-abdominal aortic aneurysm repair may become aneurysmal and ultimately

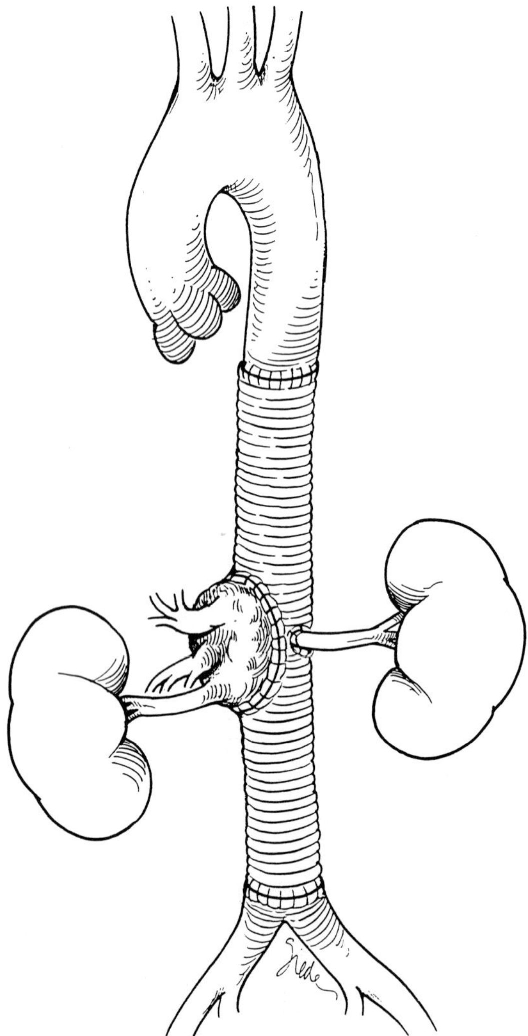

Fig. 3. Illustration of pseudo-aneurysmal dilatation of aortic cuff at site of re-implantation of the visceral vessels in a patient who underwent repair of a thoraco-abdominal aortic aneurysm.

lead to rupture, the true risk of this deadly complication remains unclear. We have not yet seen this in our patients. Based on our experience, we believe it may be safe to avoid precipitous re-operation and establish a plan of careful follow-up examinations, preferably with serial computed tomographic scans. If continued dilation can be documented, one may be justified in elective surgical intervention. Perhaps the most important aspect of this, however, relates to prevention. In general, we try to minimize as much as possible the amount of aortic cuff re-implanted by placing the suture line as close as possible to the orifices of the vessels arising from the aorta.

GRAFT INFECTION

One of 130 patients (0.8%) who underwent repair of an atherosclerotic thoraco-abdominal aortic aneurysm developed a documented graft infection with *Staphylococcus* aureus. Additionally, we treated two other patients who developed thoraco-abdominal aortic graft infections, one following repair of a mycotic thoraco-abdominal aortic aneurysm secondary to *Mycobacterium avium intracellularis* and one with a supracoeliac graft infection due to *Candida albicans*. The atypical mycobacterium was treated with appropriate antimicrobial agents and had no further graft complications, although he did develop neurologic dysfunction secondary to the chemotherapeutic agent. The other two patients underwent CT guided aspiration of the perigraft fluid with documentation of the antibiotic sensitivity of the organism causing the infection; subsequent repeat aspiration was performed with instillation of organism-specific antibiotics in each case. Additionally, a 30-day course of intravenous systemic antibiotics was given and the patients were placed on lifetime suppressive antibiotic therapy. One patient died of a stroke a year later but had no intervening signs of infection; the other patient remains alive with no sign of infection 4½ years later.

Although graft removal and extra-anatomic replacement is considered standard treatment for infrarenal aortic graft infections, replacement of a thoraco-abdominal aortic graft is less easily accomplished. Thus, our approach to late infections associated with thoraco-abdominal aortic aneurysm grafts is to initially use systemic intravenous antibiotics and direct instillation of organism-specific antibiotics in the perigraft space. If initial control of the septic process can be achieved, the patient is maintained on lifetime antibiotics.

GRAFT–PULMONARY FISTULA

One 56-year-old woman with severe chronic obstructive pulmonary disease underwent repair of an extensive type II thoraco-abdominal aortic aneurysm. Her postoperative course was complicated by respiratory insufficiency necessitating ventilatory support for more than 30 days. She ultimately went home requiring only nasal oxygen intermittently. One year later, she returned with massive haemoptysis. Endoscopy showed no intrinsic pathology. Angiography was inconclusive but a CT scan suggested an erosion of the medial segment of the left lobe of the lung by the Dacron graft. The operative report confirmed that the sac of the aneurysm had inadequately covered the graft after completion of the aneurysm repair. Re-operation disclosed the lung to be intimately adherent to the upper portion of the graft, though the aortic suture line was not involved. There was no evidence of infection and there was not active bleeding. The graft was irrigated with antibiotic solution and covered by suturing a bovine pericardial patch to the edges of the opened aneurysm sac wall. The patient's postoperative course was uncomplicated and she has had no further episodes of haemoptysis.

Since that case, we always ensure complete coverage of the graft in every case. We attempt to do this as much as possible by sewing the aneurysm sac around the graft. Whenever this is not possible, we complete coverage of the graft using a sheet of Gore-Tex® membrane, suturing it tightly to the edges of the aortic sac (Fig. 4). This not only provides a nonadherent coverage for the graft, but also aids in effective tamponade of any bleeding or continued oozing from the graft in the immediate postoperative period.

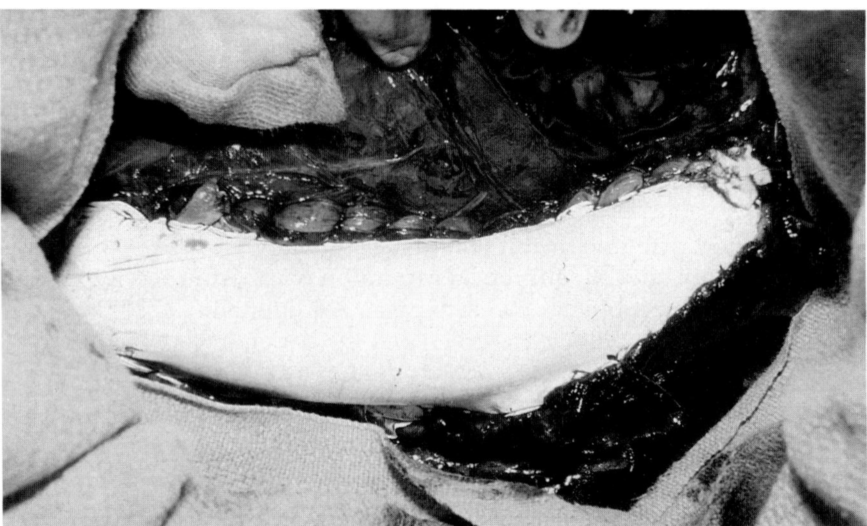

Fig. 4. Operative photograph demonstrating graft coverage by means of a Gore-Tex® membrane (reprinted with permission from B. C. Decker, Inc., Philadelphia).

AORTOGASTRIC FISTULA

We were consulted to see a 30-year-old woman who had undergone an aorto-aortic graft for aortic co-arctation at the level of the coeliac axis several years previously. She now had a painful epigastric mass that on CT scan proved to be a large perigraft mass just behind the stomach. She was scheduled for elective repair the next morning, but 1 hour prior to operation she developed severe abdominal and back pain and became mildly hypotensive. She was hurriedly moved to the operating theatre and prepared for operation. Immediately after taping the endotracheal tube in place, the anaesthesiologist noted the patient to exhibit pulsatile cheeks and pulsatile bleeding came from both nostrils. The thoraco-abdominal aorta was rapidly exposed and the aorta was clamped. An aortogastric fistula was evident, with the graft having eroded through the posterior wall of the stomach. Direct graft replacement was performed after irrigating the area copiously with antibiotic solution. After debriding the edges of the defect in the wall, the stomach was repaired primarily and an omental pedicle was interposed between the stomach and the graft. The cultures exhibited no growth and the patient made an uneventful recovery.

CHYLOUS LEAK AND DELAYED RETROPERITONEAL HAEMATOMA

Chylous leak following repair of abdominal aortic aneurysm is associated with significant mortality as evidenced by published reports.[6,7] We have managed one patient who developed a retroperitoneal chylous leak following repair of a large thoraco-abdominal aortic aneurysm. This 77-year-old woman had an extraperitoneal repair of her thoraco-abdominal aortic aneurysm but required re-operation several days after surgery because of a slowly expanding retroperitoneal haematoma. The haematoma was evacuated and all oozing sites were cauterized or oversewn; closed suction drainage was instituted. Within 48 hours a significant chylous leak

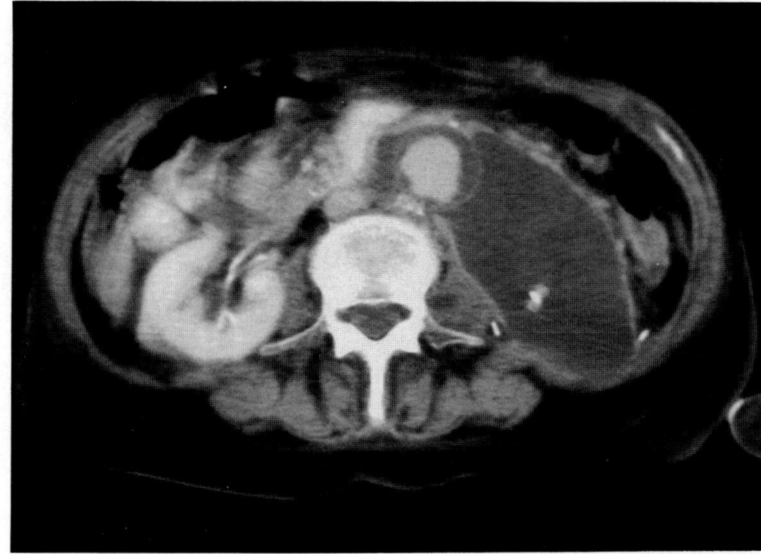

Fig. 5. CT scan showing retroperitoneal collection of chylous fluid despite suction drainage.

became evident and despite suction a retroperitoneal collection again developed (Fig. 5). An attempt to oversew the chylous fistula was unsuccessful. Closed suction drainage was continued and, after a prolonged hospital stay the drainage ceased and the suction catheter was removed. The patient was discharged with a small retroperitoneal fluid collection evident on CT scan that remained stable with no further expansion.

The patient remained asymptomatic for several months after which she started to

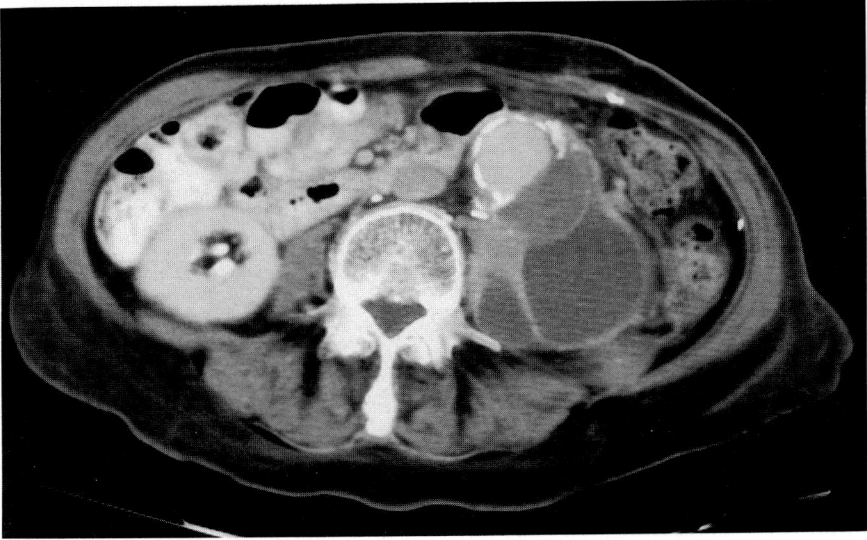

Fig. 6. CT scan on same patient with late development of multiloculated retroperitoneal haematoma causing left femoral neuropathy.

complain of pain and numbness in her left leg. Repeat CT scan showed an expanded mass in the left retroperitoneal area extending down into the left pelvis (Fig. 6). CT density was compatible with areas of old firm haematoma and other areas of fluid. CT guided aspiration removed liquified haematoma and the patient reported relief of her leg pain. Unfortunately, she has had re-accumulation of fluid and recurrent symptoms and needs intermittent re-aspiration. Re-operation may be necessary in the future.

We have seen three other patients who have developed postoperative retroperitoneal bleeding that required re-operation and evacuation of the haematoma. A specific single bleeding point cannot generally be identified. Two of these patients have required repeat operation weeks later because of slow re-accumulation of retroperitoneal haematoma.

Bleeding in the immediate postoperative period following thoraco-abdominal aortic aneurysm repair occurs in about 10% of cases.[3] Most often we have found it to be due to bleeding from injury to an intercostal artery at the site of rib transection, from an unrecognized splenic injury, or from continued diffuse bleeding from the extensive raw surface of the area of retroperitoneal dissection. While the first two problems can be easily corrected, the latter problem can be vexing. Any associated DIC or fibrinolysis obviously needs to be corrected and meticulous suture ligation of the multiple bleeding points is recommended. In rare cases, gauze packs may be needed to control this continued bleeding. In our experience topical thrombin and fibrin glue have been relatively ineffective for this problem.

SUMMARY

Late survival following thoraco-abdominal aortic aneurysm repair is impressive, particularly when one compares it with the poor survival of patients with unoperated thoraco-abdominal aortic aneurysms. Nevertheless, late problems do occur frequently. It is important that all patients who undergo thoraco-abdominal aortic aneurysm repair be followed closely thereafter. Serial CT scans are the most reliable method of identifying any late complications and provide a good basis from which to plan subsequent treatment.

REFERENCES

1. Crawford ES: Thoracoabdominal and abdominal aortic aneurysms involving renal, superior mesenteric, and celiac arteries. Ann Surg 179:763–772, 1974
2. Crawford ES, Crawford JL, Safi HJ *et al*: Thoracoabdominal aortic aneurysms: Preoperative and intraoperative factors determining immediate and long-term results of operations in 605 patients. J Vasc Surg 3:389–404, 1986
3. Hollier LH, Symmonds JB, Pairolero PC *et al*: Thoracoabdominal aortic aneurysm repair: Analysis of postoperative morbidity. Arch Surg 123:871–875, 1988
4. Hollier LH, Marino RJ: Thoracoabdominal aortic aneurysms. *In* Vascular Surgery: A Comprehensive Review, 3rd edn, Moore WS (Ed.). Philadelphia: W. B. Saunders, pp. 295–303, 1991
5. Gloviczki P, Pairolero P, Welch T *et al*: Multiple aortic aneurysms: The results of surgical management. J Vasc Surg 11:19–28, 1990
6. Williams RA, Vetto J, Quinones-Baldrich *et al*: Chylous ascites following abdominal aortic surgery. Presented at the 9th Annual Meeting of the Southern California Vascular Surgical Society, Newport Beach, California, 22 September 1990
7. Ablan CJ, Littooy FN, Freeark FJ: Postoperative chylous ascites: Diagnosis and treatment. Arch Surg 125:270–273, 1990

Complications from Defects in Prosthetic Grafts

George Johnson Jr

Prosthetic grafts have been used to replace the arteries with increasing frequency since Voorhees *et al.*[1] reported in 1952 using Vinyon 'N' after resecting the aorta for an aneurysm. The early history is well documented in a monograph by Edwards published in 1957.[2] Synthetic threads that have been used to construct the woven or knitted grafts include nylon, Teflon, Orlon and Dacron. The threads themselves have been modified to create special effects. Expanded Teflon or polytetrafluoroethylene (PTFE) was developed to create a less wettable surface, and the knit has been altered to improve longevity and resistance to infection, to decrease blood loss at time of surgery, and to give characteristics that make for easy sewing. Many of the modifications have led to improvements, but some have led to serious complications. There were early concerns regarding incorporation of the graft by fibrous tissue, so that it became a 'part of the body' and did not act as a foreign body. Thus the porous knitted graft was developed that needed to be 'clotted' with the patient's blood before being used. Velour grafts were developed to aid in this incorporation. In 1985 Robicsek[2] reported a series of patients in which one limb of a bifurcation graft was woven and one was knitted. In the follow-up period, from 2 months to 2 years, there were no differences in the patency rate between the two types of prostheses. In the last few years, manufacturers have made the woven prosthesis more like the knitted as far as handling characteristics are concerned. Some recent refinements in the knitted graft have made it less likely to bleed without preclotting before it is inserted.

In an attempt to define problems with the Dacron graft years after insertion, we reviewed all abdominal aortic aneurysms operated upon at the UNC Hospitals from 1957 to 30 September, 1990. Data from all vascular patients have been maintained in a vascular registry, periodically updated, and stored on a personal computer. In an attempt to isolate our attention on defects in the graft, only intra-abdominal grafts inserted for abdominal aortic aneurysms were reviewed. All of these were made of Dacron threads. The increased risk of groin infection and femoral-anastomotic aneurysms was not a part of this study.

The data were obtained by chart review of clinic visits or personal telephone calls. Since few deaths are followed by autopsies, the cause of death was usually based on information obtained from the private physician or family.

RESULTS

From 1957 to 30 September, 1990 725 patients had repair of an abdominal aortic aneurysm at the UNC Hospitals. Repairs performed more than 4 years ago totalled 613; 164 patients expired within 30 days of the operation (105 of these had ruptured aneurysms). None of these deaths was thought to be due to failure of the graft.

Of the 449 patients surviving the 30-day postoperative period, 100 died less than 4 years after the operation; 20 are lost to follow-up at present.

We have therefore followed 329 who survived longer than 4 years after aneurysm repair and thus were exposed to risk of graft complications. There was no problem that could be attributed specifically to failure of the Dacron graft.

During this period we operated on a number of patients not included in the above group who had complications due to defects in the graft. In one, an aorto-enteric fistula developed from the middle of an aorto-iliac bypass placed several years previously. The small hole in the graft could have been caused by failure of the prosthesis. In another, the patient expired several years after an aortofemoral graft had been inserted for severe claudication. The patient was asymptomatic and died of a heart attack. At autopsy, it was found that the Teflon had completely eroded through, exposing a well-incorporated fibrous capsule that was not aneurysmal. In a third patient, an ultralightweight knitted Dacron graft was inserted between the common femoral and popliteal artery. A year later, he returned with multiple aneurysms where the graft had deteriorated. It was successfully replaced. In 1988, an 8 mm external supported PTFE axillobifemoral bypass graft was placed after an aorto-enteric fistula was repaired. Two years later, the patient was operated upon at another institution for massive bleeding in the right side along the course of the graft. At operation, a portion of the graft on the side of the abdomen had disintegrated and the two ends distracted. More recently, one of the newly developed prostheses was inserted with the expectation that it would not bleed even if it had not been preclotted. However, it bled profusely. Although these are anecdotes, they demonstrate that vascular centres do see a few complications directly associated with failure of the prosthetic material.

DISCUSSION

A group of 725 patients who had their abdominal aorta replaced with an intra-abdominal Dacron prosthesis for aneurysm was followed for up to 30 years, looking for complications that could be attributed to failure of the prosthesis; none could be identified in this group of patients. In addition to this, a few isolated cases of graft failure from a different group of patients are briefly presented.

As soon as it became obvious that synthetic materials were going to be used to replace vessels, vascular surgeons appropriately assumed the responsibility of evaluating the grafts. The Society of Vascular Surgery in 1956 appointed a committee for the study of vascular prostheses. Creech *et al.*,[4] after an extensive review, reported to the society in 1957. Interestingly, even at this early time they concluded that Dacron or Teflon were the most satisfactory materials available.

Since then there have continued to be a number of isolated case reports of prosthesis failure. O'Hara and Nakano[5] in 1958 reported dilation and a small defect in an amylan-polyethylene (nylon-6) prosthesis inserted to replace an abdominal aortic aneurysm 1 year previously. Eastcott and Robinson[6] in 1962 described failure of an Orlon prosthesis used to replace an abdominal aortic aneurysm 6 years after insertion. The patient developed an aorto-enteric fistula and died. Hayward and White, 1971[7] reported an aneurysm in a woven Teflon graft and in 1975,[8] three instances of severe degeneration of knitted Dacron grafts supplied prior to 1969. Perry[9] in 1975 reported a 3-mm rent in a knitted Dacron bifurcation graft, a friable femoral limb knitted Dacron bifurcation graft, and a 12-mm circular hole in the anterior surface of a knitted bifurcation graft inserted from the aorta to the external iliac artery. Ottinger[10] in 1976 reported 11 cases in which the use of the ultralightweight Dacron arterial graft was complicated by interstitial haemorrhage, dilatation, or both. Campbell *et al.*[11] in 1976 reported aneurysmal dilatation in three of 50 patients with femoropopliteal bypass grafts using expanded PTFE.

In the mid 1970s the concept of making velour grafts with inner and outer velour surfaces was presented by the industry. Velour is a fabric with a pile like velvet. This allowed more platelet deposition, stimulated more fibrous tissue ingrowth, and thus improved incorporation of the prosthesis into the body. It was hoped this would strengthen the graft and decrease the chance of infection.[12]

Blumenberg and Gelfand[13] in 1977 reported five cases of defects in graft material, one in a 'Milliknit' Dacron graft developed by Wesolowski and manufactured by Golaski, two in a knitted lightweight Dacron manufactured by United States Catheter and Instrument Company, one in a 'weave-knit' Dacron graft by Meadox, and one in a Golaski knitted Dacron graft. Yashar *et al.*[14] in 1978 noted that 24 cases of arterial prosthetic failure had been described in the literature, and reported two additional failures of knitted Dacron prostheses. In 1978, May and Stephen[15] noted multiple aneurysms in a Dacron knitted internal velour graft used for a femoropopliteal bypass. Nucho and Gryboski[16] in 1984 reported multiple aneurysms 6 years after implantation in a double velour Dacron graft. Macroscopic and electron microscopic examination revealed multiple disrupted textile fibres.

Nunn *et al.*[17] in 1990 reported on 32 patients with an aortic Dacron knitted prosthesis, who were followed an average of 175 months. The mean percent dilation for the aortic portion was 67%. Three patients had to have their grafts replaced.

This review suggests that since 1980, roughly the time most of the grafts had velour in their inner or outer surface, there have been very few complications derived from the graft fabric or configuration. Among the 329 intra-abdominal Dacron grafts inserted for abdominal aortic aneurysm at this institution which were followed longer than 4 years, there were no graft failures. Thus, the incidence of graft failure from one institution, followed at least 4 years, is very low. Although Nunn has had to remove 10% of the grafts he has followed with ultrasound, this experience has not as yet been reported from other centres. Even though complications such as infection, anastomotic aneurysm, and aorto-enteric fistulae are still reported, they do not seem to be specifically related to a defect in the prosthetic material.

REFERENCES

1. Voorhees AB Jr, Jaretski A III, Blakemore AH: Use of tubes constructed from Vinyon-N cloth bridging arterial defects. Ann Surg 135:332, 1952
2. Edwards WS: Plastic Arterial Grafts. Springfield, Ill: C. C. Thomas, 1957
3. Robicsek F, Daugherty HK, Cook JC *et al*: Patency rate of bifurcated aortic grafts: comparative analysis of woven versus knitted prostheses in the same patient. Ann Thoracic Surg 40:172–174, 1985

4. Creech O Jr, Deterling RA Jr, Edwards S *et al*: Vascular prostheses: Report of the committee for the study of vascular prostheses of the society for vascular surgery. Surgery 41:62–80, 1957
5. O'Hara I, Nakano S: Rupture of arterial plastic prosthesis (Amylan-Polyethylene Tube). Arch Surg 77:55–60, 1958
6. Eastcott HHG, Robinson SHG: Rupture of Orlon aortic graft after six years. Lancet i:75–76, 1962
7. Hayward RH, White RR: Aneurysm in a woven Teflon graft. Angiology 22:188–190, 1971
8. Hayward RH, Korompai FL: Degeneration of knitted Dacron grafts. Surgery 79:581–583, 1976
9. Perry MO: Early failure of Dacron prosthetic grafts. J Cardiovasc Surg 16:318–321, 1975
10. Ottinger LW, Darling RC, Wirthlin LS *et al*: Failure of ultralightweight knitted Dacron grafts in arterial reconstruction. Arch Surg 111:146–149, 1976
11. Campbell CD, Brooks DH, Webster MW *et al*: Aneurysm formation in expanded polytetrafluoroethylene prostheses. Surgery 79:491–493, 1976
12. Sato O, Tada Y, Takagi A: The biologic fate of Dacron double velour vascular prostheses: A clinicopathological study. Jap J Surg 19:301–311, 1989
13. Blumenberg RM, Gelfand ML: Failure of knitted Dacron as an arterial prosthesis. Surgery 81:493–496, 1977
14. Yashar JJ, Richman MH, Dyckman J *et al*: Failure of Dacron prostheses caused by structural defect. Surgery 84:659–663, 1978
15. May J, Stephen M: Multiple aneurysms in Dacron velour graft. Arch Surg 113:320–321, 1978
16. Nucho RC, Gryboski WA: Aneurysms of a double velour aortic graft. Arch Surg 119:1182–1184, 1984
17. Nunn DB, Carter MM, Donohue MT *et al*: Postoperative dilation of knitted Dacron aortic bifurcation graft. J Vasc Surg 12:291–297, 1990

Long-term Results of Straight and Bifurcated Aortic Grafts for Abdominal Aortic Aneurysm Repair: A Population-based Experience

John W. Hallett and David Calcagno

Following successful elective repair of an abdominal aortic aneurysm, the patient faces late graft-related complications, new aneurysmal and occlusive disease, and other cardiovascular events. Periodic long-term surveillance for these problems is ideal, but many patients subsequently avoid doctors, die, or are lost to follow-up. This difficulty with complete follow-up can compromise both the recognition and management of late graft complications. To effectively develop long-term maintenance programs for both the patient and the graft, we have attempted to delineate the incidence of these problems, their characteristics, and their time of occurrence.

We have had the unusual opportunity of health-care maintenance for essentially all aneurysm patients in a defined community over the past 39 years. This community-based experience minimizes the bias inherent in a referral population and allows complete follow-up of patients. It provides a unique look at long-term health maintenance in the patient who has undergone a straight or bifurcated Dacron graft for abdominal aortic aneurysm repair.

METHODS

All medical care provided for residents of Rochester, Minnesota (population 62 000), and the surrounding Olmsted County (total population of city and county 90 000) is indexed, and the original medical records are retrieved readily for review. The index covers care delivered at the Mayo Clinic and its two large affiliated hospitals (Saint Marys and Rochester Methodist) as well as other institutions serving the community, including Olmsted Medical Group, Olmsted Community Hospital, Rochester State Hospital, the Veterans Administration, and the University of Minnesota Hospitals in Minneapolis, and other hospitals and practitioners in the vicinity. These indices incorporate the diagnosis made among outpatients seen in office or clinic consultation, emergency room visits, house calls, nursing home visit, as well as diagnosis and operation recorded for hospital inpatients, on death certificates, and autopsy. The potential of this data retrieval system for population-based studies has been described previously.[1] The general characteristics (age, gender, etc.) are comparable to the overall population of the USA.

All community residents with an abdominal aortic aneurysm newly diagnosed from 1951 to 1984 have been identified. This cohort of 432 patients has allowed us to identify all patients who underwent repair of their abdominal aortic aneurysm in this time period and to follow them long enough to identify late graft-related problems and new aneurysm disease. To compare the late results of aortic tube vs bifurcated grafts, we matched all patients who underwent successful repair with a straight aortic prosthesis with a group of patients with bifurcated aortic grafts matched for age and year of operation with a tube-graft group. We determined all patients with subsequent graft-related complications, new symptomatic occlusive or aneurysmal disease, and additional vascular operations to maintain the first graft or correct new occlusive or aneurysmal lesions.

Following this study, 100 subsequent abdominal aortic aneurysm repairs were examined to ascertain recent trends in straight vs bifurcated Dacron grafts based on the findings and influence of this population-based experience.

RESULTS

Of the 432 patients diagnosed with an abdominal aortic aneurysm between 1951 and 1984, 206 (48%) eventually underwent repair of their aneurysm (Table 1).

Tube grafts

Only 39 (18.9%) patients had a straight graft. The average follow-up for this group was 6 years: 5-year survival was 58%. Complete autopsy and clinical records to 1988 *did not* reveal any subsequent iliac aneurysms or iliac occlusive disease to that point of follow-up. Graft-related complications affected 5% in this group (Table 2). One patient disrupted the proximal aortic anastomosis 1 month postoperatively. A second proximal aortic anastomotic pseudoaneurysm became symptomatic 15 years post-operatively. Another 5% of this group developed aneurysmal disease proximal to the

Table 1. Abdominal aortic aneurysms (AAA) in Rochester, Minnesota 1951–1984

	Number
Total AAA diagnosed	432
Surgical repair	206 (48%)
Straight aortic grafts	39 (18.9%)
Bifurcated aortic grafts	167 (81.1%)

Table 2. Matched control study of straight vs bifurcated aortic grafts*

	Straight $n = 39$	*Bifurcated* $n = 39$
Graft-related complications	2 (5.0%)	5 (12.5%)
New aneurysms	2 (5.0%)	2 (5.0%)
Thoracic aortic dissection		1 (2.5%)
New distal occlusive disease	1 (2.5%)	4 (10.0%)
Total	5 (12.5%)	12 (30.0%)

*Matched for age, gender and year of operation. Mean follow-up was 6 years.

aortic graft at 8 and 13 years postoperatively. Only 2.5% developed claudication due to distal femoropopliteal arterial occlusive disease at 15 years postoperatively. Thus, only 10% of patients with tube grafts developed late graft-related or new clinically recognized aneurysm disease. Most of these problems were recognized between 5 and 15 years postoperatively.

Bifurcated aortic grafts

The matched control group with bifurcated aortic grafts developed more (five patients, 12.5%) graft-related problems than the tube-graft subset (Table 2). The reasons for selecting a bifurcation graft in the first place were iliac aneurysms (59%) followed by iliac occlusive disease (21%) and surgeon's technical preference (21%). Mean follow-up was likewise 6 years with a 5-year survival of 78%, higher than the tube-graft group but *not* a statistically significant difference. Graft-related complications (12.5%) included groin lymphocele, aortic suture-line dehiscence 6 years postoperatively, rupture of an iliac anastomosis at 16 years, and two femoral false aneurysms at 4 and 8 years. The ruptured proximal aortic anastomosis resulted in haemorrhagic shock and death.

In addition, seven (17.5%) patients with bifurcated grafts developed new arterial disease at other anatomic sites (Table 2). These problems included femoropopliteal occlusive disease requiring operation (5%) at 4 months and another 6 years postoperatively, claudication treated conservatively (5%), a proximal abdominal aortic aneurysm at 6 years (2.5%), (Figs 1 and 2), iliac aneurysm at 14 years (2.5%), and a descending thoracic aortic dissection at 4 years (2.5%). In total, therefore, graft-related (12.5%) and other vascular disease (17.5%) affected 30.0% of patients with bifurcated grafts.

Following completion of this study, we prospectively recorded the type of graft used in 100 recent, consecutive abdominal aortic aneurysm repairs. Straight grafts were used in 43% while 57% received a bifurcated Dacron prosthesis (aorto-iliac in 49% and aortofemoral in only 8%).

DISCUSSION

This type of population-based analysis offers certain advantages over our previously reported selected referral experience.[2] The first advantage is inclusion of our entire community-based experience rather than the potential selection bias of our referral population. The differences between our community-based and referral populations have been noted previously.[1] Second, the close and complete long-term follow-up of these patients allows detection of at least clinically apparent or autopsy-proven aneurysm or occlusive disease. This type of study, however, does have several limitations. The first has been the relatively low number of patients who have undergone aortic tube grafts. Second, relying solely on clinical presentations of problems or autopsied evidence of aneurysm or occlusive disease may have underestimated the detection of some of these problems. Although CAT scans and ultrasounds have been used for follow-up of selected community patients, they are not available in every patient. Nonetheless, autopsy did not reveal any graft complications or aneurysms in this population that we had not recognized clinically prior to death.

Straight grafts

The potential benefits of tube grafts include less periaortic and iliac dissection which may decrease the likelihood of injury to associated structures such as iliac veins or ureters. There also may be less disruption of periaortic sympathetic nerve fibres, although our current study could not substantiate this benefit. Another benefit is only two anastomoses instead of three. On the other hand, the main technical disadvantage of a tube graft is the difficulty of the distal anastomosis when the aortic bifurcation is very diseased or calcified.

In this long-term review of our early population-based experience, we were impressed with the relatively infrequent use of straight Dacron aortic tube grafts compared to other reports in the literature.[3–7] Our very selected use of tube grafts may account partially for the excellent late results. Other surgical series using a larger proportion of tube grafts have also found relatively few late iliac aneurysms (Table 3). Our own larger referral series of 1087 patients undergoing elective abdominal aortic aneurysm repair revealed only six (0.6%) with subsequent iliac aneurysms. A recent Canadian study using serial postoperative CT scans has confirmed the low risk of subsequent iliac aneurysm development following tube grafts, at least in early follow-up (5 years).[8]

When we did encounter graft-related problems with tube grafts, a proximal suture-line complication was the primary culprit. Likewise, the most common subsequent type of aneurysm in a patient with a tube graft was another aortic aneurysm proximal to the straight graft. These proximal suture-line and aortic aneurysm problems generally manifest themselves relatively late, i.e. after 5 years. The development of distal iliac or femoropopliteal occlusive disease is uncommon following tube grafts. Consequently, patients with straight grafts need long-term surveillance primarily of the proximal abdominal aorta and the tube graft. One could debate whether these patients need yearly ultrasound or CAT scanning. We currently suggest an aortic ultrasound 1 year after graft placement and then every 2–5 years with a CT scan for any graft or proximal aortic abnormality noted on ultrasound. A chest X-ray also seems reasonable since a thoracic aneurysm is the most common type of late aneurysm after repair of an abdominal aortic aneurysm (2–3%) in some series.[2]

Table 3. Late results of straight tube grafts for abdominal aortic aneurysm

Author	*n*	*Late iliac aneurysm development*	*Re-operation for distal occlusive disease*
Snellen[4]	110	1 (0.9%)	—
Glickman[6]	86	0	2 (2.3%)
Nash[7]	43	0	0
Current series	39	1 (2.5%)	0
Total	278	2 (0.7%)	2 (0.7%)

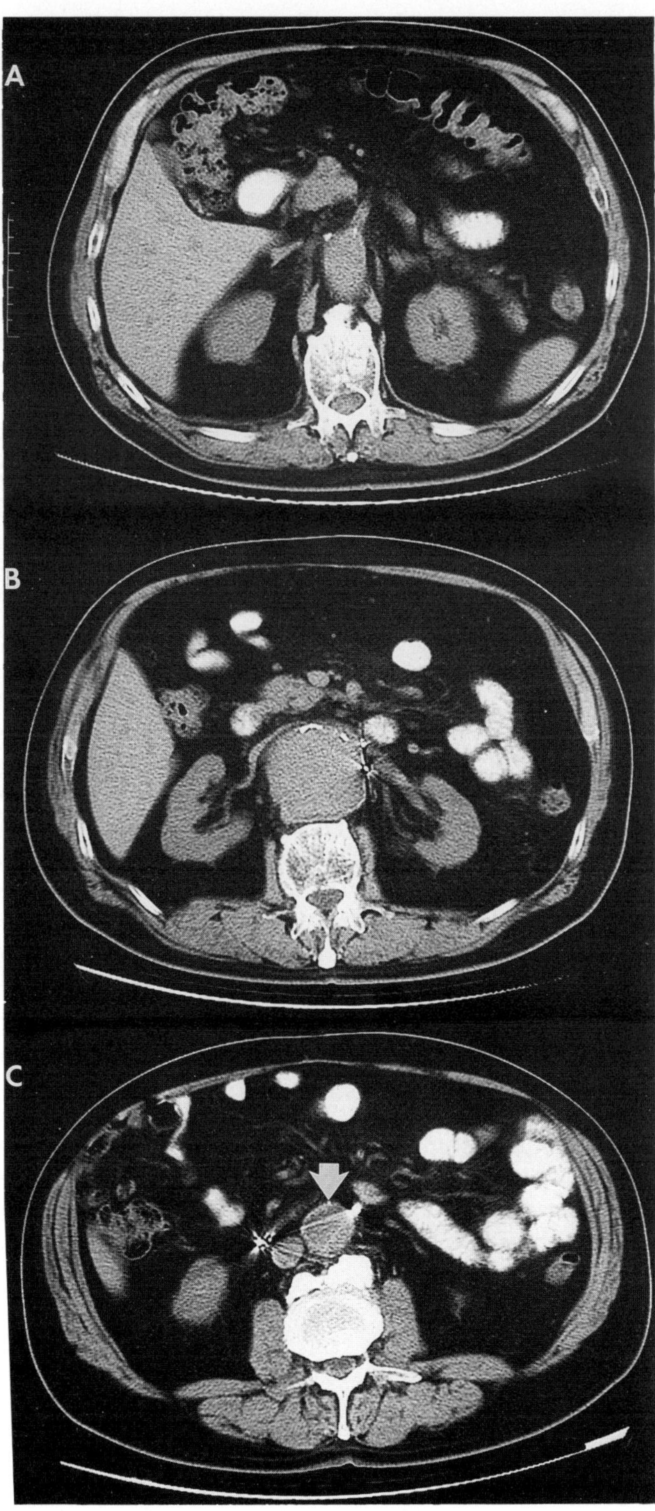

Fig. 1. Computerized abdominal tomography of a new abdominal aortic aneurysm that was recognized 6 years after an aorto-iliac graft for an abdominal aortic aneurysm. A. Normal sized aorta at the level of the superior mesenteric artery. B. 6 cm juxtarenal true aortic aneurysm. C. Proximal trunk of previous aorto-iliac graft (arrow).

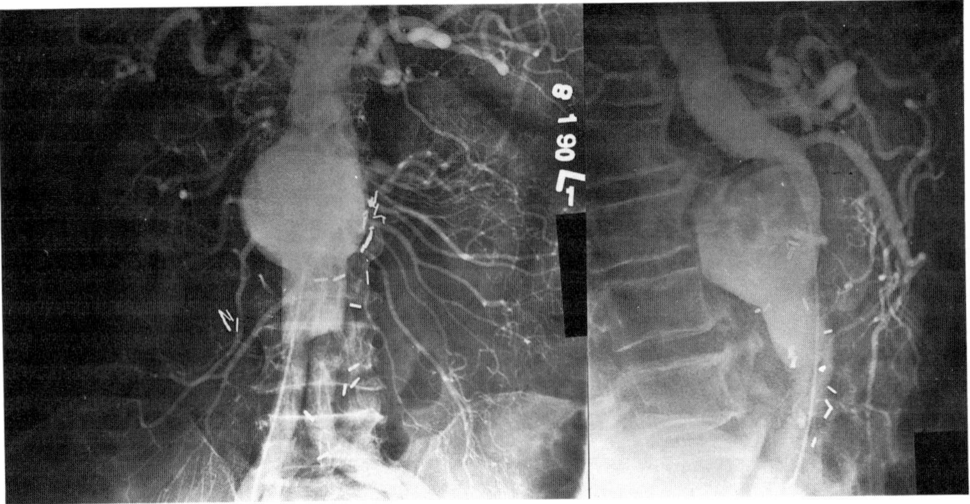

Fig. 2. Biplane aortogram of 6 cm juxtarenal aortic aneurysm shown in Fig. 1.

Bifurcated grafts

This population-based experience clearly demonstrates the higher trend of subsequent graft-related complications as well as new aneurysm or occlusive disease in the patients who received bifurcated grafts. These findings certainly do not implicate causality with the use of bifurcated grafts but may indicate that the bifurcated grafts are performed in patients with more advanced or progressive arterial disease. Bifurcated grafts have a propensity for both proximal and distal suture-line disruption or aneurysm formation. In addition, patients with bifurcated grafts tend to develop other true arterial aneurysms as well as distal occlusive disease causing both claudication and severe ischaemia. Like tube grafts, these graft-related complications and other vascular problems appear relatively late and support the need for long-term surveillance of the graft beyond 5 years.

Late monitoring of patients with bifurcated grafts should include both surveillance of the abdominal graft as well as femoral anastomoses and the femoropopliteal arterial segments. Periodic ultrasound or CT scanning will be sufficient for the aortic portion of the graft while a good physical examination and selective femoropopliteal ultrasound or Doppler-derived lower-limb pressures should detect problems below the inguinal ligaments.

CONCLUSION

The long-term findings of both our population-based and referral-based practices confirm that straight aortic grafts for abdominal aortic aneurysm have excellent results. In our own recent experience, more tube grafts (43%) are being inserted when the aneurysm disease is localized to the abdominal aorta and when no significant iliac occlusive disease is present. However, our recent experience continues to show that the majority (57%) of patients with abdominal aortic aneurysms have enough aneurysmal or occlusive disease of the common iliac segments to justify a bifurcated graft. In most cases, this bifurcated graft can be limited to an aorto-iliac prosthesis with only a small percentage of patients requiring extension of the graft to the aortofemoral level. Minimizing the extension of bifurcated grafts to the aortofemoral level for abdominal aortic aneurysm disease should reduce significantly the number of late graft-related problems at the distal femoral anastomoses.

ACKNOWLEDGEMENTS

The author gratefully acknowledges the editorial assistance of Gail Prechel and the epidemiologic and statistical expertise of Dr David J. Ballard.

REFERENCES

1. Kurland LT, Molgaard CA: The patient record in epidemiology. Sci Am 245:54–63, 1981
2. Plate G, Hollier LH, O'Brien PC: Recurrent aneurysms and late vascular complications following repair of abdominal aortic aneurysms. Arch Surg 120:590–594, 1985
3. Orr WM, Davies M: Simplified repair of abdominal aortic aneurysms using nonbifurcated (straight) inlay prosthesis. Br J Surg 61:847–849, 1974
4. Snellen JP, Terpstra OT, VanUrk H: The use of a straight tube graft decreases blood loss and operation time in patients with an abdominal aortic aneurysm. Neth J Surg 36:45–47, 1984
5. Van Uroonhaven TH JMV: Tube-inlay graft for abdominal aortic aneurysms. Arch Chir Neurol 30:164–168, 1978
6. Glickman MH, Julian CC, Kimmins S, Evans WE: Aortic aneurysm: to tube or not to tube. Surgery 9:603–605, 1982
7. Nash T: Abdominal aortic aneurysm: experience with the use of the straight tube method of treatment. Med J Aust 2:85–88, 1975
8. Provan JL, Fialkov JA, Ameli FM, St Louis EL: Is 'tube' prosthetic repair of abdominal aortic aneurysm followed by postoperative dilatation of the common iliac arteries? Abstract. 36th Scientific Program, The International Society for Cardiovascular Surgery, 1988

Popliteal Aneurysms

Anthony Chant

Recent articles on the maintenance of arterial reconstructions have emphasized the importance of radiological and ultrasound postoperative surveillance techniques.[1–3] To an extent, this focus of attention has tended to blinker vascular surgeons to other relevant factors, both before and after the reconstruction. A review of the management of popliteal aneurysms provides an excellent model to concentrate on some of the wider issues. In particular, it draws attention to the relationship between the timing of operative intervention and its eventual success.

Following arterial reconstruction for either occlusive or aneurysmal disease, there is a progressive fall-off in patency rate. The characteristic curves, illustrated in Fig. 1 are comprised of two parts, the attrition due to technical error and that due to disease progression. Successful, surgery should reduce the early attrition rate, such that any fall-off in patency is more related to disease progression than technical error. In the case of popliteal aneurysm, because disease progression is minimal, surgery *should* be curative. The difference then, between what we achieve in the way of patency rates and what nature prevents us achieving is therefore theoretically reclaimable. Such a reclamation should be possible by concentrating on the factors between the two curves.

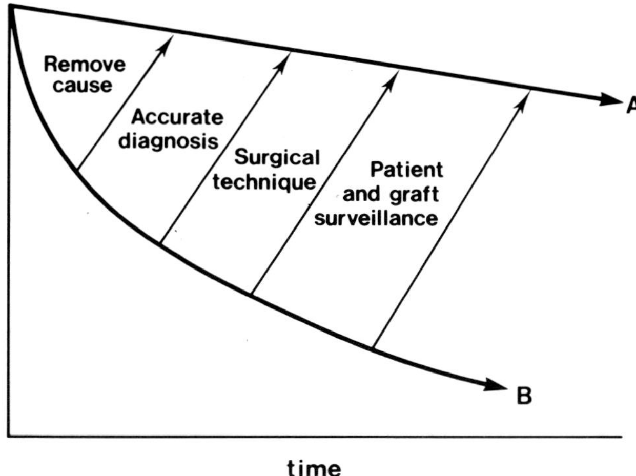

Fig. 1. Limb salvage. The area between curves A and B represents limbs which, using the techniques described in the text, could have been saved. Curve A represents the optimal results obtained by prophylactic surgery using autogenous vein. Limb salvage rates under these conditions are nearly 100%. Curve B represents those patients who present late. Late diagnosis and poor surgery are important contributory factors.

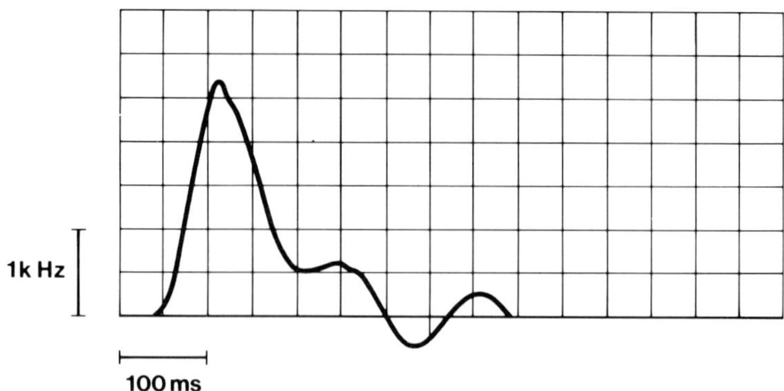

Fig. 2. Maximum frequency envelope for proximal dilatation. Characteristic wave form recorded in arteria magna. (After Humphries *et al.*, 1982.)

PREOPERATIVE CONSIDERATIONS

Removal of cause

The exact aetiology of most aneurysms remains obscure. Various observations, for example its reputed high prevalence in cavalry men and post boys, its relationship to the adductor opening and its documented association with popliteal entrapment syndromes[4] suggest that muscle compression and poststenotic dilation are relevant factors. The characteristic wave form of arteria magna[5] (Fig. 2) and possible genetic factors described in relation to aneurysms in general[6] suggests an underlying predisposition. Occasionally rare associated diseases are described as for example, Stinnet's report of fibromuscular hyperplasia causing bilateral aneurysms in a 10-year-old girl.[7] Trauma too has its role.[8] With the exception of the latter however, it seems that because popliteal aneurysms are frequently bilateral and because they normally present as a unilateral problem, the possibility of preventative treatment arises. Such treatment (prior to possible distal vessel embolization) maximizes the run-off possibilities and should theoretically therefore, enhance long-term patency rates.

Accurate diagnosis

The clinical diagnosis is usually not difficult. The size of the aneurysm and the nature of its contents require definition. Importantly, the inflow and outflow vessels also need outlining. Starting with size, it seems to me that the only reasonable definition of an aneurysm is as a ratio of it to a proximal artery (Fig. 3). Statements using absolute measurements such as 'all popliteal aneurysms greater than 2 cm require surgery' are vacuous. Conclusions based on retrospective surveys which espouse such courses of action should be viewed with caution. Although ultrasound[9] and ultrasound plus DSA[10] have their proponents, the use of computerized tomography[11] seems most promising in that, as well as defining the aneurysm and any associated thrombus, it also reveals muscular abnormalities and associated

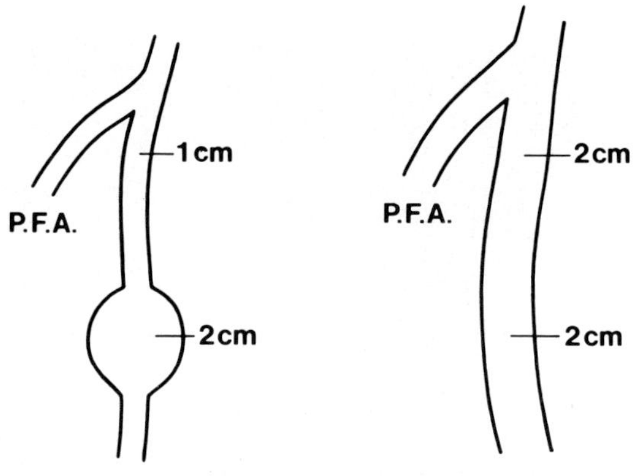

Fig. 3. Working definition of an aneurysm. If the suspect area is larger than the feeding vessel's take-off point, then an aneurysm is the likely diagnosis. Large arteries *per se* (as in the right-hand drawing) are simply large arteries. Size *per se* is therefore not too important.

entrapment syndromes. Colour duplex is also extremely useful, having the additional benefit of being able to define the inflow and to an extent, the outflow characteristics of the associated arteries.

If reconstruction is contemplated, adequate arteriography is required. Figure 4 illustrates bilateral popliteal aneurysms. The vessel on the right was occluded and the patient's consequent rest pain treated with a femorotibial bypass; the aneurysm on the left was subsequently treated prophylatically at a later date.

Surgical technique

Clearly this is important. Factors such as endothelial hyperplasia, platelet inhibitory drugs etc, are dealt with elsewhere in this volume and are all relevant to the treatment of popliteal aneurysms. Readers interested in the surgical technique of popliteal reconstruction are referred to a recent review by Kenyon and Greenhalgh.[12]

Graft and patient surveillance

Popliteal reconstructions like other femorodistal reconstructions should theoretically benefit from the kind of graft surveillance programmes mentioned earlier.[1–3] In the case of aneurysmal disease however, it is particularly important that the clinician follows up *the whole patient*. My results section confirms the findings of others (for example Haimovici[13]) that there is a high incidence of associated aneurysmal disease. The incidence of contralateral disase is high; small abdominal aneurysms grow. Just how aggressive vascular surgeons should be with respect to associated early disease is controversial but it is noteworthy that even though recent reports suggest that for example, abdominal aneurysms <5 cm in size may be observed, these reports often fail to stress that the complication rate in treating aneurysms

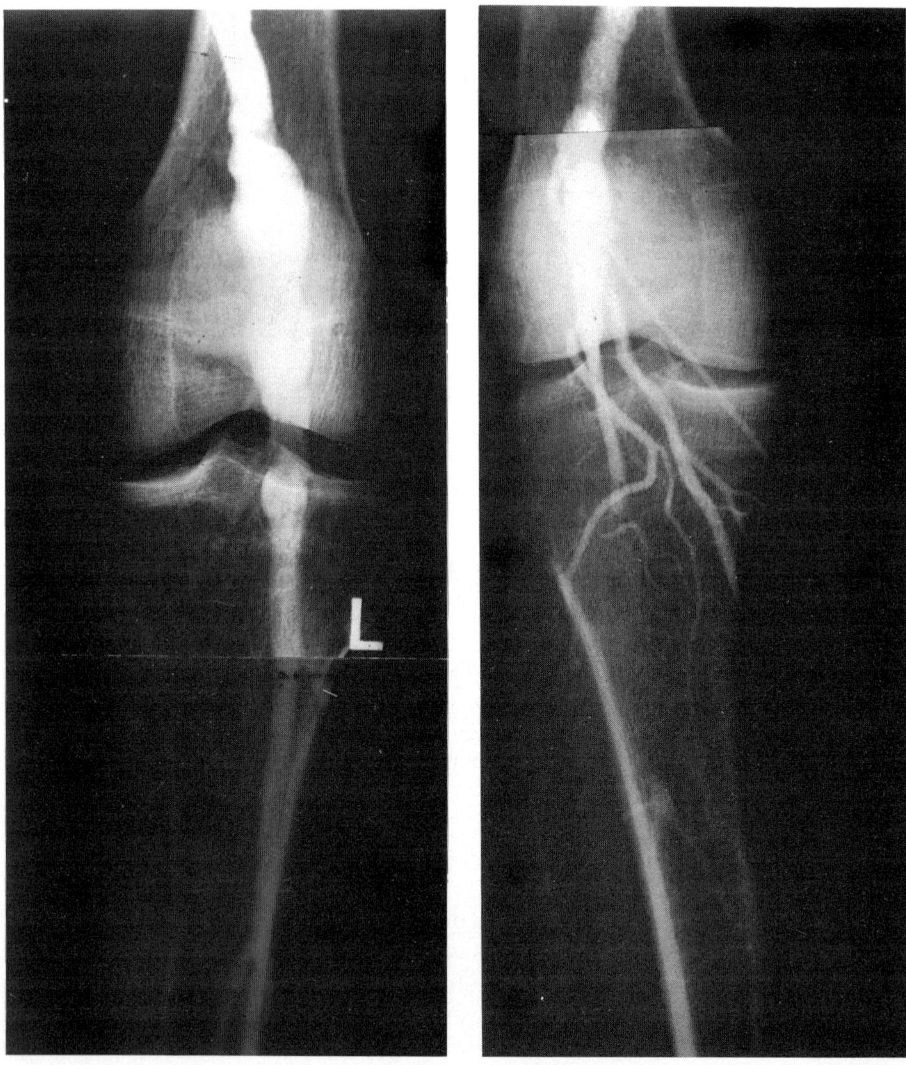

Fig. 4. Common presentation, one aneurysm (R) thrombosed, the other asymptomatic. (X-Rays courtesy of Dr S. Birch.)

>5 cm is significantly greater.[14] The possible presence of other small aneurysms should therefore not be overlooked or if found, ignored.

TREATMENT OPTIONS

The aims in treating patients with popliteal aneurysms are;

(i) To improve symptoms.

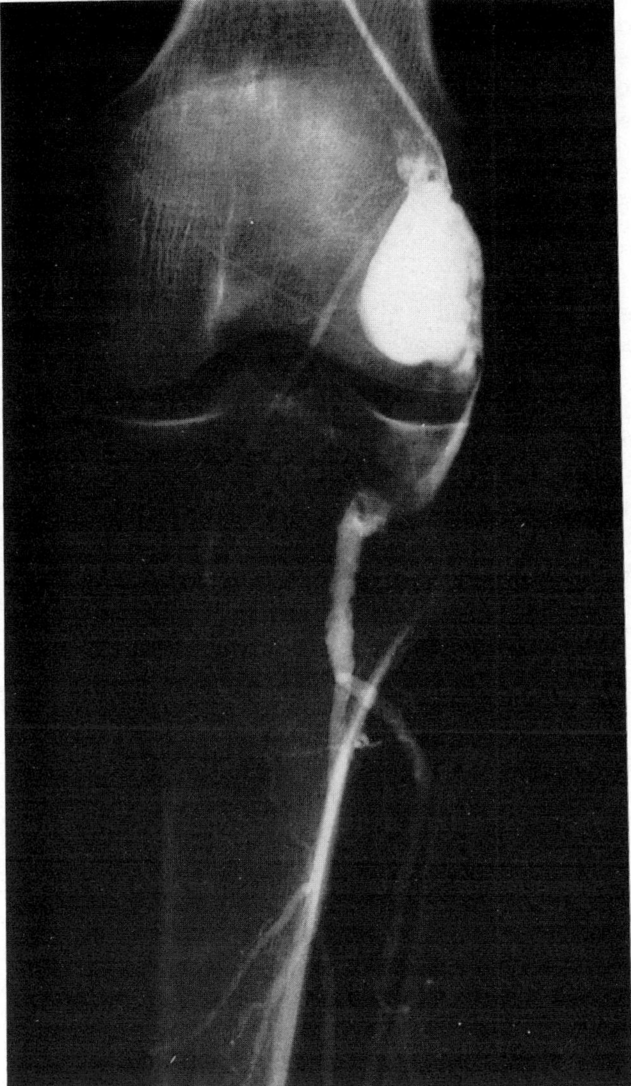

Fig. 5. Thrombosed aneurysm in the process of lysis.

(ii) By careful observation of the *complete patient* to prevent complications from either the aneurysm itself or associated aneurysms.

The treatment options relate directly to these simple aims. Starting with symptoms, in the case of rupture (rare), thrombosis, rest pain and claudication, the decision to treat is relatively easy. Given a reasonable run-off, simple bypass grafting suffices. If time permits (even following thrombosis) clot lysis with streptokinase[15] (or equivalent recombinant version) often improves run-off sufficiently (as in Fig. 5) to enable reconstruction. Asymptomatic aneurysms probably *should* be treated but, clearly, a balanced judgement of the relative risks of surgery has to be undertaken.

A review of the recent literature helps the practising surgeon take this decision but as is often the case with modern surgery, technique has outstripped our knowledge of the natural history of the disease. As far as I am aware, there is no complete epidemiological study based on objective evidence in the literature, nor now is there likely to be.

RESULTS

There is a degree of consistency in the literature in the mode of presentation, Haimovici's review[13] of the literature prior to 1980 being similar to more recent series.[16,17] Over 95% of patients are male, the reported age range varies from infancy to the late 90s. Approximately half the cases described are bilateral and between one-third and two-thirds have aneurysms elsewhere in the body. Thrombosis is probably the most common presentation, occurring in about two-fifths of all reported cases; however, differences in style of reporting makes comparison between series difficult. Less than 5% rupture. Vascular surgeons therefore, are faced during any one year, with a sporadic small number of male patients with one leg already critically ischaemic, and the other containing an asymptomatic aneurysm. In my view, unless there are significant medical contra-indications, both should be treated.

Symptomatic leg

Treatment of the symptomatic leg should follow the usual criteria adopted for peripheral ischaemia. Inevitably the quality of the distal run-off and technique will determine the outcome. The results of Lilly *et al.*[18] 1988, confirm this. In their well documented series of 48 aneurysms, only 10% had three vessel run-off and more than 50% had either zero or only one vessel remaining. Thrombus was clearly a factor for, of the 28 vessels that had CT scans, 19 had thrombus and of the 13 patent aneurysms, no less than eight had either zero or one vessel run-off. Obviously this is the high risk group where limb salvage is going to be most difficult.

The overall patency rates of both the Cleveland[19] and Chicago[18] series are similar over comparable periods of time, being of the order of 55% at 5 years, with a limb salvage rate somewhat higher.

Asymptomatic aneurysms

In contrast to symptomatic aneurysms (somewhat gloomily referred to in one British series as Harbinger of Doom[20]), asymptomatic aneurysms carry a consistently better prognosis. This is especially the case when vein grafts are used, 5-year patency rates are usually obtained in the order of 90–95%.[18,19] Prima facie therefore, the case seems conclusively in favour of prophylactic surgery especially when thrombus is identified on CT scanning. The advent of thrombolysis has however clouded the issue once more, for not only can symptomatic aneurysms be snatched from the

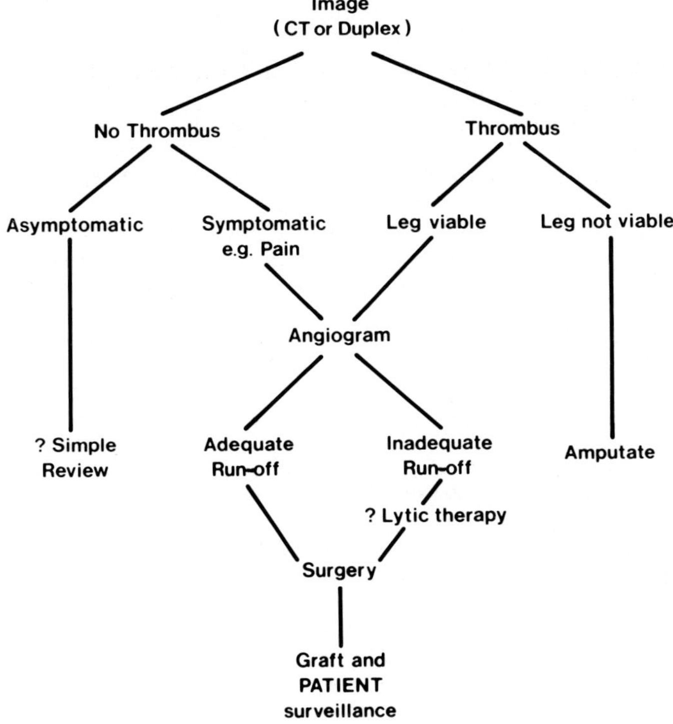

Fig. 6. Popliteal aneurysms. Suggested decision pathway.

brink of disaster, impaired run-off can be improved and patency restored; importantly the technique *may* allow a more expectant policy to be adopted in the really elderly.[21] In other words, a case *can* be made in the unfit for a watch and wait policy knowing that should the aneurysm occlude, thrombolysis may well achieve limb salvage. Clearly a greater experience of this technique is required before any firm policy could be formulated.

CONCLUSION

Of all peripheral vascular problems, it seems to me that popliteal aneurysms offer the vascular surgeon the greatest chance of success (Fig. 6). Modern imaging techniques allow exact identification of the problem and (importantly) associated problems such as other aneurysms. In the emergency situation, thrombolysis can often improve matters by improving run-off; indeed in the elderly there is now the possibility of even avoiding surgery. In younger patients however, particularly in the small subgroup of patients with associated entrapment syndromes, surgery remains the best option, prophylactic vein bypass of asymptomatic aneurysms giving the patient the best chance of long-term success.

REFERENCES

1. Wolfe JHN, Lea Thomas M, Jamieson CW *et al*: Early diagnosis of femoro-distal graft stenosis. Br J Surg 74:268–270, 1987
2. Gazzard VM, Clifford PC, Humphries KN *et al*: The role of Duplex scanning in the long-term follow-up of arterial grafts. Br J Radiol 59:732–733, 1986
3. Bandyk DF, Cato RF, Towne JB: A low flow velocity predicts graft failure. Surgery 98:700–709, 1985
4. Gyftocostas D, Koutsoumbelis C, Matheou T, Bouhoutsos J: Post-stenotic aneurysms in popliteal artery entrapment syndrome. J Cardiovasc Surg (in press)
5. Humphries KH, Hames TK, Chant ADB: Detection of arterial dilatation using continuous wave ultrasound. Cardiovasc Res 16:474–482, 1982
6. Powell JT and Greenhalgh RM: Cellular, enzymatic and genetic factors in the pathogenesis of abdominal aortic aneurysm. J Vasc Surg 9:297–304, 1989
7. Stinnett DM, Graham JM, Edwards WD: Fibromuscular dysplasia and thrombosed aneurysm of the popliteal artery in a child. J Vasc Surg 5:769–772, 1987
8. Hamza N, Marath A, Al-Fakhry MR: The management of aneurysms and arterio-venous fistulae of the popliteal artery arising from war trauma. J Cardiovasc Surg 31:457–461, 1990
9. MacGowan SW, Saif MF, O'Neill G, Fitzsimors P, Bouchier-Hayes D: Ultrasound examination in the diagnosis of popliteal artery aneurysms. Br J Surg 72:528–529, 1985
10. Turnipseed WD, Archer CW, Detmer DE *et al*: Digital subtraction angiography and B-mode ultrasonography for abdominal and peripheral aneurysms. Surgery 92:619–626, 1982
11. Rizzo RJ, Flinn WR, Yao JS *et al*: Computed tomography for evaluation of arterial disease in the popliteal fossa. J Vasc Surg 11:112–119, 1990
12. Kenyon JR, Greenhalgh RM: Popliteal aneurysm and entrapment. *In* Vascular Surgical Techniques, Greenhalgh RM (Ed.). Surrey UK: Butterworth, pp. 177–181, 1984
13. Haimovici H: Peripheral artery aneurysms. *In* Vascular Emergencies. New York: Appleton-Century-Crofts, pp. 399–413, 1982
14. Johansson G, Nydahl S, Olofsson P *et al*: Survival of patients with abdominal aortic aneurysms. Eur J Vasc Surg 4:497–502, 1990
15. Ferguson LJ, Faris I, Robertson A, Lloyd JV, Miller JH: Intra-arterial streptokinase therapy to relieve accute limb ischaemia. J Vasc Surg 4:205–210, 1986
16. Whitehouse WM Jnr, Wakefield TW, Graham LM, Kazmers A *et al*: Limb-threatening potential of arteriosclerotic popliteal artery aneurysms. Surgery 93:694–699, 1983
17. Vermillion BD, Kimmins SA, Pace WG, Evans WE: A review of 147 popliteal aneurysms with long term follow up. Surgery 90:1009–1014, 1981
18. Lilly MP, Flinn WR, McCarthy WJ *et al*: The effect of distal artery anatomy on the success of popliteal aneurysm repair. J Vasc Surg 7:653–660, 1988
19. Anton GE, Hertzer NR, Bevan EG, O'Hara PJ, Krajewski LP: Surgical management of popliteal aneurysms. Trends in presentation, treatment, and results from 1952 to 1984. J Vasc Surg 3:125–134, 1986
20. Guvendik L, Bloor K, Charlesworth D. Popliteal aneurysm: sinister harbinger of sudden catastrophe. Br J Surg 67(4):294–296, 1980
21. Bowyer RC, Cawthorn SJ, Walker WJ, Giddings AEB. Conservation management of asymptomatic popliteal aneurysm. Br J Surg 77:1132–1135, 1990

Aortic Bifurcation Grafting for Stenosing Disease

J. Fernandes e Fernandes, Angélica Damião
and C. Hilário Almeida

Atherosclerosis is the commonest arteriopathy in the Western world causing dilatation or occlusion of the main arteries. The severity of the clinical manifestations in the occlusive forms is dependent upon the degree of narrowing, its location and extension and the functional capability of the collateral circulation.

Stenosing arterial disease most frequently affects the superficial femoral artery, but involvement of the aorta and iliac arteries can occur in a significant number of patients, either as an isolated form or in association with more diffuse and widespread disease, and it represents a major determinant in clinical outcome. Its management requires correct assessment of the extension of the occlusive process i.e. the degree of haemodynamic impairment, particularly in those patients with multilevel disease, in order to establish correct therapeutic strategy for each individual patient.

Reconstructive arterial procedures for the treatment of aorto-iliac occlusive disease were established in the 1950s and were shown to be effective and durable for the relief of ischaemic symptoms.

This chapter will deal with the role of bifurcation grafts for the treatment of stenosing disease in the aorto-iliac segment and will discuss relevant aspects concerning selection of patients for this procedure and the factors that may affect their performance and long-term efficacy.

HISTORY

An early description of occlusive disease in the abdominal aorta was given by Hunter who collected autopsy specimens that demonstrated atherosclerotic involvement of both common iliac arteries[1]; these can be seen in the Royal College of Surgeons in London. However, it was Cruvheilier,[2] in the mid-nineteenth century, who established for the first time a link between diseased arteries and 'spontaneous' or 'senile' gangrene of the lower extremities.

Functional impairment with walking seen in association with aorto-iliac disease was described by Charcot,[3] in 1858, in a man with an occluded iliac artery after a gunshot wound; he 'could only walk a quarter of an hour without experiencing a feeling of weakness in his right lower limb, followed by dull pain and tingling, symptoms manifesting first in his buttocks, than in the thigh, leg and foot'.[4] Charcot did give credit to a previous observation by Barth,[5] in 1835, of a patient with hip and thigh claudication caused by an occluded abdominal aorta and common iliacs, recognized at autopsy.

Detailed description of the clinical manifestations of aorto-iliac occlusive disease was produced by Leriche in 1923[6] (Fig. 1), almost a century later, and he suggested

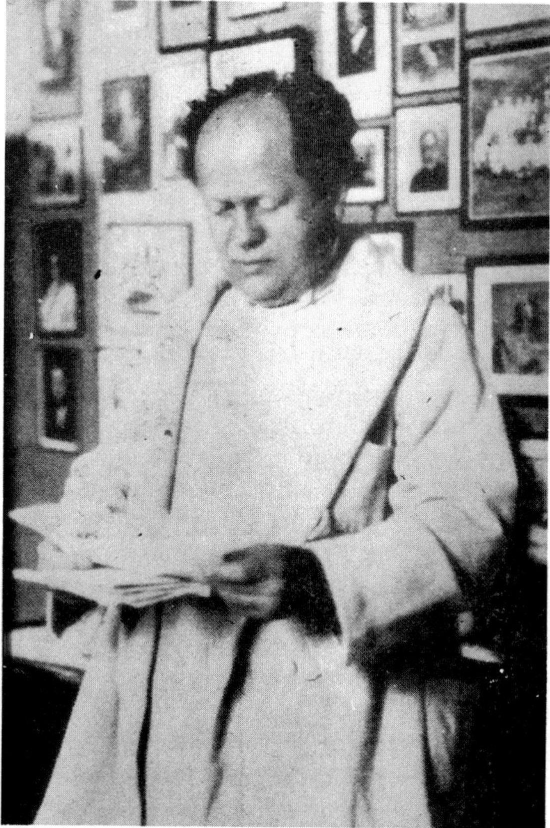

Fig. 1. René Leriche.

lumbar sympathectomy as a form of treatment to improve collateral circulation. Ten years later he promoted resection of the obstructed segment of the aorta[7] in association with lumbar sympathectomy in order to remove a noxious stimulus that would provoke peripheral vasoconstriction. Although the therapeutic suggestions of Leriche were of questionable benefit, his clinical descriptions were complete, encompassing all the symptoms associated with occlusion of the aorta, a clinical syndrome usually referred to nowadays as Leriche syndrome.

The *in vivo* visualization of occlusive disease became possible only after the development of translumbar aortography by Reynaldo dos Santos (Fig. 2) in 1927,[8] who adapted to the peripheral arteries, the concept of Moniz for arterial visualization of the cerebral circulation. Developments such as intra-arterial catheterization contributed to identify aortography as an essential diagnostic tool in the assessment of patients with lower limb ischaemia.

Surgical treatment of chronically occluded arteries was initiated by João Cid dos Santos in 1947,[9] with the introduction of endarterectomy, thus starting a new era in modern vascular surgery. The initial operations were performed in the subclavian–axillary arteries and in the iliofemoral segment, providing long-term patency and relief of ischaemic symptoms.

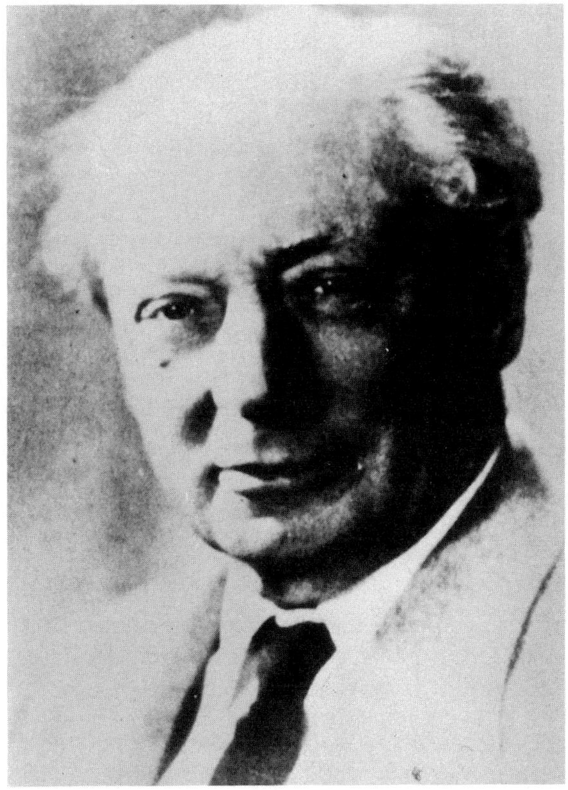

Fig. 2. Reynaldo dos Santos.

The dos Santos technique of endarterectomy was modified by several authors, with the introduction of ring disobliterators by Cannon,[10] adoption of single arteriotomy throughout the length of the obstruction, as suggested by Bazy *et al.*,[11] and the development of the 'overpass' concept by Cid dos Santos.[12]

Replacement of abdominal aorta and iliac arteries by preserved homografts[13] was another attempt to treat occlusive disease. The first case was reported by Oudot[14] in 1951, when a homograft was used to replace the aorta and common iliac through a retroperitoneal approach, the procedure complemented by a retroperitoneal 'crossover' graft to the right iliac artery.

Bypassing the lesions instead of removing them became an attractive principle that seems to have emerged in several centres in the early 1950s, and constituted a turning point in modern vascular surgery. Homografts had a short life span because of complications inherent in their structure and they were soon abandoned in favour of new plastic materials. Vorhees *et al.*[15] in 1953 introduced an allograft made of plastic (the vinyon-N graft); this was followed by others made from nylon, Orlon and Teflon. The major step forward was the development by DeBakey *et al.*[16] of the knitted Dacron graft, a more resistant and well tolerated fabric which brought a tremendous impulse to reconstructive arterial surgery.

Endarterectomy and bypass grafting became established techniques for the treatment of occlusive disease in the aorto-iliac segment, and arguments for and against each of these techniques appeared abundantly in the medical literature. Bypass grafting became widely used within the vascular community because of its being technically easier to perform, resulting in less blood and shorter operative times and also because long-term results of extensive endarterectomies of the external iliac and femoral arteries were found to be less satisfactory.[17]

The development of extra-anatomical procedures in the 1960s[18,19] made possible surgical treatment in higher risk patients and increased the surgical armamentarium for the treatment of aorto-iliac occlusive disease.

The extensiveness of the atherosclerotic process in the aorto-iliac segment, usually bilateral and its progressive nature, reduced the use of limited or unilateral reconstructive procedures, and aortofemoral bifurcation grafts became a procedure of choice in many centres,[20] with excellent long-term patency rate and reduced morbidity.

Refinements in graft materials in order to reduce porosity or to facilitate incorporation by surrounding tissues made bifurcation grafts for aorto-iliac occlusive disease one of the commonest procedures in vascular surgical practice. However, their limitations are well recognized and will be covered in this chapter. Risk of infection (inherent in the use of prosthetic material) degradation of the fabric with dilatation of the grafts, development of anastomotic aneurysms and the occurrence of late thrombosis all deserve special consideration for adequate selection of surgical procedures for the treatment of aorto-iliac occlusive disease.

Extent of disease and diagnosis

Several theories have been advanced to explain the susceptibility of the abdominal aorta and iliac arteries to atherosclerosis. Increase in arterial wall stiffness due to a reduction in the content of elastic fibres and a higher proportion of collagen associated with a particular nutritional pattern of the medial layer, may represent relevant factors that promote plaque formation in the aorto-iliac segment.[21] In fact, nutrition of the arterial wall in the distal aorta and iliac arteries is more dependent upon diffusion of elements from the circulating blood. Because of the reduced number of vasa-vasorum that penetrate the medial layer when compared with the thoracic aorta, focal areas of ischaemia are created within the media, resulting in alterations of the metabolic functions of the smooth muscle cells and leading to their proliferation and to increase in collagen production.

The pattern of flow in the aorto-iliac segment may also play an important role in plaque formation and extension; the reversal of flow in late systole in the abdominal aorta and iliac arteries can affect the normal alignment and overlapping of endothelial cells, thus increasing permeability and favouring the deposition of lipids in the subintimal space.[22] Low shear stress occurs in the posterior aspect of the aortic wall in the infrarenal segment and near the bifurcation[23] and the sudden reduction of flow distal to the renal arteries contributes to enhance particle deposition in the arterial wall and reduce clearance of atherogenic substances. Turbulence at the bifurcation leads to disruption of the endothelial lining and exposure of the subintimal layer, a factor known to promote blood cell aggregation and thrombus formation.

Biplane angiography and operative examination of diseased aorto-iliac segments confirm that atherosclerosis affects predominantly the posterior half of the arterial wall, both in the terminal aorta and iliac arteries. This fact accounts for the difficulties in accurate assessment of the extent of the occlusive process and degree of stenosis on single plane angiography.

Brewster and Darling[24] classified the atherosclerotic involvement of the aorto-iliac segment in three types according to its extension: Type I when the disease was confined to the distal aorta and common iliac vessels, present in approximately 10% of the patients, Type II if there was disease in the external iliac and femoral arteries, without infra-inguinal occlusion, present in 25 to 30% and Type III when there was simultaneous occlusions in the infra-inguinal vessels, that is, multilevel disease, which represented the majority of the patients. This classification could be correlated with clinical outcome and helped to standardize surgical approach. Type I disease was present in younger patients and had a prognosis and less progression of the occlusive process; the lesions were usually amenable to endarterectomy; Type II and III corresponded to more severe forms of lower limb ischaemia, occurring in older patients and requiring aorto-iliac or aortofemoral bifurcation grafts. Other attempts to classify the occlusive disease in the aorto-iliac segment in order to include single vessel disease, unilateral stenosis or occlusion and to contemplate the role of collateral circulation,[25] have no significant advantage.

Clinical evaluation is sufficient to establish the presence of aorto-iliac disease in the vast majority of patients. Intermittent claudication of the thigh and hip muscles, reduced erectile function in males, diminished or absent femoral pulses and the presence of bruits audible along the iliac arteries are of diagnostic value. Localized distal ischaemia in the foot[26] can be associated with proximal aorto-iliac disease and is often due to repeated embolization from atheroesclerotic plaques with adherent thrombus or ulceration.

Impotence due to thrombotic obliteration of the aorta was first recognized by Leriche in 1940, and more recent reports suggest that it can occur in as many as 30% of the patients,[27] may precede the symptoms of lower limb ischaemia[28] and can be associated either with bilateral common iliac occlusion or involvement of both internal iliac arteries.

More advanced forms of lower limb ischaemia (rest pain and critical ischaemia) usually require the presence of multilevel occlusive disease, and are evident because of the functional inability of the collateral circulation to sustain adequate flow (Fig. 3) in the presence of infra-inguinal disease.

Femoral pulse palpation may be difficult in obese patients or in those with previous groin operations, and its limitations to recognize minor stenosis (<50%) in the aorto-iliac segment have been established.[29] Disappearance of femoral pulses after exercise may improve the diagnostic accuracy of clinical examination in less severe forms of occlusive disease, but it is subjective and observer dependent.

Aortography has been the established diagnostic procedure in arterial occlusive disease of the lower limbs; development of new nonionic contrast media helped to reduce the risk of adverse reactions associated with angiography. We favour translumbar aortography (Fig. 4) because of the risk of plaque dislodgment or

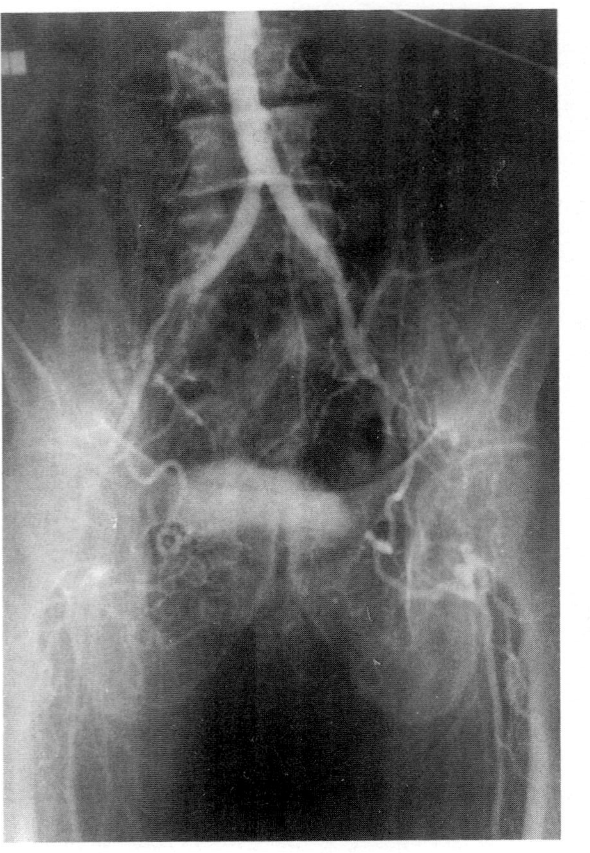

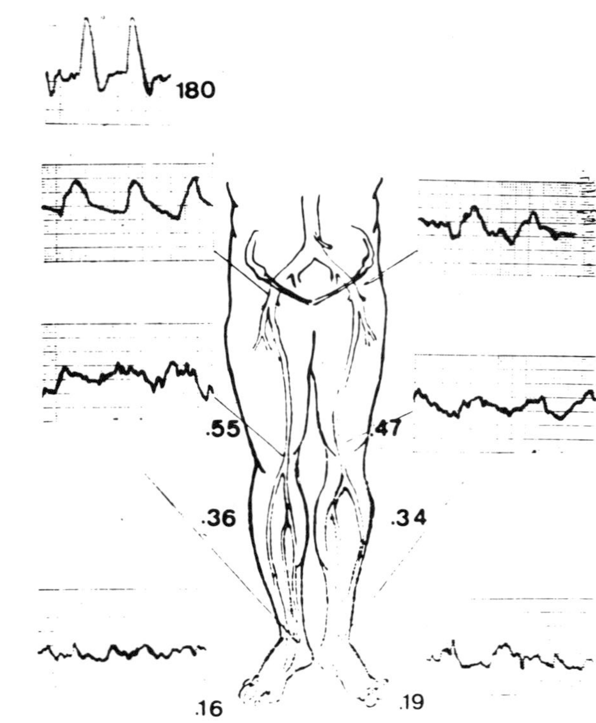

Fig. 3. A (Left): Translumbar aortogram: multisegmental involvement in aorto-iliac and femoropopliteal disease. B (Right): Severe haemodynamic impairment with low resting pressure indices.

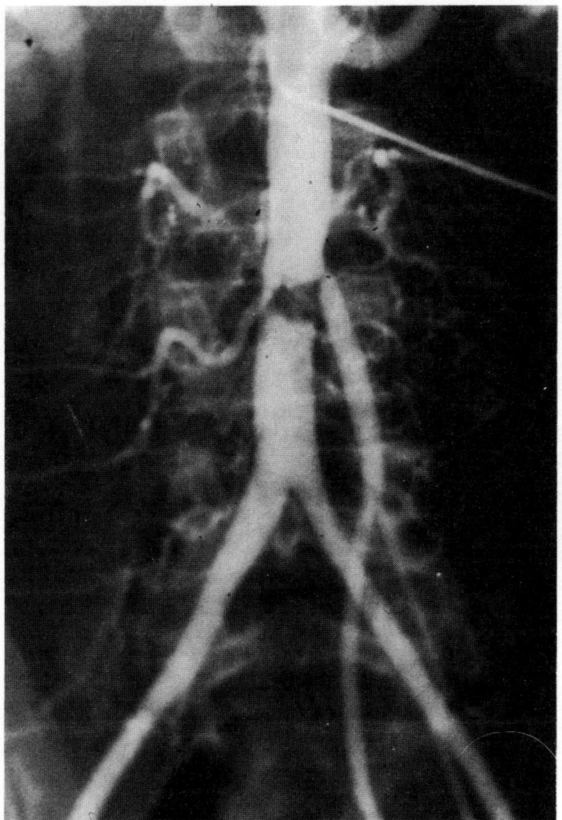

Fig. 4. Translumbar aortogram: localized stenosis of the abdominal aorta treated by endarterectomy.

embolization during retrograde catheterization, and we aim to position the tip of the needle near the renal arteries in order to obtain visualization of the visceral branches of the aorta. Morphologic aspects of the occlusive lesions, including the presence of thrombi adherent to plaque surface (Fig. 5), can be obtained with single plane views, but a clear delimitation of the extension of the disease and correct assessment of the severity of stenosis requires biplane or oblique views.[30] Angiographic information is qualitative and difficulties in identifying the 'critical lesion', that is stenosis producing a pressure-gradient, were reported in the early 1970s.[31] Pressure measurements obtained proximal and distal to an iliac stenosis,[32,33] were suggested to complement angiographic information, particularly in patients with multilevel occlusive disease. Precise functional assessment of the haemodynamic impairment of an iliac stenosis is essential for correct surgical management in this subset of patients with extensive disease.

Femoral artery pressures measured in resting conditions and during hyperaemia following vasodilation obtained by direct injection of papaverine were reported as a useful method to identify significant iliac disease,[34] the criteria for a positive test being a gradient between common femoral and radial artery pressures equal to or

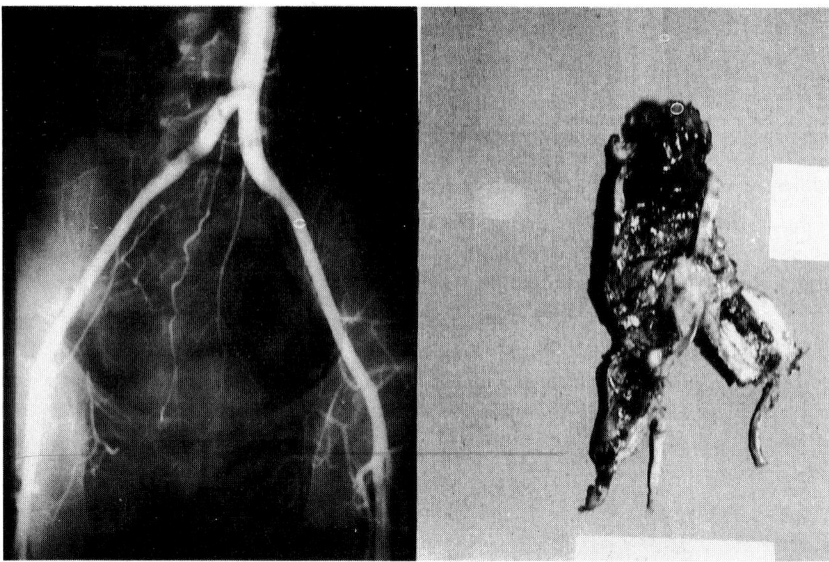

Fig. 5. Translumbar aortogram: plaque visualization with adherent thrombus and operative specimen in a patient with distal foot ischaemia and embolization into crural arteries.

greater than 10 mm Hg or a 15% pressure reduction after papaverine injection. These criteria seem to have a good predictive value for clinical and haemodynamic improvement following proximal reconstructive procedures.

Noninvasive technology has played an increasingly important role in the assessment of peripheral occlusive disease. Analysis of Doppler velocity waveforms of the femoral arteries, determinations of pulsatility index, damping factor and spectral analysis were shown to have diagnostic value for the presence of aorto-iliac occlusive disease.[35–37] Objective assessment of pulse rise time of the femoral pulse correlated well with angiography even for minor degrees of stenosis,[38] but its predictive value for the efficacy of proximal reconstructions in multilevel disease, needs further research.

Froneck *et al.*[39] suggested that low thigh brachial pressure indices obtained by segmental pressure measurements and failure to increase femoral velocity measured with directional Doppler during the initial hyperaemic phase after induced ischaemia, were of diagnostic value to identify significant iliac stenosis.

An example is shown in Figs 6, A, B and C: failure to increase femoral velocity associated with remarkable turbulence at peak systole and low thigh pressures in a patient with diffuse aorto-iliac stenosing disease and bilateral superficial femoral occlusions, were highly suggestive of haemodynamic significance of the iliac disease, which was confirmed by direct femoral artery pressure measurements and the use of the papaverine test.

Duplex scan examinations with direct visualization of the aorta and the iliac arteries may improve noninvasive diagnosis of aorto-iliac disease and assessment of its haemodynamic severity as reported recently.[40]

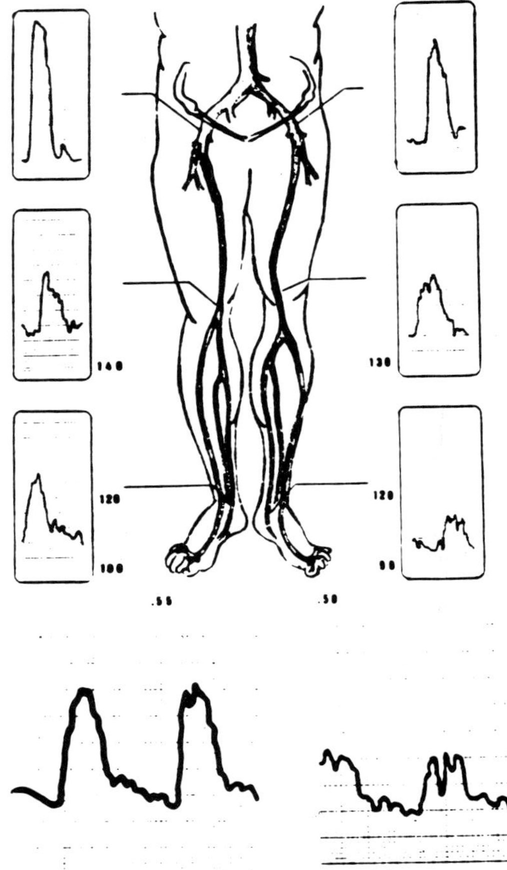

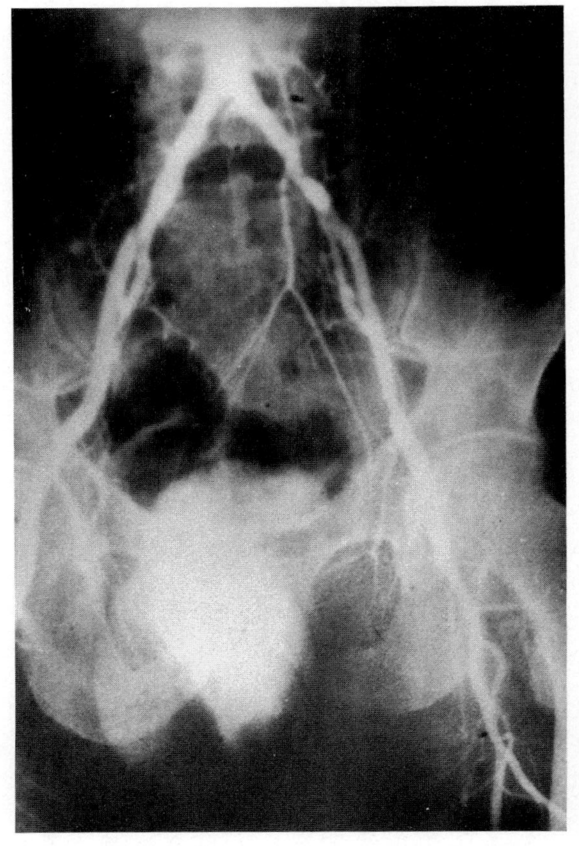

Fig. 6. Patient with disabling claudication and multilevel disease. A (Left, upper): Doppler velocity tracings and segmental pressure measurements. B (Left, lower): Velocity tracings in both femoral arteries in the initial hyperaemic phase postinduced ischaemia. Note absence of increase in velocity and turbulence at peak systole. C (Right): Translumbar aortogram: diffuse aorto-iliac disease.

SURGICAL MANAGEMENT

Conservative treatment with control of risk factors associated with atherosclerotic occlusive disease (dyslipidaemia, diabetes, control of hypertension), and cessation of smoking are essential steps in management of patients with lower limb ischaemia. The effect of exercise training programmes, in patients with intermittent claudication, on improving collateral circulation has been recognized.[41,42] However, in the presence of more extensive disease with proximal and distal occlusions, sustained benefits are uncommon and a significant percentage will require surgical treatment. Advanced forms of lower limb ischaemia (rest pain and cutaneous throphic lesions) are absolute indications for surgical repair of occlusive disease.

From 1978 to 1990, 284 consecutive patients required aorto-iliac reconstructive surgery (255 males and 29 females, mean age 56 years ranging from 37 to 79 years). The indications for surgery are listed in Table 1: 41.5% (118 patients) had disabling claudication, despite a period of medical management, 58.4% (166 patients) had severe ischaemia—Stages III and IV—and required operative treatment for limb salvage.

The presence of atherosclerotic risk factors (Table 2) did not differ from other series reported in the literature.

Table 1. Indications for aorto-iliac surgery

Claudication (Stage IIB)	118 (41.5%)
Rest pain (Stage III)	46 (16.2%)
Rest pain + throphic cutaneous lesions (Stage IV)	120 (42.2%)

Table 2. Risk factors in patients having aorto-iliac surgery

Hypertension	55%
Coronary artery disease (clinical + ECG changes)	52%
Diabetes	26%
Dyslipidaemia	28%
Smoking	89%

Coronary artery disease is the major cause of operative mortality in aorto-iliac reconstructive surgery,[43–46] and its diagnosis and treatment deserves special consideration. Improved diagnostic procedures with greater accuracy to assess the severity of coronary disease in patients with claudication were described[47,48] allowing for a better patient selection and reduction of surgical risk. Prophylactic coronary artery reconstructions were advocated[49,50] to improve operative mortality and morbidity and to increase survival after reconstructive aorto-iliac surgery.

Better medical management of cardiac disease, improved anaesthetic techniques and postoperative surveillance and the use of extra-anatomical reconstructions for higher risk patients, have limited the scope of coronary artery reconstructive surgery, in particular in patients with more advanced lower limb ischaemia. In our experience remote or extra-anatomic reconstructions represented 18% of the total number of procedures and were exclusively reserved for patients with poor cardiac and pulmonary functions.

Noninvasive studies with directional Doppler were obtained for quantitative assessment of the degree of lower limb ischaemia and to assist surgical decision in patients with multilevel occlusions by evaluation of the haemodynamic significance of proximal stenosis and infra-inguinal obstructions, as already mentioned in this chapter.

Aortography was systematically performed and the translumbar method preferred; careful assessment of the extension of the occlusive process was required for the correct choice of surgical reconstructive procedure. Multilevel disease was predominant (Table 3): 228 patients had extensive aorto-iliac and distal infra-inguinal disease and only 56 (19.7%) had limited aorto-iliac involvement. In 19 patients significant stenosis or occlusion was present in the renal and mesenteric vessels and in 32 there were focal dilatations or aneurysmal changes in the abdominal aorta.

Table 3. Extension of the occlusive disease assessed by aortography

Proximal segment (A-I only)	56
Multilevel disease (F/P and/or crural)	228
Visceral occlusive disease	19
renal	12
superior mesenteric and/or coeliac axis	3

Table 4. Aorto-iliac reconstructive surgery: procedures performed in 284 patients

Thromboendarterectomy	21
Aortofemoral bifurcation grafts	202
Unilateral reconstructions (Iliofemoral)	9
Extra-anatomical (F-F and/or Ax.-F)	52
Total	284

Reconstructive procedures used are listed in Table 4; thromboendarterectomy was reserved for localized stenosis or occlusions, not extending into the external iliac and/or femoral arteries, or in the presence of plaques acting as embolic sources (Figs 7 and 8). 'Necessity' endarterectomies were performed in combination with bypass procedures to achieve adequate inflow, as in juxtarenal aortic occlusions (Fig. 9), or to improve outflow through the profunda femoris in patients with femoropopliteal occlusion.

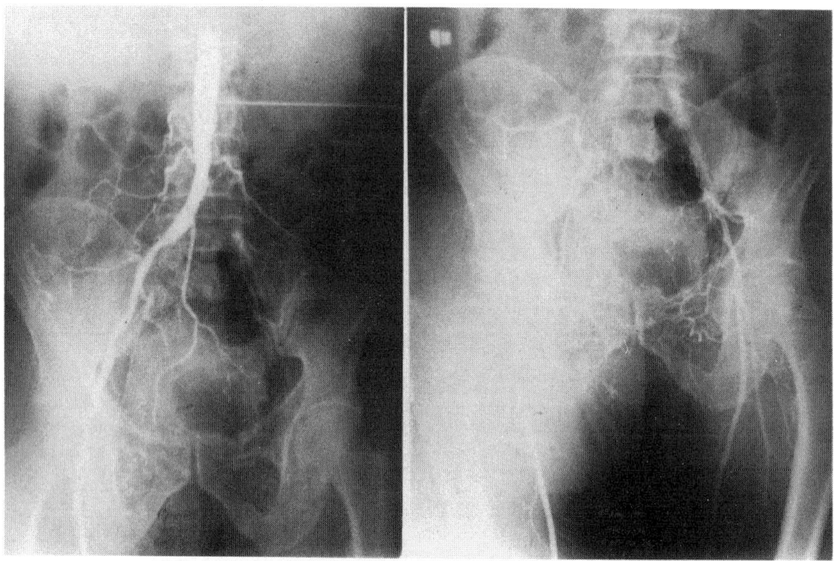

Fig. 7. Aortogram: Patient with Type I disease treated by endarterectomy and γ-patch angioplasty.

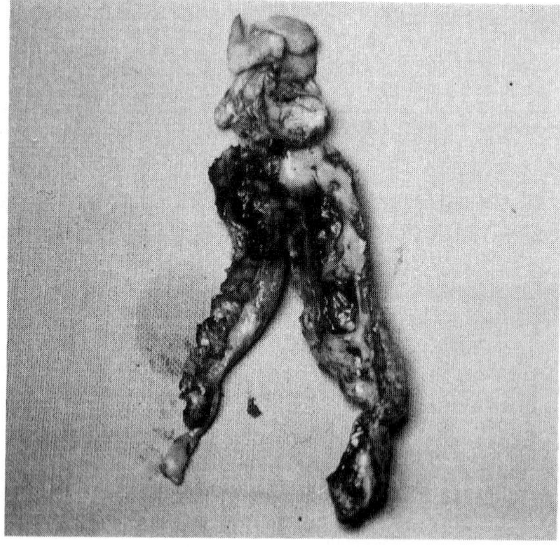

Fig. 8. Endarterectomy: Atherosclerotic plaque with ulceration and thrombus, acting as embolic source.

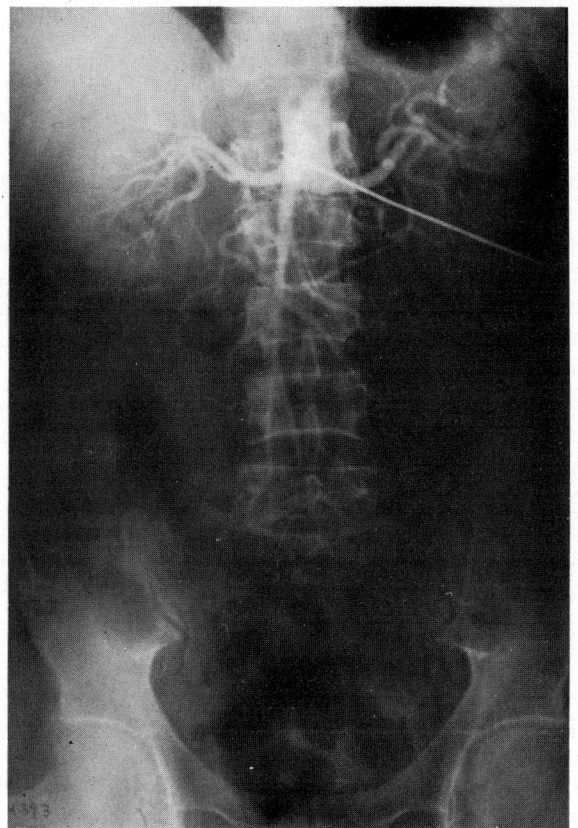

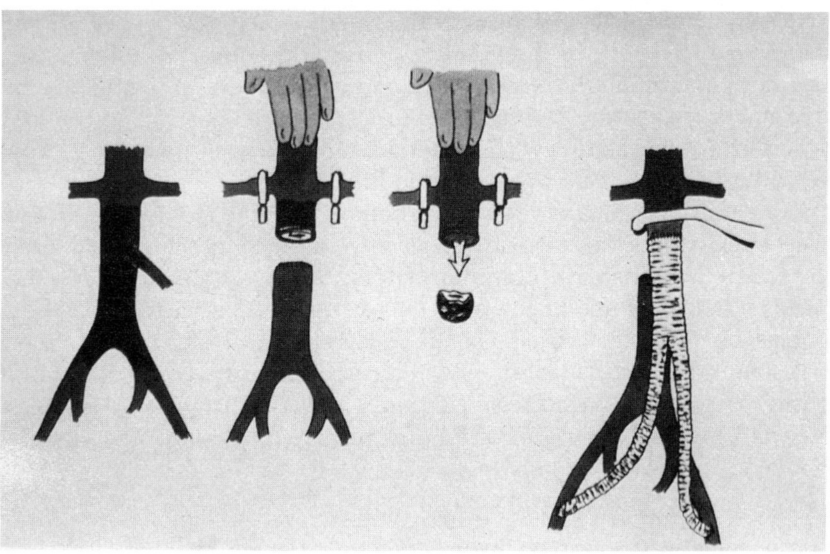

Fig. 9. A (Upper): Juxtarenal aortic occlusion. B (Lower): Schematic representation of treatment: endarterectomy is required to obtain inflow for a bifurcated graft.

Aortofemoral bifurcation grafts were the procedure of choice in 202 patients (71%) because of the extension and severity of occlusive disease.

In the presence of aneurysmal disease confined to the common iliacs without occlusive process in the remaining aorto-iliac segment it is preferable to proceed with intra-abdominal reconstructions with distal anastomosis of bifurcated grafts performed in an end-to-end fashion at the common iliac bifurcation, to preserve internal iliac perfusion, and reduce the risk of prosthetic infection.

A midline incision was routinely used and minimal dissection of the aorta was carried out to avoid injury to the peri-aortic nerve plexus; tunnelling through the retroperitoneal space into the groins was performed carefully to prevent twisting of the graft limbs, to avoid excessive tension in the anastomosis and to prevent ureteral obstruction by positioning the graft under the ureter. Systemic heparinization was not used, except in patients with extensive occlusive disease with poor outflow tracts and when longer clamping times were anticipated, but distal flushing with heparinized saline was systematically performed. Prophylactive antibiotics were always given and continued for the initial 2 or 3 postoperative days.

Proximal and distal anastomosis were constructed preferably in an end-to-side fashion, except if there was evidence of focal dilatation or aneurysmal changes in the aorta, when end-to-end anastomosis were chosen to exclude the dilated segments. Advantages of end-to-end anastomosis are based on theoretical grounds: better haemodynamics with less turbulence, anatomic position of the graft in the aortic bed which would reduce the risk of adhesion and erosion of the duodenum, and avoidance of competitive flows at the site of distal anastomosis. Evidence of turbulence in end-to-side aortic anastomosis of bifurcation grafts was not demonstrated in a group of patients studied with colour flow duplex scan (Fig. 10) and protection from the duodenum can be achieved with correct positioning of the shaft of the graft and adequate cover with retroperitoneal tissue. Preservation of the 'native' circulation to a patent inferior mesenteric artery by use of end-to-side anastomosis, may be helpful in avoiding pelvic and colonic ischaemia in patients with external iliac occlusion, which could prevent adequate retrograde perfusion of the internal iliac system. Re-implantation of one internal iliac in the limb of the graft may be useful in patients with bilateral internal iliac stenosis to improve penile perfusion pressure and treat vasculogenic impotence.[51]

The use of external iliac artery for construction of distal anastomosis in bifurcated grafts was suggested by Crawford *et al.*[52] to reduce infection and aneurysmal formation, complications more common when grafts were positioned in the groins. The higher incidence of re-occlusion reported seems to be associated with the presence and progression of arterial disease in the femoral artery. Our practice has been to perform distal end-to-side anastomosis of bifurcated grafts at the common femoral artery in the absence of distal occlusive disease or in a profundoplasty fashion (Fig. 11) if there is occlusion of the superficial femoral artery. Arteriotomy is extended in the

Fig. 10 (facing page). Colour flow duplex assessment of a bifurcated 18 × 9 mm Dacron graft of 4 years. A (Upper): Proximal anastomosis end-to-side. No evidence of turbulence in velocity tracings. B (Lower, left) and C (Lower, right): Right and left limbs of the graft with anastomosis at the profunda. Normal triphasic velocity tracings.

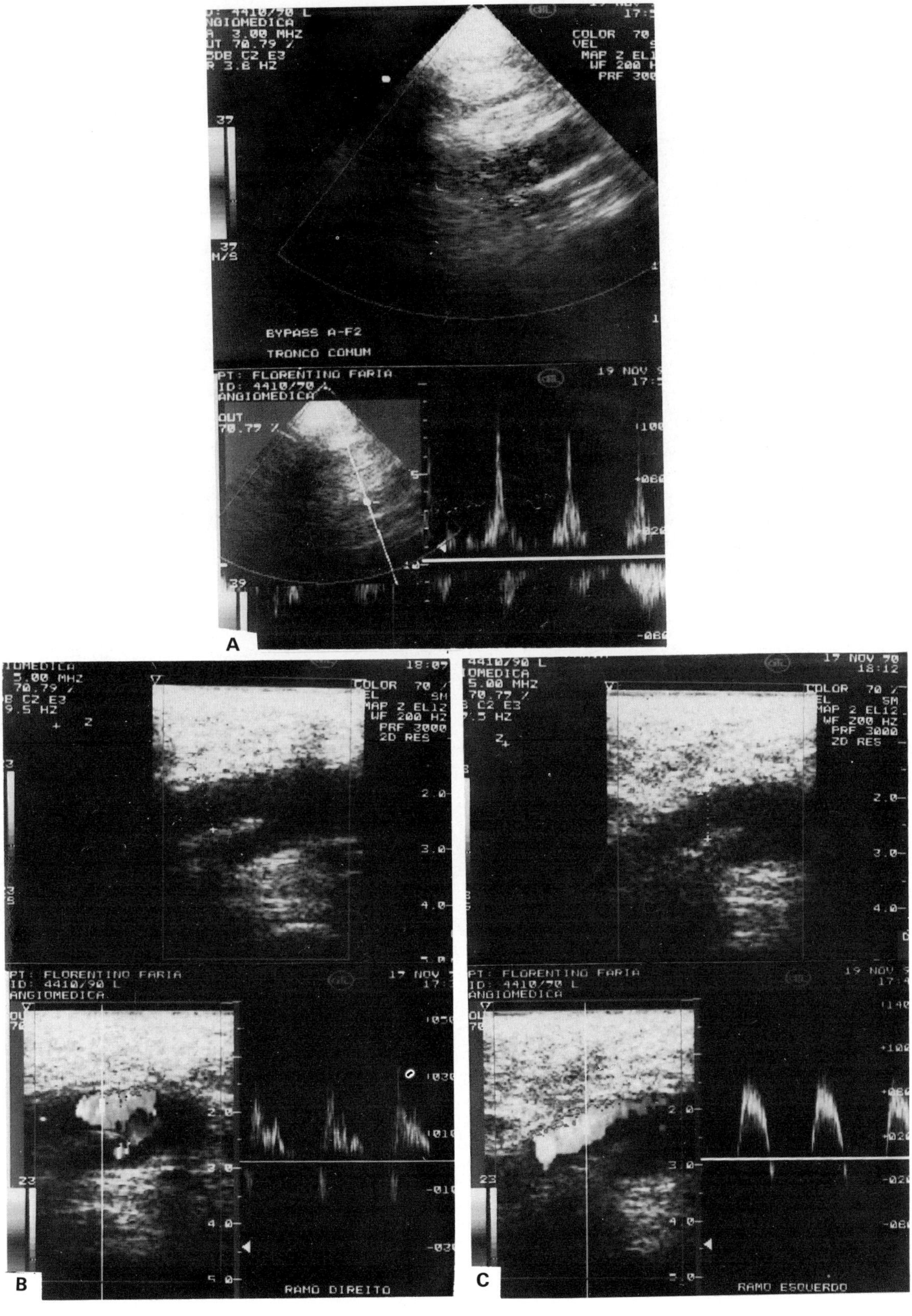

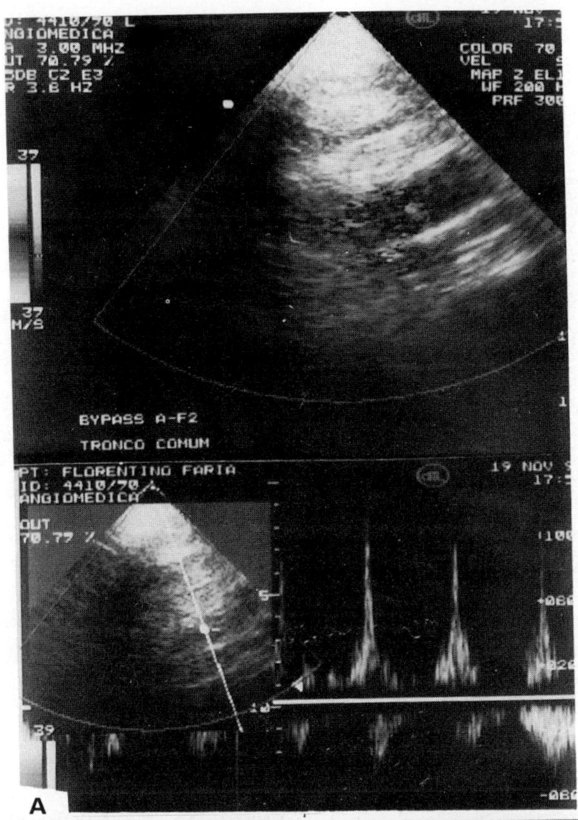
BYPASS A-F2
TRONCO COMUM
PT: FLORENTINO FARIA
ANGIOMEDICA
A

PT: FLORENTINO FARIA
ANGIOMEDICA
RAMO DIREITO
B
RAMO ESQUERDO
C

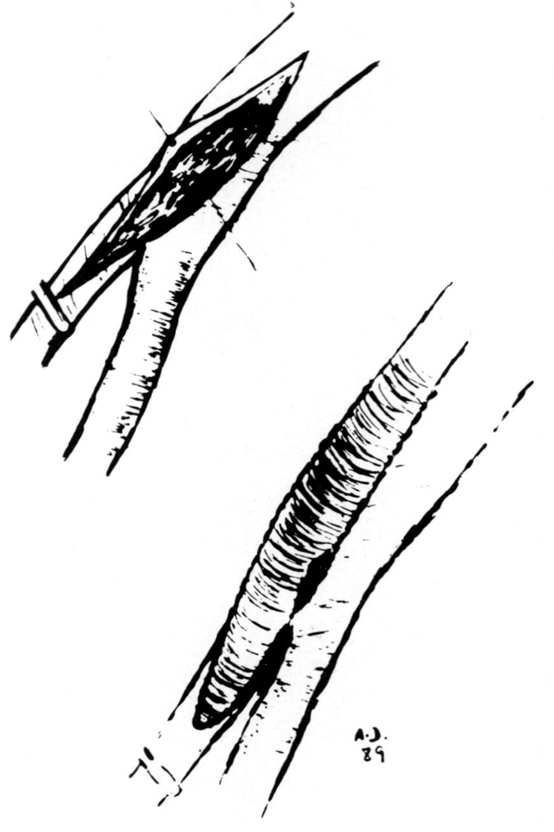

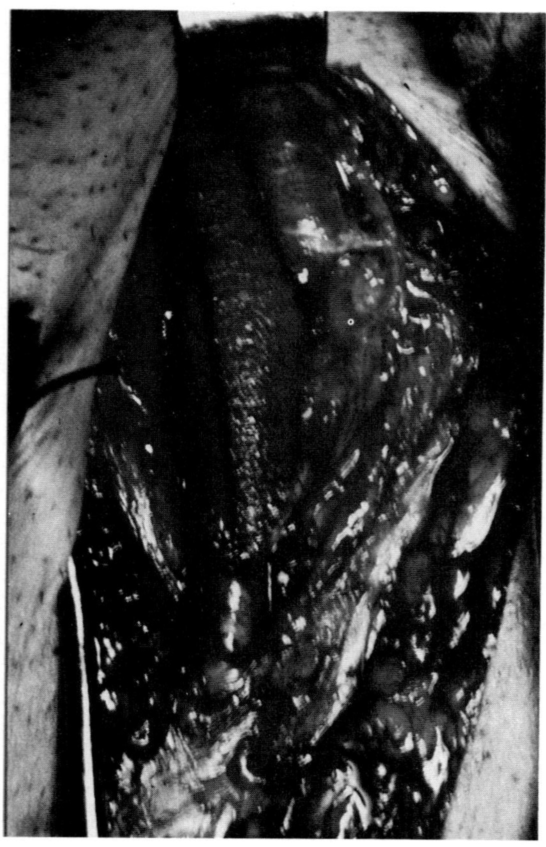

Fig. 11. Technique for performing end-to-side distal anastomosis. A (Left): Schematic representation: endarterectomy is required to restore adequate patency to the profunda. B (Right): Completed anastomosis.

initial segment of the profunda and endarterectomy is avoided unless there is ulceration or extensive plaques that would prevent the construction of an adequate anastomosis. Success of profunda femoris revascularization is dependent upon the functional capability of this collateral system and requires adequate re-entry into the mainstream popliteal artery.[53]

Failure to achieve satisfactory improvement with proximal reconstructions in multilevel disease has been reported in selected series[54,55] with an appreciable number of patients requiring subsequently femoropopliteal reconstructions. Identification of these patients preoperatively is difficult and controversial. Moderate proximal occlusive disease in combination with distal femoropopliteal complete obstructions, haemodynamic evidence of poor outflow tract assessed by segmental pressure measurements and the presence of advanced ischaemia are considered as predictors of clinical and haemodynamic failure of isolated aorto-iliac reconstructions.[54] Untreated femoropopliteal occlusive disease was reported to determine poor long-term patency rates of aortofemoral bifurcation grafts.[56,57]

Combined proximal and distal procedures can be performed at the same operation without increasing the risk of surgery.[58–60] In our series, 47 patients had simultaneous aorto-iliac and femoropopliteal procedures. The selection criteria were the presence of nondemarcated, progressive necrosis in the foot, angiographic evidence of inadequate run-off through the profunda femoris as a consequence of diffuse disease, or poor re-entry in the popliteal artery associated with high thigh-leg pressure gradient greater than 60 mm Hg, an indicator of high resistance outflow.

Saphenous vein graft was the choice for this combined procedure because of the need for extending this procedure to the lower popliteal artery or to its trifurcation; proximal anastomosis of the femoropopliteal bypass was usually constructed in the limb of the prosthetic graft, as shown in Fig. 12; short endarterectomies in the superficial femoral artery to obtain an inflow source for these grafts are not recommended.

The efficacy of lumbar sympathectomy by improving skin perfusion in association with revascularization procedures has not been proven; we performed sympathectomy in 25 patients with severe ischaemia at the time of aorto-iliac surgery, but this procedure has been progressively abandoned in our practice.

Because of atherosclerotic involvement of other arteries 16 patients required concomitant surgical procedures. The indication for carotid endarterectomy was based on clinical evidence of symptomatic carotid disease or the presence of bilateral severe asymptomatic stenosis.

Concomitant renal revascularization was performed because of severe hypertension or evidence of renal failure related to stenosis of the renal arteries. Endarterectomy, by the transaortic route was performed in three patients associated with juxtarenal aortic occlusions, but our preference is for aortorenal bypass with saphenous vein.

Superior mesenteric artery and coeliac axis occlusive disease is uncommon in our experience, in association with aortic and iliac occlusive disease. Collateral compensation through the inferior mesenteric artery and the marginal artery of Drumond is adequate in many patients; but if aorto-iliac surgery is going to be performed, it is our conviction that simultaneous reconstruction of the superior mesenteric artery should be performed. Occlusion of the distal aorta may compromise

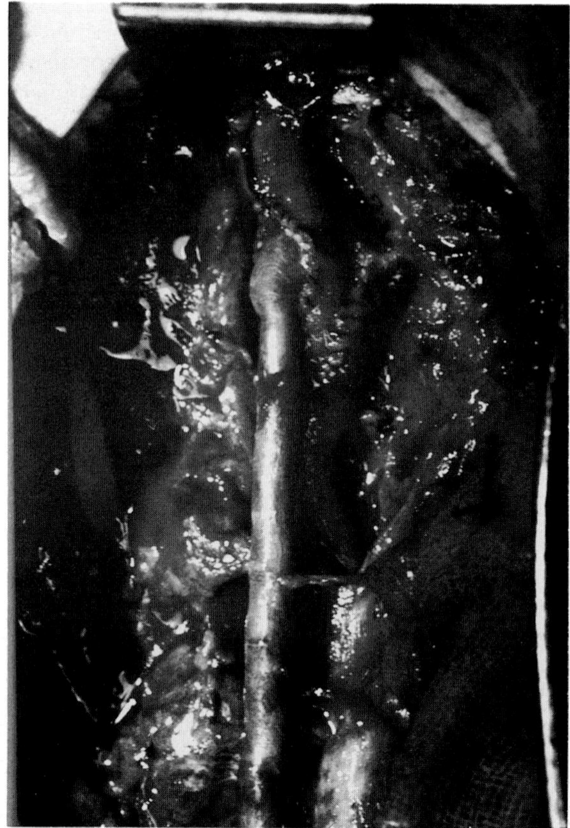

Fig. 12. Combined proximal and distal revascularization: detail of anastomosis of the venous bypass to the limb of the prosthesis.

flow through the inferior mesenteric artery and thus result in severe intestinal ischaemia in the presence of uncorrected mesenteric artery occlusion.

The choice of graft material for aorto-iliac surgery was initially the knitted Dacron graft for occlusive disease and woven prosthesis in abdominal aortic aneurysms. New coated prostheses with very low porosity have the advantage of reducing blood loss during operation without apparently affecting the long-term performance of the grafts. In the last 2 years we have routinely used coated grafts for aorto-iliac reconstructive surgery.

RESULTS

Improvement on surgical techniques, better intra-operative anaesthetic management and adequate surveillance in intensive care units during the inital postoperative period have contributed to a significant reduction in morbidity and mortality associated with aorto-iliac reconstructive surgery. Published mortality rates range from 2–6% in many series, and high long-term patency rates with sustained clinical and haemodynamic benefits were reported.[61–64]

A total of 202 patients had bifurcation grafts placed for occlusive disease involving the aorto-iliac segment, and they will be the subject of further analysis. In this group, 32 patients (15%) had concomitant aneurysmal changes in the aorta, but they were included because the aneurysm was either an incidental finding on aortography or during surgery or because the indication for surgery was lower limb ischaemia due to occlusive aorto-iliac disease, the aortic aneurysm being coincidental.

Early mortality rate was 2.9%; six patients died during the first 30 days after surgery and causes of death are listed in Table 5. Myocardial infarct accounted for 50% of the deaths, thus representing the single most common cause of operative mortality. Two patients died suddenly on the second week after bifurcation aortofemoral grafts because of pulmonary embolism, confirmed by autopsy in one, and in the other following clinical evidence of deep vein thrombosis in the lower limbs. Prophylactic subcutaneous heparin was not routinely used, although some evidence with isotopic studies suggested a significant incidence of DVT after aorto-iliac surgery.[65]

Early postoperative morbidity is represented in Table 6. Re-operation for bleeding occurred in five patients and acute thrombosis of one or both limbs of the graft in 13 patients (6.4%) but in eight, patency was restored by thrombectomy with Fogarty catheter and associated femoropopliteal bypass in three to ensure a better outflow. Two patients required laparotomy because of intestinal obstruction and one patient developed crural paralysis after a bifurcation graft and subsequently had a fatal myocardial infarct; no explanation other than embolization during aortic manipulation was found for the unilateral paralysis. Persistent lymphorrhea for 2 weeks was present in five patients, but none required surgical exploration. Superficial wound sepsis happened in 12 patients, without clinical evidence of early prosthetic infection, and was successfully treated with antibiotherapy; dehiscence of laparotomy occurred in four patients and subsequent closure carried no further hinderance for the patients.

Deterioration of renal function, without need for dialysis, occurred in one patient with severe occlusive disease in both renal arteries and aortic aneurysm. Two patients had renal bypass and bifurcation grafts because of severe hypertension and renal failure, in association with severe lower limb ischaemia due to extensive

Table 5. Early mortality in 202 patients after aortic bifurcation grafts

Cause of death	*No*	*%*
Myocardial infarct	3	50
Pulmonary embolism	2	33
Multiorgan failure	1	17
Total	6	2.9

Table 6. Early morbidity in 202 patients after aortic bifurcation grafts

	No	*%*
Bleeding	5	2.4
Thrombosis	13	6.4
successful thrombectomy: 8		
Intestinal occlusion	2	1
Renal failure	2	1
haemodyalisis: 1		
Lymphorrhea	5	2.4
Wound sepsis	12	5.9
Evisceration	4	1.9
Stroke	1	0.5
Amputation (major)	5	2.5

multilevel occlusive disease. They did not show the expected improvement in kidney function, despite patency of the renal grafts. Nonfatal myocardial infarct occurred in four patients; one patient had a stroke with partial recovery, but there was no evidence of extracranial occlusive disease on preoperative duplex scan assessment.

Five patients (2.5%) required major amputation because of early thrombosis of the graft, despite attempts to restore patency through thrombectomy or associated distal reconstruction procedures.

In all, 191 patients (97.5%) survived the operation with patent reconstructions at 1 month and experienced significant clinical improvement with relief of ischaemic symptoms. This group will constitute the basis for further analysis of durability and incidence of late complications associated with aorto-iliac reconstructive surgery.

LONG-TERM RESULTS

In all, 191 patients survived the operation at 1 month and were subsequently followed to a period extending to 132 months, with average duration of 62 months. Clinical evaluation was performed and patency of the grafts assessed by palpation and in doubtful cases by noninvasive technology. Surveillance programmes for proximal procedures have not been adopted with the same enthusiasm as for the infra-inguinal reconstructions, probably because failure of a proximal bypass can be reasonably tolerated in some patients without risk of severe ischaemia or limb loss and also because occlusions are not so common. Distal pressure measurements, at rest or after exercise, may not be adequate predictors of failure, because they are affected by the development and/or progression of disease distal to the aortofemoral bifurcation graft. Duplex scan examination provides the best noninvasive method to study arterial reconstructions. Morphologic alterations along the entire length of the graft and at the anastomosis as well as haemodynamic parameters of flow disturbance allow early detection of dilatation and/or aneurysms and restenosis, particularly at the femoral anastomosis. Figure 13 shows a moderate degree of dilatation of limbs of the graft, a condition that could lead to anastomotic aneurysms, in a patient who underwent a bifurcation graft 16 months previously.

Survival after aorto-iliac surgery is mainly influenced by coronary artery disease; 41 patients died during the period of follow-up and the major cause of death was myocardial infarction in 22.

Thrombotic occlusions occur mainly at the femoral anastomosis; neointimal fibroplasia and progression of underlying disease are the main causes of late failure of bifurcation grafts. This series provided 377 limbs at risk, and femoral anastomoses, to be analysed during follow-up. Results of patient survival, patency of reconstructions and limb preservation are shown in the actuarial form, using life table analysis (Fig. 14). Survival at 5 and 10 years was respectively 66.2% and 43%, and the major cause of death was myocardial infarction. Occlusions occurred in 33 graft anastomoses with a higher incidence in the first 36 months, a fact that may point out to the relevance of fibroplasia as a major cause of occlusion. Figure 15 shows an example of a patient who developed claudication 12 months after a bifurcation graft; angiography demonstrated occlusion of the right limb and stenosis at the left femoral anastomosis due to intense fibroplasia, confirmed at the time of

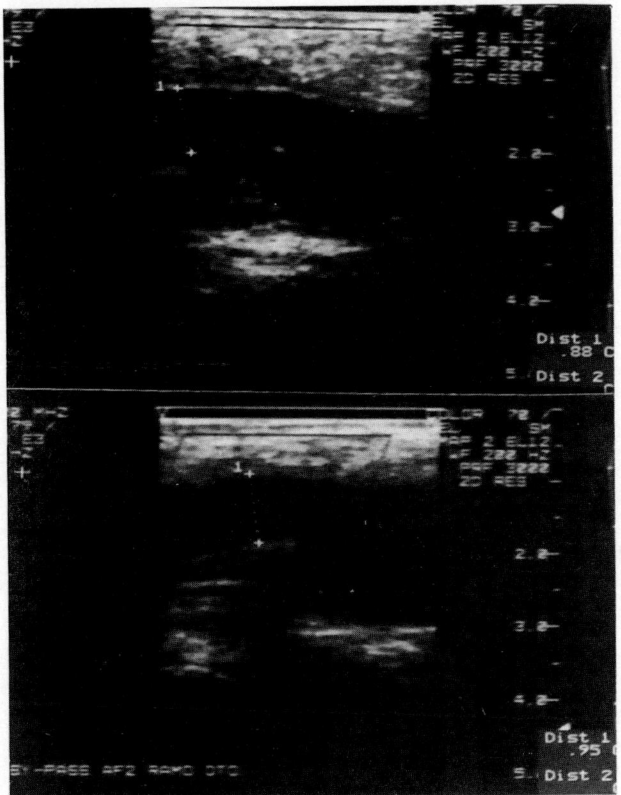

Fig. 13. Duplex scan assessment in a patient with 16×8 mm bifurcated graft 16 months previously: there is evidence of dilatation in both graft limbs measured in transverse diameter.

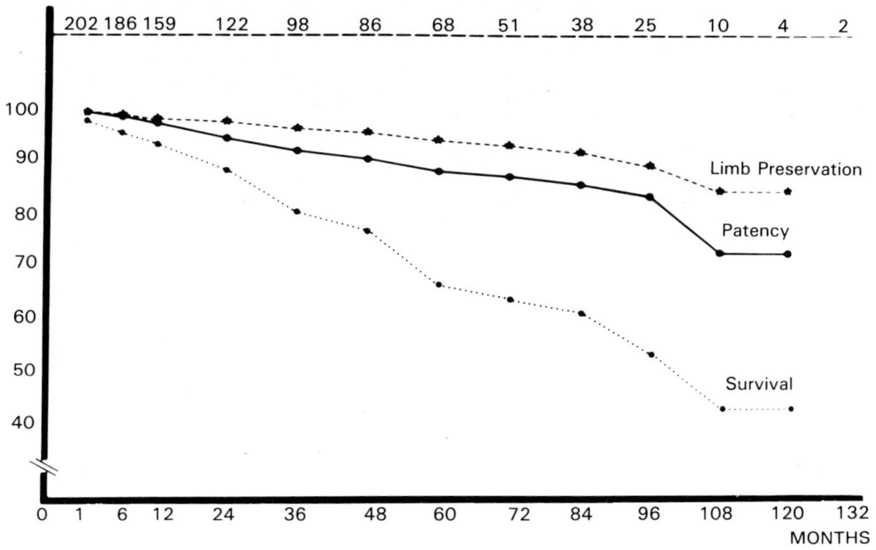

Fig. 14. Life table analysis of long-term patient survival, patency and limb-preservation, in patients submitted to bifurcated grafts for occlusive disease.

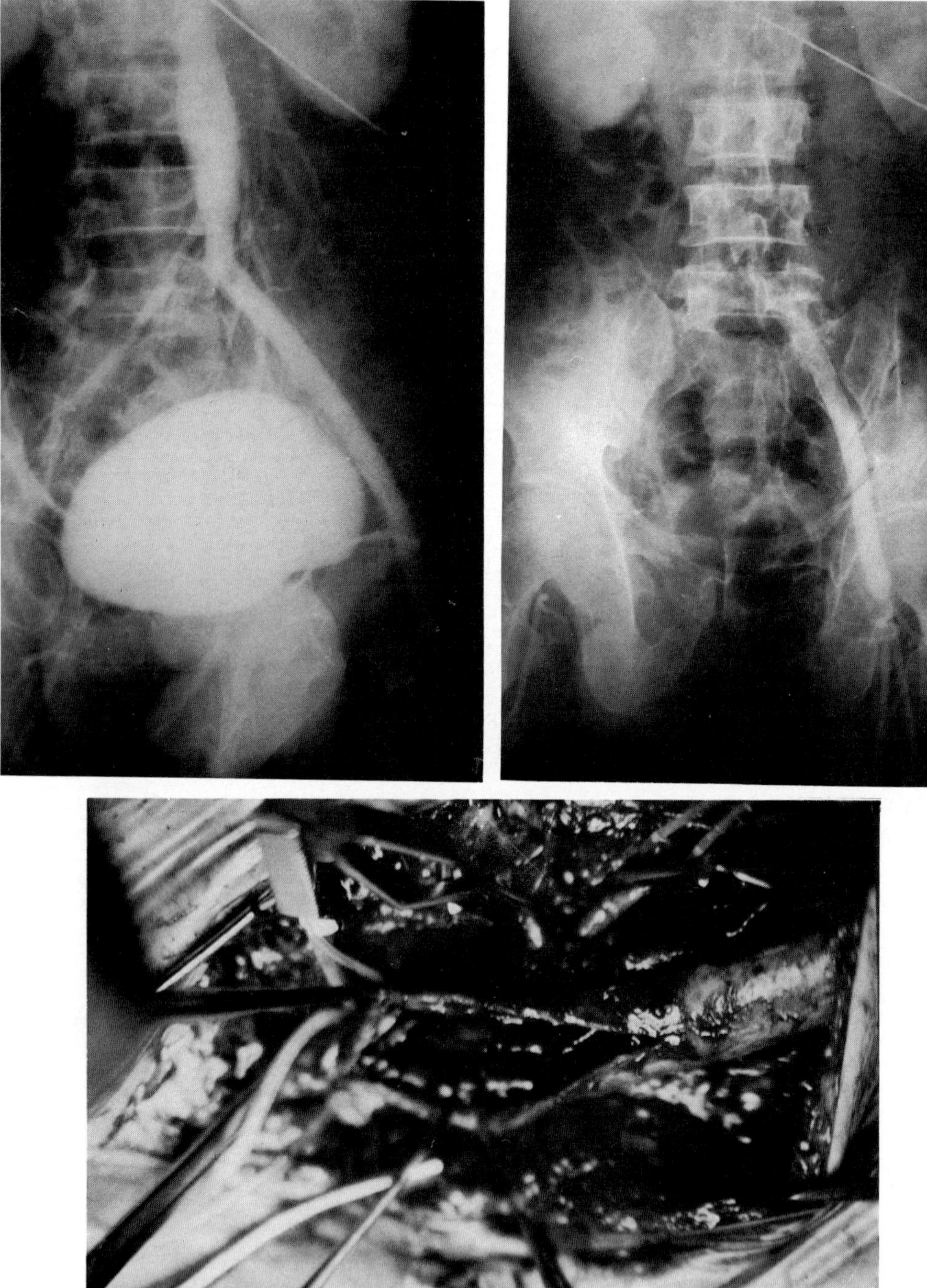

Fig. 15. A (Upper): Aortogram confirming right limb graft thrombosis 12 months after implantation; the left anastomosis shows marked stenosis or an oblique view.
B (Lower): Operative view: thrombus inside the graft and evidence of fibroplasia at the anastomosis.

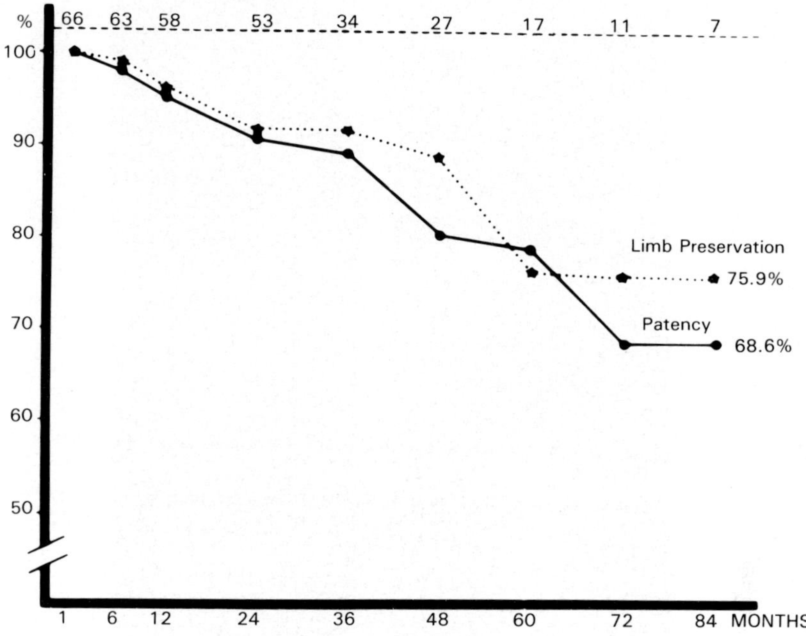

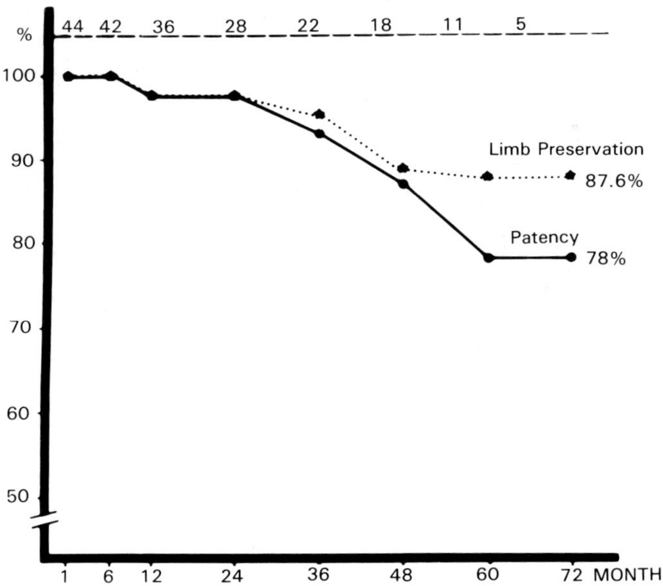

Fig. 16. Late patency and limb preservation of aorto-iliac procedures in patients with severe lower limb ischaemia: A (Upper): Patients having proximal reconstructions. B (Lower): Patients having simultaneous procedures.

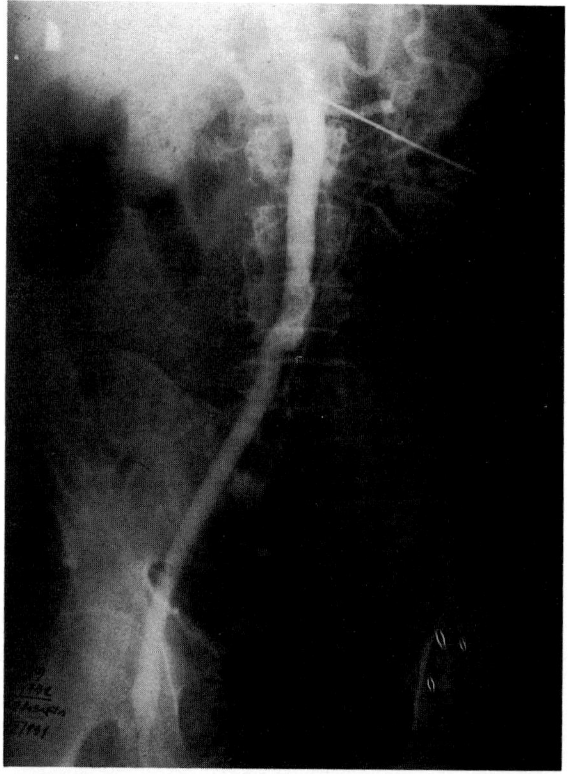

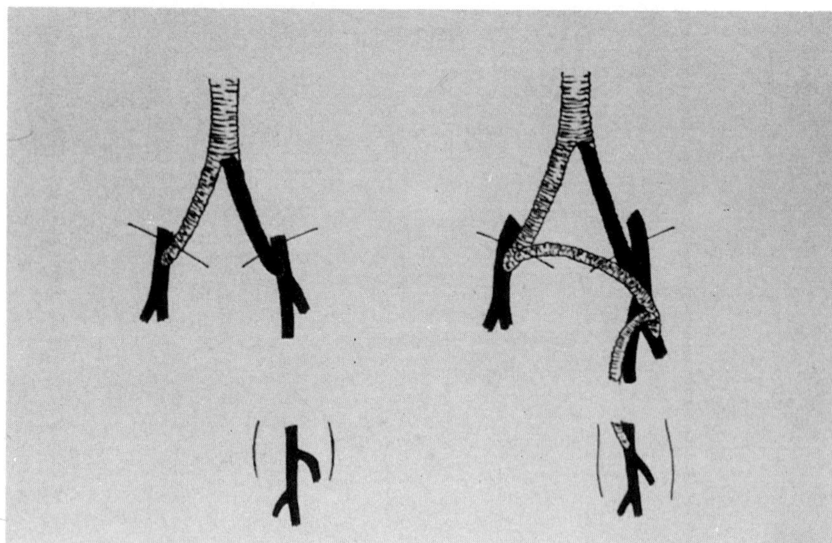

Fig. 17. A (Upper): Aortogram showing a limb of occlusion a bifurcated graft implanted 6 years previously. B (Lower): Treatment requiring crossover graft and femoropopliteal bypass because of progression of infra-inguinal disease (schematic representation).

surgery. Patency rates at 5 and 10 years, were respectively 87.8% and 72.7%, which are comparable to reported series (Table 7).

The presence and extension of infra-inguinal disease has been pointed out as a major negative factor in long term patency of aorto-iliac reconstructive procedures—the worst results being in patients with profunda femoris disease.

Table 7. Late patency in aortic reconstructions for stenosing disease

Ref.	*No of patients*	*Success (%)* 5 years	*Success (%)* 10 years
46	949	87	79
45	710	88	78
57	352	80	62
24	464	88	75
55	1649	84	78
56	180	82	66
Present study	202	88	73

Routine use of profundaplasty and combined proximal and distal reconstruction procedures in more severe ischaemia, precludes any significant analysis of the influence of infra-inguinal disease on late patency of aorto-iliac reconstructions. However, in simultaneous combined procedures, late patency of proximal reconstructions and preservation of lower limbs are slightly better than those obtained in patients submitted only to proximal reconstructions (Fig. 16) as previously reported[66] in patients with severe lower limb ischaemia. We believe this justifies an aggressive surgical approach for these patients with extensive occlusive disease.

Need for subsequent distal reconstructions because of haemodynamic failure despite a patent bypass is probably related to the progression of infra-inguinal disease. In our experience, distal bypass has been used only if there is advanced ischaemia with risk of limb loss, and rarely, for patients with claudication. However, distal revascularization may also be required for treatment of unilateral limb graft occlusion to provide a suitable run-off for the proximal reconstruction, as shown in Fig. 17.

Excluding the amputations in the early perioperative period, 14 limbs required late major amputation. The limb preservation rate in the whole series was 84.1% at 10 years.

ANASTOMOTIC ANEURYSMS

In spite of improvements in surgical techniques and routine use of antibiotics, the incidence of false aneurysms seems to occur in all series with longer follow-up periods. The aetiology is multifactorial: there is compliance mismatch between rigid grafts and host artery, mechanical stress upon the suture line, technical imperfections at the time of the anastomosis, weakness of the recipient artery, particularly if

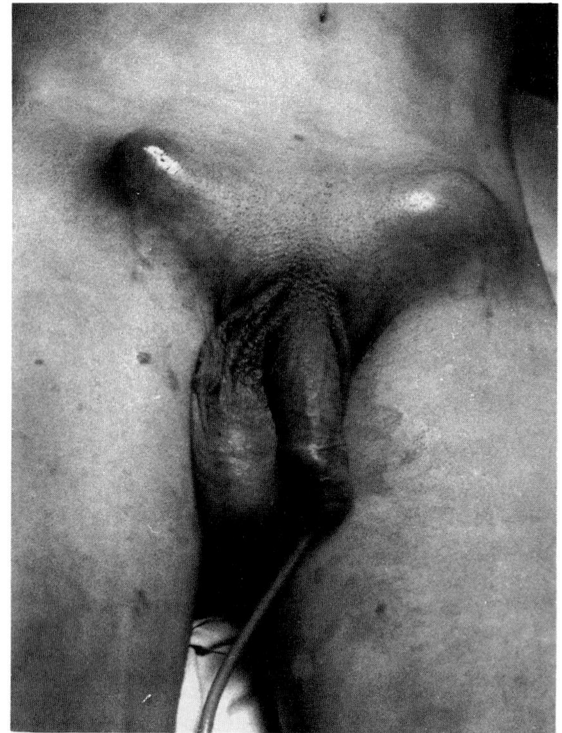

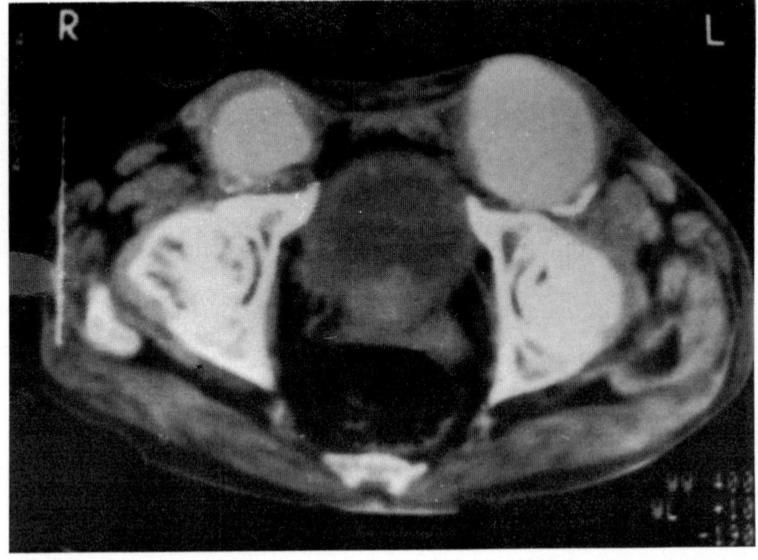

Fig. 18. A (Upper): Bilateral anastomotic aneurysms and B (Lower): CT-scan examination.

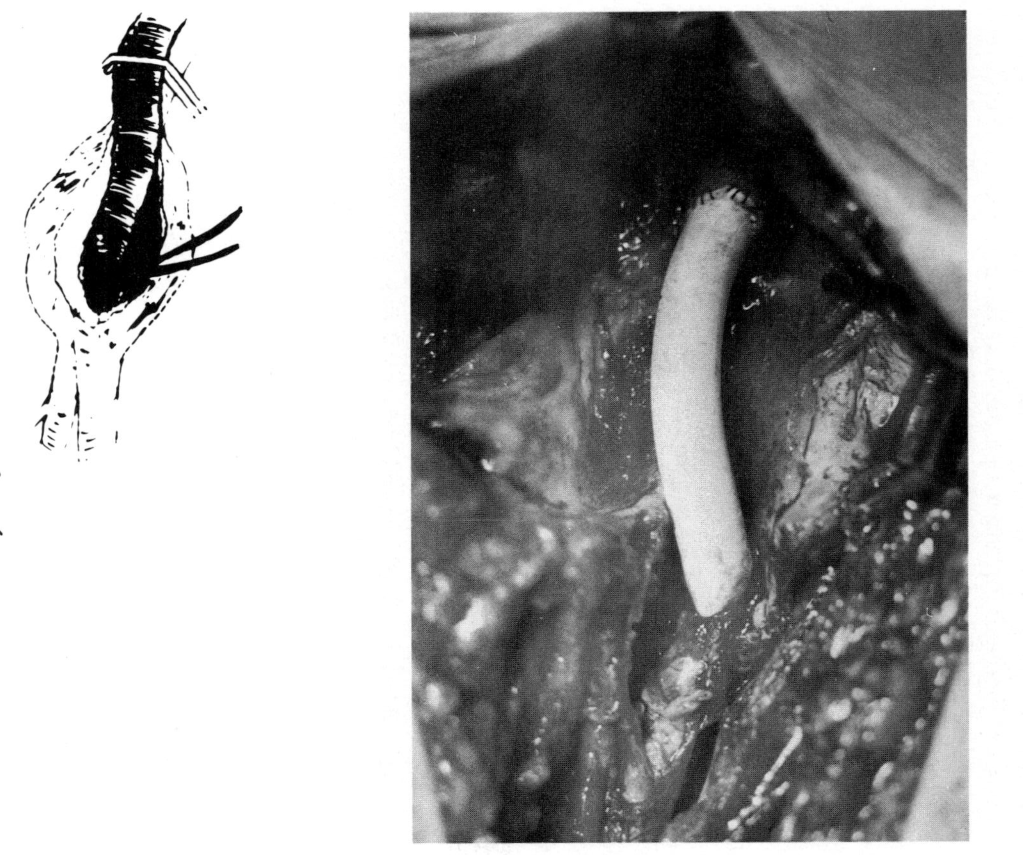

Fig. 19. A (Left): Schematic representation of surgical repair of anastomotic aneurysm. B (Right): Operative picture: PTFE graft was used.

endarterectomy was performed and occult infection. Dilatation of grafts[67] were extensively reported and already documented in Fig. 13, but its significance in the aetiology of false aneurysms is not yet fully understood. Rupture of the suture line with extravasation of blood and formation of a pulsatile haematoma is the end-result, a condition that requires prompt surgical correction. The incidence of false aneurysms is higher in the femoral anastomosis, and rare in the aortic area, where end-to-side anastomosis has been considered a predisposing factor.[68]

In our series, 10 patients (5.3%) developed 13 false aneurysms, 12 being located at the femoral area; two patients developed proximal aneurysms with aortoduodenal fistulae. Figure 18 shows anastomotic aneurysms in both groins, occurring 9 years after a bifurcation graft; CT-scan showed an intact proximal anastomosis without evidence of abnormality. Treatment required only partial resection of the graft limbs as shown in Fig. 19 and reconstruction with a new prosthetic segment using polytetrafluoroethylene (PTFE). The occurrence of anastomotic aneurysms according to time interval after initial surgery is shown in Fig. 20; eight (66%) became apparent after 36 months and four (33%), in the initial 3 years after the operation. Predisposing factors were hypertension, present in nine patients (75%), bleeding at the time of initial surgery in three patients, while previous endarterectomy at the site of femoral anastomosis in four patients, and infection in five patients. Clinical evaluation is sufficient to diagnose the presence of anastomotic aneurysms in the groins but is of limited value to assess the abdomen. Computerized tomography has been routinely used to screen these patients for the presence of proximal false aneurysms and also to identify signs suggesting prosthetic infection.

Management of anastomotic aneurysms requires excision of all tissue surrounding the anastomosis and extensive periprosthetic debridement; limited graft resection has been adopted in the absence of overt infection of the entire prosthesis and

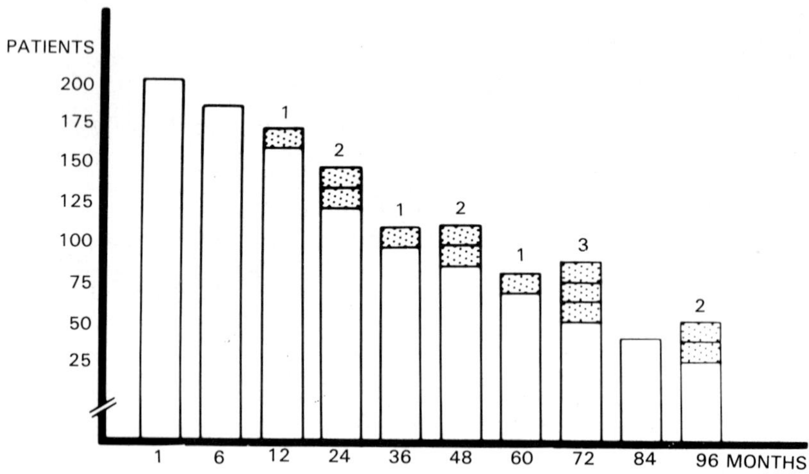

Fig. 20. Incidence of anastomotic aneurysms according to time interval after bifurcated graft.

revascularization was attempted in all our patients. The confirmation of infection is difficult, because in many instances bacteriology of resected specimens has been negative. Cultures from the excised graft, host artery wall, clots and surrounding tissues were positive in only five patients, and the pathogens identified were *Escherichia coli* in two patients and *Staphylococcus epidermides* in three patients. Two patients had recurrence of false aneurysms; they subsequently developed extensive prosthetic infection, proximal aortic aneurysms and aortoduodenal fistula.

Recognition of active infection is of paramount importance for surgical decision. Absence of signs of infection in the CT scan and good incorporation of the remaining graft as assessed during operation may support the decision to do partial resection of the prosthetic graft and *in situ* revascularization.

Mortality occurred only in the two patients with proximal anastomotic aneurysms, but one survived 2 years after the initial resection of the graft and repair of the intestinal defect and died after recurrence of aneurysm with an aortoduodenal fistula from the aortic stump.

Careful performance of the anastomoses without excessive tension, strict avoidance of contamination during surgery, routine perioperative antibiotics, and prompt treatment of any infection occurring after surgery are major factors to be considered in the prevention of false-aneurysm formation and prosthetic infection.

INFECTION IN BIFURCATION GRAFTS

The incidence of graft infection is greater when the procedure is extended to the groin and seems higher in patients with aneurysmal disease than in those with occlusive arterial disease.[69,70]

This complication represents the main disadvantage of bypass procedures when compared with endarterectomy, where infectious complications are extremely rare. The sources of prosthetic infection are mainly three: inadequate preparation of patients with unrecognized and untreated infections at the time of operation, contamination during surgical manipulation and haematogenous seeding in the postoperative period following remote infection. *Staphylococcus aureus* has been the leading pathogen in aortofemoral graft infection, but other bacteria, such as *Escherichia coli, Streptococci* and anaerobes have been found in some cases of graft infection.

Diagnosis is often extremely difficult; evidence of wound purulence at the groins, history of wound sepsis in the immediate postoperative period, persistence of unexplained fever and malaise or evidence of intestinal bleeding because of aortoenteric fistulae should lead to exhaustive investigations to confirm prosthetic infection.

Computerized tomography, and more recently magnetic resonance imaging are essential methods that provide direct and indirect diagnostic information. Presence of air along the shaft of bifurcation grafts some weeks after surgery is of diagnostic value for the presence of infection, as shown in Fig. 21. Perigraft fluid collection may be confusing and is not specific for infection. However, its persistence or increase in patients with unexplained fever have diagnostic value. Scintigraphic methods with labelled leucocytes may be useful to confirm and localize sepsis.[71]

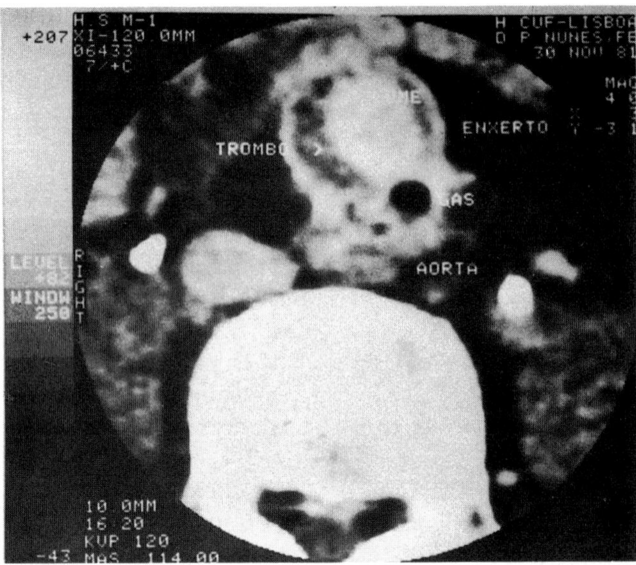

Fig. 21. CT-scan with late infection of a bifurcated graft: evidence of air and fluid surrounding the prosthesis.

Aorto-enteric fistula is a rare complication of bifurcation grafts associated with infection. Usually it involves the third and fourth portions of the duodenum, occurring at the level of the aortic anastomosis or along the shaft of the graft, and rarely, at the left colon. Diagnosis is often difficult; suspicion is raised in patients with recurrent gastro-intestinal bleeding and a previous history of bypass grafting. Confirmation of diagnosis requires CT-scan with the use of intravenous contrast, and endoscopy to exclude other causes of haemorrage. Two physiological mechanisms can account for the aortoduodenal fistula; first, infection at the anastomosis can lead to the formation of a false aneurysm that subsequently erodes the duodenum. The second, is adherence of the duodenum to the graft and secondary erosion of the wall by the pulsating bypass, leading to the formation of a paraprosthetic enteric fistula. Four patients, 2.0% of the total of 191 bifurcated grafts, developed overt infection, with aortoduodenal fistula in three and aortocolonic fistula in the fourth patient.

Treatment consists of total resection of the infected prosthesis, repair of the intestinal wound and maintenance of perfusion of the lower limbs through remote reconstructions. These procedures are associated with high morbidity and mortality and detailed discussion is beyond the scope of this chapter. In our series three patients with aorto-enteric fistulae were treated by resection of the graft and extra-anatomic bypass; one survived, but 2 years later developed recurrent aortoduodenal fistula from the aortic stump and died from aortic rupture, despite careful closure and reinforcement of the stump. The fourth patient developed renal failure and died of massive haemorrhage before surgical treatment.

Adequate coverage of the prosthesis by the retroperitoneal tissue, with correct positioning to avoid prominence of the shaft of the graft immediately distal to the aortic anastomosis, are essential steps to prevent adherence of the duodenum and secondary fistulization.

CONCLUSIONS

Aortofemoral bifurcation grafting is one of the commonest and safest procedures in the armamentarium of the vascular surgeon. Its durability and reduced incidence of serious complications in more recent series made the procedure the first option for treatment of aorto-iliac stenosing disease in the majority of vascular centres.

New developments in prosthetic graft materials, such as gelatin or albumin coating or impregnation with collagen appear promising since they reduce porosity and blood loss at the time of operation, without increasing long-term complications, such as infection or aneurysm formation.

New endovascular procedures, covered in other chapters, will change management of occlusive disease in the aorto-iliac segment. Laser assisted devices and angioplasty can now be used for treatment of complete occlusions and the introduction of stents to prevent restenosis show promising results. However, for more extensive disease, with calcification and advanced ischaemia, placement of a bifurcation graft will still be required, and continue to represent one of the most gratifying surgical procedures in the vascular field.

REFERENCES

1. Hunterian Museum of the Royal College of Surgeons, London: Specimens 1177, 1178 (Antoiliac Obstruction)
2. Cruvheilier J: Senile gangrene. *In* Anatomie Pathologique du Corps Humain, Sect 27 (Maladie des Artéres). Paris, pp. 1–8, 1835–1842
3. Charcot JM: Obstruction artérielle et claudication intermittente dans le cheval et dans l'homme. Mem Soc Biol 1:225–238, 1858
4. Barker WF: Transcription from Charcot. *In* Surgery of the Aorta: An Historical Perspective in Aortic Surgery, Bergan JJ, Yao JST (Eds). Philadelphia and London: W. B. Saunders, 1989
5. Barth: Observation d'une oblitération compléte de l'aorte abdominal, recuillie dans le service de M. Louis, suivie de refléctions. Arch Gen Med (2nd series) 8:26–53, 1835
6. Leriche R: Des obliterations artérielles hautes (obliteration de la termination de l'aorte) comme causes des insuffisances circulatoires des membres inférieurs. Bull Mem Soc Chir (Paris) 49:1404–1406, 1923
7. Leriche R: De la réssection du carrefour aortoiliaque avec double sympathectomie lombaire pour thrombose artéritique de l'aorte. Presse Med 48:601–604, 1940
8. Dos Santos R, Lamas A, Caldas J: L'artériographie des membres, de l'aorte et de ses branches abdominales. Bull Mem Soc Natl Chir (Paris) 55:587–601, 1929
9. Dos Santos JC: Sur la désobstruction des thromboses artérielles anciernes. Mem Acad Chir 73:409–411, 1947
10. Cannon JA, Barker WF: Successful management of obstructive femoral arteriosclerosis by endarterectomy. Experience with a semiclosed technique in selective cases. Surgery 38:48–60, 1955
11. Bazy L, Hugier J, Reboul H *et al*: Technique des ''endarterectomies'' pour artérites oblitérantes chroniques des membres inférieures, des iliaques, et de l'aorte abdominale inférieur. J Chir 65:196–210, 1949

12. Cid dos Santos JC: From embolectomy to endarterectomy or the fall of a myth. J Cardiovasc Surg 17:113–128, 1976
13. Hufnagel CA: Rapid freezing technique for preserved homologous arterial transplants. Bull Am Coll Surg 32:231, 1947
14. Oudot J: La greffe vasculaire dans les thromboses du carrefour aortique. Presse Med 59:234–236, 1951
15. Voorhees AB Jr, Janetzki A III, Blakemore AH. Use of tubes constructed of Vinyon-''N'' cloth in bridging arterial defects. Ann Surg 135:332–336, 1952
16. DeBakey ME, Cooley DA, Crawford ES, Morris GC Jr: Clinical application of a new flexible knitted Dacron arterial substitute. Arch Surg 77:713–724, 1957
17. Szilagyi DE: Ten years experience with aorto-iliac and femoro popliteal arterial reconstruction. J Cardiovasc Surg 5:502–509, 1964
18. Vetto RM: The treatment of unilateral iliac artery obstruction utilizing femoro-femoral graft. Surgery 52:342, 1962
19. Blaisdell FW, Hall AD: Axillary–femoral artery bypass for lower extremity ischemia. Surgery 54:563, 1963
20. Darling RC, Brewster DC, Hallett JW Jr: Aorto-iliac reconstruction. Surg Clin North Am 59:565, 1979
21. Wolinsky H, Glagov S: Nature of species differences in the medial distribution of aortic vasa-vasorum in mammals. Circ Reg 20:409, 1967
22. Clark JM, Glagov S: Luminal surface of disturbed arteries by scanning electron microscopy. Eliminating configurational artifacts. Br J Exp Path 57:129–135, 1976
23. Friedman MH, Hutchins GM, Bargeron CB *et al*: Correlation between intimal thickness and fluid shear in human arteries. Atherosclerosis 39:425–436, 1981
24. Brewster DC, Darling RC: Optimal methods of aorto-iliac reconstruction. Surgery 84:739, 1978
25. Volmar JF, Heyden B: Experiences with reconstructive surgery of the aorto-iliac segment. *In* Surgery of the Aorta and its Body Branches, Bergan JJ, Yao JST (Eds). London and New York: Grune & Stratton, pp. 243–261, 1979
26. Karmody AM, Powers FR, Monaco VJ *et al*: Blue toe syndrome: An indication for limb salvage surgery. Arch Surg 11:1263, 1976
27. Queral LA, Flinn WR, Bergan JJ, Yao JST: Sexual function and aortic surgery. *In* Surgery of the Aorta and its Body Branches, Bergan JJ, Yao JST (Eds). London and New York: Grune & Stratton, pp. 263–274, 1979
28. Scheer A: Impotence as a symptom of arterial vascular disorder in the pelvic region. Munch Med Wochenschr 102, 1713, 1960
29. Myers KA: Preoperative assessment of lower limb ischemia. *In* Diagnostic Techniques and Assessment Procedures in Vascular Surgery, Greenhalgh RM (Ed.). London and New York: Grune & Stratton, 1985
30. Grummy AB, Rankin R, Turnipseed WD *et al*: Biplane arteriography in ischemia of the lower extremities. Radiology 126:11, 1978
31. Moore WS, Hall AD: Unrecognized aorto-iliac stenosis. A physiologic approach to the diagnosis. Arch Surg 103:633, 1971
32. Brenner BJ, Rainls JK, Darling RC: Measurement of systolic femoral artery pressure during reactive hyperemia: an estimate of aorto-iliac disease. Circulation 49 (Suppl. 2):258, 1974
33. Brewster DC, Waltman AC, O'Hara PJ *et al*: Femoral artery pressure measurement during aortography. Circulation 60 (Suppl. 1):120, 1979
34. Flannigan DP, Williams LR, Schwartz JA *et al*: Hemodynamic evaluation of the aorto-iliac system based upon pharmacologic vasodilation. Surgery 93:709, 1983
35. Johnston KW, Kassam M, Cobbold RSC: Relationship between Doppler pulsatility index and direct femoral pressure measurements in the diagnosis of aorto-iliac occlusive disease. Ultrasound Med Biol 9:271, 1983
36. Gosling RG, Key DH: Arterial assessment by Doppler shift ultrasound. Proc Roy Soc Med 67:447, 1974
37. Baker JD, Machleder HI, Bkidmore R: Analysis of femoral artery Doppler signals by Laplace transform damping method. J Vasc Surg 1:520, 1984

38. Green IL, Greenhalgh RM: Objective evaluation of the femoral pulse. *In* Diagnostic Techniques and Assessment Procedures in Vascular Surgery, Greenhalgh RM (Ed.). London and New York: Grune & Stratton, p. 241, 1985
39. Froneck A, Coel M, Bernstein EF: The importance of combined multisegmental pressure and Doppler flow velocity in the diagnosis of peripheral occlusive disease. Surgery 84:840, 1978
40. Langsfeld M, Nepult J, Hershey FB *et al*: The use of deep Duplex Scanning to predict hemodynamically significant aorto-iliac stenoses. J Vasc Surg 7:363, 1988
41. Larsen OH, Lassen NA: Effect of daily muscular exercise in patients with intermittent claudication. Lancet ii:1093, 1966
42. Sorlie D, Myhre K: Effects of physical training in intermittent claudication. Scand J Clin Lab Invest 38:217, 1978
43. DeBakey ME, Crawford ES, Morris GC *et al*: Late results of vascular surgery in the treatment of artherosclerosis. J Cardiovasc Surg 5:473, 1963
44. Malone JM, Moore WS, Goldstone J: Life expectancy following aortofemoral arterial grafting. Surgery 81:551, 1977
45. Martinez BD, Hertzer NR, Beven EG: Influence of distal arterial occlusive disease on prognosis following aortofemoral bypass. Surgery 88:795, 1980
46. Crawford ES, Bomberger RA, Glaser DH *et al*: Aorto-iliac occlusive disease: Factors influencing survival and function following reconstructive operation over a twenty-five year period. Surgery 90:1055, 1981
47. Salmasi AM, Nicolaides AN, Vecht RY *et al*: Electrocardiographic chest wall mapping in the diagnosis of coronary artery disease. Br Med J 2:9, 1983
48. Bodenheimer MW, Bauka VS, Fooshee CM *et al*: Comparative sensitivity of the exercise electrocardiogram, thallium imaging and stress radionuclide angiography to detect the presence and severity of coronary heart disease. Circulation 60: 1270, 1979
49. Crawford ES, Morris GC Jr, Howell JF: Operative risk in patients with previous coronary bypass. Ann Thorac Surg 26:215, 1978
50. Hertzer NR, Beven EG, Young JR *et al*: Coronary artery disease in peripheral vascular patients: A classification of 1000 coronary angiograms and results of surgical management. Ann Surg 199:223, 1984
51. De Palma RG, Levine SB, Feldman S: Preservation of erectile function after aorto-iliac reconstruction. Arch Surg 113:958, 1978
52. Crawford ES, Manning LG, Kelly TF: "Redo" Surgery after operations for aneurysm and occlusion of the abdominal aorta. Surgery 81:41, 1977
53. Fernandes e Fernandes J, Nicolaides AN, Angelides NA *et al*: An objective assessment of common femoral endarterectomy and profundoplasty in patients with superficial femoral occlusion. Surgery 83:313, 1978
54. Brewster DC, Perler BA, Roknison JG *et al*: Aortofemoral graft for multilevel occlusive disease. Predictors of success and need for distal bypass. Arch Surg 117:1593, 1982
55. Szilagyi DE, Elliott JP Jr, Smith RF *et al*: A thirty-year survey of the reconstructive surgical treatment of aorto-iliac occlusive disease. J Vasc Surg 3:421, 1986
56. Malone J, Moore WS, Goldstone J: The natural history of bilateral aortofemoral bypass grafts for ischemia of the lower extremities. Arch Surg 110:1300, 1975
57. Nevelsteen A, Suy R, Daenen W *et al*: Aortofemoral grafting: factors influencing late results. Surgery 88:642, 1980
58. Charlesworth D: Simultaneous proximal and distal reconstruction. *In* Aortic Surgery, Bergan JJ, Yao JST (Eds). Philadelphia and London: W. B. Saunders, p. 373, 1989
59. Harris PL, Cane-Bigley DJ, MaSweeney L: Aorto-femoral bypass and the role of concomitant femoro-distal reconstruction. Br J Surg 22:317, 1985
60. Fernandes e Fernandes J, Damião A, Almeida CA *et al*: Simultaneous proximal and distal reconstructions in lower limb ischemia. Paper presented at the meeting of the European Society of Cardiovascular Surgery, Abstracts, p. 171, 1984
61. Lyons JH Jr, Weismann RE: Surgical management of late closure of aorto-femoral reconstruction grafts. N Engl J Med 278:1035, 1968

62. Najafi H, Dye WS, Javid H *et al*: Late thrombosis affecting one limb of aortic bifurcation graft. Arch Surg 110:409, 1975
63. Vantinnen E, Imberg MV: Aorto-ilio femoral arterial reconstructive surgery. Acta Chir Scand 141:600, 1975
64. Stanton PE Jr, Lamis PA, Gross WS *et al*: Correction of late aortic-bifemoral failures. Am Surg 43:497, 1977
65. Angelides NS, Nicolaides AN, Fernandes e Fernandes J *et al*: Deep Venous Thrombosis in patients having aorto-iliac reconstructions. B J Surg 64:517, 1977
66. Fernandes e Fernandes J, Damião A, Almeida CH: Severe lower limb ischemia: The value of proximal and distal simultaneous revascularizations. Paper presented at the inaugural meeting of the European Society for Vascular Surgery, London, 1987
67. Berger K, Sauvage LR: Late fiber deterioration in Dacron arterial grafts. Ann Surg 193:477, 1981
68. Millini JJ, Lanes JS, Nemir P Jr: A study of anastomotic aneurysms following aorto femoral prosthetic bypass. Ann Surg 192:69, 1980
69. Bernhard VM: Management of graft infections following abdominal aortic aneurysm replacement. World J Surg 4:679, 1980
70. Lorentzen JE, Nielsen OM, Arendrup H *et al*: Vascular graft infection: an analysis of sixty-two graft infections in 2411 consecutively implanted synthetic vascular grafts. Surgery 98:81, 1985
71. Serota AI, Williams RA, Rose JG *et al*: Uptake of radiolabelled leucocytes in prosthetic graft infection. Surgery 90:35, 1981

The Surgical Management of Occluded Aortobifemoral Grafts

Simon G. Darke

Occlusions of aortobifemoral grafts in the immediate or early postoperative period (within 30 days) are due to inappropriate case selection, thrombotic disorders, but most commonly operative technical error.[1] These problems are outside the remit of this chapter and are thus not considered further.

Late graft occlusion is fortunately not a common problem because in general, direct reconstruction for aorto-iliac occlusive disease gives durable long-term results as shown in the preceding chapter. When it does occur it is in the order of 10% after 5 years and 15–30% for patients followed up for 10 years or more.[2] Only rarely is this attributable to progression of atheroma above the proximal anastomosis causing embarrassment to the other arterial run-in, and if this is the case it is usually because the previous surgeon has failed to secure an adequate juxtarenal anastomosis.[1] There may be problems within the graft itself, but this again is an uncommon cause attributable to dilatation or graft degeneration.[2] False aneurysm formation at the lower anastomosis probably accounts for between 5 and 10% of occluded graft limbs.[1] The cause may be uncertain, perhaps due to an embolic episode, hypercoaguable states as a result of tumours or myeloproliferative disorders or low output due to cardiac or other causes.[1] The most common problem, however, is failure of run-off due to anastomotic intimal hyperplasia or progression of disease in the distal vasculature.

That this factor should be the most significant is not surprising because patients undergoing aortofemoral bypass may have had dual level disease at the time of the original surgery. The dilemma or co-existent occlusive disease in the aorto-iliac and femorodistal segment remains a problem for vascular surgeons. The conventional approach in this situation is to revascularize the groin alone;[3–6] usually the deep femoral artery. This is of fundamental importance to the long-term patency because not only is it difficult to predict the immediate relief of the symptoms of critical ischaemia, and claudication by this procedure but it runs the risk of subsequent occlusion.[3–17] The restoration and maintenance of patency therefore is very likely to mandate improvement of the outflow vessels; either the profunda or by sequential distal bypass, or both.

A second fundamental consideration is how vascular inflow can be restored. The common situation, however, is that a single limb of the graft is occluded[1] and under these circumstances most contemporary authors would agree that graft thrombectomy can be achieved with reasonable safety in the majority of cases. If this fails the alternative lies in extra anatomic axillofemoral or femorofemoral bypass; direct replacement of the graft itself *in situ*,[18] or more rarely by bypassing from the supracoeliac or intrathoracic aorta.[19,20] It is less common for both limbs of the aortofemoral graft to occlude but essentially the approach is similar.

PRE-OCCLUSIVE IDENTIFICATION

Much has been written recently on the regular and systematic surveillance of femorodistal vein bypass and the contents of other chapters within this book will bear testimony to this contemporary interest. Is the same philosophy applicable to the aortofemoral bypass? There seems little doubt that the timely pre-emptive revision of any graft that would seem to be failing would have distinct advantages over undertaking procedures on one that has already occluded. It can be under ideal circumstances as an elective procedure. It will be possible to obtain angiograms under optimal conditions which will give maximum information; in this instance regarding the state of the circulation in the groin and vessels round the knee. Once a bypass has thrombosed this information may be difficult to obtain and be misleading. Propagated thrombus may extend into vessels which are potentially salvageable, and poor tissue perfusion may limit imaging.

However, against these conceptual considerations are differences in comparing surveillance with the femorodistal situation. The latter is much more likely to occlude and to do so within a limited time frame; usually in the first year. Thus the returns for invested effort are substantially greater. Femorodistal bypasses develop graft stenoses which are a specific problem and remediable by angioplasty or timely surgery. Finally, distal grafts are easily accessible by duplex scanners which makes sensitive and noninvasive follow-up a feasible objective. These important factors therefore are reflected in limited interest in systematic follow-up to identify the 'failing graft' for aortofemoral bypass. In practical terms long-term surveillance is likely to be restricted to careful documentation of ankle pressures before and after exercise. A fall may indicate the need for angiography and re-assessment.

CLINICAL PRESENTATION

Occlusion most commonly affects one limb of the graft. Only rarely are both affected synchronously.[2]

At this stage one of three clinical situations exist:

(i) A reversion of the circulatory state within the affected leg which approximates to the same situation that existed prior to the original surgery. Usually this will be a noncritical or at the very worst a critical state but undemanding of immediate action. It is, however, unusual for this situation to be the case—probably in less than 20%.[1]

(ii) A worse situation than existed prior to previous surgery with critical ischaemia but with immediate preservation of limb viability as witnessed by continued sensation and motor function in the foot and the presence of venous circulation on Doppler insonnation at ankle level.

(iii) A state of acute critical ischaemia with an anaesthetic paralysed limb demanding emergency intervention to achieve limb salvage.

Unfortunately it is the situations ii and iii that are the most common (80%).[1]

FURTHER EVALUATION

For these reasons mentioned above, time is rarely an available luxury. When a noncritical state does exist then clearly the need for further investigation and surgical intervention at all must be given consideration. In an elderly patient with the return of modest symptoms of claudication a conservative course may be entirely appropriate. However, if attempted restoration of flow is contemplated then it should be undertaken expeditiously. Although late thrombectomy of the graft is possible,[22] the fresher the thrombus the more easily will it be extracted.

The more common situation demands immediate and decisive action if the limb is to be salvaged. If available, the original operative notes and angiograms should be scrutinized. At that time was there a profunda femoris of reasonable quality? If still patent was there a superficial femoral artery stenosis? It is worth assessing the extent of the previous groin dissection and the precise anatomical site of the anastomosis, to common femoral, superficial femoral or more likely down on to the origin of the deep femoral artery. Valuable information may be available regarding the state of the more distal circulation. Was there a popliteal artery above or below knee of reasonable quality or were there only calf vessels available? Although the situation may well have deteriorated since those angiograms it gives a base line from which to work.

At this stage three principal decisions need to be made. On the basis of the previous angiograms and the patient's general state it may be felt that further operative measures are inappropriate and a primary amputation should be considered. Decisions of this nature are made on the basis of multiple factors involving philosophical and practical considerations. Depending on the patient's life quality, expectation and fitness in terms of further surgery a careful judgement needs to be made. Balanced against this must be the likely benefits of a further procedure (see below).

The second point is whether a further angiogram is required. If at all possible this should be considered if redo surgery is anticipated to be feasible. However, if the patient's limb is immediately critical and time has already elapsed before arriving at hospital then the further albeit small delay may be outweighed by the need of expeditious action. In these circumstances on-table angiography is often a better option anyway because it is quicker and it is definition of the run-off into the deep femoral and more distal vessels that is required.

The final point is the patient's fitness for surgery. Although a relatively minor surgical approach is likely to be necessary, an assessment must be made as to whether major reconstruction would be feasible in the event it became necessary. If this is deemed to be an option, even if unlikely, then adequate preoperative provisions must be made for this.

OPERATIVE TACTICS

The skin preparation and anaesthetic technique must take into account the uncertainties that may now prevail. Although a simple graft thrombectomy and extended profunoplasty are the aim, provision must be made

(i) for failure to unblock the graft
(ii) extension of the bypass into the distal limb circulation, or both.

The first objective is to restore inflow. The old groin incision is re-opened. The degree of scarring varies but care must be taken not to damage the saphenous vein because this may well be required if not at this juncture then at some future date. Anatomical orientation may be difficult second time in. A helpful point is to extend the incision a few centimetres more distally into virgin ground. It is usually then quite easy to find the distal superficial femoral artery. Having found the periadventitial plane, this vessel can be followed proximally up to the point at which the Dacron graft is attached. (If the artery is explored directly through scar tissue, there is a risk for an inexperienced operator to develop a 'plane' within the artery wall itself between adventitia and muscle and dissect up in the belief that this is correct.)

The extent of tissue reaction round the Dacron will depend on the type of graft previously employed. Knitted grafts will be more densely incorporated than woven grafts which tend to have a very well-defined 'capsule' around them. In either event, as the graft is approached, preferably by cautious sharp dissection, the Dacron will be visualized glistening through the surrounding tissues.

HOW TO UNBLOCK THE GRAFT

The graft 'capsule' is incised thus entering a clear plane twixt host tissues and Dacron. This should be orientated vertically at a site at which it is anticipated the Dacron will be opened (see below). This is because it is easy to damage the Dacron whilst attempting to identify this plane. Once the margins of the graft have been defined within its 'capsule' it is usually quite easy to develop this plane proximally to give room for graft clamping. The prosthesis may well have elongated since implantation and gentle traction can often deliver several useful extra centimetres into the wound. Careful dissection should now be undertaken distally to define the origin of the original anastomosis. This may be difficult and care should be taken to minimize damage to the host vasculature and if possible the original suture line. The dissection in the host vessel should be continued with the objective of obtaining control of the common femoral artery behind the graft if still patent and the distal deep femoral artery down to a healthy and disease-free area. This facilitates complete clamping before attempting to unblock the graft and break into the patent distal circulation. However, if comprehensive dissection proves to be difficult it may be prudent to abandon this attempt and resort to the use of blocking Fogarty catheters as necessary.

A vertical incision is now made in the centre of the graft immediately above the previous anastomosis which is likely but not necessarily to have been originally extended down on to the deep femoral artery origin. The first priority must be to try and unblock the graft by removing the contained thrombus and pseudo intima (see Fig. 1). This concept is a now well established technique in contemporary vascular surgical practice. Malone *et al*[21] were successful in 68 out of 71 limbs, Bernhard[20] was successful in 30 of the 37 limbs in which it was attempted. MacPherson and Bell[22] had comparable experience. More recent reports by Brewster,[1] unblocking was successful in 80 of the 84 grafts in which this was undertaken. This procedure may also be successful several months after occlusion.[1,22,23]

Within the lumen of the occluded graft will be a combination of the central core of recent thrombus and the long established 'skin' of pseudo intima smoothly lining

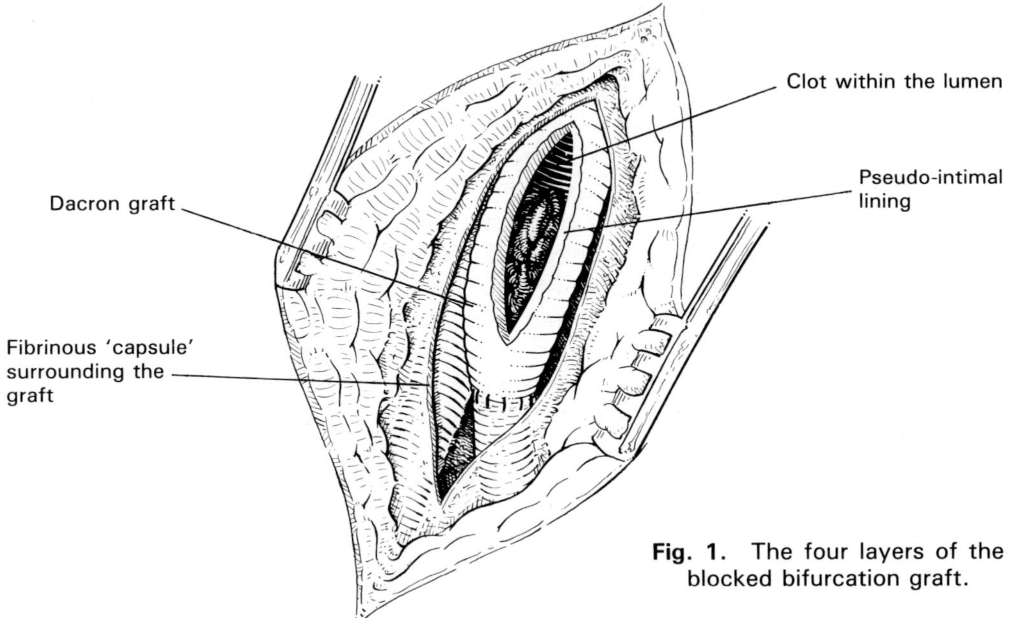

Fig. 1. The four layers of the blocked bifurcation graft.

the wall of the graft. Sometimes it is only necessary to extract the thrombus alone if the pseudo intima is thin but this is not usually the case. This 'intima' is loosely adherent and can be removed surprisingly easily.

Its thickness probably develops to approximate the lumenal size of the prosthetic inflow tract to the size of the native run-off vessel; in this case the profunda femoris.[24] Where graft failure has occurred from deterioration of run-off, the native vessel size is thus small and the 'compensatory' thickness of the pseudo intima therefore that much greater.

The technique requires a combination of the use of a long sucker, Fogarty emobolectomy catheters and intimal ring stripper to be inserted under the pseudo intima to dislodge it. By a combination of these techniques it is possible in the majority of cases to completely remove the intraluminal debris to achieve a satisfactory inflow. Care should be taken in dislodging these contents from the region of the upper graft bifurcation because of the risks of dislodgement causing occlusion or embolism down the good limb of the graft. This eventuality can perhaps be minimized by appropriately applying digital pressure on the femoral pulse of the opposite patent side.[22] However, in practical terms the chances of this happening are surprisingly small.[1,2,22]

It is important to get complete clearance of the pseudo intima because fragments can dislodge and rotate or embolize in the early postoperative period. How can the adequacy of this removal and restoration of inflow be confirmed? This may be an awkward yet vital point on which to be certain. Arterioscopy, on-table angiography or direct pressure measurements of the graft itself may be considered and all of these have their uses.

In the relatively unlikely event that these direct unblocking measures should prove unsuccessful then inflow needs to be re-established via a number of alternative techniques that are outside the detailed remit of this chapter. They include direct replacement of the limb of the graft in its entirety, or by extra anatomic bypass by axillo or femorofemoral crossover.

RE-ESTABLISHMENT OF RUN-OFF

Essentially one of three situations will be encountered.

(i) There is a relatively localized area of disease either due to fibromuscular intimal hyperplasia, or atheroma, immediately below the original anastomosis. This is fortunately the commonest situation[1,2,25] because it is the easiest with which to deal. The vertical opening in the graft is extended down into the profunda through the diseased area and into healthy vessel (see Fig. 2). Intimal hyperplasia is usually adherent and no attempt should be made to remove it. Loose superficial atheromatous plaques can sometimes be picked off quite easily without disturbing the main intimal layer. A formal endarterectomy should be considered with care. If the atheroma is seen to extend into the distal deep femoral vessel it may be best to leave the diseased intima undisturbed because of the problems of securing the distal intimal flap.

Whichever of these options have been employed, however, some sort of patch is now required. If the profunda revascularization is to be complemented by a more distal graft, (see below) then the top anastomosis of the latter, whether vein or prosthesis can be applied to this area to form a synchronous patch. Otherwise, a direct patch is applied either with vein or a further piece of Dacron (see Fig. 3). Some authors feel that vein gives better results.[21] A large tributary of the long saphenous should be used thus saving the main trunk for some future contingency. The technical aspects of application of the patch are self evident

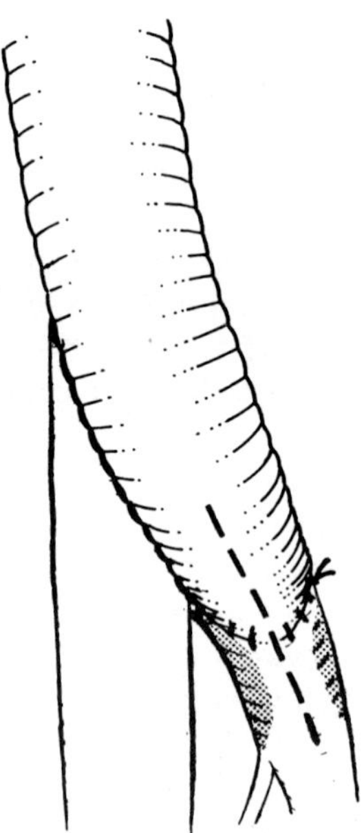

Fig. 2. Line of incision through graft and stenosed segment of profunda into healthy vessel.

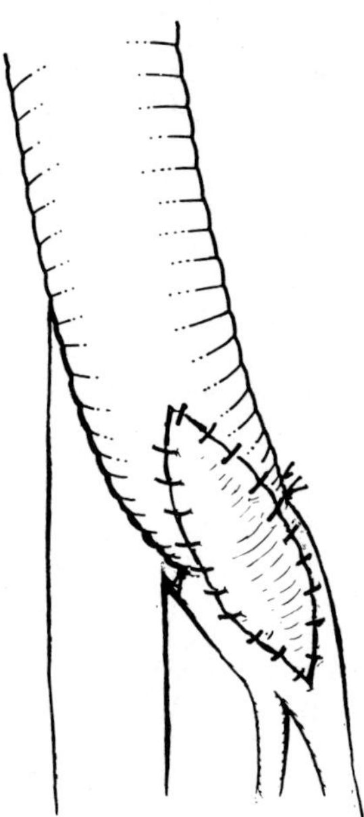

Fig. 3. Vein patch applied to 'grabbing' arteriotomy.

but it is probably advisable to secure the divided pre-existing suture line by underrunning it with the newly inserted sutures. More than this seems unnecessary because the pre-existing anastomosis should be well healed.

If healthy profunda is several centimetres down from the site of the original anastomosis it may be simpler to re-anastomose the graft directly at this level with a further piece of Dacron anastomosed to give extra length (see Fig. 4).

(ii) A deep femoral artery remains but is now extensively diseased. Although it may be possible to restore perfusion through this vessel to some extent by employing the measures described above, the question then arises as to whether this will be adequate both to maintain future graft patency and achieve limb salvage. This may pose difficulties in decision making and delicate judgement may be required in determining what more if anything should be done. Pre-operative or on-table angiograms will give information regarding the collateral circulation and the state of the vessels round the knee and in the calf. Comparison with previous films may indicate that major deterioration has occurred in the deep femoral since the original surgery which may favour a complementary procedure. Alternatively, if the original situation has essentially been restored then no further procedure would seem to be required. The final decision is a question of clinical judgement but if doubt exists it is best to complement this procedure with an extension to the popliteal or infracrural vessels preferably with vein. This is likely to be judged advisable in about one-third of cases.[1] One option is to wait for 24 hours to evaluate the effect of profunda revascularization alone before deciding.

(iii) The deep femoral artery and all other vessels in the groin are either occluded or too diseased to be utilized as an outflow tract. Fortunately this is an uncommon situation.

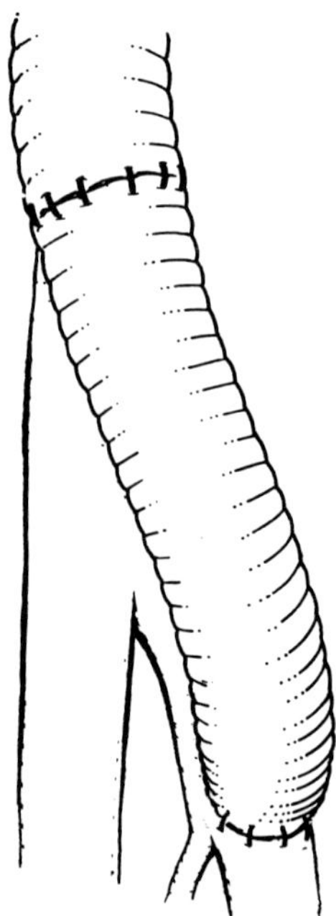

Fig. 4. Extension of Dacron taken down to distal healthy profunda.

The options for further procedures now clearly depend on the availability of vessels further down the limb. In the absence of a popliteal artery in the author's view, no further operation is appropriate and amputation is likely to be necessary.

However, bypasses direct to the popliteal particularly above knee can give reasonable results. What is now effectively an aortopopliteal bypass can when done as a primary procedure give 3-year patency rates of 65%.[25] This is probably easiest accomplished above knee by the addition of a further prosthetic length of graft; either Dacron or polytetrafluoroethylene (PTFE).

If extension is to below the knee and a usable long saphenous vein is available then the best chance of salvage is probably by utilizing this with a direct anastomosis of vein to the Dacron at groin level.

LONG-TERM PATENCY OF RE-OPENED AORTOBIFEMORAL GRAFTS

Patency rates of re-operated limbs are about 70%, 60% and 45% at 1, 3 and 5 years respectively. Some of these that do fail can be maintained by appropriate further surgery; after distal bypass grafting. If this 'extended' cumulative patency is considered the rates rise to 75%, 75% and 55% respectively.[1] It will be appreciated therefore from these data that although this form of surgery may be difficult and require varied and innovatory procedures, the results fully justify the effort involved.

REFERENCES

1. Brewster DC, Meier GH, Darling RC *et al*: Reoperation for aorto femoral graft limb occlusion: optimal methods and long term results. J Vasc Surg 5:363–374, 1987
2. Brewster DC: Direct reconstruction of aorto-iliac occlusive disease. *In* Vascular Surgery, Rutherford CB (Ed.). Philadelphia and London: W. B. Saunders, 3rd edn, pp. 667–691, 1989
3. Edwards WH, Wright RS: A technique for combined aorto femoral popliteal arterial reconstruction. Ann Surg 179:572–579, 1974
4. Royster TS, Lynn R, Mulcare RJ: Combined aorto iliac and femoro popliteal occlusive disease. Surg Gynaecol Obstet 143:949–952, 1976
5. Garrett WY, Slaymaker CC, Heintz SE, Barnes RW: Intra operative prediction of symptomatic results of aorto femoral bypass from changes in ankle pressures index. Surgery 82:504–509, 1977
6. Hill DA, McGrath MA, Lord RS, Tracy GD: The effect of superficial femoral artery occlusion on the outcome of aorto femoral bypass for intermittent claudication. Surgery 87:133–136, 1980
7. Richardson JV, Slaymaker EE, Wright CB: Distal reconstruction following aorto bifemoral bypass grafting: predictability of early haemodynamic results. Ann Surg 46:477–480, 1980
8. Satiani B, Hayes JP, Evans WE: Prediction of distal reconstruction following aorto femoral bypass for limb salvage. Surg Gynaecol Obstet 151:500–502, 1980
9. Martinez BD, Hentzer HR, Bevan EG: Influence of distal arterial occlusive disease on prognosis following aorto bifemoral bypass. Surgery 88:795–805, 1980
10. O'Donnell TF, McBride KA, Callow AD *et al*: Management of combined segment disease. Am J Surg 141(4):452–459, 1981
11. Satiani B, Liapis CD, Evans WE: Aorto femoral bypass for severe limb ischaemia. Long term survival and limb salvage. Am J Surg 141(2):252–256, 1981
12. Crawford ES, Bomberger RA, Glaesen DH *et al*: Aorto-iliac occlusive disease; factors influencing survival and function following reconstructive operation over a twenty five year period. Surgery 90:1055–1067, 1981
13. Brewster DC, Porter BA, Robison JG, Darling RC: Aorto femoral graft for multi level occlusive disease. Predictors for success and need for distal bypass. Arch Surg 117:1593–1600, 1982
14. Harris PL, Cane Bigley DJ, McSweeney L: Aorto femoral bypass and the role of concomitant femoro distal reconstruction. Br J Surg 72:317–320, 1985
15. Poulias GE, Polemis L, Skoutas B, *et al*: Bilateral aorto femoral bypass in the presence of aorto iliac occlusive disease and factors determining results. Experience and long term follow up with 500 consequential cases. J Cardiovasc Surg (Torino) 26:527–538, 1985
16. Simma W, Bassiouny H, Hartl P, Brucke P: Evaluation of profundoplasty in reconstructions of combined aorto iliac and femoro popliteal disease. J Cardiovasc Surg (Torino) 27:141–145, 1986
17. Eidt J, Charlesworth D: Combined aorto bifemoral and femoro-popliteal bypass in the management of patients with extensive athersclerosis. Ann Vasc Surg 1:453–459, 1986
18. Crawford ES, Manning LG, Kelly TF: Redo surgery after operations for aneurysm and occlusion of the abdominal aorta. Surgery 81:41–46, 1977
19. Baird RJ, Feldman P, Miles JT *et al*: Subsequent downstream repair after aorto iliac and aorto femoral bypass operations. Surgery 82:785–792, 1977
20. Bernhard VM, Ray LI, Towne JB: The reoperation of choice for aorto femoral graft occlusion. Surgery 82:867, 1977
21. Malone JM, Goldstone J, Moore WS: Artogenous profundoplasty: the key to long term patency in secondary repair of aorto femoral graft occlusions. Ann Surg 188:817–823, 1978
22. MacPherson DS, Bell PRF: The unblocking of occluded dacron grafts. *In* Extra Anatomic and Secondary Arterial Reconstruction, Greenhalgh RM (Ed.). London: Pitman Books Ltd, 1982
23. Ernst CB, Daugherty ME: Removal of a thrombotic plug from an occluded limb of an aorto femoral graft. Arch Surg 113:301, 1978

24. Horton RE, Bird DR, Baird RN, Giddings AFB: Long grafts in the treatment of critical ischaemia. Ann Roy Coll Surg (Engl) 63:181–185, 1981
25. Darke SG: Aorto popliteal and ilio popliteal bypass. *In* Surgical Management of Vascular Disease, Bell PRF, Jamieson CW, Ruckley CV (Eds). Philadelphia and London: W. B. Saunders, 1990

Femorofemoral Crossover Bypass

Henner Müller-Wiefel

Extra-anatomic bypass procedures are used whenever a special local situation (e.g. infection, radiation, multiple previous operations, stoma) or an unfavourable general condition of the patient precludes a direct reconstructive approach to the occluded arterial segment, or when a minimum stress operation without opening a large body cavity must be performed.

Whether or not an extra-anatomic bypass procedure is indicated will largely depend on its value for the specific vascular region involved, as established by comparing the mortality, patency rates and functional results with those of the classical procedures.

Aortofemoral bypass with synthetic grafts as well as iliac thrombendarterectomy are the classical and well established techniques for revascularization of a leg suffering from ischaemia by an obliterative process of the pelvic pathway. Recently, newer endovascular procedures such as balloon angioplasty have been added.

Apart from this the vascular surgeon's amamentarium alternatively offers crossover femorofemoral grafting for those patients with a unilateral iliac arterial obstruction and a sufficiently patent contralateral pelvic pathway.

It was in 1953 when Oudot and Beaconfield[1] first described the technique of femorofemoral crossover grafting while using homologous conduit material. Freeman and Leeds[2] then, in 1952, made use of the crossover principle choosing an endarterectomized superficial femoral artery as a bridge between the left groin and the right common femoral artery.

Subsequently Vetto[3] popularized this operation by describing his first successful experience with 10 patients in 1962, and the basic technique has not changed since that time.

SURGICAL TECHNIQUES

The crossover principle for revascularization of a leg with a bypass originating at the contralateral donor side can be realized in different ways.

The most important alternative is the suprapubic bridge from the iliofemoral vessels of the one side to the inguinal region of the other side. Depending on local findings the distal anastomosis is constructed with the common femoral artery or the origin of the profunda femoris. The central anastomosis at the donor limb may be pointed either in the direction of blood-flow and then created with the external iliac artery, or against the direction of flow and here be done with the common femoral artery or its bifurcation (Figs 1 and 2).

According to this the course of the graft will resemble a cranial-convex 'C' or form a somewhat 'S'-shaped configuration (Figs 3 and 4). The latter obviously should have

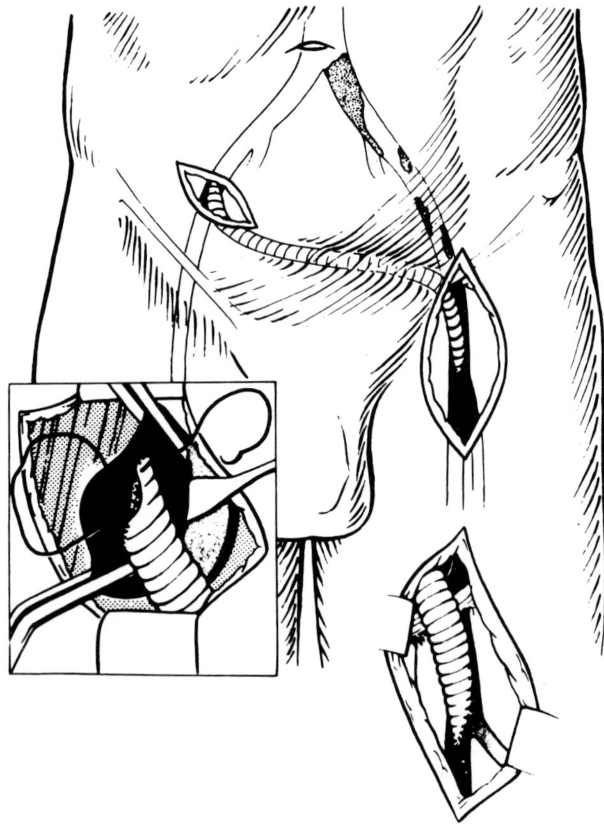

Fig. 1. Suprasymphyseal crossover bypass with favourable haemodynamic conditions due to a central anastomosis with the external iliac artery. Taken from Müller-Wiefel.[18]

some advantages for haemodynamic reasons and therefore is preferred by us to the original C-shaped graft described by Vetto.[3]

The second alternative is realized whenever an axillobifemoral bypass is constructed. The suprapubic bridge here, however, does not originate from the patient's own vasculature but from the long conduit at the lateral aspect of the trunk. The crossover graft may originate with an acute angle or in a 90°-position, as shown in Fig. 5.

The third variation in the crossover principle is given when the bypass runs through the obturator foramen. This may be done at the recipient side or at the side of the proximal anastomosis with the donor artery (Fig. 6). In the latter case the crossover conduit has to cross the perineum subscrotally and will be anastomosed at the anteromedial part of the thigh to the superficial femoral artery.

INDICATIONS

As for other vascular surgical reconstructions in the aortoiliac segment the indications for a femorofemoral crossover bypass are ischaemic rest pain,

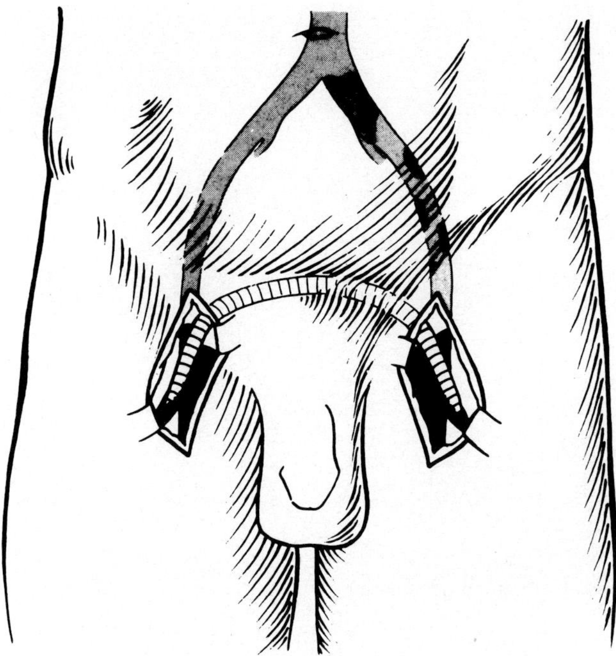

Fig. 2. Femorofemoral crossover bypass from one common femoral artery to the opposite one, combined with a bilateral profundaplasty. Taken from Müller-Wiefel.[18]

ischaemic tissue loss, and severely disabling claudication due to unilateral iliac artery occlusive disease (Fig. 7).

In particular, the femorofemoral bypass has proven to be an effective and durable way of treating high-risk patients when avoidance of a transabdominal operation is desired. It may also be considered when one limb of an aortobifemoral graft has occluded and cannot be disobliterated by thrombectomy.

In addition, femorofemoral crossover may be an option in very obese patients; in cases with infections; and in young males in order to preserve sexual function by avoiding injury to the hypogastric plexus under surgical dissection in this area.

PATIENT SELECTION AND PREOPERATIVE CONSIDERATIONS

The fundamental rule for any arterial reconstruction is that blood inflow to the endarterectomized or bypassed segment has to be haemodynamically adequate in order to prevent premature thrombotic occlusion and this, of course, also applies for the crossover bypass.

All patients requiring arterial reconstruction for lower limb revascularization need preoperative angiography in order to evaluate the extent and degree of the obliterative process and to estimate the run-off and the inflow conditions. It is, however, interesting to read that Vetto, who originally popularized the

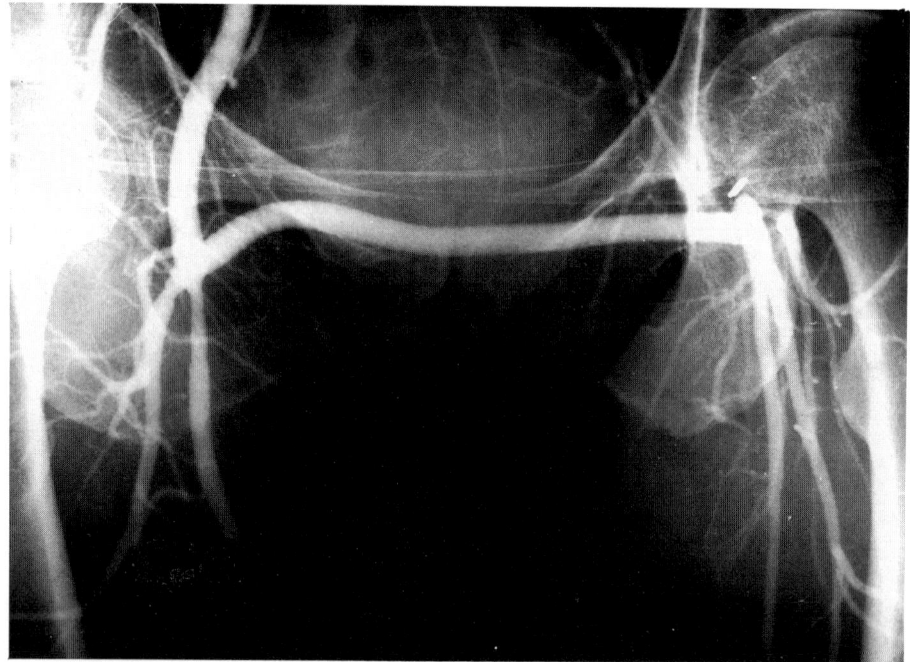

Fig. 3. Postoperative angiogram after a crossover bypass construction in a modified 'C'-configuration.

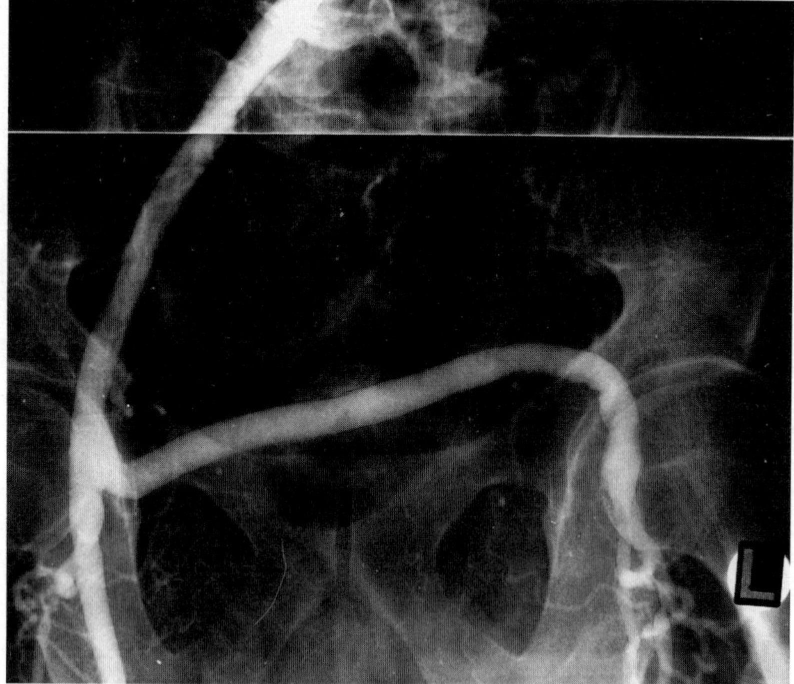

Fig. 4. Suprasymphyseal crossover bypass in a modified 'S'-configuration.

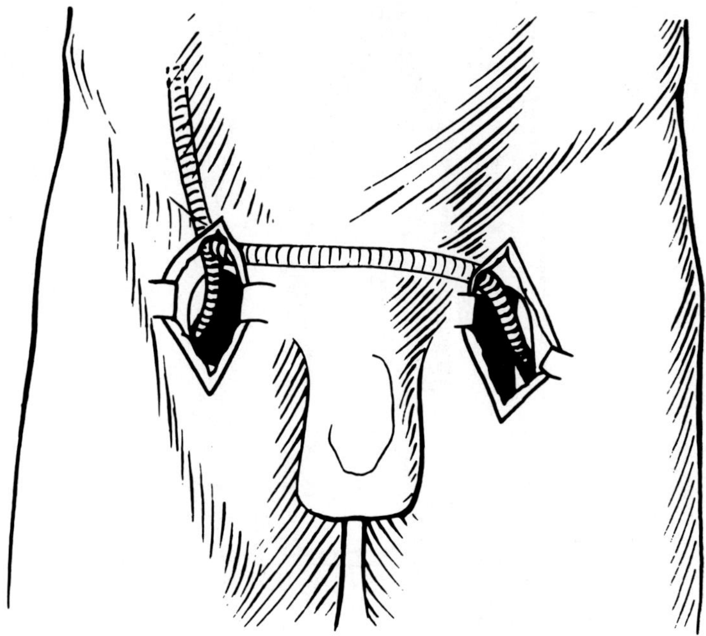

Fig. 5. Femorofemoral crossover bypass originating not from an iliac or femoral artery but from an axillofemoral conduit. Taken from Müller-Wiefel.[18]

femorofemoral crossover bypass, rarely used arteriography at that time and felt that a palpable pulse in one groin was sufficient to permit the corresponding common femoral artery to be used as a donor vessel to bypass the iliac occlusion of the opposite side.[3,4]

It is certainly true that if the femoral pulse is diminished, it is unlikely that blood flow through that iliofemoral segment will be adequate to support limb revascularization with use of a femoropopliteal or a femorofemoral crossover bypass. However, a normal femoral pulse at rest and a normal Doppler-derived high-thigh pressure do not necessarily indicate an adequate inflow, since a subcritical stenosis in the ipsilateral iliofemoral system may still be present.[5–7]

Therefore all patients should undergo preoperative angiography except in circumstances of utmost emergency. We emphasize that we are in agreement with the statements of Blaisdell and Carson[4] and Ellenby and Schuler[8] on this point.

Angiography will not only provide the surgeon with detailed anatomic information but also will give some functional data if pressure measurements at different levels can be included with the catheter angiography. Additionally the angiographic examination will provide the surgeon with detailed data in order to decide whether a simultaneous catheter dilatation of a stenosed iliac segment might be indicated in order to improve the inflow to the crossover graft (Fig. 8).

Function tests with pressure measurement and papaverine application will, furthermore, be helpful in predicting the suitability of the pelvic pathway on the

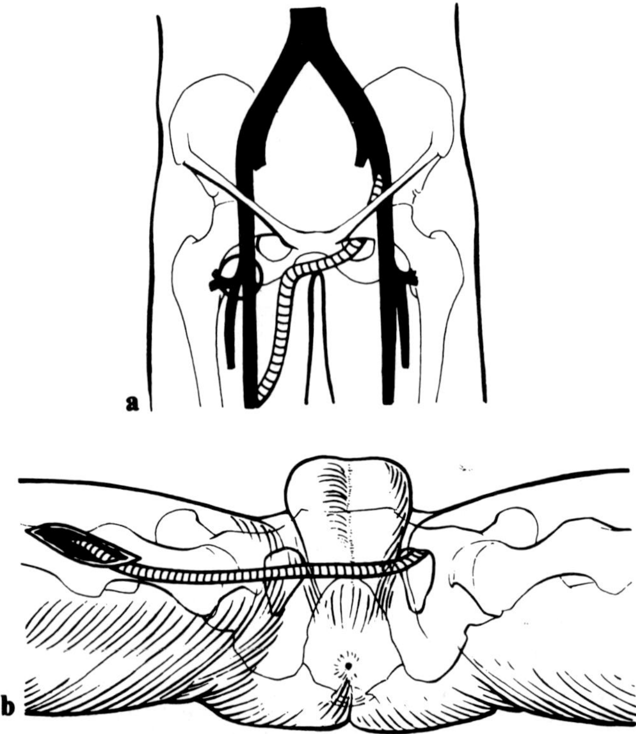

Fig. 6. Modification of the femorofemoral crossover technique by graft passage through the obturator foramen and a subscrotal perineal course to the contralateral limb. Taken from Müller-Wiefel.[18]

donor side and the reader's attention must be drawn to the communications of Flanigan *et al.*[6,7,9] and Ellenby and Schuler.[8]

The situation is similar when one limb of an aortobifemoral graft has occluded. A major stenosis within the graft limb remaining patent is usually not to be expected and the inflow for the suprapubic bridge should be fine.

RESULTS

Early (<30 days) results as reported in the literature give a favourable impression. Depending on the selection of patients the mortality rate ranges between 0%[10] to 8%,[11] mostly about 3–4%.[12,13] Our own mortality is 5.1% and thus reflects the great portion of very high-risk cases in this cohort of reconstructions.

Early failures by re-occlusion of the femorofemoral bridge has very seldomly been observed in the literature; however, Lamerton *et al.* reported a 13% incidence.[13] Our own rate was 1.1%.

More importantly, however, are the follow-up results. Long-term patency compares favourably with the classical *in situ* correction of the iliac pathway by endarterectomy

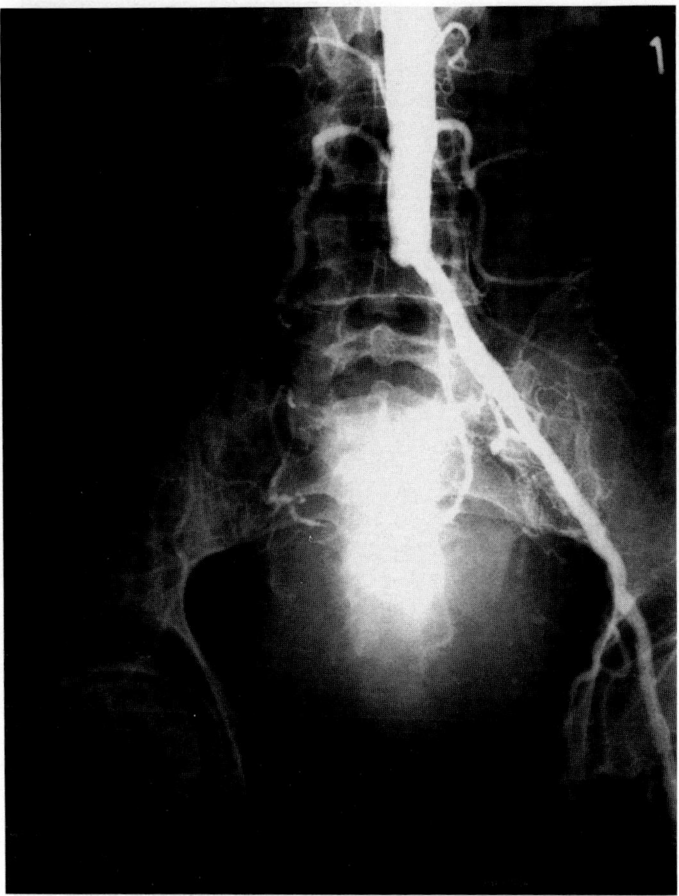

Fig. 7. Unilateral iliac arterial occlusion and almost completely patent pelvic pathway at the opposite side are the classical angiographic indications for a femorofemoral crossover bypass.

or aortofemoral bypass. As listed in Table 1 the 5-year values vary from 60% up to 82.4% according to different reports in the literature.[4,9,11,13–16]

Eight-years results are given at 80.8% by Brief *et al.*[14] and 82.4% by Schweiger and Raithel[16] whereas Plecha and Plecha[15] report a lower success of only 55% patency. The same patency also was found after 10 years.[15]

Our own results (Fig. 9) are evaluated from the experience with 187 patients that were operated on between September 1975 and August 1990. The male : female ratio was nearly 3 : 1 and the average age was 64 ± 11 years with a range of 36–85 years.

As seen in Table 1, the patency rates were 83% for the 5-year period, 73% for 8-year follow-up and 69% for the 10-year interval.

Numerical details concerning indication, donor site and location of the peripheral anastomosis of the crossover graft in our series are given in Table 2.

A wound infection occurred in 3.4% of the cases, whereas a lymph fistula developed in 1.7% of the operations. Repeat operations during the postoperative

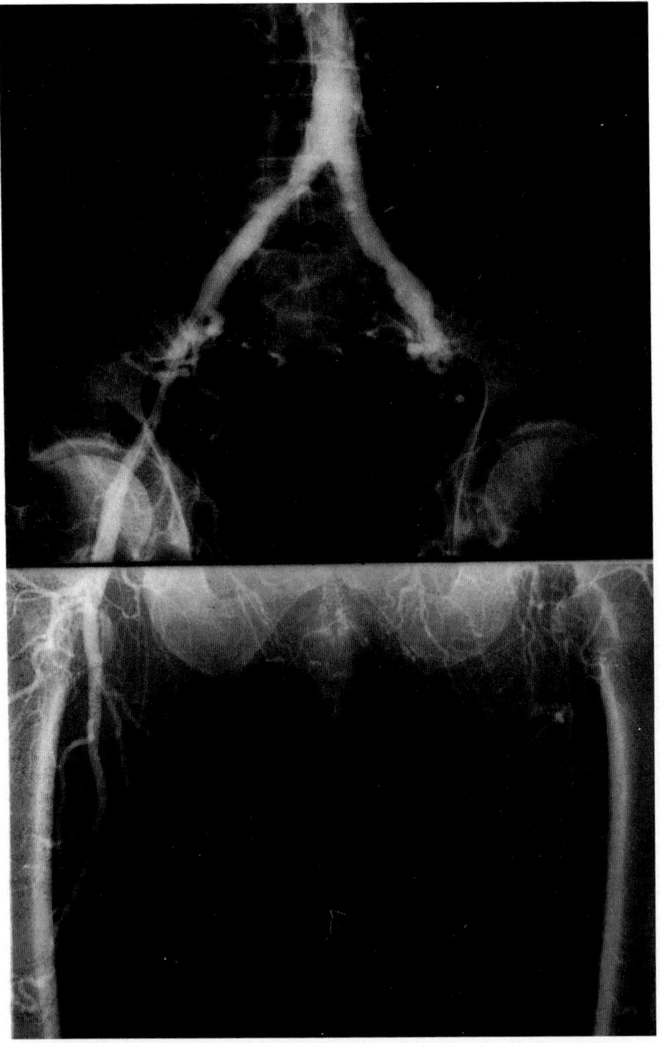

Fig. 8. Stenotic section in the external iliac artery of the donor side may need an intra-operative balloon dilatation.

course were thrombectomy (10%), correction of the distal anastomosis because of a progressive stenosis and impairment of the run-off condition (8%) and finally the additional construction of a femoropopliteal or femorocrural bypass to improve the outflow situation on the recipient limb.

DISCUSSION AND CONCLUSIONS

Femorofemoral crossover bypass is a well accepted procedure with surprisingly high patency rates, especially when compared with the axillofemoral or bifemoral leg revascularization as another extra-anatomic technique for this purpose.

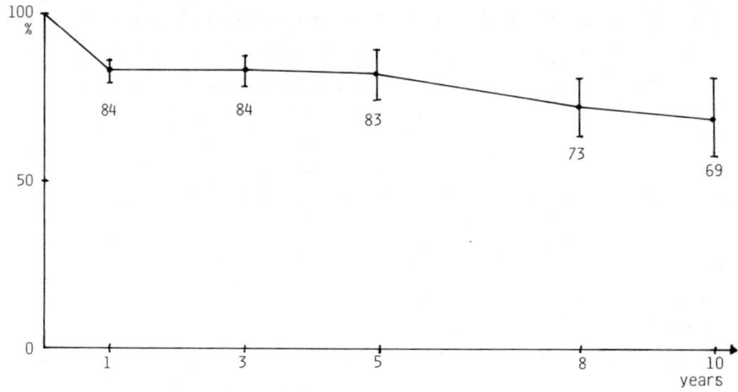

Fig. 9. Patency rates during follow-up of 187 patients between September 1975 and August 1990 according to the life table method.

Table 1. Long-term results after femorofemoral crossover bypass (patency rates, %)

Years: *Author*	*3* *(%)*	*5* *(%)*	*8* *(%)*	*10* *(%)*	*Total no.* *of cases*
Brief *et al.*	84	80.8	80.8	—	57
Flanigan *et al.*	74	74	—	—	134
Vetto	—	74	—	—	59
Plecha *et al.*	83.3	72.2	55	55	119
Schweiger *et al.*	82.4	82.4	82.4	—	192
Kalman *et al.*	67	—	—	—	82
Pietri *et al.*	75	71	—	—	50
Müller-Wiefel	84	83	73	69	187

These favourable long-term results permit the extension of the indication also to 'non high-risk' situations, one of them being the avoidance of a local iliac arterial repair in young male patients with a unilateral obliteration in order to protect sexual function.

There are, of course, different factors which influence the long-term patency of the suprapubic conduit. From isolated reports in the literature it is not always clear if, and by which method, antithrombotic or antiaggregation treatment was given. Our own policy is to treat all our patients with a femorofemoral crossover bypass with aspirin provided that no intolerance or contra-indications exist.

Similar to the experiences with the inguinal anastomoses of an aortobifemoral graft, there does also develop over the course of time in crossover bypass anastomoses a reduction in calibre. This may become a tight stenosis and may require a typical surgical correction. However, with these repeat operations, the patency and full function of the crossover bypass can be maintained. On the other hand we observed that stenosis of the anastomosis at the donor side is extremely less frequent, especially when the bridging conduit originates from the external iliac artery.

This underlines the observation of Vetto[3] who reported the very slow development of iliac atherosclerosis at the donor side during the postoperative years.

Table 2. Femorofemoral crossover bypasses in 187 patients between September 1975 and August 1985 (%)

Indication			
Chronic ischaemia	81.9	acute ischaemia	11.2
Stage IIb	9.6	infection	4.3
Stage III	44.8	false inguinal aneurysm	2.6
Stage IV	27.5		
Donor site			
External iliac artery	49.2		
Femoral bifurcation	30.1		
Limb of bifurcation graft	20.7		
Peripheral anastomosis at:			
Deep femoral artery	53.4		
Femoral bifurcation	42.2		
Proximal popliteal artery	4.4		

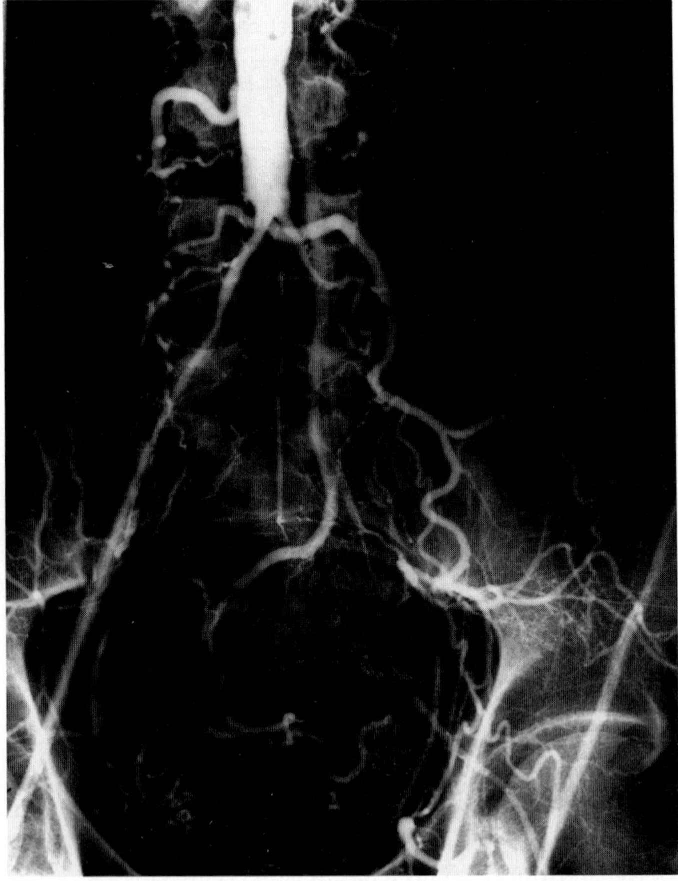

Fig. 10. Angiographic findings, as shown here, exclude a partial patent iliac artery from being used as a donor site. A reconstruction by a transluminal endovascular operation has to preceed the crossover bypass construction.

This may be caused by an increased blood-flow in the donor artery when the crossover graft works as an additional outflow tract.

As already mentioned, we regularly perform preoperative angiography except in very urgent cases and would like to state that this should be a general rule. Information on inflow-tract as well as outflow conditions are of the utmost importance for our strategic planning. Despite the increased iliac bloodflow in the donor system a haemodynamically significant stenosis may result in a decrease of the distal donor vessel flow.[17] Clinical judgement of the pulse quality in the groin alone is often difficult and unreliable. Functional tests and measurements are helpful or mandatory in all doubtful situations[4,6,7,9,10,15] and thus may be regarded as the basis for a good long-term success.

In addition to graft patency, clinical results are an important criterion. Some patients have continued symptoms despite a patent femorofemoral bypass. This usually will happen when there are additional blocks in the arterial vessels of the thigh or calf but also when the iliac inflow from the donor side is insufficient. This may be avoided by intra-operative measurements and, if indicated, a simultaneous intra-operative catheter dilatation as an endovascular procedure (Fig. 10).

As a general rule one may follow Flanigan *et al.*[9] who stated that a femorofemoral bypass should never be expected to give satisfying results when a stenosis of the donor iliac artery of 50% or above exists.

Additional emphasis has to be given to the anastomotic technique. Since the femoral bifurcation is a location of predominance for chronic arteriosclerotic occlusion it is advisable to construct the peripheral anastomosis of the crossover graft not only to the common but also to the deep femoral artery as we do in most cases also with the classical aorto-bifemoral bypass. This will prevent an early increase of outflow resistance and thus contribute positively to better long-term patency.

REFERENCES

1. Oudot J, Beaconfield P: Thrombosis of the aortic bifurcation treated by resection and homograft replacement. Arch Surg 66:365–374, 1953
2. Freeman NE, Leeds FH: Operations on large arteries. Calif Med 77:229–233, 1952
3. Vetto RM: The treatment of unilateral iliac artery obstruction utilizing femoro-femoral graft. Surgery 52:342–345, 1962
4. Blaisdell FW, Carson SN: Alternatives to direct surgery and aortoiliac disease. *In* Surgery of the Aorta and its Body Branches, Bergan JJ, Yao JST (Eds). New York and London: Grune & Stratton, 1979
5. Sobinsky KR, Borozan PG, Gray B *et al*: Is femoral pulse palpation accurate in assessing the hemodynamic significance of aortoiliac occlusive disease? Br J Surg 68:423–425, 1981
6. Flanigan DP, Pratt DG, Goodreau JJ *et al*: Hemodynamic and angiographic guidelines in selection of patients for femorofemoral bypass. Arch Surg 113:1257–1262, 1978
7. Flanigan DP, Gray B *et al*: Correlation of Doppler-derived high-thigh pressure and intra-arterial pressure in the assessment of aorto-iliac occlusive disease. Br J Surg 68:423–425, 1981
8. Ellenby MI, Schuler JJ: Femorofemoral grafts and distal variations. *In* Techniques in Arterial Surgery, Bergan JJ, Yao JST (Eds). Philadelphia and London: W. B. Saunders, 1990
9. Flanigan DP, Yao JST, Bergan JJ: Crossover femorofemoral grafting in patients with severe lower extremity ischemia. *In* Gangrene and Severe Ischemia of the Lower Extremities, Bergan JJ, Yao JST (Eds). New York and London: Grune & Stratton, 1978

10. Kalman PG, Hosang M, Johnston KW *et al*: The current role for femorofemoral bypass. J Vasc Surg 6:71–76, 1987
11. Pietri P, Pancrazio F, Adovasio R *et al*: Long term results of extra anatomical bypasses. Inter Angio 6:429–433, 1987
12. Pratschke E, Schäfer K, Becker HM: Der gekreuzte suprapubische femoro-femorale Bypass. Angio 1,2:31–36, 1980
13. Lamerton AJ, Nicolaides AN, Eastcott HHG: The femorofemoral graft. Arch Surg 120:1274–1278, 1985
14. Brief DK, Brener BJ, Alpert J, Parsonnet V: Crossover femorofemoral grafts followed up five years or more. Arch Surg 110:1294–1299, 1975
15. Plecha FR, Plecha FM: Femorofemoral bypass grafts: Ten-year experience. J Vasc Surg 1:555–561, 1984
16. Schweiger H, Raithel D: Der femoro-femorale Bypass beim einseitigen Beckenarterienverschluss: Alternative oder Verfahren der Wahl? Vasa 13:147–152, 1984
17. Sumner DS, Strandness DE Jr: The hemodynamics of the femorofemoral shunt. Surg Gynecol Obstet 134:629–633, 1972
18. Müller-Wiefel H: Extraanatomic bypasses in chronic arterial occlusive disease (Infections, patients at risk). *In* Vascular Surgery, Heberer G, Van Dongen RJAM (Eds). Berlin: Springer, 1989

Single Sided Iliac Reconstruction

Paolo Fiorani

In recent years, aortofemoral reconstruction by means of bypass technique has proved completely satisfactory because of steady improvements in patient selection, surgical techniques, anaesthesiological assistance and perioperative monitoring.

Many authors have reported that early morbidity and the mortality rate have decreased continuously during the last decades, declining from 9% to 2%, while long-term patency up to 99% has been reported.[1–12]

Although aortobifemoral bypass is considered the operation of choice in patients with extensive atherosclerotic lesions of the infrarenal aorta or the iliac arteries, the ideal choice in cases with unilateral iliac artery occlusion without significant stenotic lesions of the contralateral side is still controversial.[3,13–16]

Several alternative procedures have been proposed such as aortofemoral, iliofemoral, femorofemoral bypass, thromboendarterectomy and, more recently, endovascular procedures (percutaneous transluminal angioplasty (PTA), laser assisted angioplasty).[17–20]

However, frequently it is difficult to compare the validity of these different methods because of the heterogeneity of the series, particularly the patient selection and the indications for surgery.

Furthermore, these four methods have some disadvantages: when performing iliofemoral bypass, the evolution of atherosclerotic lesions in the donor artery may frequently occur; when the femorofemoral procedure is carried out, also when an 'asymptomatic groin' has to be operated, the thromboendarterectomy, usually performed in young patients, may cause impotence; finally, the results of the PTA are still controversial.

Similarly, in these patients, the decision to perform aortobifemoral bypass seems to be ill-advised because severe complications, such as ischaemia or prosthetic graft infection, may occur in the asymptomatic side.

On the other hand, the unilateral aortofemoral procedure, although showing high late patency rate, does not afford any kind of protection against evolution of atherosclerotic lesions on the contralateral iliac artery. This unfavourable aspect may actually be minimized if future improvement in pharmacological therapy proves capable of delaying the evolution of atherosclerotic lesions; additionally, one has the possibility of performing several alternative procedures.

The aim of this study is to evaluate, based on our experience and a review of the literature in terms of early and late complications, mortality and patency rates, the efficacy of unilateral aortofemoral bypass and the chance of unfavourable evolution on the contralateral asymptomatic side.

CASE MATERIAL

A consecutive series is considered of 58 patients submitted to aortofemoral unilateral bypass (AF) during the period between 1979 and 1989, in the Vascular Surgery Department of the University of Rome 'La Sapienza'.

Of the patients, 54 (93%) were male while four (7%) were female, and the mean age was 57 years (range 25–77 years).

The risk factors included cigarette smoking in 53 patients (92%), arterial hypertension in 12 patients (20%) and diabetes in eight cases (14%) (of which three were insulin-dependent).

Regarding other vascular disease, we observed previous myocardial infarction in three patients (5%), ischaemic heart disease in nine patients (15%) and cerebrovascular insufficiency in three cases (5%).

Thirty-six patients (62%) suffered from severe claudication, 14 patients (24%) had rest pain and in eight patients (14%) ulceration or gangrene were present.

All patients were submitted to conventional angiography (according to Seldinger or dos Santos technique) or, during the last years, digital subtraction angiography (DSA). In 20 patients (23%) we observed a concomitant occlusion of the superficial femoral artery.

Haemodynamic tests were performed in all the patients in order to evaluate the Winsor Index and, in case of occlusion of the superficial femoral artery, the Profunda-Popliteal Collateral Index and the Residual Resistance Index. Additionally, in order to evalute the haemodynamic characteristics of the iliac artery haemodynamic (postischaemic hyperaemia test) and pharmacological (papaverine test) studies were performed.

A Dacron graft (knitted or double velour) was the prosthetic material routinely utilized.

RESULTS

No case of early death was observed among the 58 patients who underwent a unilateral aortofemoral bypass.

The primary early patency rate (30 days) was 94.8% (55 patients); in three cases, because of early graft thrombosis, a redo surgery was performed resulting in a secondary early patency rate of 98.2% (57 patients). In one case, after failure of redo surgery, a major amputation was required.

Early complications included groin lymphorrea in three patients, pneumonia in one patient and partial intestinal obstruction in one patient.

The mean follow-up was 60 months (range 6–124 months) with a late patency rate of 87% (51 patients). In three patients with late graft thrombosis a re-operation was performed successfully while in one patient (1.7%) the failure of this procedure led to major amputation.

Long-term survival rate was 82.5% (49 patients); late deaths were due to myocardial infarction in three cases, stroke in two cases and cancer in four cases.

Evolution of atherosclerotic lesions in the contralateral iliac artery was observed in seven patients (12%); five of these patients underwent other surgical procedures (three femorofemoral bypass, one axillofemoral bypass and one endarterectomy).

Late complications included graft infection in two cases (3.4%) and false aneurysm in one case (1.7%); there was no case of aorto-enteric fistula in this group of patients.

DISCUSSION

Surgery of the aortofemoral area has been performed for about 40 years and is continuously evolving with improved results. Mortality rate has decreased from 9% to 2% and less, and long-term patency rates have been reported up to 99%, mainly due to improvements in patient selection, surgical techniques, anaesthesiological assistance and perioperative monitoring.[1–12,15–16]

Moreover, in the last 10 years, several selected cases of aorto-iliac occlusive diseases have been treated by means of interventional radiological techniques (PTA, laser assisted angioplasty, atherectomy, etc.) with short-term satisfactory results.[17–20] However, at the present time it is not possible to give a definitive judgment on long-term results of these techniques.

A particular problem is related to the choice of treatment in cases of isolated iliac artery occlusion. Such a situation was not infrequent in our experience (35% of cases in the present series). In such cases, several limited reconstructions (aortofemoral, iliofemoral, femorofemoral bypasses, iliac thromboendarterectomy) and more extensive procedures (aortobifemoral bypass) have been advocated.[11,21–23]

Regarding long-term patency, our experience and the literature show better results for aortic procedures rather than for extra-anatomic or iliofemoral bypasses.[10,11,13,14,22] This can be explained by the better haemodynamic performance of a graft in an anatomic rather than in an extra-anatomic or iliofemoral position.

Iliofemoral grafts, although anatomically situated in the retroperitoneal space, take the inflow from an artery in which atherosclerotic lesions frequently occur, so that unfavourable results often occur.

There are not, however, significant differences, in terms of long-term patency between unilateral or bilateral aortofemoral bypasses (respectively 87% and 82% in our experience).

Apart from late thrombosis, which is quite rare and usually correctable with low surgical risk and a secondary patency rate of about 95%, there are two main problems which can impair the long-term results of aortofemoral unilateral bypasses: graft infection and contralateral iliac artery occlusion.[2,4,5,24,25]

Graft infection in the aortofemoral area is reported in the literature in 0.6 to 6% cases, comparing well with our own incidence of 2.4%.[26–30] The most catastrophic manifestation of this complication is represented by aorto-enteric fistula (0.6–2.4% of cases in the literature) that in our experience occurred in 2.1% of patients.[31–33] The literature review shows that the mortality rate of this complication reaches 25–88% (48% in our experience).

In our general experience aorto-enteric fistula was observed more frequently ($p=0.041$) in aortobifemoral procedures than in unilateral aortofemoral bypass. That could be explained by the anatomical and technical differences in these two procedures; during the bilateral procedure, the proximal anastomosis is performed in proximity to the renal arteries with more extensive mobilization of the duodenum, with the common tract of the graft protruding anteriorly firmly adherent to the third portion of the duodenum. It is well known that in 90% of cases this portion represents the critical area for the development of an aorto-enteric fistula.[28]

On the other hand, an important advantage of performing a unilateral aortofemoral bypass is that we use a small calibre graft overlying the aorta behind the duodenum, with proximal anastomosis on the anterolateral aspect of the aorta with minimal periaortic tissue dissection. Another benefit is the ability to easily approach the aorta by an extraperitoneal access, reducing the operating time and the blood loss, and preserving the contralateral groin.

The second problem in performing a unilateral aortofemoral bypass concerns the possible evolution of atherosclerotic lesions on the contralateral iliac axis.[3,11,13,14]

The role of the groin in the aetiopathogenesis of a graft infection is well recognized. In the groin area there are many lymphatic vessels, which drain the lower limbs and the perineal area, potentially exposing the graft to pathogenic bacterial flora of the skin.

Regarding the haemodynamic and angiographic indications for unilateral procedure, the preoperative study of the contralateral iliac artery is very important. In fact, in the literature and in our experience, it is not unusual to find patients with unilateral occlusive lesions of the iliac artery and satisfactory patency of the contralateral iliac arteries.

Clinical, haemodynamical and morphological methods have been proposed to evaluate the presence of contralateral iliac artery lesions. The clinical criteria include the recognition of a valid femoral pulse and the absence of femoral arterial bruit.

The instrumental evaluations include Doppler findings to identify and quantify the presence of pressure gradients and echotomography to recognize eccentric lesions which have to be confirmed by an angiographic exam. Sometimes a direct measurement of femoral artery blood pressure, using pharmacological tests (papaverine), can be helpful.[23]

The literature suggests that an iliac artery can be considered normal if the pressure gradient between brachial and femoral pressure does not exceed 15 mmHg. In our experience, among the 58 patients with unilateral iliac artery lesions, the measurement of the femoral artery blood pressure showed a gradient less than 15 mmHg in all cases.

The most reliable instrumental evaluation is angiography which, in the oblique and lateral projections, allows identification of aortic bifurcation lesions otherwise obscured by the skeleton in conventional projections.

With regard to the fate of the contralateral iliac artery, in our experience, the clinical and instrumental tests performed during the follow-up period suggest an evolution of atherosclerotic lesions in 12% of cases (seven patients, which compares with a 6–17% incidence in the literature[3,11,13,14] (Figs 1, 2).

It seems that the most appropriate action, in patients with unilateral iliac artery lesions and with a good contralateral femoral arterial pulse, is not to proceed with bilateral grafting but to do a unilateral aortofemoral bypass.

For several years, haemodynamical studies have shown the significance of competitive flow between prosthetic and host arterial flow.[34] The competitive flow,

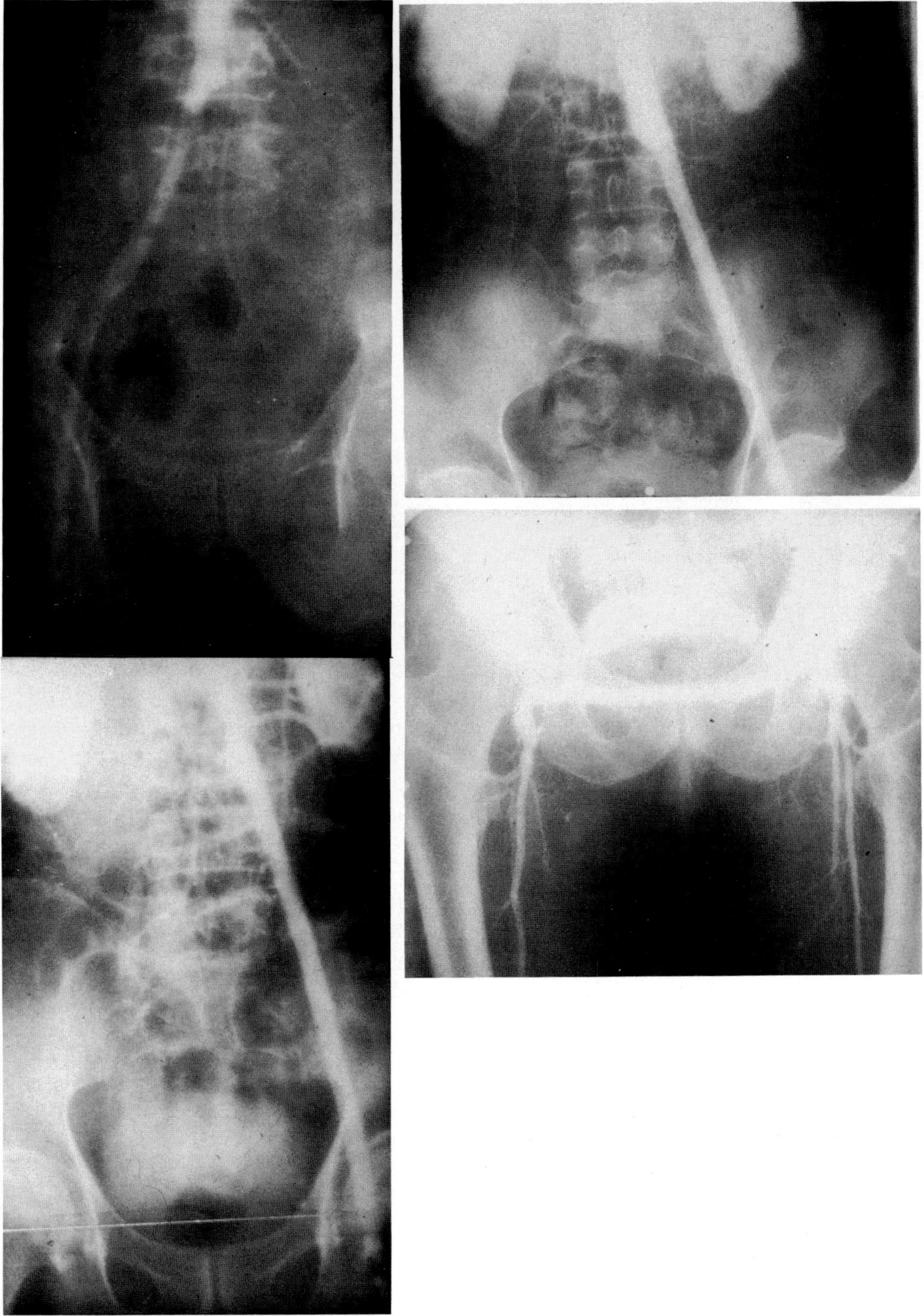

Fig. 1. Unfavourable evolution of contralateral iliac artery 6 years after unilateral aortofemoral bypass (left) treated by femorofemoral bypass (right).

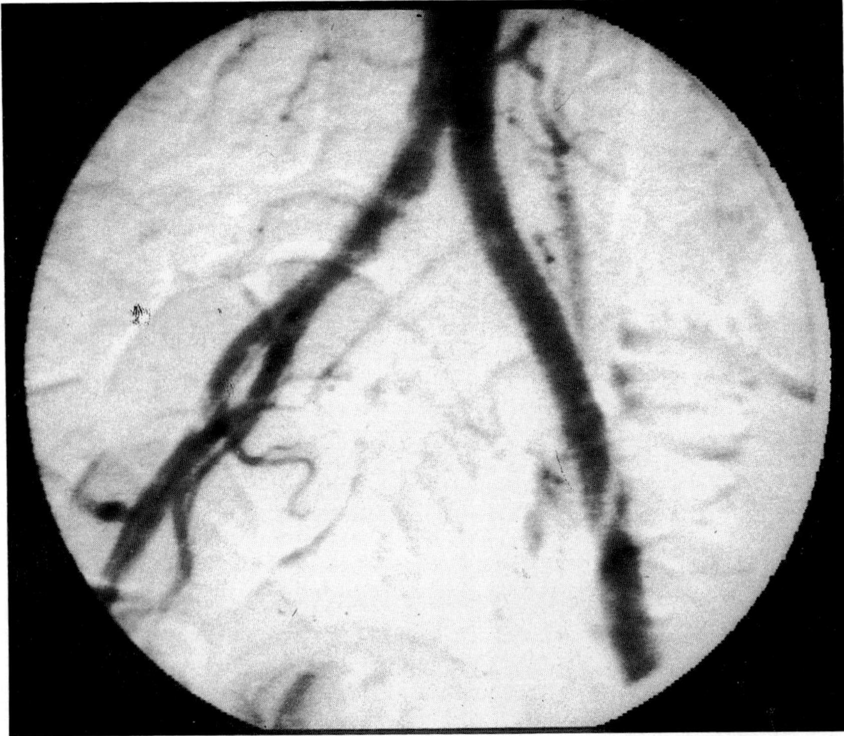

Fig. 2. Maintenance of patency of the contralateral iliac artery 12 years after unilateral aortofemoral bypass.

reducing the blood flow through the patent iliac artery, causes a progressive lumen reduction and a more rapid evolution in thrombosis.[35] Furthermore, competitive flow caused by turbulence at the femoral anastomotic site, (especially when performed as end-to-side), may provoke intimal hyperplasia and an arterial wall weakening with onset of false aneurysm due to wall vibration.[36] We observed some complications of the asymptomatic side such as one thrombosis, one false aneurysm and two graft infections; these events could have been avoided, perhaps, by a unilateral surgical procedure.

During the follow-up period, an early finding by noninvasive methods of an initial iliac arterial lesion can be easily corrected, even in high risk patients, with endovascular procedures (PTA, laser angioplasty etc.). In these selected cases the possibility of performing an endovascular procedure may offer better long-term results (60–90% according to the literature).

CONCLUSIONS

Considering the results of our experience, and from a review of the literature, the treatment of choice for the revascularization of the aortofemoral area seems to be the anatomic bypass procedure.

In cases of unilateral iliac occlusion, an accurate preoperative screening by clinical, haemodynamical and angiographic studies, allows correct selection of the type of surgical treatment required.

Although unilateral or bilateral aortofemoral bypass techniques result in quite similar long-term patency, more extensive utilization of unilateral surgical procedures may avoid, or at least reduce, the incidence of graft infection which, even if rare, influences significantly the results in terms of morbidity and mortality.

In addition, with accurate surveillance of the contralateral iliac artery, through serial noninvasive tests or DSA, further improvement of long-term results can be obtained by performing endovascular procedures in selected cases.

REFERENCES

1. De Bakey ME, Crawford SE, Cooley DA, Morris GC Jr: Surgical considerations of occlusive disease of the abdominal aorta and iliac and femoral arteries: Analysis of 803 cases. Ann Surg 148:306–324, 1958
2. Lyons JH Jr, Wiesmann RE: Surgical management of late closure of aortofemoral reconstruction grafts. N Engl J Med 278:1035–1037, 1968
3. Mozersky DJ, Sumner DS, Strandness DE: Long term results of reconstructive aortoiliac surgery. Am J Surg 123:503–509, 1972
4. Najafi H, Dye WS, Javid H *et al*: Late thrombosis affecting one limb of aortic bifurcation graft. Arch Surg 110:409–412, 1975
5. Malone J, Wesley SM, Goldstone J: The natural history of bilateral aortofemoral by-pass graft for ischemia of lower extremities. Arch Surg 110:1300–1306, 1975
6. Brewster DC, Darling RC: Optimal methods of aortoiliac reconstruction. Surgery 84:739–749, 1978
7. Neverlsteen AS, Suy R, Daenen W, Boel A, Staelpaert G: Aortofemoral grafting: Factors influencing late results. Surgery 88:642–653, 1980
8. Crawford SE, Bomberger R, Glaeser DH, Saleh AS, Russell WL: Aortoiliac occlusive disease: factors influencing survival and function following reconstructive operation over a twenty five years period. Surgery 90:1055–1067, 1981
9. Szilagyi E, Joseph PE Jr, Smith RF, Reddy DJ, McPharlin M. A thirty years survey of the reconstructive surgical treatment of aortoiliac occlusive disease. J Vasc Surg 3:421–436, 1986
10. Taurino M, Speziale F, Faraglia V, De Santis F, Rizzo L, Guerricchio R, Fiorani P: How is the femoral artery revasculirized and when a profunda repair is essential. *In* Limb Salvage and Amputation for Vascular Disease, Greenhalgh RM, Jameson CW, Nicolaides AN (Eds). London and Philadelphia: W. B. Saunders, 1988
11. Piotrowski J, Pearce WH, Jones DN *et al*: Aortobifemoral by-pass: the operation of choice for unilateral iliac occlusion. J Vasc Surg 8:211–218, 1988
12. Sterpetti A, Feldhaus RJ, Schultz RD: Combined aortofemoral and extended deep femoral artery reconstruction. Arch Surg 123:1269–1273, 1988
13. Levinson SA, Levinson HJ, Holloran G: Limited indication for unilateral aortofemoral or iliofemoral vascular grafts. Arch Surg 107:791–796, 1973
14. Kalman PG, Hosang M, Johnston KW, Walker PM: Unilateral iliac disease: The role of iliofemoral bypass. J Vasc Surg 6:139–43, 1987
15. Hill DA, McGrafth MA, Tracy GD: The effect of superficial femoral artery occlusion on the outcome of aortofemoral by-pass for intermittens claudication. Surgery 87:133–136, 1980
16. Martinez BB, Hertzer NR, Beven EG: Influence of distal arterial occlusive disease on prognosis following aortobifemoral by-pass. Surgery 88:759, 1980
17. Gallino A, Mahler F, Probst P, Nachbur B: Percutaneous transluminal angioplasty of the arteries of the lower limbs: A five year follow up. Circulation 70:619–623, 1981

18. Schneider E, Gruntzig A, Bollinger A: Long term patency rates after percutaneous transluminal angioplasty for iliac and femoropopliteal obstructions. *In* Percutaneous Angioplasty, Dotter CT *et al*: (Eds). Berlin: Springer-Verlag, pp. 175–180, 1983
19. van Andel GJ, van Erp WFM, Krepel VM, Breslau PJ: Percutaneous transluminal dilatation of the iliac artery: Long term results. Radiology 156:321–323, 1985
20. Jorgensen B, Henriksen LO, Karle A *et al*: Percutaneous transluminal angioplasty of iliac and femoral arteries in severe lower-limb ischemia. Acta Chir Scand 154:647–652, 1988
21. Blaisdell RW, Hall AD, Lim CR Jr, Moore WC: Aortoiliac arterial subcutaneous grafts. Ann Surg 172:775, 1970
22. Devolfe C, Adelaine P: Ileo-femoral and femoro-femoral cross-over grafting. Analysis of 11 years experience. J Cardiovasc Surg 24:634–640, 1983
23. Flanagan PD, Ryan TJ, William LR, Schwartz JA, Gray B, Shuler JJ: Aortofemoral or femoro-popliteal revascularization? A prospective evaluation of papaverine test. J Vasc Surg 1:215, 1984
24. Crawford SE, Manning LG, Kelly TF: Redo surgery after operations for aneurysm and occlusion of the abdominal aorta. Surgery 81:41–45, 1977
25. Malone J, Moore SM, Goldstone J: Life expectancy following aortofemoral grafting. Surgery 81:551, 1977
26. Szilagyi E, Smith RF, Elliott JP: Infection in arterial reconstruction with synthetic grafts. Ann Surg 176:321, 1972
27. Jamieson GG, De Weese JA, Rob CG: Infected arterial graft. Ann Surg 181:850, 1975
28. Fiorani P *et al*: L'addome acuto nel paziente con protesi arteriosa. Arch Soc It Chir 82 Congr Rome 1980, pp. 573–588
29. Bunt TJ, *et al*: Synthetic vascular graft infection. Surgery 93:733–746, 1983
30. Speziele F *et al*: Le infezioni protesiche in chirurgia vascolare. Atti del 3 Corso Agg Chir Vasc Trieste, pp. 74–92, 1988
31. Shepard AD, Ernst CB: Aortoenteric and aortocaval fistulae. *In* Vascular Surgical Emergencies. London and New York: Grune & Stratton, 1987
32. Thomas WE, Baird RN: Secondary aorto-enteric fistulae: towards a more conservative approach. Br J Surg 73:875–878, 1986
33. Walker WE, Cooley DA, Duncan JM *et al*: The management of aortoduodenal fistula by *in situ* replacement of the infected abdominal aortic graft. Ann Surg 205:727–732, 1987
34. Brief DK, Brener BJ, Alpert J, Parsonnet V: Crossover femorofemoral grafts followed up five years or more. Arch Surg 110:1294–1299, 1975
35. Ernst CB: Axillary-femoral bypass graft patency without aorto-femoral pressure differential. Ann Surg 181:424–427, 1975
36. Schultz RD, Hokanson DE, Strandness DE Jr: Pressure-flow relation of the end-side anastomosis. Surgery 62:319–324, 1967

Long-term Patency After Reconstructive Surgery and PTA for Renal Artery Stenosis

S.-E. Bergentz, H. Weibull and D. Bergqvist

Reconstructive surgery and percutaneous transluminal renal angioplasty (PTRA) are the two techniques used for active treatment of renovascular hypertension and renovascular uraemia caused by renal artery stenosis (RAS). The literature on the results, and particularly on the long-term results, of these treatment modalities is very difficult to evaluate. There are several reasons for this:

The patient group is heterogeneous, varying from infants and children to elderly patients, sometimes with severe generalized atherosclerosis.

The location of the lesions is variable, and so is the definition of RAS.

The pathology varies and is often not known or reported.

The patient selection can be very different. In many reports it is only stated that the patients had hypertension, and an angiographically demonstrated renal artery stenosis. Such a selection will mean that many of the patients do not have a renovascular hypertension, i.e. a hypertension caused or worsened by RAS, but rather an essential hypertension occurring coincidentally with an insignificant RAS.

The criteria for *technical* success vary. There are very few reports where long-term technical success is documented with studies on renal vascular anatomy or perfusion.

The criteria for *clinical* success are often not defined. Repeated blood pressure measurements under standardized conditions before and at various times after treatment are rarely reported. The use of antihypertensive drugs before and after the treatment is often not stated.

For these reasons it is not surprising that the problem with active treatment of RAS using PTRA or reconstructive surgery is controversial. It is the purpose of this paper to critically review the available knowledge of long-term results after active treatment for renovascular hypertension and/or uraemia in the three large patient groups, those with atherosclerosis, those with fibrous dysplasia and children, with emphasis on selecting the best method of treatment appropriate to each patient.

CRITERIA FOR SUCCESS

The criteria for success after active treatment of renovascular hypertension should be based on three different types of parameter: the technical result, the blood pressure response and the effect on renal function.

Documentation of the degree of technical success is essential for evaluation of the results. The definition of technical success varies. Some authors define it as a residual stenosis not exceeding 50%,[1,2] others have no definition but report the technical results in terms of success, improvement, failure or deterioration.[3] Weibull *et al.*[4] define it as absence of a significant stenosis, a concept which is strictly defined by the authors. Conventional angiography is the most reliable method to document the rate of technical success and should, if possible, be used whenever there is any doubt. Recent reports indicate that duplex sonography can be used as a surveillance procedure;[5] DSA has also been recommended for follow-up. Schwarten[6] reported that the DSA findings agreed with the findings after conventional arteriography in 26 out of 30 patients undergoing both types of examination (87%).

With regard to blood pressure response the patients are usually reported as cured, improved or failures, according to the criteria recommended by the US Cooperative Study of Surgery for Renovascular Hypertension.[7] A patient is cured if the diastolic pressure is 90 mmHg or less in the absence of antihypertensive medication. If the decrease in diastolic pressure is at least 15%, but medication still is required, the patient is considered improved. A failure means a smaller fall in blood pressure or no decrease at all. Several authors use modifications of these criteria.[4,8,9] Data on the need for antihypertensive drugs before and after treatment are essential for a proper evaluation of the blood pressure response. Blood pressure must be measured repeatedly and under standardized conditions before and at different periods after the treatment. Such data are lacking in many publications.

Blood pressure fluctuations may occur for various reasons and are not always related to the degree of technical success. Immediately after a PTRA or reconstructive surgery there is often a short temporary rise in blood pressure, which may be due to a renin washout from the kidney, followed, at least in the operated group, by a drop for several months, which may be part of a general response seen after any type of major surgery. After that the blood pressure may rise again. Brawn and Ramsay[8] have pointed out that improvement of blood pressure after active treatment of RAS may be 'spurious' and not always a consequence of the treatment. According to these authors cure of the hypertension is the only reliable criteria for successful treatment. On the other hand a successful technical result may be accompanied by a lack of clinical response. Failure of blood pressure response may in these cases be due to an erroneous patient selection, to a parenchymatous lesion of the kidneys, to a stenosis of the contralateral kidney, or to a recurrency of the treated stenosis.

The effect of the treatment on kidney function is rarely reported. This may be acceptable in series where the kidney function is satisfactory and the indication for the treatment mainly is to correct or improve a severe hypertension, as is often the case in fibrous dysplasia. Today, however, many patients, particularly the elderly and atherosclerotic group, are treated mainly to save or restore kidney function.[10] In these patients early and late data on serum creatinine, and preferably also creatinine clearance, are mandatory.

There are no generally accepted criteria for the duration of follow-up. Five years appears to be an acceptable time, but it should, if possible, be much longer in the young patients.

ATHEROSCLEROTIC RENOVASCULAR HYPERTENSION

Patient characteristics

Atherosclerotic RAS is usually, but not always, a sign of generalized atherosclerotic disease. The patients therefore often have such risk factors as hyperlipoproteinaemic disorders, diabetes, smoking, and essential hypertension.[11,12] They are usually men above 50 years of age. There is, however, a considerable difference between patients with documented signs and symptoms of extrarenal atherosclerotic disease, as signified also by bilateral renal artery stenosis, and patients without such signs.[12,13] The latter group has signs of local atherosclerosis of the renal artery, and therefore the short- and long-term blood pressure response is better and the mortality is lower. There may also be a difference between patients with atherosclerosis localized to the aorta, and those with stenosis in the renal artery, usually its proximal part. The former type is called ostial stenosis,[1,2,14] origin stenosis[3] or isthmus stenosis,[4] the latter postostial,[2,14] nonostial[1] or juxta-aortic stenosis.[4] Isthmus stenosis is localized to the aorta and therefore often a sign of a more generalized atherosclerotic disease, which may make the prognosis worse than in patients with juxta-aortic stenosis strictly limited to the renal artery.[15] Furthermore, the localization of the atherosclerosis might also be of importance for the choice of treatment (see below).

Reconstructive surgery

A large number of techniques has been used to reconstruct atherosclerotic RAS.[16] The preference varies from centre to centre. Thromboendarterectomy (TEA) either

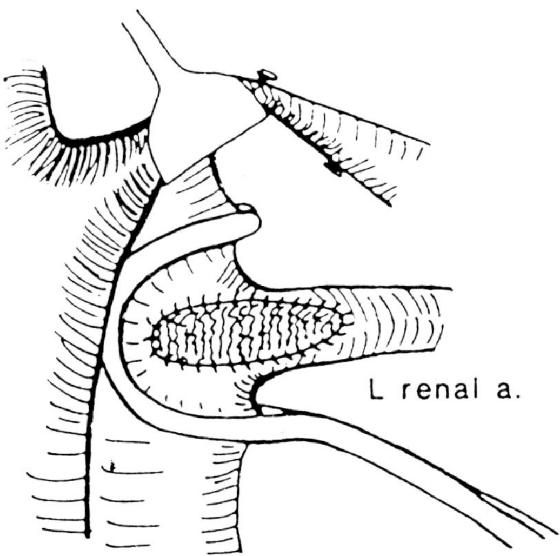

Fig. 1. For atherosclerotic RAS a thromboendarterectomy and Dacron patch is a satisfactory procedure. Since the stenosis often is localized to the aortic wall rather than the renal artery, it is important to extend the patch into the aorta.

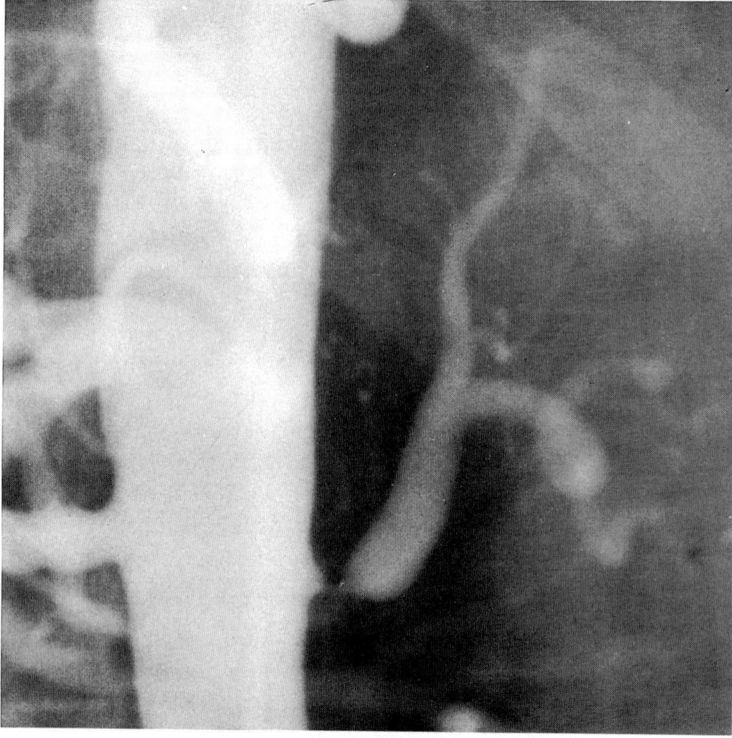

Fig. 2A. Athersclerotic renal artery stenosis treated with thromboendarterectomy and patch: before surgery.

transaortic with a longitudinal incision, or a transverse incision with extension to the first part of the renal artery, seems to be the most commonly used technique. We prefer the latter variety, as illustrated in Fig. 1, since it gives a guarantee that the critical first part of the renal artery really is widely open. The arteriotomy is closed with a patch, preferably of Dacron. The critical part of this reconstruction is the distal tip of the patch, where it is recommended to use interrupted stitches to avoid a stricture.[16] The arteriography of a patient with a TEA and patch graft before and at a 4-year follow-up is shown in Figs. 2A and B.

Aortorenal bypass does not seem to offer any advantages in atherosclerotic RAS over a TEA and patch. If the aorta is severely diseased, splenorenal, hepatorenal or gastroduodenorenal reconstructions have been recommended.[17,18] A prerequisite for these procedures is a normal coeliac axis, which must be demonstrated on a high-quality angiography with side projection. Even if the coeliac axis looks normal at the time of surgery, there must be a potential risk for late atherosclerosis in this patient category. Only anecdotal reports on the long-term results by using this technique are available.[17] In experienced hands, using a satisfactory technique, the long-term (more than 5 years) *technical success rate* after reconstructive surgery for atherosclerotic renal artery stenosis should exceed 90%.[16,19] The *blood pressure* response varies since it depends not only on technical success, but also on patient selection and other factors, as stated above.

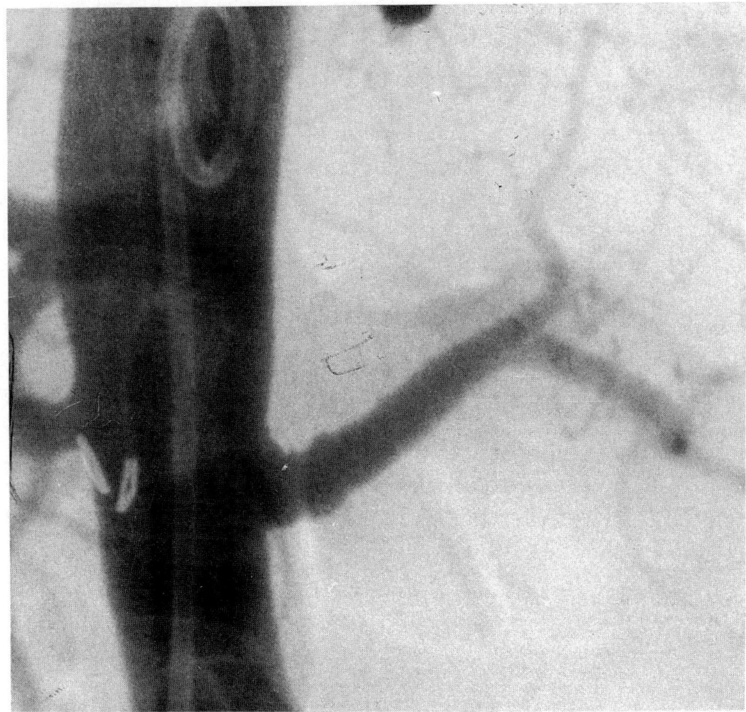

Fig. 2B. Atherosclerotic renal artery stenosis treated with thrombendarterectomy and patch: 4 years after surgery.

PTRA

It is quite clear that PTRA in atherosclerotic renovascular disease has a much higher failure rate than surgery, both initially and late.[1,3,4,20,21] It is also clear that PTRA in this patient group is much less successful than in some types of fibrous dysplasia.[1–3,8] It is, however, disturbing that both initial and late results reported from different centres are extremely variable. This is true also for experienced and well established centres. Sos *et al.*[1] report an initial technical success rate of 57% in unilateral atheromatous stenosis, but only 10% in bilateral stenosis. Baert *et al.*[3] report an initial success rate of 95% in unilateral atheromatosis and 76% in bilateral. In several reports a distinction is made between isthmus (ostial) and juxta-aortic (postostial) types of stenosis. The former has been reported to give less satisfactory results,[5,14] but this has not been confirmed by others.[3,4] Complete occlusions, or very narrow stenoses, are also difficult to dilate, and the technical success rate is low.[2,4,16] With regard to the results of PTRA in the treatment of renovascular uraemia we know very little about the rate of success, since most of the reported data are anecdotal.

Regarding the long-term results there are few hard data in the literature, and usually limited to the blood pressure response. Since the majority of the patients are in the groups of 'improvement', or 'failures', a restenosis may pass unnoticed unless objective studies on vascular anatomy and/or renal blood flow have been performed. In the vast majority of the published series, such studies have not been reported and very little is therefore known about long-term technical success. When only 'documented restenoses'[2] are counted, it is not surprising that they appear to be few. In most series the figure is between 10 and 30%,[2,21,22] but varies between 0 and 100% after 1–2 years.[3,4,19] Our restenosis frequency in carefully followed patients is around 40%, and equal in stenoses of isthmus and juxta-aortal type.[4] The restenoses practically always appear during the first 12 months after the initial PTRA, and a new PTRA is often successful. If this is not the case, reconstructive surgery can be performed. We have therefore come to the conclusion that PTRA can be recommended as the initial treatment of most patients with atherosclerotic renal artery stenosis, provided that the follow-up is intensive, particularly during the first year, and indications for re-intervention liberal. PTRA should, however, not be used in the treatment of very narrow or occluded arteries, in patients with a severely impaired renal function, severe atherosclerosis in the aorta or iliac arteries, or when the atherosclerotic stenosis is localized close to a branch. With this policy, close to 25% of the originally PTRA-treated patients need a re-PTRA, and 20% need surgery,

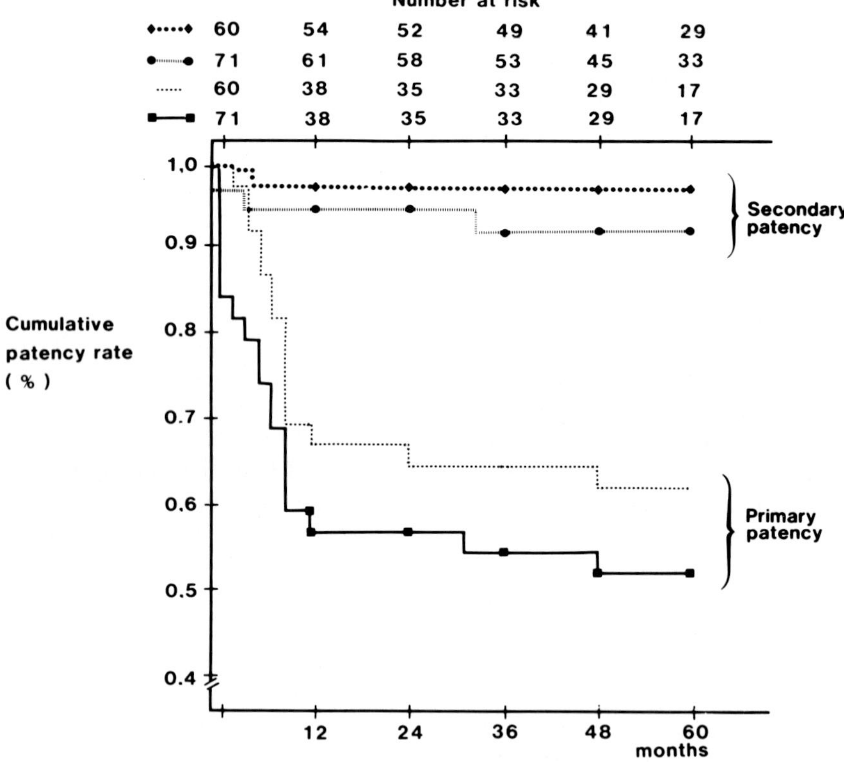

Fig. 3. Primary and secondary patency after PTRA of atherosclerotic RAS during a 5-year follow-up period. Data are given with initial technical failures excluded ($n = 60$) and included ($n = 71$). The different procedures performed to achieve the secondary patency are reported in Fig. 4.

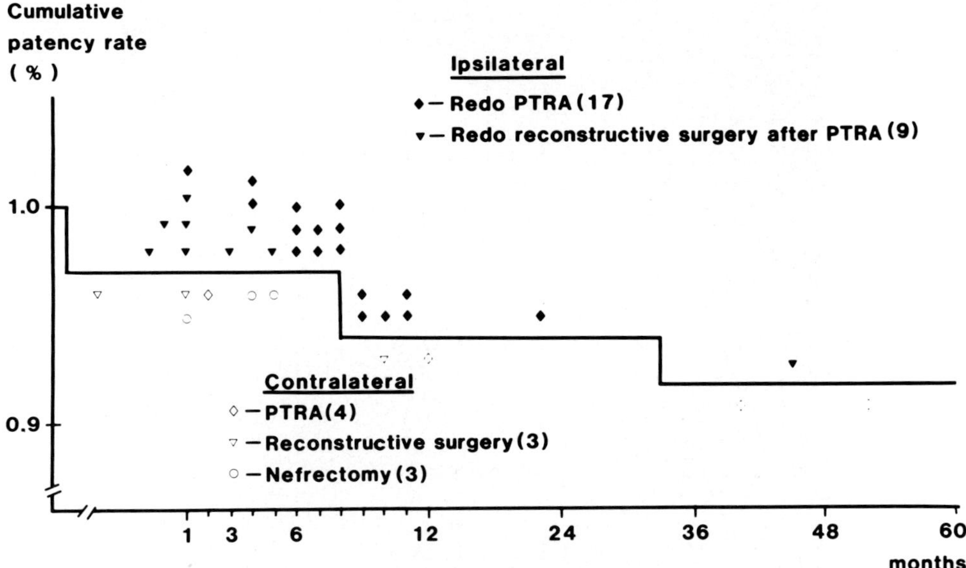

Fig. 4. The same patient series as in Fig. 3: 17 redo PTRAs and nine interventions with reconstructive surgery were performed to achieve the 93% 5-year patency after the initial PTRA. Note that almost all re-interventions were made during the first 12 months. It can also be seen that not less than ten interventions were required on the contralateral kidney to achieve a satisfactory blood pressure control.

but in the remaining patients one single PTRA treatment will be sufficient.[4] Figure 3 depicts cumulative patency rates during 5 years without (primary patency) and with (secondary patency) re-interventions. Patency is defined as patent without significant stenosis. In Fig. 4 is shown the types of re-interventions that have been applied.

In summary, PTRA in atherosclerotic RAS is in most series accompanied by a relatively high initial failure rate, and a high rate of restenoses, particularly during the first year. It can still be used as the initial treatment in most cases, but only if surgical expertise is available, the patients are followed intensively, and re-intervention with new PTRA or reconstructive surgery is used aggressively. When reconstructive surgery is necessary, a TEA with a patch gives satisfactory long-term results.

STENOSIS DUE TO FIBROUS DYSPLASIA

Patient characteristics

These patients are between 16 and 60 years old, and about 85% are females. The most common type of renal artery fibrous dysplasia (or fibromuscular dysplasia) is medial fibroplasia, which dominates among young and middle-aged women.[3,23] A relatively long segment of the mid- and distal renal artery is usually diseased, and the alternating stenoses and micro-aneurysms give the classical 'string of beads'

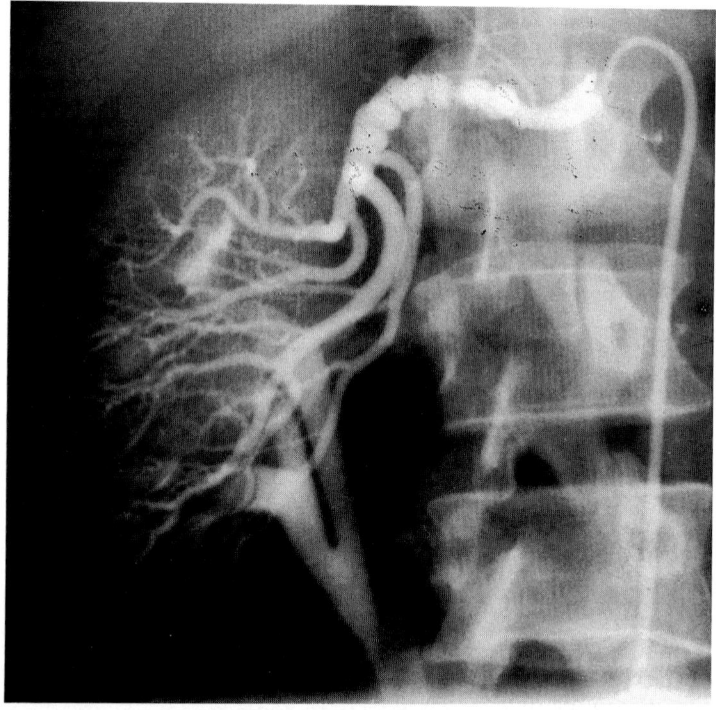

Fig. 5A. A typical case of medial fibroplasia in the right renal artery of a young female patient: before PTRA.

appearance on the arteriogram. Other less common types of fibrous dysplasia are intimal fibroplasia, characterized by accumulation of fibrous tissue within the internal elastic membrane, and subadventitial fibroplasia characterized by severe fibroplasia between the adventitia and media.[23] These lesions sometimes appear in children, and probably have a different pathogenesis than medial fibroplasia.

Reconstructive surgery

Reconstructive surgery for fibrous dysplastic lesions has been reported extensively, but again only few series document a long-term follow-up. Since these patients have a long expected survival, requirements for durable reconstructions must be high. Synthetic material should therefore be avoided if possible. Resection and direct anastomosis is rarely possible, particularly when long segments of the artery are diseased. The use of saphenous vein as a graft for renal artery reconstruction has been discussed extensively.[24,25] It is now well known that such grafts dilate, probably due to the high flow in the renal artery, but also that aneurysm formation is rare in adults as opposed to children.[26] The only case of an aneurysmatic dilatation we have seen was caused by a stenosis proximal to the graft at its anastomosis to aorta.[16] Therefore, the use of a saphenous vein for reconstruction is an acceptable alternative in adults. The use of autologous artery, mainly the

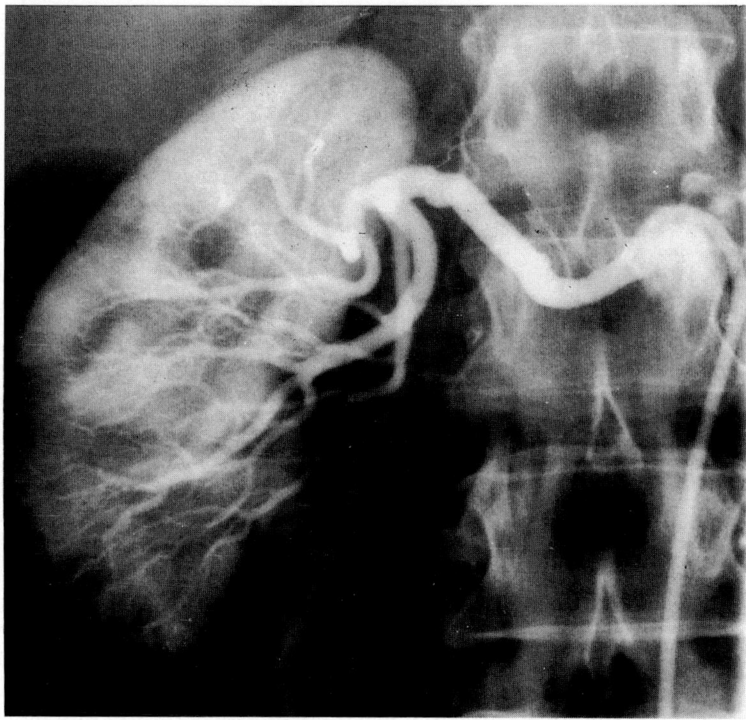

Fig. 5B. A typical case of medial fibroplasia in the right renal artery of a young female patient: 6 years after PTRA.

hypogastric artery, is now an established technique, with an excellent long-term patency documented.[27]

Extracorporeal surgical reconstruction with autotransplantation of the kidney may be required in a few cases, mainly where the lesion is located in the branches of the renal artery. Satisfactory long-term results have been documented.[28]

PTRA

Only the medial fibroplasia seems to be possible to dilate with acceptable initial technical results. A well-known complication to PTRA in these cases is perforation of the renal artery, where it is very thin and micro-aneurysms have been formed.[29] Larger series with long-term results of PTRA treatment in this particular group of patients are few, but the results appear to be satisfactory.[1,2,6] A typical case of medial fibroplasia, with late result after PTRA, is seen in Figs 5A and B.

The other types of fibrous dysplasia, i.e. intimal fibroplasia and subadventitial fibroplasia, are usually difficult or impossible to dilate. Although the results may be successful initially, the recurrence rate is very high in the few reported cases.[23]

In summary, PTRA can be recommended as the initial standard treatment in medial fibroplasia. Reconstructive surgery is necessary in other types of fibrous dysplasia, and in situations where PTRA of medial fibroplasia is unsuccessful. For reconstructive surgery the use of autologous material can be recommended. It cannot be considered proved that autologous artery is superior to saphenous vein in adults.

RENOVASCULAR HYPERTENSION IN CHILDREN

Patient characteristics

Hypertension is uncommon in children. However, more than half of all children less than 10 years of age with hypertension have a renovascular cause for their disease.[30] The pathology is very heterogeneous, and often not well defined. The midaortic syndrome (co-arctation of the abdominal aorta), neurofibromatosis, intimal fibroplasia and subadventitial fibroplasia are the most common types. Medial hyperplasia with micro-aneurysm formation, resulting in a 'string of beads' formation on the arteriogram, is not seen in children.[23,31]

Reconstructive surgery

Reconstructive surgery has been reported in a number of cases, but long-term results are largely unknown. In the midaortic syndrome the aorta must be reconstructed, which makes the use of synthetic graft necessary in most cases.[32] The critical lesion in this syndrome is, however, in the vast majority of cases a stenosis at the origin of the renal arteries, requiring implantation of the renal arteries in the reconstructed aorta, sometimes with the use of a graft. In all other situations requiring reconstruction of the renal artery in children, only autologous material should be used. It is now well established that the saphenous vein should be avoided in the paediatric age group, probably due to an unsatisfactory maturity of the vessel wall and therefore a tendency for the graft to dilate.[33] The use of tubular Dacron mesh to externally support the vein graft has been recommended, but no long-term results are available.[34] The best documented long-term results have been reported with the use of autologous artery, either hypogastric artery or, if necessary, external iliac artery.[27,35] In the latter case a reconstruction of the iliac artery with a synthetic graft is necessary. No early or late harmful effects have been reported from sacrificing one or both hypogastric arteries or from replacing external iliac artery with a synthetic graft.

Renal autotransplantation has been used in difficult cases of renovascular hypertension in children but without documentation of long-term results.[36]

PTRA

Initially successful PTRA in children has been described in a few cases.[37,39] A number of unsuccessful attempts are also known, particularly in complex lesions, associated with neurofibromatosis, aortic anomalies, stenosis located to the renal artery ostium, and in intimal or subadventitial hyperplasia. Complications requiring emergency surgery are not uncommon.[38]

Late results are remarkably few and disappointing. Simunic *et al.*[39] reported in 1990 on four patients treated between 1982 and 1984. Two were lost to follow-up, the other two had recurrency. The authors' conclusion is that PTRA can give a temporary effect on the hypertension and therefore make it possible to postpone surgical correction until a suitable age is reached.

In summary, PTRA of RAS has at the best only a temporary effect in the paediatric age group, and the risk for complications is high. Knowledge of the long-term results of reconstructive surgery is still limited. Synthetic material is usually necessary for aortic reconstruction in the midaortic syndrome. In all other situations, synthetic material, as well as saphenous vein grafts, should be avoided. Autologous artery is probably the graft material of choice in these patients, and is the only material for which reasonably long-term results have been documented.

CONCLUSIONS

Patients with renovascular hypertension and/or uraemia from RAS represent a heterogeneous group of different ages, with a number of different types of pathology and different indications for intervention. For active treatment with reconstructive surgery or PTRA there is no standard procedure which can be recommended for all patient categories. Although short-term results are relatively well known, the results of long-term follow-up are largely unknown, particularly in the paediatric age-group. Long-term studies should include documentation of the anatomy of the renal arteries, or perfusion of the renal parenchyma, careful recording of blood pressure under standardized conditions and, in selected cases, also data on kidney function.

REFERENCES

1. Sos TA, Pickering TG, Sniderman K *et al*: Percutaneous transluminal renal angioplasty in renovascular hypertension due to atheroma or fibromuscular dysplasia. N Engl J Med 309: 274–279, 1983
2. Klinge J, Mali WPTM, Puijlaert CBJAJ *et al*: Percutaneous transluminal renal angioplasty: Initial and long-term results. Radiology 171: 501–506, 1989
3. Baert AL, Wilms G, Amery A *et al*: Percutaneous transluminal renal angioplasty: initial results and long-term follow-up in 202 patients. Cardiovasc Intervent Radiol 13: 22–28, 1990
4. Weibull H, Bergqvist D, Jonsson K *et al*: Long-term results after percutaneous transluminal angioplasty of atherosclerotic renal artery stenosis: The importance of intensive follow-up. Eur J Vasc Surg (in press).
5. Eidt JF, Fry RE, Clagett GP *et al*: Postoperative follow-up of renal artery reconstruction with duplex ultrasound. J Vasc Surg 8: 667–673, 1988
6. Schwarten DE: Percutaneous transluminal angioplasty of the renal arteries: intravenous digital subtraction angiography for follow-up. Radiology 150: 369–373, 1984
7. Maxwell MH, Bleifer KH, Franklin SS, Varady PD: Cooperative study of renovascular hypertension: demographic analysis of the study. J Am Med Assoc 220: 1195–1204, 1972
8. Brawn LA, Ramsay LE: Is 'improvement' real with percutaneous transluminal angioplasty in the management of renovascular hypertension? Lancet ii: 1313–1316, 1987
9. Whitehouse WM, Kazmers A, Zelenock GB *et al*: Chronic total renal artery occlusion: Effects of treatment on secondary hypertension and renal function. Surgery 89: 753–763, 1981.

10. Bergentz S-E, Berqvist D, Weibull H: Changing concepts in renovascular surgery. Leading article. Br J Surg 76: 429–430, 1989
11. Bergentz S-E, Kjellbo H, Hood B: Renal artery stenosis. Prog Surg 9: 1, 1971
12. Wollenweber J, Sheps SG, Davis GD. Clinical course of atherosclerotic renovascular disease. Am J Cardiol 21: 60, 1968
13. Ernst CB, Stanley JC, Marshall FF, Fry WJ. Renal revascularization for arteriosclerotic renovascular hypertension: Prognostic implications of focal renal arterial vs overt generalized arteriosclerosis. Surgery 73: 859–867, 1973
14. Cicuto KP, McLean GK, Oleaga JA *et al*: Renal arrtery stenosis: anatomic classification for percutaneous transluminal angioplasty. Am J Roent 137: 599–601, 1981
15. Andersson I, Bergentz S-E, Dymling JF, Ericsson BF, Hansson B-G: Bilateral renal artery stenosis/occlusion and renovascular hypertension. Correlation of angiographic findings with blood pressure response after surgery. Acta Chir Scand 145: 535–543, 1979
16. Bergentz S-E, Bergqvist D, Weibull H: Optimal reconstruction of the renal arteries. Acta Chir Scand (Suppl) 555: 227–235, 1990
17. Moncure AC, Brewster DC, Darling RC *et al*: Use of the splenic and hepatic arteries for renal revascularization. J Vasc Surg 3: 196–203, 1986
18. Moncure AC, Brewster DC, Darling RC, Abbott WM, Cambria RP: Use of the gastroduodenal artery in right renal artery revascularization. J Vasc Surg 8: 154–159, 1988
19. Weibull H, Bergqvist D, Jendteg S *et al*: Clinical outcome and health care costs in renal revascularization—percutaneous transluminal renal angioplasty versus reconstructive surgery. Br J Surg (in press)
20. Grim CE, Luft FC, Yune HY *et al*: Percutaneous transluminal dilatation in the treatment of renal vascular hypertension. Ann Intern Med 95: 439–442, 1981
21. Beebe HG, Chesebro K, Merchant F, Bush W: Results of renal artery balloon angioplasty limit its indications. J Vasc Surg 8: 300–306, 1988
22. Geyskes GG, Puylaert CBAJ, Oei HY, Dorhout Mees EJ: Follow up study of 70 patients with renal artery stenosis treated by percutaneous transluminal dilatation. Br Med J 287: 333–336, 1983
23. Wise KL, McCann RL, Dunnick NR, Paulson DF: Renovascular hypertension. J Urol 140: 911–924, 1988
24. Stanley JC, Ernst CB, Fry WJ: Fate of 100 aortorenal vein grafts: characteristics of late graft expansion, aneurysmal dilatation, and stenosis. Surgery 74: 931–944, 1973
25. Dean RH, Wilson JP, Burko H, Foster JH: Saphenous vein aortorenal bypass grafts: serial arteriographic study. Ann Surg 180: 469–477, 1974
26. Stanley JC, Whitehouse WM, Graham LM *et al*: Operative therapy of renovascular hypertension. Br J Surg (Suppl) 69: 63–66, 1982
27. Stoney RJ, De Luccia N, Ehrenfeld WK, Wylie EJ: Aortorenal arterial autografts. Long-term assessment. Arch Surg 116: 1416–1422, 1981
28. van Bockel JH, van Schilfgaarde R, Felthuis W *et al*: Long-term results of *in situ* and extracorporeal surgery for renovascular hypertension caused by fibrodysplasia. J Vasc Surg 6: 355–364, 1987
29. Weibull H, Bergqvist D, Jonsson K, Carlsson S, Takolander R: Analyses of complications after percutaneous transluminal angioplasty of renal artery stenosis. Eur J Vasc Surg 1: 77–84, 1987
30. Lawson JD, Boerth R, Foster JH, Dean RH: Diagnosis and management of renovascular hypertension in children. Arch Surg 112: 1307–1316, 1977
31. Benjamin SP, McCormack LJ, Dustan HP *et al*: Stenosing renal artery disease in children. Clinicopathologic correlation in 20 surgically treated cases. Cleveland Clin Quart 43: 197–206, 1976
32. Bergentz S-E, Bergqvist D, Ericsson BF, Esquivel CO: Coarctation of the abdominal aorta associated with renal hypertension. Vasa 12: 133–138, 1983
33. Stanley JC, Fry WJ: Pediatric renal artery occlusive disease and renovascular hypertension. Etiology, diagnosis and operative treatment. Arch Surg 116: 669–676, 1981

34. Berkowitz HD, O'Neill Jr JA: Renovascular hypertension in children. Surgical repair with special reference to the use of reinforced vein grafts. J Vasc Surg 9: 46–55, 1989
35. Stoney RJ, Cooke PA, String ST: Surgical treatment of renovascular hypertension in children. J Pediatr Surg 10: 631–639, 1975
36. Jordan ML, Novick AC, Cunningham RL: The role of renal autotransplantation in pediatric and young adult patients with renal artery disease. J Vasc Surg 2: 385–392, 1985
37. McCook TA, Mills SR, Kirks DR *et al*: Percutaneous transluminal renal artery angioplasty in a 3½-year-old hypertensive girl. J Pediatr 97: 958–960, 1980
38. Guzzetta PC, Potter BM, Kapur S, Ruley EJ, Randolph J: Reconstruction of the renal artery after unsuccessful percutaneous transluminal angioplasty in children. Am J Surg 145: 647–651, 1983
39. Simunic S, Winter-Fuduric I, Radanovic B *et al*: Percutaneous transluminal renal angioplasty (PTRA) as a method of therapy for renovascular hypertension in children. Eur J Radiol 10: 143–146, 1990.

ASSOCIATED PROCEDURES AFFECTING LONG-TERM RESULTS

Can Preoperative Assessments Influence Long-term Patency of Intra-Inguinal Bypass Grafts?

Martin G. Veller, Charles M. Fisher and Andrew N. Nicolaides

Graft patency is dependent on the inflow, the type, length and flow characteristics of a graft and the run-off. In addition factors that affect clotting, rheology, the progression of atherosclerosis and the development of intimal hyperplasia will influence long-term results.

The noninvasive vascular laboratory provides important predictive information to the clinician about the potential benefit and likely long-term result of a bypass graft. This knowledge, if it is correct and suitably acted upon, can be expected to result in prolonged graft patency and therefore improved limb survival rates. It is in the treatment of occlusive disease of the superficial femoral artery in which the predictive facilities of the noninvasive vascular laboratory are of most benefit to those vascular surgeons managing patients with limb threatening ischaemia.

The aim of this chapter is to review those factors, mentioned here, that can be assessed preoperatively. This will include first, a summary of the methods currently used to assess the arterial inflow and outflow of infra-inguinal bypass grafts and secondly, a survey of haematological and biochemical factors which should be assayed preoperatively and which are known to affect the eventual outcome.

EVALUATION OF AORTO-ILIAC INFLOW

Introduction

The majority of patients with superficial femoral artery occlusion also have atherosclerotic lesions in the aorto-iliac segment, and are therefore often at risk of also having haemodynamically significant stenoses in this region. This association results in a significant incidence of infra-inguinal bypass graft occlusion.[1]

In the presence of haemodynamically significant atherosclerotic disease in both the aorto-iliac and superficial femoral arteries, only one lesion requires bypass grafting and it is uncommon that both segments will need to be addressed. A proximal procedure is usually enough to improve claudication or to relieve rest pain and only when this does not realize the desired effect, is a more distal bypass undertaken. However, this is not always the best approach and an evaluation of the individual contribution of the disease in each segment is required before choosing the appropriate operation.

More commonly, angiographic lesions of the aorto-iliac segment are underestimated, and haemodynamically significant stenoses may even go unrecognized. This is highlighted by Gupta and his colleagues[2] who report that 10% of patients undergoing femorofemoral or femoropopliteal bypass grafting have significant aorto-iliac pressure gradients that are only recognized at the end of the operation despite the use of extensive pre- and intra-operative investigations.

The diagnosis of aorto-iliac inflow disease is made by either imaging the diseased segments, or by observing changes in blood flow or pressure produced by the stenoses. The haemodynamic changes can be summarized into the following steps:

1. *Increased flow velocity through the stenosis which is in proportion to the reduction of the cross-sectional area*: According to Bernoulli's theorem, an increase in velocity (kinetic energy) reduces the lateral pressure (potential energy). This is specified by:

$$V_1 * \text{cross-sectional area}_1 = V_2 * \text{cross-sectional area}_2$$

2. *Energy loss distal to the stenosis due to turbulence and a subsequent reduction in pressure:* If this stenosis were in an ideal system, in which there is laminar flow, there would be complete transfer of kinetic to potential energy after the stenosis. An artery with atherosclerosis, is, however, not an ideal system, and a narrowing causes disturbed (turbulent) flow distal to the stenosis. Energy loss resulting from turbulence is not regained, and this together with losses due to viscous drag and fluid inertia through the stenosis cause changes in the pressure and velocity waveform well before there is reduced peripheral perfusion.[3] The maintenance of distal peripheral perfusion is temporarily achieved by a reduction in peripheral resistance which raises the pressure gradient across the stenosis.
3. *The haemodynamic effect*: As the artery continues to narrow, there comes a point when the energy loss from turbulence is sufficient to cause a fall not only in pressure but also of flow in the distal vessels because at this stage the peripheral vascular bed is maximally vasodilated and the peripheral resistance cannot be reduced any further. The decrease in flow is proportional to the degree of the stenosis,[4] the length of the stenosis,[5] and the number of stenoses.[6]

The changes described above can be accentuated by increasing the flow across a stenosis. Exercise, the intra-arterial injection of a vasodilator such as papaverine, or artificially induced ischaemia all cause vasodilation of the peripheral vascular bed and therefore stress the proximal inflow system. This effect can be combined with one of a number of tests,[7] such as intra-arterial pressure measurements.

Clinical assessment

A careful clinical assessment is a prerequisite to the successful investigation of a patient, particularly in resolving whether treatment is indicated for the presenting problem. In addition some of the problems mentioned previously can be resolved to some degree. For example, a very weak or absent pulse is clearly indicative of aorto-iliac disease. On the other hand, determining whether a normal or slightly reduced pulse is indicative of a haemodynamically significant stenosis, even in the presence of a bruit is not accurate. The ability of a number of clinicians to agree whether a pulse is normal or reduced in amplitude has been shown to be poor, and the interobserver agreement is not better than that expected from chance.[8] Other causes for errors are the stronger pulse felt in the presence of a distal occlusion, and a weaker pulse felt when there is a reduced cardiac output or when the subject is obese. Therefore, it is prudent to investigate the aorto-iliac inflow using noninvasive techniques.

Doppler ultrasound

Noninvasive vascular investigations use Doppler ultrasound extensively to study the changes in blood flow characteristics associated with atherosclerotic abnormalities proximal to the common femoral artery. The methods commonly used are segmental blood pressure measurements, analysis of Doppler velocity wave form changes, and duplex scanning.

Segmental pressure measurements

This technique was initially described by Yao and his colleagues.[9] Sphygmomanometer cuffs are placed over the thigh, calf, ankle or toe. Doppler ultrasound is then used to detect the pulse velocity in any vessel distal to the cuff. These systolic pressures are lower than the brachial systolic pressure if there is a haemodynamically significant stenotic lesion proximal to the cuff. It has been suggested that in the absence of associated superficial femoral artery occlusion, the ratio of thigh systolic blood pressure to the systolic brachial blood pressure is a measure of the severity of aorto-iliac disease.[10–12] However, Sumner and Strandness[13] found that there was no significant difference between the preoperative thigh pressure index in patients with successful compared with failed aorto-iliac grafts even in the presence of a patent superficial femoral artery. In addition further attempts to improve the accuracy of this test, by for example using a wide thigh cuff, have not been effective.[14] By performing experiments comparing these indirectly measured pressures with pressures measured intra-arterially it has been demonstrated that this is a good screening test with low false negative but many false positive values.[15] Therefore segmental pressures can exclude significant proximal disease if the results are normal but are of little value in patients with multisegment disease and are not really helpful in predicting graft outcome.

Doppler velocity waveform changes

Evaluation of the Doppler velocity waveform derived from the common femoral artery using directional Doppler can give information concerning the presence, site and severity of the arterial disease.[16] The normal triphasic waveform has a sharp upstroke (acceleration) followed by a downstroke (deceleration), reversal of flow, and finally a third small component representing forward flow. In regions distal to a stenosis, a damped monophasic velocity waveform occurs and these changes occur before blood flow to the limb is reduced.[17] In diagnosing proximal stenoses many vascular surgeons use pattern recognition, yet analysis of several aspects of the velocity profile can numerically estimate the severity of proximal stenosis. At present the most commonly used methods are:

The pulsitility index (PI). This is a ratio which is independent of the angle of insonation. It is defined as:

PI = Peak to peak velocity/mean velocity through the pulse cycle.[18,19]

Normally the PI increases from central to peripheral arteries. It is reduced in the presence of a proximal stenosis, but also if the patient is warm and vasodilated. In the clinical setting there are some laboratories that use the PI as a method of detecting stenosis of 50% or greater and report that it is better than other indices in evaluating such proximal stenoses.[12,20,21] However, others have found that the PI does not become abnormal until the stenosis is sufficient to cause a clinically obvious reduction in peripheral perfusion, and that the PI on its own is not sufficiently discriminating to make clinical decisions in borderline lesions ranging from 30 to 70% diameter stenosis.[22–24]

Laplace transform. The Laplace transform method of characterizing velocity waveforms was developed by Skidmore and Woodcock.[25–27] By using a third order Laplace transform polynomial the Doppler velocity waveform at the common femoral artery could be fitted to a formula that was related amongst others to a proximal damping factor (δ), arterial wall stiffness (ω), and inversely related to the peripheral vascular resistance (γ). The evidence presented by these authors showed that the damping factor correlates well to proximal arterial narrowing. Using $\delta = 0.6$ as the cut-off for the damping factor, 50% or greater diameter stenoses could be separated from lesser lesions with a 95% accuracy (sensitivity 100%, specificity 93%) even in the presence of superficial femoral artery occlusion. The problem with this method in the past has been the need of a special computer program that had not been readily available so that the above results could not be easily reproduced by others.[21] Several groups have used this technique in patients with concomitant aorto-iliac and superficial femoral artery occlusive disease and have been able to accurately distinguish significant stenosis greater than 50%.[20,24,28,29] The problem related to the complex computer assisted calculation has now been solved with commercially available equipment that can do this analysis simply and automatically.

Velocity waveform shape. Nicolaides and his colleagues[30] studied several parameters of the velocity waveform of the common femoral artery in patients with angiographically proven aorto-iliac disease. Using multivariate analysis, an equation was developed using peak velocity, initial acceleration time from the onset of the upstroke, disturbance of the peak velocity after exercise, and a modification of the PI. This was a sensitive screening method of determining 10% or greater diameter stenosis and preventing patients with normal or near normal aorto-iliac segments from unnecessarily being subjected to arteriography. Many clinicians however, find that visual interpretation of the velocity waveform gives just as good discrimination as these more complex indices.[31]

Mean power frequency index. Sawchuck and his colleagues[32] have developed a technique to quantify the frequency transfer function between duplex Doppler ultrasound derived velocity waveform patterns of the aorta and the common femoral artery. Using this technique they have been able to separate patients with normal arteries, from those with subcritical and critical stenosis with an accuracy similar to intra-arterial pressure measurements (accuracy of 92–100% depending on the degree of stenosis). This is the first report of this technique, but the study did not include patients with multisegment disease. It therefore remains to be seen whether this technique will be of clinical use in the latter group of patients.

Duplex scanning

Duplex scanning can be used to both visualize the aorto-iliac segment (B-mode ultrasound) and assess the blood flow characteristics through the region of disease (Doppler ultrasound). The benefits are that the morphological characteristics of the lesion can be appraised, and that the velocity and turbulence of blood flow in the region of, and just distal to the stenosis can be evaluated.[33] This information has been condensed into a method of grading[34,35] by categorizing the degree of spectral broadening of the velocity waveform, and combining this with the peak systolic frequency (or velocity if the angle of insonation can be determined). Using this method the accuracy of duplex scanning in identifying aorto-iliac disease is similar to that of angiography. In lesions with 50% diameter stenosis or more on angiography, duplex scanning has a sensitivity of 82% and a specificity of 92%. Further methods of more accurately evaluating the degree of stenosis have been described by relating peak systolic flow velocity to flow just proximal to the stenosis.[36] These techniques may in the future be enhanced by applying the Bernoulli principle to calculate the pressure gradient across the stenosis.[37] Cardiologists are now using a simplified formula to calculate the pressure gradient across a stenotic valve:

$$P = 4V^2$$

(where P represent the pressure gradient, and V the maximum velocity of the jet passing through the stenosed valve).

Duplex scanning is a most effective method to investigate the aorto-iliac segment but does have some drawbacks which include the expertise required by the operator, the relatively long scanning time, and the limitations in visualizing the aorto-iliac vessels due to obesity or overlying bowel gas.

Isotope clearance studies

Nicolaides and Angelides[38] used the simultaneous clearance of a radio-isotope (^{99m}Tc) from the thigh and calf at rest during and after exercise. By evaluating the isotope clearance curves they were able to calculate the muscle blood flow in both the thigh and calf and grade both proximal and distal disease with an accuracy at least as good as two plane angiography. This test, although accurate, is complicated to perform, is invasive and has now been superseded by duplex scanning.

Angiography and pressure gradients

Under ideal circumstances biplane angiography can provide an unrivalled view of arterial occlusive disease and is the definitive investigation in patients being considered for vascular reconstruction. Prior noninvasive investigations are of benefit because firstly they can help anticipate the likely angiographic appearances and secondly, because they can supplement the anatomical details provided by the angiogram with functional information.

Monoplanar angiography is unreliable. Slot and his colleagues[39] found that interobserver agreement in regard to the degree of narrowing in the aorto-iliac segment was little better than that expected from chance, although occlusions were well recognized by all participants. The benefits of biplanar angiography are, first that the latter provides separation of overlapped and unfolded tortuous vessels, second that it improves vessel image quality by realignment away from an unsuitable background and third the profile of atheroma is outlined more accurately (atherosclerosis has a predisposition for posterior walls in the proximal limb vessels which therefore makes it better shown in oblique and lateral views).

Measuring pull-through arterial pressures during angiography in diseased vessels maximizes the benefits of the investigation. In addition, the intra-arterial injection of papaverine will produce vasodilatation and increase the pressure gradient across a stenosis simulating the effect of exercise.[7] The criteria usually used to diagnose a 50% or greater diameter occlusion are a pressure gradient across the stenosis of 10 mmHg or more at rest and 20 mmHg or more after the injection of papaverine. The value of these investigations is highlighted by Breslau and his colleagues[40] who recommend that this procedure is performed in all patients.

Conclusions

Both invasive and noninvasive techniques are accurate in evaluating arterial occlusive disease when the disease involves only one segment. However, in the presence of multisegment disease these tests are less reliable. As previously mentioned, this is reflected in the experience of Gupta *et al.*[2] who at the end of the operation found a 15 mmHg or greater gradient between the central systolic blood pressure and that measured in the common femoral artery in 16 of 87 patients undergoing femorofemoral bypass and 43 of 510 patients undergoing infra-inguinal bypass grafting. This occurred despite extensive preoperative evaluation of the aorto-iliac segment as well as the use of early intra-operative pressure measurements and the augmentation of flow with papaverine. This eventuality should always be borne in mind and every patient should be adequately prepared for possible balloon angioplasty or bypass surgery of the iliac arteries, when being subjected to an infra-inguinal graft.

EVALUATION OF RUN-OFF

The evaluation of the distal outflow bed in bypass surgery to arteries in the calf, foot or ankle is difficult and remains the most elusive of goals, in the quest for improved graft patency rates. Although many questions regarding the run-off in patients undergoing femoropopliteal or femorocrural bypass grafting, are still unanswered, there is general agreement that in the presence of a high peripheral resistance (that is poor run-off determined intra-operatively), grafts have been shown to have a high incidence of early occlusion.[41–43] It is now possible to measure peripheral resistance preoperatively by measuring flow (for example by using air pletysmography) and pressure, but it has not been applied in the prediction of infra-inguinal bypass graft outcome.

Follow-up studies have indicated that the following criteria, determined by angiography, influence long-term patency:

1. The number of patent vessels (i.e. anterior tibial, posterior tibial or peroneal arteries) in the distal run-off. This is directly related to the peripheral resistance.[41]
2. The presence of patent arch vessels. The physiological importance of this vascular configuration is its value as a low resistance outflow bed between the anterior and posterior tibial vessels.[44]
3. The isolated popliteal segment. The vascular resistance provided by the isolated popliteal segment is comparable to the outflow of a single calf artery, but has a much higher resistance than a popliteal artery with patent run-off.[45] This is reflected in the successful bypass to an isolated segment in many patients, but the patency and salvage rates are inferior when compared to bypass to crural vessels.[46]

Doppler ultrasound

A number of techniques have been described using Doppler ultrasound in the evaluation of patent vessels in the distal vascular bed.

Examination by Doppler ultrasound

Roederscheimer and his colleagues[47] have shown that by using Doppler ultrasound in its simplest form they could establish whether there is arterial blood flow in the peroneal or tibial arteries, and the perforating branches of the plantar arch with a good correlation to angiography (r=0.96). Other groups have confirmed these results.[48]

Some authors state that the patency of the distal popliteal artery and its major branches can be easily evaluated using duplex scanning.[49] However, the evaluation of the vessels distal to the popliteal artery appears to be more difficult, and no evidence is presently available to indicate that the use of colour duplex imaging will make this investigation any easier.

Ankle brachial pressure index (ABI)

Dean and his colleagues[50] found that 91% of the femoropopliteal grafts in patients with an ABI of less than 0.2 had early graft thrombosis and that a low ABI correlated with low postoperative graft flow rates. They suggested that bypass in such patients was futile. Samson and his colleagues[51] also found that the early and late patency rates after femoropopliteal bypass grafts were related to the preoperative ankle pressure indices. If the index was less than 0.2 there was approximately twice the risk of both early and late failure, although the patency rate was still 39% at 2 years. Further support was reported by O'Donnell and his colleagues.[52] They found that polytetrafluoroethylene (PTFE) grafts that failed within 6 months had a significantly lower preoperative ankle pressure index than those which remained patent.

A low distal pressure and ABI is the result of a high resistance proximal to the ankle and therefore this index is linked to the severity of the atherosclerotic disease. Using the same principles, the pressure gradient from the knee to the ankle has been suggested as an index of distal resistance[15] yet this method has not been widely applied.

Pulse generated run-off (PGR)

Quantification of Doppler ultrasound waveforms of the circulation distal to an occlusion is inappropriate as these tracings are severely damped; PGR overcomes this problem by generating a new pulse wave by rapidly inflating a sphygmomanometer cuff placed over the upper calf. The resultant waveform can then be quantified using the pulsatility index or Laplace transform analysis. Scott and his colleagues[53] analysed the PGR by assigning a score for good, bad, or intermediate waveforms and called this the PGR score. In 35 limbs they compared this preoperative score to resistance measured intra-operatively by the infusion of blood at a constant pressure, and found a moderate correlation (Spearman ranks $rs = -0.39$; $p < 0.02$). If the status of the pedal arch was added to the score, then the correlation was even better ($rs = -0.44$; $p < 0.01$). This exciting new technique will require further validation in relation to long-term graft patency.

Arteriography

The pattern of lower limb arterial occlusion seen in advanced atherosclerosis was described in detail by Dible.[54] Performing angiography on 140 legs amputated for ischaemia he found that the majority had occlusions of the main below knee arteries (88% anterior tibial arteries, 83% posterior tibial arteries) but that peroneal artery occlusion was less common (59%). However, further distally the small arteries remained patent (medial plantar arteries 82%, digital arteries 92%). This has emphasized the fact that the ischaemic process in the foot is due to proximal inflow disease.

Many methods to enhance the visualization of these distal vessels by using delayed exposures, reactive hyperaemia, contralateral limb occlusion, and others[55] have been described with apparently good results. However, many surgeons have found that preoperative angiography does not visualize the distal vascular anatomy sufficiently to enable them to proceed to primary ablation without first performing a bypass graft.[56] The use of intra-arterial digital subtraction arteriography has been suggested to improve the rate of distal vessel visualization.[57]

Most authors now suggest that the best quality angiograms are performed peroperatively with clamping of the artery proximal to the site of injection, which may be at any level of the limb.[58] The features that are found to be important in evaluating the run-off (and therefore the peripheral resistance) on angiograms (performed prior or during operation) have already been discussed.

Conclusion

In general, the available preoperative tests underestimate the quality of the distal run-off (especially when arterial perfusion pressures are very low) and limbs should therefore not be dismissed as inoperable on the basis of preoperative investigations alone. This observation is best reflected in the results of St Mary's hospital[59] were an aggressive policy of infra-inguinal bypass grafting for critical ischaemia, has resulted in only 3% of patients undergoing primary amputation and that only 15% had a subsequent major limb amputation in up to 34 months of follow-up.

DETECTION OF ADVERSE BIOCHEMICAL AND HAEMATOLOGICAL STATES

In recent years, causes of graft failure other than technical considerations and progression of atherosclerotic lesions have been recognized. Those conditions that can be manipulated by pharmacological or other methods include the hypercoagulable states, abnormalities of lipid metabolism and the effects of smoking. By addressing these, prolonged graft patency can be achieved.

Detection of hypercoagulable states

The hypercoagulable states (Table 1) refer to a group of conditions that predispose patients to thromboembolic complications.[60] With the exception of low fibrinolytic activity, they can be divided into familial and acquired disorders. The diagnosis of an inherited abnormality is made after systemic diseases have been excluded and the abnormality is found in other members of the family. Examples of acquired deficiencies are: protein C and S which are vitamin K dependent and can be reduced in the presence of liver disease; protein loosing enteropathy or nephropathy; oestrogen therapy which may reduce antithrombin II. Ahn[60] in a comprehensive review, suggests that the incidence of graft failure attributable to these hypercoaguable states is unknown and probably underestimated.

Eldrup-Jorgensen and his colleagues[61] have prospectively studied all their young patients (20 patients aged 50 years or less), undergoing revascularization of the lower limb. They measured protein C, protein S, factor VIII-related antigen, lupus-like anticoagulant, and platelet aggregation profiles and assessed the early outcome

Table 1. The hypercoagulable states

Antithrombin III deficiency
Heparin cofactor II deficiency
Protein C deficiency
Protein S deficiency
Factor XII deficiency
Lupus-like anticoagulant
Decreased fibrinolytic activity
plasminogen activator deficiency
plasminogen deficiency
increased plasminogen activator
Combination of two or more of the above

after the operation. Only four of 17 patients (24%) in whom all parameters were tested had normal profiles, and hypercoagulability (plasminogen deficiency, protein S deficiency, and hypercoagulable platelet profiles) was found in all patients whose grafts thrombosed within 30 days of the operation. Donaldson and his colleagues[62] reported on their prospective investigation of 158 patients presenting with a variety of vascular problems. Of these patients 15 (9.5%) had detectable abnormalities (antithrombin III deficiency, protein C deficiency, lupus-like anticoagulant, heparin induced platelet activation), and graft thrombosis occurred in 27% of these patients compared with 1.6% if no abnormality was detected. In a subsequent report they found that 33% of early graft failures were attributable to hypercoaguable states and that 14% of all vascular surgical patients had such abnormalities.[63] Each report concludes that the routine investigation for hypercoagulable states in patients about to undergo bypass grafting is now warranted.

Given preoperative warning of the presence of a hypercoagulable state, preventive measures are available. For example, regulatory protein and plasminogen deficiencies can be treated with replacement by fresh frozen plasma or with careful anticoagulation by means of heparin and coumadin. In the case of heparin induced platelet activation, aspirin reduces the platelet aggregation.

Hyperlipidaemia

A close relationship between atherosclerosis and elevated plasma levels of cholesterol and triglycerides has been observed in the Framingham study.[64] Many subsequent reports have further highlighted the relationship between peripheral vascular disease and abnormalities of lipid metabolism.[65] Seeger and his colleagues[66] studied the lipid risk factors in 144 patients with peripheral atherosclerosis and 61 age matched control subjects. Patients with atherosclerosis had higher levels of very low density lipoprotein cholesterol (VLDL) and lower levels of high density lipoprotein (HDL) than control subjects, yet the serum cholesterol and low density lipoprotein (LDL) were similar. Peripheral atherosclerosis below the inguinal ligament was strongly predicted by low HDL and increased VLDL but not by increased cholesterol or LDL levels. They conclude that the risk factors for infra-inguinal atherosclerosis are different to more central disease, and that attempts to limit graft failure by lowering lipid levels should be directed towards these lipoproteins.

In fact, no evidence exists at present to show that the treatment of hyperlipidaemia improves infra-inguinal graft patency rates. However, some indirect evidence may indicate that this may well be the case. It has for example been demonstrated in a controlled randomized trial that treating hyperlipidaemia does retard the progression of atherosclerosis in peripheral vascular disease.[67] In addition, the Cholesterol-Lowering Atherosclerosis Study (CLAS)[68] which was also a randomized, controlled trial in patients with previous coronary bypass surgery, showed that the treatment group had significantly fewer atherosclerotic lesions that formed or had progressed in the native coronary vessels as well as in the venous grafts. Graft patency was also higher in the treated group. Furthermore, regression of the atherosclerotic disease, as perceived by improvement in the overall coronary status, occurred in 16.2% of treated patients compared to 2.4% in the placebo group.

The vascular surgeon is fully aware that at least a third of his patients have severe three-vessel coronary disease. Therefore, the aggressive treatment of hyperlipidaemia would be in the patient's interest from the coronary artery point of view. The likelihood of retarding the progression of peripheral arterial lesions also after bypass grafting would be a bonus. However, it is necessary to establish that this is so by performing prospective studies.

Smoking

Smoking is the greatest risk factor for atherosclerotic occlusive disease of the peripheral circulation and well over 90% of patients with aorto-iliac and superficial femoral artery stenoses smoke tobacco.[69] The adverse influence of smoking on graft patency is also well established. Wiseman and her colleagues[70,71] found that vein and PTFE graft patency rates were significantly higher in non-smokers than in smokers (84% vs 63% at 1 year, $p<0.02$ for vein grafts; 78% vs 57% at 2 years, $p<0.05$ for PTFE grafts). These studies were based on detecting smoking markers, and significantly higher levels of blood carboxyhaemaglobin, plasma thiocyanate, plasma fibrinogen, and plasma apolipoprotein levels were found in patients with occluded graft than in those whose grafts remained patent for at least 1 year. This analysis of serum markers also indicated that 26% of patients were untruthful in their claims to have stopped smoking. Powell and Greenhalgh[72] in a further report conclude that the cheapest and perhaps most effective advice that they can give their patients is to stop smoking.

CONCLUSIONS

Under the present circumstances the following strategy is recommended to evaluate a patient preoperatively:

1. A careful history and clinical examination will suggest whether an operative procedure is justified. An evaluation of the pulse status and the presence or absence of necrotic tissue can also predict to a degree what procedure would be required to correct the presenting abnormality.

2. In evaluating the aorto-iliac segment (inflow) the suggested approach would be initially to use a good screening technique, such as Doppler velocity waveform analysis using pattern recognition or Laplace transform. If this test is normal there is only a small (about 10%) chance that a significant haemodynamic lesion in the aorto-iliac segment will be missed on the subsequent angiogram. If on the other hand an abnormality is detected by the screening test, then the aorto-iliac segment should be investigated with duplex Doppler prior to performing angiography combined with pull through pressure measurements (this should also include the injection of papaverine). In the presence of a haemodynamically significant iliac stenosis the radiologist, who will have been forewarned by the noninvasive investigations, should be prepared to proceed to balloon angioplasty.
3. The evaluation of the distal run-off is the area in which there is at present most uncertainty, and the general consensus is that despite using many of the previously described techniques, acceptable results can be achieved with a global policy of bypass grafting even in limbs with an apparently hopeless prognosis. The described tests, however, do help in finding the most suitable site into which the graft should be placed. High quality distal angiography pre- or intra-operatively remains the key for success. Screening by using PGR or simple Doppler insonation will also help choose the appropriate vessel for femorocrural grafting.
4. A serum lipid profile, and a full screen for hypercoaguable states (including tests for antithrombin III, protein C, and protein S deficiencies, lupus anticoagulant, fibrinogen activity, and platelet aggregation profiles) should be evaluated in each patient. This is particularly so if the subject has a strong family history, has particularly aggressive disease, or if a graft has failed previously in the absence of an obvious mechanical cause. It may be argued that such a policy is expensive, but then the cost of a failed graft is also expensive.
5. The patient should be encouraged to stop smoking.

REFERENCES

1. Nicolaides AN, Yao JST: General considerations and conclusions. *In* Investigation of Vascular Disorders, Nicolaides AN, Yao JST (Eds). New York: Churchill Livingstone, pp. 600–616, 1981
2. Gupta SK, Veith FJ, Kram HB, Wengerter KA: Significance and management of inflow gradients unexpectedly generated after femorofemoral, femoropopliteal, and femoro-infrapopliteal bypass grafting. J Vasc Surg 12:278–283, 1990
3. Young DF, Cholvin NR, Roth AC: Pressure drop across artificially induced stenoses in the femoral arteries of dogs. Circ Res 36:735–743, 1975
4. Teague SM, Van Ramm OT, Kisslo JA: Pulsed Doppler spectral analysis of bounded fluid jets. Ultrasound Med Biol 10:435, 1984
5. Teirstein PS, Yock PG, Popp RL: The accuracy of Doppler ultrasound measurement of pressure gradients across irregular, dual and tunnellike obstructions to blood flow. Circulation 72:577–584, 1985
6. Flanigan DP, Tullis JP, Streeter VL *et al*: Multiple subcritical arterial stenosis: Effect on poststenotic pressure and flow. Ann Surg 186:663–668, 1977
7. Flanigan DP, Williams LR, Schwarz JA, Schuler JJ, Gray B: Hemodynamic evaluation of the aortoiliac system based on pharmacologic vasodilation. Surgery 93:709–714, 1983

8. Myers KA, Scott DF, Devine TJ *et al*: Palpation of the femoral and popliteal pulses: A study of the accuracy as assessed by agreement between multiple observers. Eur J Vasc Surg 1:245–249, 1987
9. Yao JST, Hobbs JT, Irvine WT: Ankle systolic pressure measurements in arterial disease affecting the lower extremities. Br J Surg 56:676–679, 1969
10. Lynch TG, Hobson RW II, Wright CB *et al*: Interpretation of Doppler segmental pressures in peripheral vascular occlusive disease. Arch Surg 119:465–467, 1984
11. Barringer M, Poole GV, Shircliffe AC *et al*: The diagnosis of aorto-iliac disease: a noninvasive femoral cuff technique. Ann Surg 197:204–209, 1983
12. Flanigan DP, Collins JT, Schwarz JA *et al*: Hemodynamic and arteriographic evaluation of femoral pulsitility index. J Surg Res 31:234–238, 1982
13. Sumner DS, Strandness DE: Aortoiliac reconstruction reconstruction in patients with combined iliac and superficial femoral arterial occlusion. Surgery 84: 348–355, 1978
14. Flanigan DP, Gray B, Schuler JJ *et al*: Utility of wide and narrow blood pressure cuffs in the haemodynamic assessment of aortoiliac occlusive disease. Surgery 92:16–20, 1982
15. Yao JST: Surgical use of pressure studies in peripheral arterial disease. *In* Noninvasive Diagnostic Techniques in Vascular Disease, Bernstein EF (Ed.). St Louis: C. V. Mosby Co, pp. 545–553, 1985
16. Satomura S: Study of flow patterns in peripheral arteries by ultrasonics. J Acoust Sci Jpn 15:151–158, 1959
17. Rutherford RB, Jones DN, Lowenstein D, Fleming P: The effects of changes in lumen and flow on the arterial waveform. J Surg Res 32:110–120, 1982
18. Gosling RG, King DH: Ultrasonic angiology. *In* Arteries and Veins, Harcus AW, Adamson L (Eds), Edinburgh: Churchill Livingstone, pp. 61–98, 1975
19. Johnston KW, Maruzzo BC, Cobbold RSC: Errors and artifacts of Doppler flowmeters and their solution. Arch Surg 112:1335–1342, 1977
20. Campbell WB, Cole SEA, Skidmore R, Baird RN: The clinician and the vascular laboratory in the diagnosis of aortoiliac stenosis. Br J Surg 71:302–306, 1984
21. Junger M, Chapman BLW, Underwood CJ, Charlesworth D: A comparison between two types of waveform analysis in patients with multisegmental arterial disease. Br J Surg 71:345–348, 1984
22. Flanigan DP, Collins JT, Goodreau JJ, Burnham SJ, Yao JST: Femoral pulsatility index in the evaluation of aortoiliac occlusive disease. J Surg Res 31:392–399, 1981
23. Evans DH, Quin RO, Bell PRF: The significance of blood pressure measurements in patients with peripheral vascular disease. Br J Surg 67:238–241, 1980
24. Archie JP, Feldtman RW: Determination of the hemodynamic significance of iliac stenosis by noninvasive Doppler ultrasonography. Surgery 91:419–424, 1982
25. Skidmore R, Woodcock JP: Physiological interpretation of Doppler-shift waveforms—I. Theoretical considerations. Ultrasound Med Biol 6:7–10, 1980
26. Skidmore R, Woodcock JP: Physiological interpretation of Doppler-shift waveforms—II. Validation of the Laplace transform method for characterisation of the common femoral blood velocity/time waveform. Ultrasound Med Biol 6:219–225, 1980
27. Skidmore R, Woodcock JP, Wells PNT, Bird D, Baird RN: Physiological interpretation of Doppler-shift waveforms-III. Ultrasound Med Biol 6:227–231, 1981
28. Macpherson DS, Evans DH, Bell PRF: Common femoral artery Doppler wave-forms: a comparison of three methods of objective analysis with direct pressure measurements. Br J Surg 71:46–49, 1984
29. Baker JD, Machleder HI, Skidmore R: Analysis of femoral artery Doppler signals by LaPlace transform damping method. J Vasc Surg 1:520–524, 1984
30. Nicolaides AN, Gordon-Smith IC, Dayandas J, Eastcott HHG: The value of Doppler blood velocity tracings in the detection of the aortoiliac disease in patients with intermittent claudication. Surgery 80:774–778, 1976
31. Walton L, Martin TRP, Collins M: Prospective assessment of the aorto-iliac segment by visual interpretation of frequency analysed Doppler waveforms—a comparison with arteriography. Ultrasound Med Biol 10:27, 1984

32. Sawchuk AP, Flanigan DP, Tober JC *et al*: A rapid, accurate, noninvasive technique for diagnosing critical and subcritical stenosis in aortoiliac arteries. J Vasc Surg 12:158–167, 1990
33. Myers KA, Williams MA, Nicolaides AN: The use of Doppler ultrasound to assess disease in arteries to the lower limb. *In* Cardiovascular Applications of Doppler Ultrasound, Salmasi A-M, Nicolaides AN (Eds). Edinburgh: Churchill Livingstone, pp. 289–314, 1989
34. Kohler TR, Nance DR, Cramer MM, Vandenburghe N, Strandness DE: Duplex scanning for diagnosis of aortoiliac and femoropopliteal disease: a prospective study. Circulation 76:1074–1080: 1987
35. Kohler TR, Andros G, Porter JM *et al*: Can duplex scanning replace arteriography for lower extremity arterial disease. Ann Vasc Surg 4:280–287, 1990
36. de Smet AAEA, Kitslaar PJEHM: A duplex criterion for aorto-iliac stenosis. Eur J Vasc Surg 4:275–278, 1990
37. Moneta GL, Taylor DC, Yeager RA, Porter JM: Duplex ultrasound: Applications to intra-abdominal vessels. Perspectives Vasc Surg 2(2):133–148, 1989
38. Nicolaides AN, Angelides NS: Application of isotope technology to the clinical study of arterial disease. *In* Noninvasive Diagnostic Techniques in Vascular Disease, Bernstein EF (Ed.). St Louis: C. V. Mosby Co, pp. 592–601, 1985
39. Slot HB, Strijbosch L, Greep JM: Interobserver variability in single-plane aortography. Surgery 90:497–503, 1981
40. Breslau PJ, Joering PJG, Greep JM: Assessment of aortoiliac disease using haemodynamic measures. Arch Surg 120:1050–1052, 1985
41. Parvin SD, Evans DH, Bell PRF: Peripheral resistance measurement in the assessment of severe peripheral vascular disease. Br J Surg 72:751–753, 1985
42. Cooper GC, Austin C, Fitzsimmons E *et al*: Outflow resistance and early occlusion of infrainguinal bypass grafts. Eur J Vasc Surg 4:279–283, 1990
43. Ascer E, Veith FJ: Outflow resistance measurements in infra-inguinal bypass operations by injecting saline and measuring the integral of pressure. *In* Diagnostic Techniques and Assessment Procedures in Vascular Surgery, Greenhalgh RM (Ed.). London: Grune & Stratton, pp. 269–284, 1985
44. Dardik H, Ibrahim IM, Sussman B *et al*: Morphological structure of the pedal arch and its relationship to patency of crural vascular reconstruction. Surg Gynaecol Obstet 152:645–648, 1981
45. Cooper GC, Hood JM, Barros D'Sa AAB *et al*: The "isolated" popliteal segmant: A comparative evaluation of its vascular resistance. Eur J Vasc Surg 4:493–496, 1990
46. Mason R, Lanfranchi A, Giron F: Isolated popliteal vs distal bypass for limb salvage. Surg Gynecol Obstet 155:49, 1982
47. Roedersheimer LR, Feins R, Green RM: Doppler evaluation of the pedal arch. Am J Surg 142:601–604, 1981
48. Campbell WB, Fletcher EL, Hands LJ: Assessment of the distal lower limb arteries: a comparison of arteriography and Doppler ultrasound. Ann R Coll Surg (Engl) 68:37–39, 1986
49. Jager KA, Ricketts HJ, Strandness DE: Duplex scanning for the evaluation of lower limb arterial disease. *In* Noninvasive Diagnostic Techniques in Vascular Disease, Bernstein EF (Ed.). St Louis, C. V. Mosby Co, pp. 619–631, 1985
50. Dean RH, Yao JST, Stanton PE, Bergan JJ: Prognostic indicators in femoropopliteal reconstructions. Arch Surg 110:1287–1296, 1975
51. Samson RH, Gupta SK, Veith FJ, Ascer E, Scher L: Perioperative noninvasive haemodynamic ankle indices as predictors of infrainguinal graft patency. J Vasc Surg 2:307, 1985
52. O'Donnell TF, Mackey W, McCullough JL *et al*: Correlation of operative findings with angiographic and noninvasive hemodynamic factors associated with failure of polytetrafluoroethylene grafts. J Vasc Surg 1:136, 1984
53. Scott DJA, Vowden P, Beard JD, Horrocks M: Non-invasive estimation of peripheral resistance using pulse generated runoff before femorodistal bypass. Br J Surg 77:391–395, 1990
54. Dible JH: The Pathology of Limb Ischaemia. Edinburgh, London: Oliver and Boyd Ltd, 1966

55. Imparato AM, Kim GE, Madayag M, Haveson S: Angiographic criteria for successful tibial artery reconstruction. Surgery 74:830–838, 1973
56. Leather RP, Shah DM, Karmody AM: Infrapopliteal arterial bypass for limb salvage: Increased patency and utilisation of the saphenous vein used "in situ". Surgery 90:1000–1008, 1981
57. Pomposelli FB, Jepsen SJ, Gibbons GW *et al*: Efficacy of the dorsal pedal bypass for limb salvage in diabetic patients: Short-term observations. J Vasc Surg 11:745–752, 1990
58. Flanigan DP, Williams LR, Keifer J *et al*: Prebypass operative arteriography. Surgery 92:627–633, 1982
59. Chesire NJ, Noone MA, Davies L, Drummond M, Wolfe JHN: Economic options and decision making in the ischaemic lower limb. *In* Proceedings of the First Tripartite Meeting of the British and Irish, Canadian, and Dutch Vascular Surgical Societies, London 22–23 November 1990
60. Ahn SS: The hypercoagulable states: A comprehensive review for the vascular surgeon. Sem Vasc Surg 3:6–20, 1990
61. Eldrup-Jorgensen J, Flanigan DP, Brace L *et al*: Hypercoaguable states and lower limb ischaemia in young adults. J Vasc Surg 9:334–341, 1989
62. Donaldson MC, Weinberg DS, Belkin M, Whitemore AD, Mannick JA: Screening for hypercoaguable in vascular surgical practice: a preliminary study. J Vasc Surg 11:825–831, 1990
63. Whittemore AD, Donaldson MC, Mannick JA: Detection and treatment of hypercoaguable states: Can they improve infrainguinal bypass results? *In* Proceedings of the 17th Annual Symposium on Current Critical Problems and New Horizons in Vascular Surgery, New York City 16–18 November 1990
64. Gordon T, Kannel WB: Predisposition to atherosclerosis in the head, heart, and legs. J Am Med Ass 221:661–666, 1972
65. Rapp JH: Basic data related to lipid abnormalities in peripheral vascular disease. Ann Vasc Surg 4:604–608, 1990
66. Seeger JM, Silverman SH, Flynn TC *et al*: Lipid risk factors in patients requiring arterial reconstruction. J Vasc Surg 10:418–424, 1989
67. Duffield RGM, Lewis B, Miller NE *et al*: Treatment of hyperlipidaemia retards progression of symptomatic femoral atherosclerosis. A randomised controlled trial. Lancet ii:639–642, 1983
68. Blankenhorn DH, Nessim SA, Johnson RL *et al*: Beneficial effects of combined Colestipol-Niacin therapy on coronary atherosclerosis and coronary venous bypass grafts. J Am Med Ass 257:3233–3240, 1987
69. Kannel WB, Shurtleff D: The Framingham Study: Cigarettes and the development of intermittent claudication. Geriatrics 28:61, 1973
70. Wiseman S, Kenchington G, Dain R *et al*: Influence of smoking and plasma factors on patency of femoropopliteal vein grafts. Br J Med 229:642–646, 1989
71. Wiseman S, Powell J, Greenhalgh R *et al*: The influence of smoking and plasma factors on prosthetic graft patency. Eur J Vasc Surg 4:57–61, 1990
72. Powell JT, Greenhalgh RM. Changing the smoking habit and its influence on the management of vascular disease. Acta Chir Scand (Suppl) 555:99–103, 1990

Does Combined Sympathectomy Improve Peripheral Reconstruction Patency?

Lars Norgren

Few treatments in vascular medicine have been as controversial as sympathectomy. From a historical point of view it is understandable that a transformation of a cold pale foot into a warm and bright condition[1] was rated a success. Nevertheless, in patients with claudication, today's knowledge provides evidence against any improvement on walking distance,[2] even if positive reports exist.[3]

Regarding critical limb ischaemia the situation may be different. In these patients, who for technical reasons are not suitable for reconstructive procedures and who suffer from rest pain, ulcers and gangrene, sometimes an improvement on rest pain may be achieved with a sympathetic ablation. Cross and Cotton in a randomized study[4] were able to show relief of rest pain in 83.5% vs 23.5% for placebo treatment. After 6 months 66% were still pain-free. No effect was found on haemodynamic parameters. In some cases a critical ischaemia may be transformed to a more benign condition where ulcers heal and amputation is avoided for a longer period.

EFFECTS OF SYMPATHETIC INTERRUPTION

These findings raise the question of the effects of a sympathetic interruption. Regional differences are known. Thus, Barcroft and Swan[5] were able to show the differences between the effects in the hand and in the foot, the blood flow increase of the arm being eight-fold and lasting about a week, while in the foot, the flow was less increased and less reactive. They also concluded that the blood flow increase was restricted to skin and did not involve muscles. Gillespie and Douglas[6] came to the same conclusion in patients with intermittent claudication. Masuoka and Shimomura[7] using radioisotope clearance did not achieve muscle blood flow increase after sympathectomy despite an increase of total femoral blood flow.

The main reason for flow increase seems to be an opening of arteriovenous shunts[8] reducing the arterial tone.[9] Evidently a warm and red foot may be the clinical result. The question still remains whether there is any increase in nutritive capillary flow. If not, the flow increase could even imply a steal phenomenon from sensitive structures, such as muscles.

More and Hall[10] using Xenon^{133} clearance found a 10% capillary blood flow increase. Muscle blood flow, however, does not seem to be augmented.[11] The second question is whether capillary flow increase is the only way of increasing oxygenation. In an experimental work Conlon and coworkers discussed this matter,[12] finding evidence for an increased $tcPO_2$ after sympathectomy. The other effect, relief of rest pain may be attributed to a sympathetic control of pain pathways and moreover there is also evidence that sympathetic fibres transmit pain. It also seems that an adequate pain relief is well correlated to an improved capillary flow.[29]

From this introductory point of view it can be concluded that sympathectomy may be able to increase blood flow, mainly due to the opening of arteriovenous shunts and may also relieve rest pain under certain circumstances.

ARTERIAL RECONSTRUCTIONS AND SYMPATHECTOMY

Do these modes of action support a use of sympathectomy in conjunction with arterial reconstructions? Most of the published studies concern aortofemoral reconstructions, understandable since the lumbar chain is easily accessible during surgery, but rationally not the proper situation to study, since outflow is seldom extensively restricted, and rest pain is a lesser problem in this case than distal reconstructions.

Experimental evidence exists that sympathectomy gives rise to better patency after small blood vessel anastomoses. Casten and coworkers[13] found a 1-month patency of 66 vs 26% after femoral artery suture in dogs if a sympathectomy was added.

In a more recent investigation in dogs[14] where run-off had been restricted, and arterial thrombosis induced, an adjunctive arteriovenous fistula (AVF) was compared to sympathectomy and to controls. Only AVF was capable of significantly preventing rethrombosis. No benefit was achieved using sympathectomy.

Evidently this experimental situation is far from the clinical one. Controversial results are reported with adjunctive sympathectomy to aorto-iliac and aortofemoral reconstructions. Most important, few of the studies are conducted in a controlled fashion.

When Cannon *et al.* reviewed 94 cases of aorto-iliac endarterectomy during the late 1950s[15] they found that sympathectomy increased the favourable outcome both in patients with and without restricted outflow. The study was by no means controlled. During the same period Weismann and Upson[16] clearly stated that neither aorto-iliac nor femoropopliteal operations showed a lesser incidence of early failures after sympathectomy. Van der Stricht[17] reported 30% late postoperative thrombosis vs 60% in femoropopliteal operations if a sympathectomy had been added. The findings, however, are discussed on a basis of earlier operations performed without, and later ones with, sympathectomy. Changes in technique may therefore have influenced the results.

In the investigation by Terry *et al.*[18] they found that when signs of vasoconstriction were evident, an adjunctive sympathectomy increased limb blood flow. This was apparently valid both for proximal and distal reconstructions.

Three prospective randomized studies have been reported (Table 1). Barnes and coworkers[19] were able to show that peripheral vascular resistance, plethysmographically determined, was significantly reduced in the sympathectomized leg. The study shows moreover that this increase of leg blood flow and decrease of vascular resistance has nothing to do with patency of an aorto-iliac reconstruction.

In a corresponding study on aortofemoral reconstructions performed by Shanik and coworkers,[9] sympathectomy was able to significantly reduce peripheral resistance. The authors were not able to draw any conclusions regarding early or late patency.

Table 1. Randomized controlled studies on the effect of concomitant lumbar sympathectomy

Author	*Sympathec-tomy (S)*	*Surgical procedure*	*Results of re-constructions in regard to S*	*Addendum*
Shanik *et al.* 1976 (9)	Bilateral, level?	Aorto-iliac Aortofemoral	Not known	Foot blood flow increase
Barnes *et al.* 1977 (19)	Bilateral, L2-L4	Aorto-iliac	Not influenced	Foot blood flow increase
Satiani *et al.* 1982 (20)	Bilateral, L2-L4	Aortofemoral	Not influenced	Ankle index slightly increased

In a third prospective study concerning aortofemoral reconstructions Satiani and coworkers[20] concluded at a mean follow-up of 11 months that there was no significant difference in graft patency or demand for subsequent distal bypasses between the sympathectomized and nonsympathectomized groups.

Recently, no controlled studies have been published. Rossi *et al.* concluded that sympathectomy in combination with vascular procedures was of benefit for patients over 70 years of age and not suffering from diabetes. Their conclusions are drawn on patients in Fontaine stages II and III.[21] As late as 1990 one paper has appeared advocating sympathectomy in conjunction with distal graft bypass[22].

SURGICAL OR CHEMICAL SYMPATHECTOMY

The question has not been brought up whether surgical or chemical sympathectomy shall be performed. Evidently most procedures are performed in conjunction with aortic surgery. Therefore chemical sympathectomy has seldomly been tried. Existing reports show that chemical sympathectomy has a greater failure rate than surgical sympathectomy,[4] but the opposite result has also been presented.[23,24]

CONCLUDING REMARKS

In two different reviews as close to each other as 1985 and 1988 Cotton and Cross[25] concluded with the suggestion that 'the role of sympathectomy is wider than commonly realized', while Campbell[26] carefully pointed out the need for better studies before any conclusion can be drawn.

Despite the results discussed, it would be unfair to conclude that sympathectomy is of no value. Obviously this is correct for aortofemoral reconstructions with a good outflow. For very distal reconstructions an increase of graft blood flow might be of interest, provided the vasodilatation achieved does not imply a steal phenomenon from more vulnerable structures than skin.

Such a problem can not be solved without well performed controlled studies involving as similar groups of patients as possible. Ethical consequences also have to be considered if a surgical sympathectomy is to be an alternative. The main reason

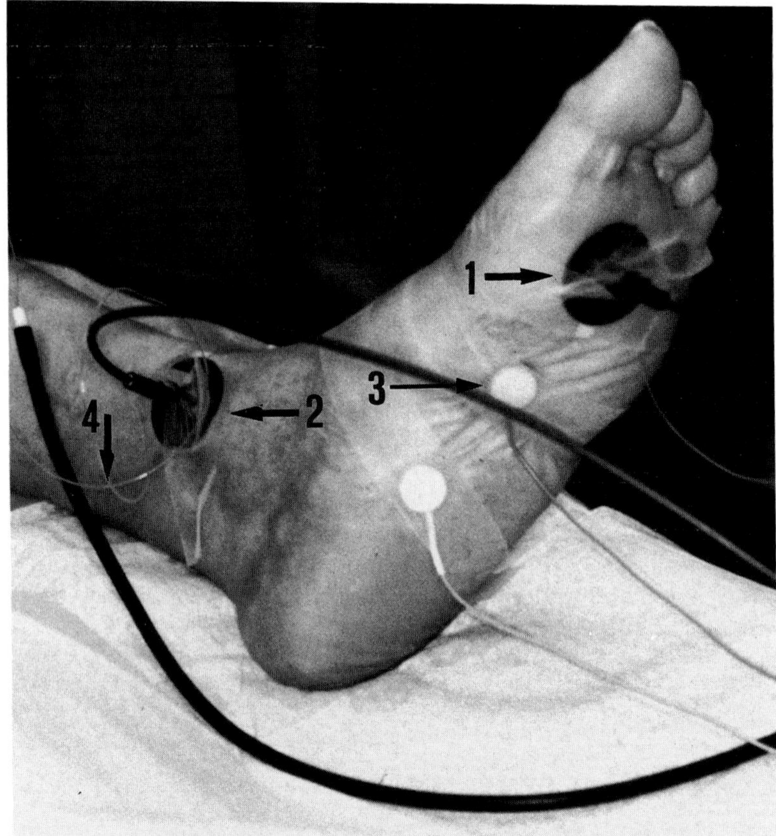

Fig. 1. Measurement of laser Doppler flux (sole of the foot = 1; ankle = 2), galvanic skin response (3) and temperature of the foot (4) during lumbar sympathetic stimulation.

for performing such studies is that there is enough evidence that in some instances sympathectomy can improve the situation for patients without technical possibilities for vascular reconstruction. It is, however, impossible to predict who will be a responder. Therefore it is reasonable to return to the original question about the sympathetic effects *per se*.

CURRENT RESEARCH

Aortic surgery gives the opportunity to investigate sympathetic activity since the lumbar chain is readily accessible. Epidural anaesthesia at least to the level of Th7 minimizes the risk for false interpretation regarding vasoactivity on the foot level.

Using two laser Dopplers (Periflux I, Perimed, Sweden) with one probe at the ankle, the other at the sole of the foot, and a device for measuring galvanic skin response (Fig. 1) as well as an electromagnetic flow measurement equipment (Cliniflow, Carolina Medicals, USA), skin vasoactivity, sweating and deep femoral artery blood flow is measured during electrical stimulation of the sympathetic chain with two

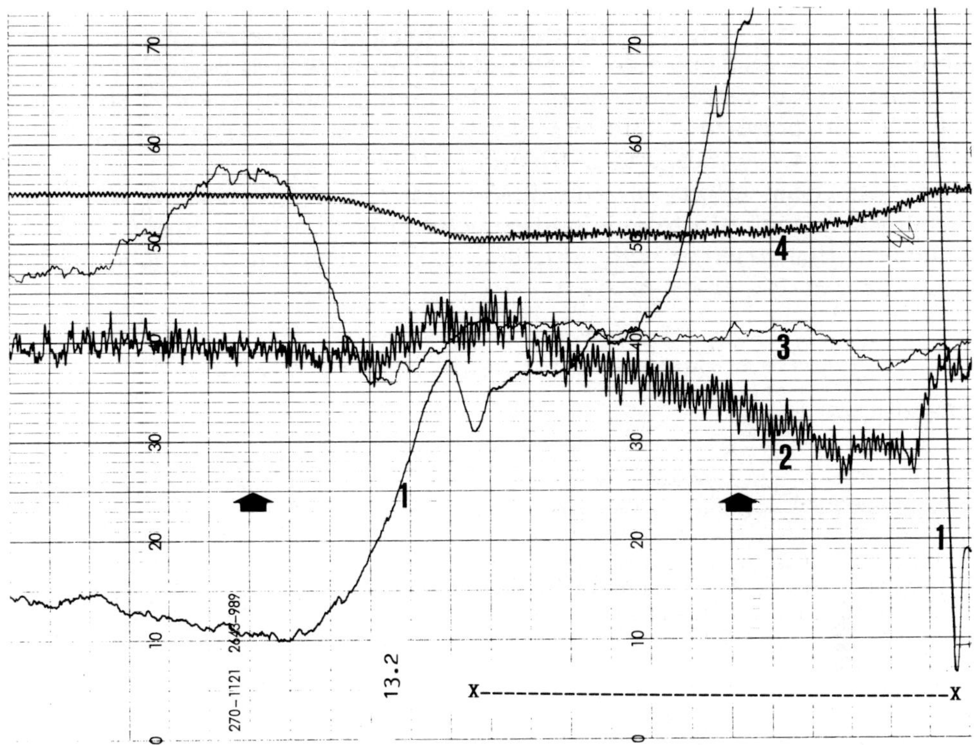

Fig. 2. Recordings from a lumbar sympathetic stimulation: x---x = stimulation period; 1 = galvanic skin response; 2 = laser Doppler response from the sole of the foot; 3 = laser Doppler response from the ankle region; 4 = electromagnetic flow measurement of the deep femoral artery. Arrows indicate the direction of increases.

needle electrodes. A constant current stimulator is used (Disa 1505 or 1507). From the beginning both frequencies and currents were varied. Now 30 second stimulation periods are delivered with intervals of 2 min and the stimulation frequency is kept at 10 Hz and the stimulation strengths are varied between 1 and 12 mA.

A galvanic skin response is considered evidence for an effective stimulation.

Briefly, our results have shown both increases and decreases of blood flow in the skin of the foot (Fig. 2). In the deep femoral artery only decreases have been found. The likely explanation that not only vasoconstriction but also dilatation occurred in the skin seems to be that stimulation causes activation of two different types of fibres. Our results thus give evidence for an active sympathetic vasodilatation of the skin of the foot.[27]

THE AUTHOR'S PHILOSOPHY

One can not easily turn these findings into evidence in favour of sympathectomy under certain circumstances. The unexpected finding of vasodilatory fibres in the ganglia may, however, suggest that measures on the sympathetic system may give a spectrum of effects, not easily predicted.

Therefore, more research in this field is essential. More evidence for sympathetic responses and possible increase of nutritional flow as well as properly performed controlled clinical studies are needed. The findings using epidural stimulation (ESES)[28,29] do point in a different direction to that commonly accepted—that ischaemic ulcers may heal and nutritional flow increase.

Thus, beneficial effects of sympathetic ablation in conjunction with distal reconstructions and restricted outflow cannot be excluded, while a simpler conclusion evidently is that together with aortofemoral reconstructions and good outflow, sympathectomy is a waste of effort.

REFERENCES

1. Royle ND: A new operative procedure in the treatment of spastic paralysis and its experimental basis. Med J Aust 1:77, 1924
2. Fyfe T, Quin RO: Phenol sympathectomy in the treatment of intermittent claudication; a controlled clinical trial. Br J Surg 62:68–71, 1975
3. Courbier R, Reggi M, Jausseran JM: Evaluation of effectiveness of lumbar sympathectomy by non invasive diagnostic techniques. J Cardiovasc Surg 20:333–337, 1979
4. Cross FW, Cotton LT: Chemical lumbar sympathectomy for ischemic rest pain. Am J Surg 150:341–345, 1985
5. Barcroft H, Swan HJC: Sympathetic Control of Human Blood Vessels. London: Arnold, 1953
6. Gillespie JA, Douglas DM: Obliterative Vascular Disease of the Lower Limb. London: E&S Livingstone, 1961
7. Masuoka S, Shimomura T: Lumbar sympathectomy and blood flow in the lower extremity. Am J Surg 136:369–374, 1978
8. Cronenwett JL, Lindenauer SM: Direct measurement of arteriovenous anastomotic blood flow after lumbar sympathectomy. Surgery 82:82–89, 1977
9. Shanik GD, Ford J, Hayes AC, Baker WH, Barnes RW: Pedal vasomotor tone following aorto femoral reconstructions. Ann Surg 183:136–138, 1976
10. Moore WS, Hall AD: Effects on lumbar sympathectomy on skin capillary blood flow in arterial occlusive disease. J Surg Res 14:151–157, 1973
11. Perry MO, Horton J: Muscle and subcutaneous oxygen tension. Arch Surg 113:176–178, 1978
12. Conlon KC, Flanagan PV, Naughton PM, O'Higgins N: The effect of lumbar sympathectomy on the ischaemic canine limb. Surg Res Comm 1:203–206, 1987
13. Casten DF, Sadler AH, Forman D: An experimental study of the effect of sympathectomy on patency of small blood vessel anastomoses. Surg Gynecol Obstet 115:462–466, 1962
14. Yoshida WB, Maffei FH, Lastoria S, Curi PR, Rollo HA: Lumbar sympathectomy and distal arteriovenous fistula as adjuncts to prevent arterial rethrombosis after thrombectomy: experimental study in dogs. J Cardiovasc Surg 29:19–25, 1988
15. Cannon JA, Kawakami IG, Barker WF: The present status of aortoiliac endarterectomy for obliterative atherosclerosis. Arch Surg 82:51–63, 1961
16. Weismann MD, Upson JF: Use of lumbar sympathectomy as an adjunct to reconstructive arterial surgery. Ann Surg 154:788–790, 1961
17. van der Stricht J: The influence of lumbar sympathectomy on the permeability of reconstructions. J Cardiovasc Surg 16:552–553, 1975
18. Terry HJ, Allan JS, Taylor GW: The effect of adding lumbar sympathectomy to reconstructive arterial surgery in the lower limb. Br J Surg 57:52–55, 1970
19. Barnes RW, Baker WH, Shanik G *et al*: Value of concomitant sympathectomy in aortoiliac reconstruction. Arch Surg 112:1325–1330, 1977

20. Satiani B, Liapis CD, Hayes JP, Kimmins S, Evans WE: Prospective randomized study of concomitant lumbar sympathectomy with aortoiliac reconstruction. Am J Surg 143:755–760, 1982
21. Rossi M, Perbellini A, Laterza E, Zorzi R, Genna M: Current state of sympathectomy in peripheral reconstructive surgery. Chir Ital 38:185–192, 1986
22. Boltax RS: Lumbar sympathectomy: a place in clinical medicine. Conn Med 53:716–717, 1989
23. Becquemin JP, Kassab M, Belloard A, Brugiere P, Melliere D: Lumbar sympathectomy in the aged subject. Surgery or phenolization? J Mal Vasc 14:327–333, 1989
24. Vulpio C, Borzone A, Iannace C *et al*: Lumbar chemical sympathectomy in end stage of arterial disease, early and late results. Angiology 40:948–952, 1989
25. Cotton LT, Cross FW: Lumbar sympathectomy for arterial disease. Br J Surg 72:678–683, 1985
26. Campbell WB: Sympathectomy for chronic arterial ischaemia. Eur J Vasc Surg 2:357–364, 1988
27. Lundberg J, Norgren L, Ribbe E *et al*: Direct evidence of active sympathetic vasodilatation in the skin of the human foot. J Physiol 417:437–446, 1989
28. Jivegård L, Augustinsson LE, Carlsson CA, Holm J: Long term results by epidural spinal electrical stimulation (ESES) in patients with inoperable severe lower limb ischaemia. Eur J Vasc Surg 1:345–349, 1987
29. Jacobs MJHM, Jörning PJG, Beckers RCY *et al*: Foot salvage and improvement of microvascular blood flow as a result of epidural spinal cord electrical stimulation. J Vasc Surg 12:354–360, 1990

When Should Arteriovenous Fistula be used with Femorodistal Bypass?

Hans O. Myhre and Ola D. Sæther

Vascular reconstruction by autologous saphenous vein bypass to the tibial or peroneal arteries is often successful in patients facing amputation for severe ischaemic disease.[1] The results following such operations have improved during recent years probably due to improved surgical technique. However, many patients with critical ischaemia are not candidates for arterial reconstruction according to conventional criteria because of poor run-off caused by an absent or insufficient pedal arch, unusually small-calibre leg arteries, and discontinuity or multiple obstructions of these arteries. Also the lack of suitable autologous vein has been regarded as a contra-indication to arterial reconstruction at this level. Several attempts have been made to obtain limb salvage in this group of patients either by pharmacological treatment or by modification of the operative technique.

The idea of using an arteriovenous shunt in the treatment of limb ischaemia is not new.[2] The combination of bypass grafting and the formation of an arteriovenous fistula (AVF) was explored experimentally and clinically in the 1960s with promising results. The purpose of this presentation is to evaluate the indication for the use of AVF as an adjunct to femorotibial bypass grafting.

THEORETICAL CONSIDERATIONS AND EXPERIMENTAL WORK

One of the most important causes of graft failure is thrombosis due to low blood flow. Sauvage *et al.*[3] have stressed that a vascular graft has its 'critical thrombotic threshold'. Below a certain critical level of blood flow re-occlusion is likely to occur. This critical flow threshold is higher for synthetic vascular grafts than for autologous vein grafts. By adding an AVF, the risk of graft thrombosis is decreased by increasing graft blood flow, which in turn could improve the patency rate for reconstructions which would otherwise have a poor prognosis.

Sumner[4] has compared an AVF with a Wheatstone bridge model for electrical current, where the distal artery corresponds to the cross-arm of the bridge (Fig. 1). Placing an AVF distal to the reconstructed segment will increase the rate of blood flow through the bypass graft, probably improving the patency rate. However, the possibility exists that the fistula could 'steal' blood from the peripheral arterial tree. This could be detrimental to the tissue increasing the risk of gangrene development. If the arterial segment proximal to the AVF has been reconstructed with a graft of sufficient diameter and the fistula is not too large, the pressure head at the level of the fistula will increase with the additional effect of improving peripheral perfusion. Referring to the Wheatstone bridge analogue, flow in the distal direction will occur as long as the ratio of the fistula resistance to the proximal artery resistance

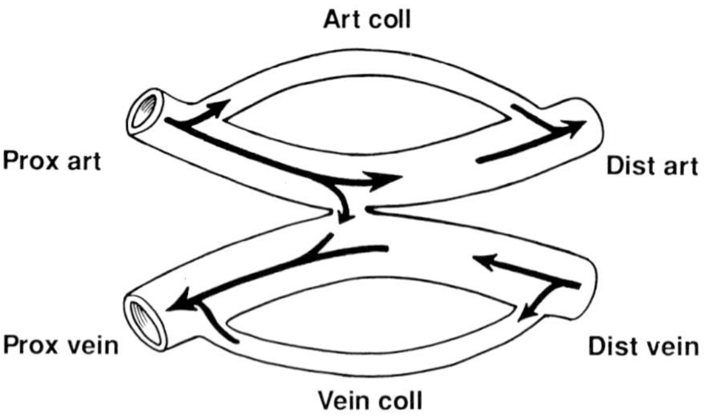

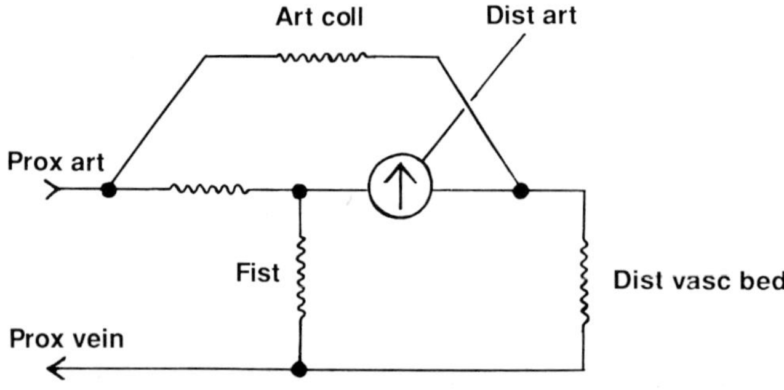

Fig. 1. The haemodynamics of an arteriovenous fistula can be compared with a Wheatstone bridge: the fistula represents the arm of the bridge and the blood flow of the distal artery is determined by the resistance of the fistula, the proximal arterial tree, the distal vascular bed and the arterial collaterals (from Ref. 4).

exceeds that of the distal vascular bed to the arterial collaterals.[4] This is likely to occur in the type of fistula used in conjunction with arterial reconstruction since they are relatively small, high resistance fistulas and with limited collateral development.

The major portion of the graft blood flow enters the venous system, and using densitometric flow estimation, the portion of blood entering the distal artery is found to be about 10% of the total graft flow.[5] However, this will often be sufficient to cure rest pain and to prevent the progression of gangrene.

The importance of the size of the fistula as regards the direction of distal blood flow has been studied experimentally showing that fistulas in the thigh region of 4 mm in length always had arterial flow directed towards the periphery, in contrast to fistulas between 15 and 19 mm where a central flow was recorded.[6] Another important factor predisposing peripheral vascular steal is a proximal arterial obstruction.[7]

Convincing evidence of the effect of AVF has been found in experimental studies where ischaemia was induced by arterial occlusion of canine hind limbs.[8,9] The ischaemia was then reversed by an end-to-side arteriovenous anastomosis. The result was evaluated by clinical examination of the extremity, by measurement of intramuscular pO_2, muscle surface pH, arterial blood pressure and pletysmographic recordings.[9,10] It is stressed that a proximal fistula may create distal venous hypertension, emphasizing that the location of the fistula is also of importance for the clinical result. Thus the fistula should probably be located as distally as possible.[11]

Although most experimental work supports the view that an AVF may be beneficial when combined with distal bypass grafting in severely ischaemic limbs,[12] the question is still controversial. Thus, Gwynn *et al.*[13] conclude that although an AVF may improve bypass graft flow, it is unlikely to benefit distal limb perfusion. Their view is based on finding flow reversal in the distal arterial tree. Controversial results from the various reports may be caused by differences in the experimental model as regards factors like methods for the induction of ischaemia, revascularization, as well as location and the size of the fistula. Finally, an experimental model can not easily imitate an ischaemic extremity of an elderly atherosclerotic patient.

CLINICAL EXPERIENCE

The first attempts at using an AVF to treat severe arterial insufficiency were based on proximal fistulas, which failed to improve the peripheral circulation.[14] Other attempts at reversing arterial blood flow via the venous system have failed partly due to competent venous valves preventing distal blood flow and partly to various complications.

Early clinical experience with AVF used in combination with revascularization procedures was presented by Blaisdell and coworkers in 1966.[15] Although their series was relatively small a certain therapeutic success was attributed to the use of AVF. They stressed the importance of making the fistula of proper size and to avoid a proximal location of the fistula, thereby avoiding decrease in distal arterial pressure.

In recent series AVF has been used as an adjunct to femorotibial reconstruction whereby graft blood flow is increased with the intention to improve the patency rate (Table 1). Especially when synthetic grafts are anastomosed to leg arteries, the patency rate is poor[16] although it may be improved somewhat by the addition of anticoagulant therapy.[17] Most presented experience is, however, not based on prospective randomized series and without proper controls.

Preliminary clinical results in 13 patients with this technique were presented by Ibrahim *et al.* in 1980.[18] The patients were selected from a group having poor run-off, calcification, multifocal stenosis or small calibre leg arteries. All had undergone previous surgery which had failed and belonged to a group where reconstruction

Table 1. Patency rates following femorotibial bypass with adjuvant arteriovenous fistula

Author	Journal	*Year*	*1-Year patency*	*2-Year patency*
Moody *et al.*	J Cardiovasc Surg	1990	39	36
Dardik *et al.*	Unpublished series	1990	—	44
Paty *et al.*	J Vasc Surg	1990	67	—
Snyder *et al.*	J Cardiovasc Surg	1985	—	≈15
Miksic *et al.*	Angio	1988	54	32
van Henegouwen *et al.*	Eur J Vasc Surg	1987	—	62 (vein)

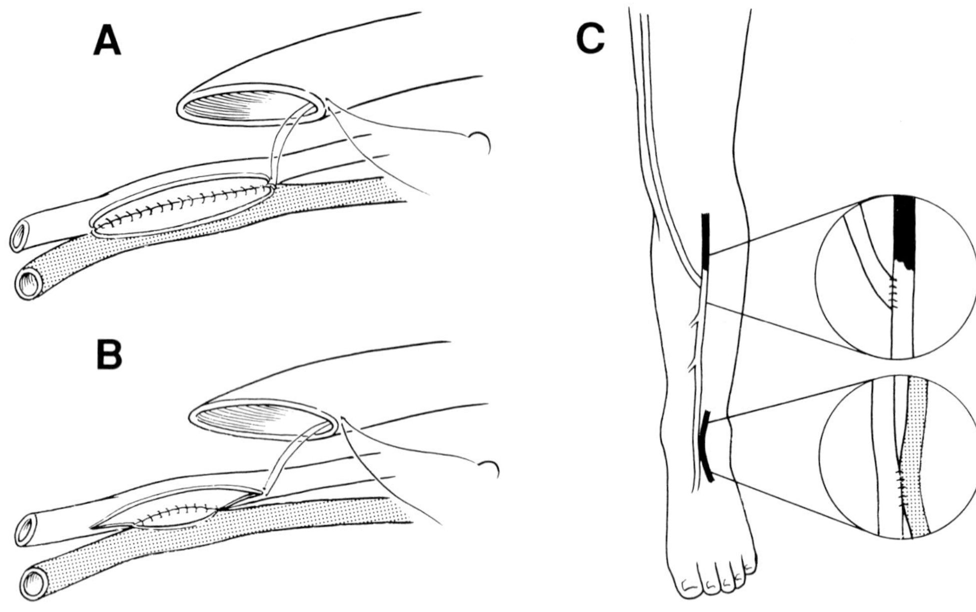

Fig. 2. Various types of arteriovenous fistulas to improve graft blood flow during femorotibial bypass grafting. The common ostium technique is shown to the left (A). The venotomy may be decreased to increase the resistance of the fistula thereby reducing the risk of peripheral arterial steal (B). A remote arteriovenous fistula is shown to the right (C).

would have most likely resulted in immediate failure with amputation as the final outcome. The group has used the so-called common ostium technique for creating the AVF. Thus, the recipient artery and one of its concomitant veins are opened longitudinally and the adjacent walls are sutured together to create a common ostium. The vascular graft is then anastomosed to this ostium (Fig. 2). In the majority of cases they have used glutar-aldehyde-stabilized umbilical vein grafts for reconstruction. The group has now an accumulated experience from a total of 210 adjunctive AVFs performed during the last decade in 203 patients, representing the greatest experience with this particular technique (H. Dardik, pers. comm.) During this period the 2-year patency rate has increased from 18% to 44%. The distal blood flow has been recorded by completion angiography or Doppler examination and no reversal of distal blood flow has been observed.[19,20]

In other series with adjunctive AVFs in femorotibial bypass grafting most of the patients were also operated by synthetic bypass-grafts having seriously compromised arterial run-off.[21,22] The results were compared with a group of better risk patients having a patent pedal arch reconstructed without an AVF. During follow-up the patency rate in the two groups was almost identical, probably indicating a beneficial effect of the AVF. In these series the AVF was created by the common ostium technique, but slightly modified since the venotomy was about 0.5 cm whereas the arteriotomy was about three times longer to increase the resistance of the fistula.[21] The authors conclude that probably most patients receiving a graft to the distal part of the leg should have an AVF irrespective of the status of the pedal arch. In a recent review of the experience of this group with 80 femorodistal reconstructions including AVF, an overall 2-year patency rate of 36% was observed. Another conclusion from this work was that shorter grafts did significantly better than longer ones.[23]

However, inconsistent and conflicting results are found in the literature even although basically the same technique has been applied. Thus, from 30 reconstructions in 27 patients, graft patency was obtained in four cases only whereas limb salvage was seen in six during a follow-up period for up to 21 months.[24] In other series the two-year patency rates have varied from 32%[25] to 62%[26]. The difference may be explained by the fact that the first series included mainly synthetic grafts while the latter included autologous saphenous vein bypass reconstructions in addition to a few homologous vein grafts.

In a similar series consisting of 37 operations mainly using synthetic grafts, a 75% limb salvage was achieved with a follow-up varying from 4 to 24 months. The authors conclude that the technique seems justified in patients resisting the idea of amputation and having extremely poor run-off, with an absent pedal arch.[27]

The possibility of using a remote side-to-side fistula distal to the anastomosis has been explored in two recent series (Fig. 2).[28,29] Bypass using synthetic grafts to the leg arteries was performed in all patients who have had one or more previously failed reconstructions. The idea was that this type of fistula to a greater extent augments blood flow between the distal anastomosis and the fistula, thereby improving distal limb perfusion in addition to increasing graft patency. Although the series are small, consisting of 12 and 16 patients only, the preliminary results are promising. Myo-intimal hyperplasia at the distal anastomosis is a problem when creating an AVF with a common ostium technique. A remote fistula could theoretically reduce this problem by minimizing turbulence at the anastomosis.

In most clinical series the use of AVF has shown no side-effects such as steal from the distal circulation or cardiac failure. Occasional leg oedema is observed, especially in patients having sequelae following previous deep venous thrombosis, which is a contra-indication to the use of an adjuvant AVF.

CONCLUSION

There is general agreement that autologous material should be used for femorotibial bypass grafting whenever possible. Refinement of the technique has improved the patency rate following these operations. Furthermore, other treatment modalities like adjuvant pharmacotherapy, endothelial cell seeding, and the use of patches and cuffs have been introduced. It is therefore possible that the need for adjuvant AVF with femorotibial bypass will decrease in the future.

At present there is not sufficient evidence to draw firm conclusions regarding the benefit of AVF as an adjunct to distal arterial reconstructions since no controlled prospective trials have been made. However, the technique of using an adjuvant AVF may be applied in patients with critical ischaemia who otherwise are faced with a major amputation, and where conventional femorotibial bypass grafting with autologous vein is impossible for a variety of reasons. These could include patients who might need a bypass to the leg arteries with a synthetic graft. Other indications could be distal bypasses where the artery is unusually small or calcified or where

Table 2. Possible indications for adjuvant arteriovenous fistula during femorotibial reconstruction

Synthetic bypass-grafting to leg arteries
Small or calcified leg arteries
Poor run-off (multiple obstructions of the leg arteries, insufficient or absent pedal arch)
High peripheral resistance measured intraoperatively
Early re-occlusion following femorotibial bypass-grafting

the run-off is deficient due to discontinuity or multiple obstructions of the leg arteries and insufficient or absent pedal arches.[30] Another indication for the application of AVF could be in patients having a high outflow resistance measured during the operation. Thus, it has been shown that reconstructions having a total outflow resistance of more than 1.2 mm Hg/ml/min have an extremely poor prognosis.[31] Finally, patients who have an early failure following femorotibial bypass grafting due to some of the factors mentioned could be candidates for an adjunctive AVF during the reoperation (Table 2).

REFERENCES

1. Leather RP, Shah DM, Chang BB, Kaufmann JL: Resurrection of the *in situ* saphenous vein bypass: 1000 cases later. Ann Surg 208; 435–442: 1988
2. Sastrustegui SMY: Chirurgie de l'appareil circulatuire; l'anastomose arterio-veneuse. Semaine Med 22; 395: 1902
3. Sauvage LR, Berger KE, Mansfield PB *et al*: Future directions in the development of arterial prosthesis for small and medium caliber arteries. Surg Clin N Am, 54; 213–228: 1974.
4. Sumner DS: *In* Collateral Circulation in Clinical Surgery, Strandness DE Jr, (Ed.). Philadelphia and London: W. B. Saunders, pp. 27–90, 1969
5. Stelzer G, van Berge Henegouwen DP: Flow estimation by DSA in bypasses with or without a distal arterio-venous fistula. Eur J Vasc Surg 1; 227–234: 1987
6. Ingebrigtsen R, Wehn PS: Local blood pressure and direction of flow in experimental arterio-venous fistula. Acta Chir Scand 120; 142–150: 1960
7. Billet A, Queral LA, Polito WF, Dagher FJ: The vascular steal phenomenon: An experimental model. Surgery 96; 923–928: 1984
8. Hyman WA, Brewer MA: The hemodynamics of arterial steal. J Biomechanics 13; 469–475: 1980
9. Johansen K, Bernstein EF: Revascularization of the ischemic canine hindlimb by arteriovenous reversal. Ann Surg 190; 243–253: 1979
10. Gerard DF, Gausewitz SH, Dilley RB, Bernstein EF: Acute physiologic effects of arteriovenous anastomosis and fistula in revascularizing the ischemic canine hind limb. Surgery, 89; 485–493: 1981
11. Bernstein EF: Physiologic basis for arteriovenous fistulas as an adjunct to lower extremity arterial reconstructions. *In* Current Problems in Vascular Surgery, Veith FJ (Ed.). St Louis, Missouri: Quality Medical Publishing, 1989
12. Dean RE, Read RC: The influence of increased blood flow on thrombosis in prosthetic grafts. Surgery 55; 581–584: 1964
13. Gwynn BR, Shearman CP, Simms MH: Anastomotic arteriovenous fistulae—are they worth it? Eur J Vasc Surg 2; 71–76: 1988
14. Szilagyi DE, Jay GD, Munnel ED: Femoral arteriovenous anastomosis in the treatment of occlusive arterial disease. Arch Surg 63; 435–451: 1951

15. Blaisdell FW, Lim RC, Jr, Hall AD, Thomas AN: Revascularization of severely ischemic extremities with an arteriovenous fistula. Am J Surg 112; 166–174: 1966
16. Veith FJ, Gupta SK, Ascer E *et al*: Six-year prospective multicenter randomized comparison of autologous saphenous vein and expanded polytetrafluoroethylene grafts in infrainguinal arterial reconstructions. J Vasc Surg 3; 104–114: 1986
17. Flinn WR, Rohrer MJ, Yao JST *et al*: Improved long-term patency of infragenicular polytetrafluoroethylene grafts. J Vasc Surg 7; 685–690: 1988
18. Ibrahim IM, Sussman B, Dardik, I *et al*: Adjunctive arteriovenous fistula with tibial and peroneal reconstruction for limb salvage. Am J Surg 140; 246–251: 1980
19. Dardik H, Sussman B, Ibrahim IM *et al*: Distal arteriovenous fistula as an adjunct to maintaining arterial and graft patency for limb salvage. Surgery 94; 478–486: 1983
20. Dardik H: Clinical evaluation of arteriovenous fistulas as an adjunct to lower extremity arterial reconstructions. *In* Current Critical Problems in Vascular Surgery, Veith FJ (Ed.). St Louis, Missouri: Quality Medical Publishing, 1989
21. Harris PL: Adjuvant arteriovenous fistula at the distal anastomosis of a femorotibial bypass graft. *In* Vascular Surgical Techniques: An Atlas, Roger M. Greenhalgh (Ed.). London and Philadelphia: W. B. Saunders, 2nd edn, 1989
22. Harris PL, Campbell H: Adjuvant distal arteriovenous shunt with femorotibial bypass for critical ischaemia. Br J Surg 70; 377–380: 1983
23. Moody AP, Fagih SA, Edwards PR, Campbell H, Harris PL: Adjuvant arterio-venous fistula in femoro-distal bypass. J Cardiovasc Surg 31; 94–95: 1990
24. Snyder SO Jr., Wheeler JR, Gregory RT, Gayle RG: Failure of arteriovenous fistulas at distal tibial bypass anastomotic sites. J Cardiovasc Surg 26; 137–142: 1985
25. Miksic K, Flis V: Die arteriovenöse Fistel bei femoro-cruralen Rekonstruktionen. Angio 10; 27–32: 1988
26. Henegouwen van Berge DP, Stelzer G, Dautzenberg T, Helmig L, Ehresmann U: Pedal and distal lower leg bypasses with a distal arteriovenous fistula. Eur J Vasc Surg 1; 251–258: 1987
27. Hinshaw DB, Schmidt CA, Hinshaw DB, Simpson JB: Arteriovenous fistula in arterial reconstruction of the ischemic limb. Arch Surg 118; 589–592: 1983
28. Shah DM, Paty PSK, Chang BB, Leather RP: Remote distal arteriovenous fistula to improve infrapopliteal bypass patency. *In* Current Critical Problems in Vascular Surgery, Veith FJ (Ed.). St Louis, Missouri: Quality Medical Publishing, 1989
29. Paty PSK, Shah DM, Saifi J *et al*: Remote distal arteriovenous fistula to improve infrapopliteal bypass patency. J Vasc Surg 11; 171–178: 1990
30. O'Mara CS, Flinn WR, Neiman HL, Bergan JJ, Yao JST: Correlation of foot arterial anatomy with early tibial bypass patency. Surgery 89; 743–751: 1981
31. Ascer E, Veith FJ, Morin L *et al*: Components of outflow resistance and their correlation with graft patency in lower extremity arterial reconstructions. J Vasc Surg 1; 817–828: 1984

Postoperative Impedance Findings

Michael Horrocks and Michael G. Wyatt

Successful arterial grafting for critical ischaemia depends on the maintenance of an adequate blood flow to the ischaemic tissue through a patent graft. Graft failure may be due to technical error at the time of surgery or to the subsequent development of graft or run-off stenoses, either due to intimal hyperplasia or to progression of atherosclerosis.[1,2]

Following correction of technical errors, the largest group of failures occur within the first year and is due to graft related stenoses.[3] These account for up to 43% of all failures occurring in the first 5 years after surgery.[4]

Szilagyi *et al.*[3] first demonstrated that graft stenoses may develop within weeks of implantation and may rapidly progress to graft failure. The value of early detection of these lesions prior to graft failure was emphasized by Whittemore *et al.* in 1981.[1] They reported 5-year patency rates of 80% for stenoses repaired before graft failure compared with rates of less than 40% for those grafts requiring thrombectomy followed by repair. Sladen and Gilmour[5] reported a series of 173 vein grafts, 20% of which developed stenoses. These were corrected resulting in a 16% improvement in the 5-year patency rate. Bandyk *et al.*[6] have 3-year primary and secondary (modified primary) patency rates of 48% and 89% for femoropopliteal grafts and 58% and 80% for femorodistal grafts respectively. Further studies have confirmed these findings and it is concluded that if stenoses can be accurately diagnosed and corrected prior to graft occlusion, 80% of grafts can be salvaged before they fail and patency rates can be improved by 15–20%.[7,8]

Sadly many limbs with graft stenoses have no symptoms of claudication prior to sudden failure. Grafts which develop stenoses are liable to occlude and can be called 'at risk'. In order to detect these at risk limbs prior to graft failure, a graft surveillance programme is required. An ideal test should be noninvasive, easy to perform, repeatable and reproducible.[9] It should detect lesions both within the graft and more distally within the run-off vessels before clinical symptoms develop. Although various methods of graft surveillance have been advocated, none has as yet fulfilled all of these requirements.

Peripheral resistance, measured at the time of operation, can predict early graft outcome.[10–12] In a pulsatile system, in addition to viscous resistance, fluid inertia and vessel compliance become important and the concept of impedance rather than resistance becomes more relevant.[13–15] Several authors have attempted to use vascular impedance measured at the time of operation to predict outcome following femorodistal bypass, but results have been disappointing.[13,16] The use of impedance analysis for graft surveillance has not been previously explored.

A new noninvasive method of assessing impedance within a femoropopliteal/distal (FPD) graft has recently been described.[17] It involves computer assisted analysis of pulsatile pressure/flow signals and utilizes Fourier waveform analysis to predict mean limb impedance values for the thigh and calf respectively (Fig. 1).[18]

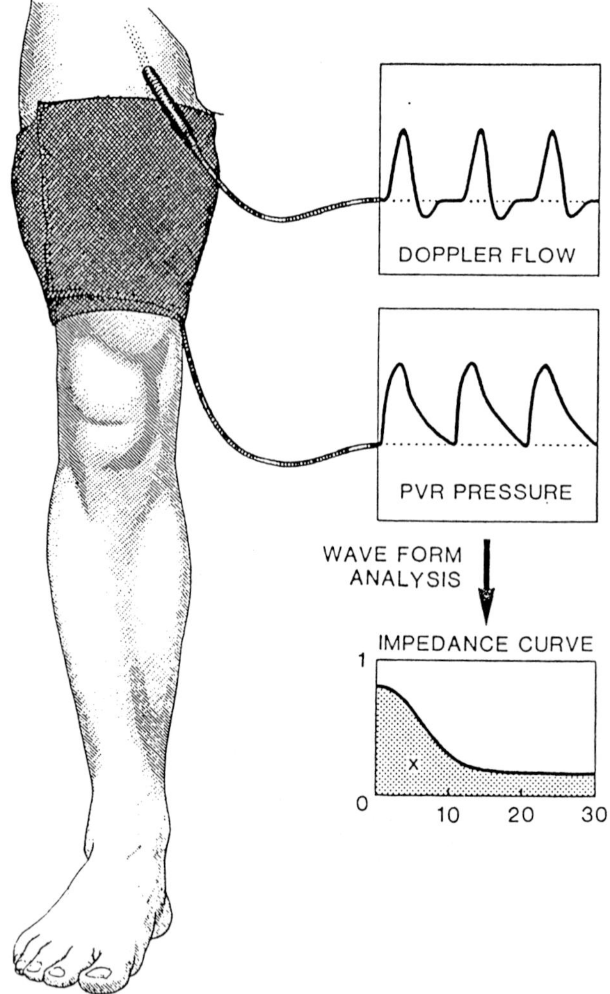

Fig. 1. Measurement of thigh impedance. A Doppler velocimeter measures pulsatile flow from the proximal graft. A pulse volume recorder measures pulsatile pressure from a cuff around the thigh. An impedance curve is produced by performing waveform analysis on the paired flow/pressure signals. The area (×) under the curve represents the mean thigh impedance and is expressed as a fraction of the total area (×/30). A similar measurement of calf impedance is made by recording Doppler flow from the lower graft and placing the cuff around the calf.

Doppler waveforms (pulsatile flow) are obtained from the upper and lower portions of the graft using a standard 8 MHz probe connected to a velocimeter (Quantascope, Vital Science, UK). Pulse volume recordings (pulsatile pressure) are obtained from segmental air plethysmography cuffs placed around the mid-thigh (20 cm cuff, 400±75 ml air) and calf (14 cm cuff, 75±75 ml air) and linked to a Pulse Volume Recorder (PVR, Life Sciences, Greenwich, Connecticut, USA).[19,20]

The means of at least 20 Doppler/PVR waveforms are stored by a portable Toshiba 2100 computer. By dividing the pressure modulus at each harmonic by the appropriate flow modulus (Fast Fourier Transfer Analysis[18]), an impedance curve can be derived for the thigh and calf respectively (Fig. 1). Errors due to inconsistency in the angle of Doppler insonation and manual manipulation of Doppler/PVR amplitudes are eliminated by 'normalization' of the vertical discrete Fourier axis (0–1). The horizontal frequency axis is limited to the first 30 radians in order to minimize errors due to reflected wave components. The area beneath the impedance curve (x) represents the mean impedance expressed as a fraction of the total available area ($\times/30$). The higher of the two impedance scores (calf or thigh) is used for subsequent data analysis. The technique is performed by a research nurse in the Vascular Studies Unit and is completed within 10–15 min.

VALIDATION STUDY

The method has been validated on 50 patients with functioning nonreversed vein grafts performed for critical ischaemia. There were 36 men and 14 women aged between 51 and 87 years (median age = 73 years). Thirty-seven grafts were performed to the popliteal artery (14 supragenicular, 23 infragenicular) and 13 to a single calf vessel. Impedance analysis was performed on all patients at a median time of 5 months postoperatively (range 1–55 months).

Following noninvasive investigation, biplaner intra-arterial digital subtraction angiography (IADSA)[21] was performed via a green needle puncture to the appropriate groin. Grafts were defined as at risk or control dependant upon the presence or absence of graft or run-off stenoses $>50\%$.

IADSA revealed 28 control grafts (no stenoses) and 22 at risk (graft/run-off stenoses $>50\%$); six lesions were within the body of the graft, six were around the distal anastomosis and ten were within the dependant run-off vessels. Control and at risk groups were evenly matched for age, sex, diabetes and smoking habit (Table 1).

Numerical results are expressed as means with 95% confidence intervals. A Kruscal–Wallace one-way analysis of variance for nonparametric data was first performed and then a Mann–Whitney U test was used to compare the individual groups. A χ^2 test with Yates correction was used for nonnumerical data analysis.

Table 1. Demographic/clinical assessment

		Controls	*At risk*
Number		28	22
Median age (range) years		71 (51–86)	73 (61–87)
Median postop (range) years		13 (1–55)	4 (1–48)
M:F		21:7	14:7
Smoking		8	5
Anastomosis	AK	6	8
	BK	17	6
	Crural	5	8
Claudication		0	5
Ulcers		3 (healing)	3
Reported improvement		28	21

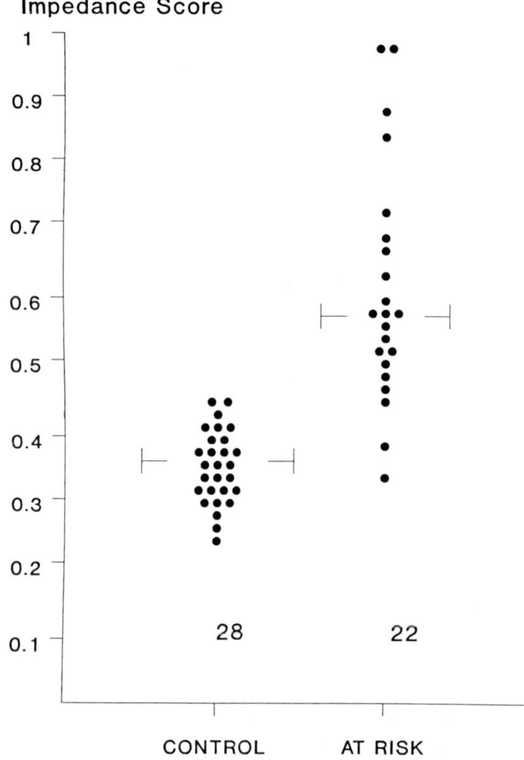

Fig. 2. Impedance scores for the 50 grafts in the validation study classified as at risk (stenoses >50%) or control (no stenoses). For each graft the higher of the two impedance scores (thigh/calf) has been used. The impedance scores for the at risk graft are significantly higher than those of the controls ($p<0.001$, Mann-Whitney U Test).

Impedance scores were significantly higher in the at risk grafts (0.58+ [0.43–0.72]) when compared with the controls (0.34+ [0.30–0.38], $p<0.001$, Fig. 2). With increasing degree of stenosis the slope of the impedance curve flattened and its enclosed area, representing the mean limb impedance, increased (Fig. 3). A calf or thigh impedance score of >0.45 was able to detect 20 of 22 stenoses (sensitivity 87%, specificity 96% and positive predictive value 93%). The two 'missed' lesions were grafts to an isolated popliteal segment.

At 1-year follow-up all control grafts were patent with no evidence of deterioration. Of the 22 'at risk' grafts, eight had occluded, seven remained at risk and seven stenoses had been successfully treated (six balloon angioplasty, one patch graft). There was a significant difference between the pre- and postangioplasty impedance values ($p<0.05$), on each occasion the impedance score returning to normal (<0.45).

GRAFT SURVEILLANCE STUDY

The noninvasive impedance technique was then applied prospectively to a graft surveillance programme. Over an 18-month period, 56 patients undergoing FPD vein

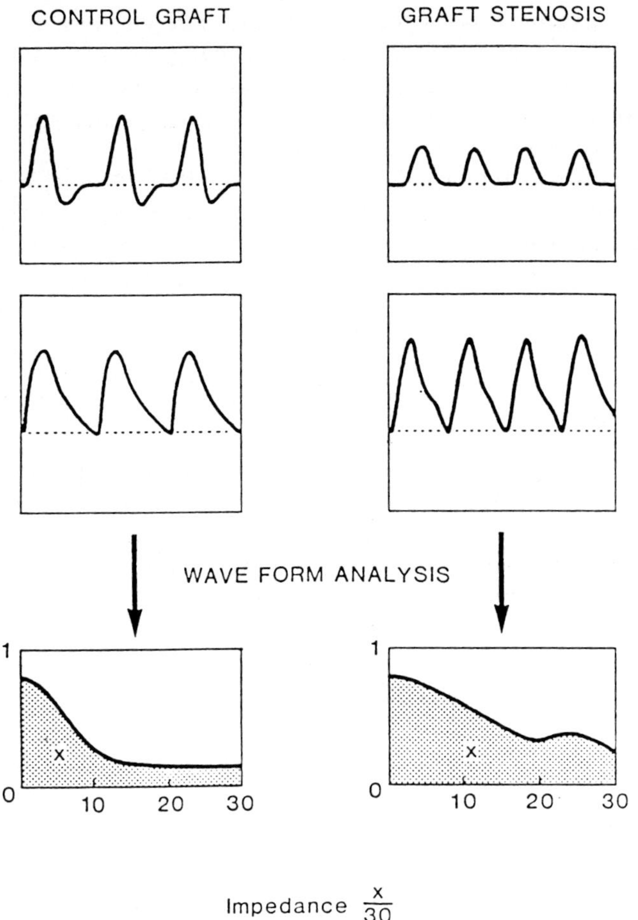

Fig. 3. Doppler, PVR and impedance curves for a normal (left) and a stenosed (right) graft. In the stenosed graft the area under the curve (x) is increased and the impedance (×/30) is high compared with the normal graft.

bypass for critical ischaemia were recruited; there were 51 men and 5 women aged between 50 and 88 years (median age=70 years). Thirty-seven veins were anastomosed to the popliteal artery (13 supragenicular, 23 infragenicular) and 19 to a single calf vessel. The following noninvasive investigations were performed at 1 week, monthly to 3 months and 3 monthly to 1 year:

Ankle brachial indices

Ankle brachial indices (ABI) were obtained from each patient at rest and following an occlusive cuff hyperaemia test.[22] Measurement of resting ankle systolic pressure was performed by the transcutaneous Doppler ultrasonographic flow-detection technique.[23] A 12-cm sphygmomanometer cuff was applied just above the ankle and a Doppler probe (8 MHz CW Huntleigh Mini Doppler velocimeter) was placed over the posterior tibial or dosalis pedis artery. The cuff was then inflated to 20 mmHg or more above the level at which flow ceases. During deflation of the cuff, a return of flow signals indicated the level of systolic pressure at the ankle. The ankle brachial index was calculated by dividing the ankle systolic pressure by the higher of the two measured brachial pressures.

The hyperaemic stress test involved placing a further 12 cm sphygmomanometer cuff around the upper calf and inflating to a pressure of 50 mmHg above systolic pressure for 2 minutes.[22] Before and immediately following deflation, the ankle and brachial pressures were measured and the posthyperaemic ankle brachial index calculated.

Duplex scanning

Each graft was examined using a 10 MHz ultrasonic duplex scanner (Autosector, Technicare Corp., Cleveland, Ohio). Real time images of the complete length of each graft were obtained and an attempt made to visualize the dependant run-off vessels. Areas of increase in the maximum frequency were noted with a frequency increase of greater than ×2 considered significant.[24] Low frequency data was not used.

Computer assisted impedance analysis

Impedance analysis was performed on each graft as described and the higher of the two values (calf/thigh) used for subsequent data analysis.

Noninvasive results were controlled using the 'gold standard' of biplaner IADSA examination[21] at 1 week and 3 monthly to 1 year. Grafts were considered to be at risk or control dependant on the presence or absence of a graft or dependant run-off stenosis >50%.

To date, serial biplanar IADSA examination has identified 22 grafts as controls (no stenoses) and 34 as at risk (graft/run-off stenoses >50%); seven stenoses were within the main body of the graft, 20 were close to the distal anastomosis and seven were within the run-off vessels.

There was a significant difference in ankle brachial indices between control and at risk grafts both at rest (0.97+ [0.95–0.99] vs 0.85+ [0.79–0.91], $p<0.05$) and following reactive hyperaemia (0.92+ [0.88–0.96] vs 0.71+ [0.61–0.81], $p<0.01$). However, whereas all control grafts had a resting ABI >0.8, there was wide variation in values recorded for the at risk grafts, with only 10 of the 34 having an ABI <0.8 (sensitivity 29%, specificity 100%, PPV 100%). The addition of a stress test (occlusive cuff hyperaemia) increased the sensitivity of ABI measurement, but despite this, 19 stenoses were missed (sensitivity 44%, specificity 91%, PPV 88%).

Duplex scanning successfully detected all seven body of graft lesions (100%), but was only able to visualize eight of 20 (40%) distal anastomotic related stenoses and none of the seven run-off lesions (0%).

Impedance scores were significantly higher in the at risk group (0.56+ [0.44–0.68]) when compared with the controls (0.38+ [0.35–0.41], $p<0.001$, Fig. 4): an impedance score of >0.45 successfully predicted 33 of the 34 lesions (97%). The single at risk

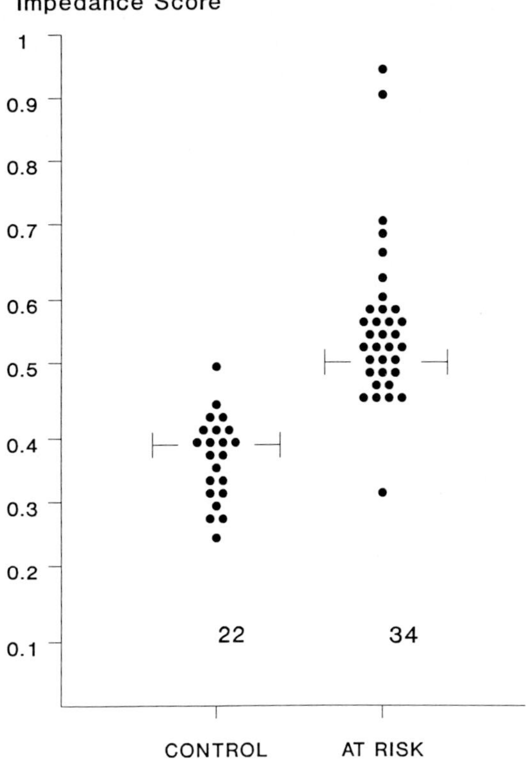

Fig. 4. Prospective graft surveillance study. The impedance scores for the at risk graft are significantly higher than those of the controls ($p<0.001$, Mann-Whitney U Test). An impedance score of >0.45 was able to predict 33 of 34 at risk grafts.

patient with a low impedance score had a kink at the knee and on subsequent examination the impedance score rose and fell as the knee was flexed and extended. The single control graft with a normal IADSA and a high impedance score utilized a very small vein (<2 mm); we would suggest that this graft is just as likely to be at risk as those with isolated stenoses.

Nine of the at risk group failed prior to intervention. In 12 at risk grafts correction was attempted (three surgical, nine balloon angioplasty). Two of the surgical revisions and seven of the angioplasties were successful; one failed angioplasty went on to successful patch revision. One control graft failed following a routine IADSA (vessel dissection). An impedance score of >0.5 successfully predicted 12 of 13 failed grafts ($p<0.001$, χ^2+Yates correction).

Following successful repair, impedance scores fell significantly from 0.56+ [0.49–0.63] to 0.38+ [0.32–0.44] ($p<0.001$, Fig. 5). In the failed intervention group ($n=5$), there was no difference between the pre- and postinterventional impedance scores (0.53+ [0.48–0.58] vs 0.50+ [0.45–0.55]).

DISCUSSION

This work has confirmed the limitations that exist if ankle pressures alone are used for graft follow-up.[25–28] Even with an occlusive cuff hyperaemic test, the sensitivity

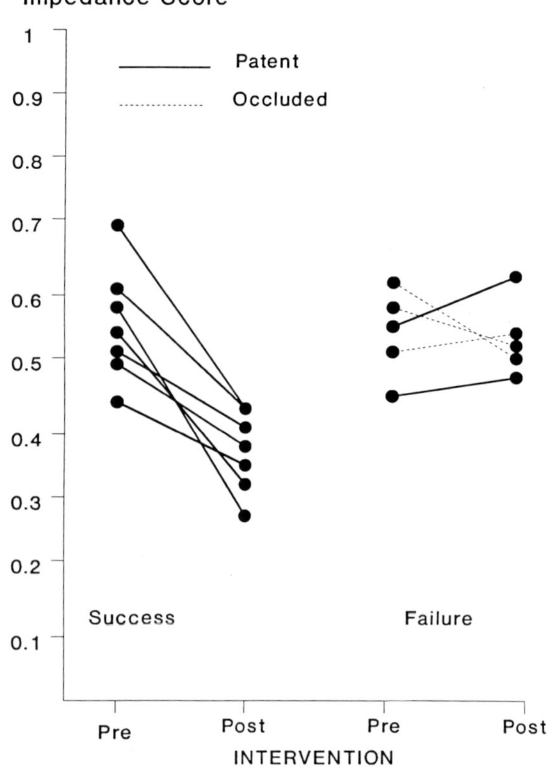

Fig. 5. Impedance scores before and after intervention for graft or run-off stenoses. Following successful repair (five angioplasty, two operative) impedance scores returned to normal (<0.45) on each occasion. For the five unsuccessful repairs (four angioplasty, one operative) the impedance scores remained high and three of these grafts have subsequently occluded. Success: $p<0.001$; failure: NS.

of ankle pressure measurement is still less than 50%. Although a standard exercise test[29] may have provided a more pronounced pressure drop than occlusive cuff hyperaemia, the difference is not significant and is compensated for by the increased patient compliance with the occlusive cuff hyperaemia test.[22]

Despite initial enthusiastic reports concerning the suitability of duplex scanning for graft surveillance,[30–33] subsequent follow-up has been disappointing and even with the introduction of colour flow techniques, as many as 10% of graft stenoses remain undetected often resulting in graft failure.[34] Although duplex scanning is excellent for body of graft lesions (100%), only one in three of distal anastomotic related and run-off lesions were successfully predicted in this study despite the use of velocity ratio criteria.[24]

Prior to impedance analysis, arteriography was the only method of detecting stenoses not visible on duplex examination in patients with normal ankle pressures.[35] Unfortunately, invasive methods of graft surveillance, including IA DSA,[31] are not without morbidity and this risk is highlighted by our single control graft which occluded following a routine IADSA. Even when IADSA is used for graft surveillance, few centres use biplanar views which must result in missed lesions. A further disadvantage of arteriography is its inability to provide haemodynamic data. Intervention should ideally be reserved for those grafts in which both an anatomical abnormality and a haemodynamic disturbance are demonstrated.

Defined as the ratio of pulsatile pressure to pulsatile flow,[18] impedance analysis considers the frequency dependant components of the arterial system and is theoretically superior to the measurement of peripheral resistance.[16] Before impedance can be calculated, both flow velocity and pressure waves must be resolved into their harmonic components. The method most widely used, and incorporated into our computer software, is harmonic analysis, in which the pulse wave is mathematically resolved by a microcomputer to a mean term and a series of sinusoidal waves (Fourier series).[18] This method has been used to calculate the impedance of vascular beds in both animals and man.[35–38] The impedance spectrum contains a large amount of information about the physical state of the vascular system and is sensitive enough to detect graft stenoses prior to significant haemodynamic deterioration.

Computer Assisted Impedance Analysis is a new, noninvasive method of estimating postoperative graft impedance. It gives an indirect indication of the relationship between pulsatile pressure and flow within the graft. The method relies entirely on the 'shape' rather than the 'amplitude' of the flow velocity and pressure waveforms, and eliminates the variability of alteration in angle of Doppler insonation and in the pressure/volume recording sensitivity.

This study has shown that following the application of 'waveform analysis' to paired Doppler/PVR waveforms, an impedance curve can be derived, which is capable of predicting the development of both graft and run-off stenoses, often before significant deterioration of peripheral pulse pressure.

The method has been validated retrospectively and an impedance score of >0.45 (calf or thigh) has been identified as the cut-off at which the function within a FPD graft begins to deteriorate. The low impedance values found in grafts to isolated popliteal segments may explain why the patency rates for these grafts are so good; many have patent geniculate vessels providing a good collateral run-off.

The application of impedance analysis to a prospective graft surveillance programme has resulted in 33 of 34 at risk grafts being successfully identified prior to arteriography.

Impedance analysis, in addition to being a very sensitive indicator of graft function, is also able to predict outcome. Grafts with an impedance score of >0.5 have a higher chance of failure than those with a lower score ($p<0.001$, χ^2). It is this group in which secondary procedures are going to improve patency rates. Furthermore, impedance analysis is able to accurately monitor graft function following successful intervention (balloon/patch angioplasty or jump graft) and may give a clear indication of stenosis recurrence. Figure 6 shows results at 1-year for intervention in a series of nonreversed femorodistal vein grafts performed for critical ischaemia.

SUMMARY

Computer assisted impedance analysis is a simple noninvasive test which can detect both graft and run-off stenoses prior to graft failure. The examination is inexpensive

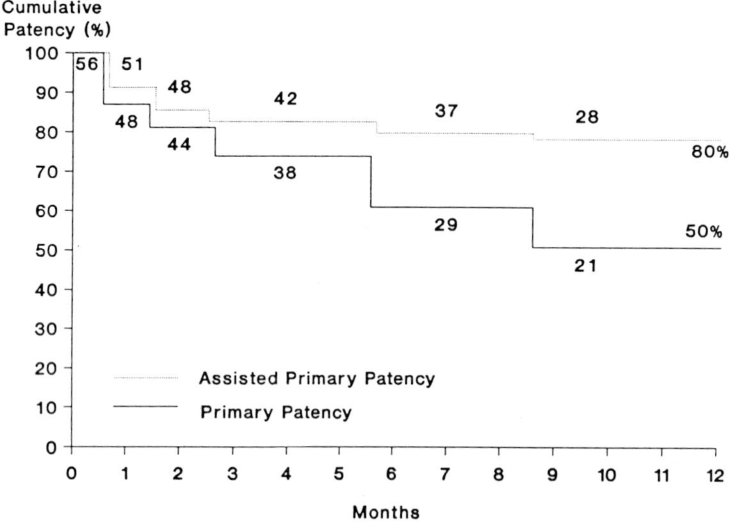

Fig. 6. Primary and assisted primary cumulative patency rates for a series of 56 FPD vein graft performed for critical ischaemia. An active policy of intervention for graft stenoses with an impedance score of >0.45 has improved the 1-year cumulative patency rate by 30%.

and quick to perform and the results are highly reproducible (coefficient of experimental error <5%). This test is now in routine use for graft surveillance in our vascular studies unit. All those patients with a high impedance score (>0.45) are examined with IADSA. This allows elective radiographic (balloon angioplasty) or surgical (patch or jump graft) intervention to be performed before graft failure. It is now policy to intervene early and this has improved our 1-year patency rate by 30%.

REFERENCES

1. Whittemore AD, Clowes AW, Couch NP *et al*: Secondary femoropopliteal reconstruction. Ann Surg 193:35–42, 1981
2. Levine AW, Bandyk DF, Bonier PF, Towne JB: Lessons learned in adopting the *in situ* saphenous vein bypass. J Vasc Surg 2:145–150, 1985
3. Szilagyi DE, Elliott JP, Hageman JF *et al*: Biologic fate of autogenous vein implants as arterial substitutes. Ann Surg 178:232–246, 1973
4. Moody P, Gould DA, Harris PL: Vein graft surveillance improves patency in femoro-popliteal bypass. Eur J Vasc Surg 4:117–121, 1990
5. Sladen JG, Gilmour JL: Vein graft stenosis: characteristics and effect of treatment. Am J Surg 41:549–553, 1981
6. Bandyk DF, Kasbnick HW, Stewart GW, Towne JB: Durability of the in-situ saphenous vein by-pass. A comparison of primary and secondary patency. J Vasc Surg 5:256–258, 1987
7. LiCalzi LK, Stanzel HC Jr. Failure of autologous reversed saphenous vein femoro-popliteal grafting: Pathophysiology and prevention. Surgery 91:352–358, 1982
8. O'Mara CS, Flinn WR, Neiman HL, Bergan JJ, Yao JST: Correlation of foot arterial anatomy with early tibial bypass patency. Surgery 89:743–752, 1981
9. Grigg MJ, Wolfe JHN, Tovar A, Nicolaides AN: The reliability of duplex derived haemodynamic measurements in the assessment of femoro-distal grafts. Eur J Vasc Surg 2:177–181, 1988

10. Beard JD, Scott DJA, Skidmore R, Baird RN, Horrocks M: Operative assessment of femorodistal bypass grafts using a new Doppler flowmeter. Br J Surg 76:925–928, 1989
11. Ascer E, Veith FJ, White Flores SA, Morin L, Gupta SK, Lesser ML: Intraoperative outflow resistance as a predictor of late patency of femoro-popliteal and infra-popliteal arterial bypasses. J Vasc Surg 5:829–827, 1987
12. Parvin SD, Evans DH, Bell PRF: Peripheral resistance measurement in the assessment of severe peripheral vascular disease. Br J Surg 72:751–753, 1985
13. Milnor WR: Pulsatile blood flow. N Engl J Med 1:27–34, 1972
14. Baird RN, Abbott WM: Pulsatile blood flow in arterial grafts. Lancet ii:948–950, 1976
15. Kidson IG: The effect of wall mechanical properties on patency of arterial grafts. Ann Roy Coll Surg (Engl) 65:24–29, 1983
16. Cave FD, Walker A, Naylor GP, Charlesworth D: The hydraulic impedance of the lower limb: It's relevance to the success of bypass operations for occlusion of the superficial femoral artery. Br J Surg 63:408–412, 1976
17. Wyatt MG, Muir RM, Tennant WG *et al*: Impedance Analysis to identify the 'at risk' femoro-distal graft. J Vasc Surg 1991 (in press)
18. McDonald DA: Blood Flow in Arteries. Baltimore: Williams and Wolkins, 1960.
19. Darling RC, Raines JK, Brener BJ, Austen WG: Quantitative segmental pulse volume recorder: A clinical tool. Surgery 72:873–887, 1972
20. Raines JK, Jaffrin MY, Tao S. A non-invasive pressure pulse recorder: development and rationale. Med Inst 7:245–250, 1973
21. Turnipseed WD, Detmer DE, Berkoff HA *et al*: Intra-arterial digital angiography: A new diagnostic method for determining limb salvage bypass candidates. Surgery 92:322–327, 1982
22. Wyatt MG, Muir RM, Tennant WG, Scott DJA, Horrocks M: An objective comparison of four stress tests in the assessment of 'at risk' femoro-distal grafts. J Cardiovasc Surg 30 (3):76–77, 1989
23. Yao JST, Hobbs JT, Irwine WT: Ankle systolic pressure measurement in arterial disease affecting the lower extremities. Br J Surg 56:675–678, 1969
24. Grigg MJ, Nicolaides AN, Wolfe JHN: Detection and grading of femoro-distal vein graft stenoses: Duplex velocity measurements compared with angiography. J Vasc Surg 8:661–666, 1988
25. Berkowitz HD, Hobbs CL, Roberts B, Freiman D, Oleaga J, Ring E: Value of routine vascular laboratory studies to identify vein graft stenoses. Surgery 90:971–979, 1981
26. Ouriel K, Zarins CK: Doppler ankle pressures—an evaluation of three methods of expression. Arch Surg 177:1297–1300, 1982
27. Cohen JR, Mannick JA, Cough NP, Whittlemore AD: Recognition and management of impending graft failure. Arch Surg 121:758–759, 1986
28. Taylor RS, Fox ND: Ultrasonic prediction of graft failure. J Cardiovasc Surg 18:309–316, 1977
29. Laing SP, Greenhalgh RM: Standard exercise test to assess peripheral arterial disease. Br Med J 1:13–16, 1980
30. Clifford PC, Skidmore R, Bird DR *et al*: Pulsed Doppler and real time duplex imaging of Dacron arterial grafts. Ultrasonic Imaging 2:381–390, 1980
31. McShane MD, Gazzard VM, Clifford PC *et al*: Duplex ultrasound assessment of femoro-distal grafts: Correlation with angiography. Eur J Vasc Surg 1:409–414, 1987
32. Bandyk DF, Cato RF, Towne JB: A low flow velocity predicts failure of femoro-popliteal and femoro-tibial bypass grafts. Surgery 98:799–809, 1985
33. Jager KA, Phillips DJ, Martin RL *et al*: Non-invasive mapping of lower limb arterial lesions. Ultrasound Med Biol 11:515–521, 1985
34. Killewich LA, Fisher CA, Bartlett ST: Color flow duplex for in situ bypass surveillance: Is the increased cost worthwhile? J Cardiovasc Surg 30 (5): 76, 1989
35. Patel DJ, De Freitas FM, Fry DL: Hydraulic input impedance to aorta and pulmonary artery in dogs. J Appl Physiol 18:134–140, 1963

36. Gabe IT, Karnell J, Porje IG, Rudewald B: The measurement of input impedance and apparant phase velocity in the human aorta. Acta Physiol Scand 61:73–84, 1964
37. Westerhof N, Elzinga G, Van den Bos GC: Influence of central and peripheral changes on the hydraulic input impedance of the arterial tree. Med Biol Eng 11:710–723, 1973
38. Mills CJ, Gabe IT, Gault JH *et al*: Pressure flow relationships and vascular impedance in man. Cardovasc Res 4:405–417, 1970

A Comprehensive Regional Vascular Registry: How is the Population Served?

D. Bergqvist, E. Einarsson, L. Norgren and T. Troëng

The results of vascular surgical procedures have progressively improved, this speciality being a fairly recent branch on the surgical tree. There has been a dramatic expansion of peripheral vascular surgery as far as number of operations is concerned.[1–3] Simultaneously, it has also been established in an increasing number of centres, the technology having been adopted by general surgeons and in some countries with the development of a speciality of its own. However, and perhaps not surprising, most clinical publications still emanate from university hospitals and the results obtained may not be true for nonuniversity institutions. From time to time there is a vivid discussion concerning volume and long-term results in surgery as a whole.[4–8]

For vascular surgery this debate has for obvious reasons been focused on prophylactic surgical interventions such as carotid endarterectomy or elective resection of nonsymptomatic abdominal aortic aneurysms.[8–16] Theoretically this is easy to accept; the results of surgery must be better than the natural course of the disease. The volume to obtain desirable results is, however, not known and may vary quite considerably because not only surgical training or volume is included in the equation but also individual skill, the decision process to accept a certain case for surgical treatment, peri- and postoperative routines including intensive care, the quality of follow-up and so on.

Also in the future it is important to present results from highly specialized centres and of new innovative ways of handling vascular diseases and follow-up after various therapeutic procedures. But it is as important also to evaluate the results of all peripheral vascular operations and the quality of vascular surgical care which can be provided to the inhabitants living in a region. This is the purpose of a clinical audit or registry.[17] Ideally it should include three components: structure (facilities and organization), process (procedures used in treatment) and outcome (results and complications). Through the registry it should be possible to identify regions and hospitals with suboptimal results and by a feedback mechanism get them corrected. It should also be possible to identify indicators highlighting poorer results than expected for the registry as a whole, also with the aim to give better care in the

***Responsible surgeons**
University hospital: Lund — Lars Norgren; Malmö — Bengt Lindblad.
County hospital: Borås — Christer Drott; Falun—Claes-Göran Björck; Halmstad — Erik Wellander; Helsingborg—Gunnar Plate; Kalmar—Åsa Molde; Karlskrona—Thomas Troëng; Karlstad — Henrik Weibull; Kristianstad—Mogens Thomsen; Växjö—Hilding Björkman; Örebro—Björn Stenberg.
District hospital: Eksjö—Eibert Einarsson; Hässleholm—Torsten Nilsson; Karlshamn — Rutger Eriksson; Landskrona — Anders Alwmark; Ljungby — Magnus Schwartz; Trelleborg — Gösta Bergman; Varberg — Lars Karlström; Värnamo — Arild Stubberöd; Ystad — Anders Evander; Ängelholm — Ingemar Hagenfeldt.

future. This is not only important for the individual patient but also has a substantial influence on the health-care costs.[18] For the surgeons involved in the registry it is important that the feedback mechanism is educational, not punitive.[19]

It must be remembered that unlike most of the other more technical methods discussed during this symposium to maintain postreconstructive patency on an individual basis, the vascular audit or registry deals with the total population of patients operated on in their peripheral blood vessels. Continuous evaluation is an ethical necessity or as Wesley S. Moore formulated the view: '. . . it is the responsibility of every surgeon. . . to monitor his experience with care. Only those surgeons with acceptable results are ultimately qualified.' However important this is from the individual point of view the aim of a vascular registry must be to cover overall results and trends, perhaps in a different way than well defined specific research projects but nonetheless important.

Vascular audits have certainly been used on a clinical basis in several centres, one model being morbidity and mortality conferences. Results from the audit of John Radcliffe Hospital in Oxford have recently been reported.[20] In the Lothian Health Board it has been part of a voluntary surgical audit with the participation of all 31 consultant general surgeons and urologists serving a population of 750 000.[21,22] The Canadian Society for Vascular Surgery has a similar audit including most surgeons.[23] In the USA vascular registries have been in use for some ten years (Upstate New York Vascular Society;[24] Cleveland Vascular Society[25–27]). In those audits and registries 30-day results have frequently been included, and they are thus dealing with registration of the surgical procedure and immediate postoperative outcome.

The aim of this chapter is to report and to discuss the experience of a population based vascular registry in southern Sweden as a means of analysing results of peripheral vascular surgery within a total population. Some aspects of it have been published previously.[28,29]

VASCULAR REGISTRY IN SOUTHERN SWEDEN

The first outline of the registry was discussed during the autumn 1985, the first half of 1986 being used to establish a protocol which turned out to be a compromise between the wish to have as many details as possible registered and to get as good compliance as possible. The protocol was to be simple without loss of important information. The aim from the very start was to cover all peripheral vascular surgery performed in the southern part of Sweden. During October 1986 a pilot study was undertaken to test the record form before starting in full scale. Only some minor changes were considered necessary and from 1 January 1987 the registry has functioned. Initially it covered the South Swedish Health Care Region with 1.4 million inhabitants as well as two hospitals with near contact to the region, making up the population basis of 1.9 million (two university hospitals, six county hospitals, nine district hospitals). By and by an increasing number of hospitals has joined, which means that the registry now covers more than 4 million of the Swedish population (8.5 million). This expansion has led to a change of name from VRISS (Vascular Registry in Southern Sweden) to Swedvasc (Vascular Registry in Sweden).

The organization is rather simple. There is a steering committee of four surgeons representing the different categories of hospitals (two from the university hospitals, one each from county and district hospitals). Every hospital has appointed one surgeon responsible for the registry. The representatives meet twice a year to discuss various problems concerning the registry as well as potential research projects. Administrative support has been provided by the board of the South Swedish Health Care Region.

When the registry started not all hospitals had personal computers available; we started with and still use record forms to be filled in and mailed to a secretary who feeds the data into the central computer. For practical and legal reasons the computer of the regional oncological centre is used. One obvious aim is the installation and use of microcomputers in every participating hospital—a goal which is near.

The variables used in the registry are summarized in Table 1. For details of layout of the record form see our first report.[28] Registration is made of all arterial surgical procedures including angio-access in the form of arteriovenous communications, percutaneous transluminal angioplasty, surgery for thoracic outlet syndrome, venous thrombectomy and venous reconstructions (but not varicose vein surgery).

From the start there have been strictly defined rules how to handle the data results from the registry and about authorship of potential publications. One aim is to use the registry as a base for prospective research projects with specific questions.

Table 1. Variables used in the vascular registry in Sweden

Preoperative	
1	Level of care
2	Risk factors
3	Operation code number (official by board of health and welfare)
4	Surgical classification (primary, secondary, elective, emergency)
5	Indication
6	Ankle brachial index
Peroperative	
7	Anatomy of inflow/outflow
8	Reconstructive procedure
9	Graft material
Outcome at 30 days	
10	Surgical complications
11	General complications
12	Nonvascular re-operations
13	Level of care
14	Function/patency
15	Ankle brachial index
16	Re-operation
Outcome at 1 year	
17	Re-operation
18	Date of amputation if any
19	Date of occlusion if any
20	Level of care
21	Function/patency
22	Ankle brachial index

ADVANTAGES AND BENEFITS WITH A REGISTRY

Consecutive registration of all peripheral vascular operations within a defined population (geographical area) creates a unique data base for assessing the value of vascular surgical technology. The health care system in Sweden is very homogenous and there are no private hospitals within the region performing peripheral vascular surgery, which means that the registry really does cover all vascular surgery in the area. With time, possible secular trends will be available for analysis.

The 1-year follow-up of such a patient series has previously not been presented, and obviously long-term results are very important.

Different aspects of quality control can be recognized, such as geographical aspects of vascular surgery, complication rates, differences between hospitals and health care levels in results of vascular surgery as well as the influence of the surgeons' training as expressed in number of operations.

Through the central computer of the regional oncological centre the registered patients are linked with the registry of causes of death. The meetings with the responsible surgeons form a basis to discuss results and serve hopefully as a feedback mechanism towards both individual surgeons and hospitals. So far, data illustrating changes on the basis of positive feed-back are lacking, but hopefully will come when the timespan of the registry is longer. Yearly reports of results from every hospital will make possible comparisons with total registry and thereby hopefully increase compliance.

PROBLEMS WITH THE REGISTRY

From the beginning one department of surgery in the southern region decided not to participate and it still does not, the reason being that this department only performs a few embolectomies a year.

One question is whether all operations really are registered. Every responsible surgeon has to decide for himself how to make the compliance as good as possible in his department. Checking against anaesthesiology registry in one university hospital showed 9% of operations to be missed (predominantly embolectomies and access procedures) and in one county hospital all procedures were registered. This is clearly more than the estimation of the approximately 80% inclusion in the Cleveland Vascular Registry.[9]

The reproducibility of the registered data has been checked by re-registration of a 10% random sample yearly during the last 3-year period. This procedure showed 90–95% agreement for most variables. However, discrepancies in some of the preoperative risk factors occurred in 42% of the cases and details in postoperative complications in 22% (Table 2). This type of validation has not been made in previous reports for registries and audits and gives important information on one weak point in registration. It also throws some doubt on the validity of retrospective data.[30]

The focus on validity problems in this form of registration is important and has not hitherto been discussed in the few available publications. The awareness of the problem will hopefully make a basis for future improvements.

Table 2. Validation of protocols. A random sample of ca 50 protocols have been refilled by the responsible surgeons at each hospital and compared with the original protocol. The majority of discrepancies are small and of minor significance only. The data shown in the table are percentage and serve as an example

	1987	*1988*	*1989*
Total protocol agreement	12	15	37
Differences in			
risk factors	42	39	17
operation code	2	0	6
indication	6	9	8
operation anatomy	4	4	8
surgical complications	22	20	10
level of care	2	0	4
ankle brachial index	6	4	8
hospitalization time	4	0	4

Another matter of concern is the uniformity of registration routines which has to do with definitions of variables in the record form. Some of them are admittedly soft and the definition is up to the surgeon filling in the record form. To simplify and unify there is written advice—and problematic issues are continuously discussed within the steering committee and twice yearly with all the responsible surgeons from each hospital. When relevant, the definitions suggested by the Ad Hoc Committee were used.[31] Concerning abdominal aortic aneurysms the clinical classification by Eriksson *et al.*[32] was adopted.

One problem, at least in Sweden, is the economic basis for such a registry. It started on the basis of individual enthusiasm and falls between the health care sector and official research funding.

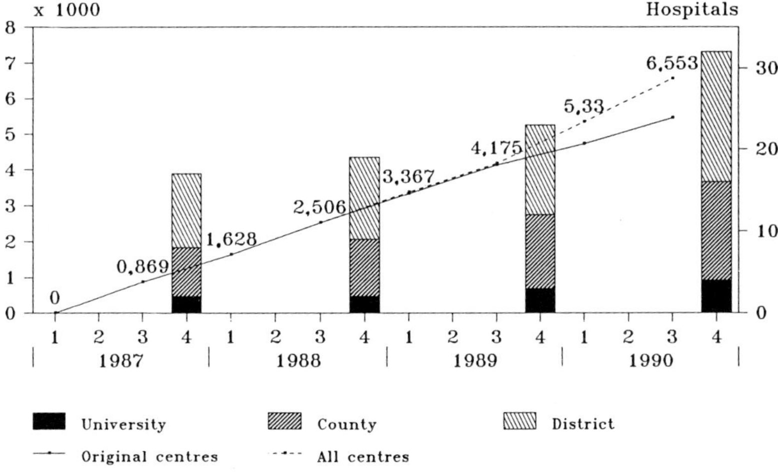

Fig. 1. The development of the Vascular Registry in Sweden in number of operations (curve) and participating centres (bar).

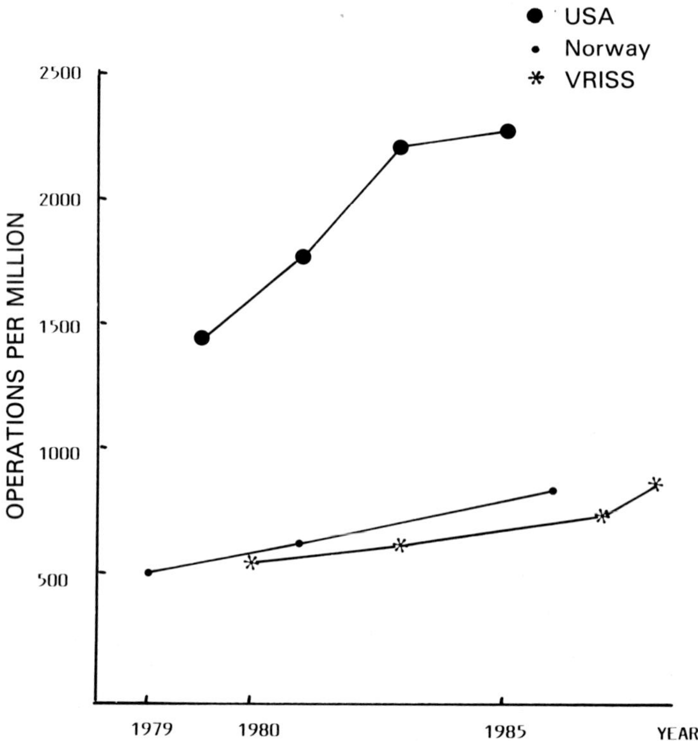

Fig. 2. The development of volume of arterial surgery per million inhabitants during the 1980s (data from 1, 2, 33, 34, VRISS).

THE VOLUME OF VASCULAR SURGERY

Figure 1 shows the recruitment speed in the VRISS, as well as the increasing number of participating hospitals. Table 3 shows the number of the most common surgical procedures performed per population unit and in those hospitals originally constituting the vascular registry of southern Sweden. In Fig. 2 the increase of vascular operations within the region is illustrated, the two first figures taken from postal questionnaires on vascular surgical performance with very high response rates (96%).[3,33,34] For the sake of interest and comparison similar curves are constructed on the basis of data from the USA[1] and Norway.[2] The number of vascular operations in the UK is of the same order of magnitude as that in Scandinavia.[35] The very large discrepancy between countries raises questions not only on possible epidemiological differences but on differences in attitudes and indications and even more important how such differences influence the results. This would indicate needs for outcome audits where uniform basic variables are registered.

Table 3. Number of some surgical procedures per million inhabitants within the original VRISS area (1.9 million)

	1987		*1988*	
Carotid endarterectomy	60		36	
Acute limb ischaemia				
embolism	114	173	109	175
thrombosis	59		66	
Chronic limb ischaemia				
claudication	127	340	168	395
critical	213		227	
Aortic aneurysm				
elective	41	69	43	71
emergent, nonrupture	8		3	
emergent, rupture	20		25	
Vascular trauma	12		9	

OUTCOME REGISTRY

From the data base of VRISS with 3417 vascular operations (in 2376 patients) 1987–1988 the most common categories dealing with infrarenal surgery were chosen to illustrate the occurrence of adverse events (complications, re-operations, amputations and mortality) and relate those to type of hospital (university, county, district), the surgeon's case load (<20, 20–50, >50 vascular procedures per year), surgical factors (level of reconstruction) and patient characteristics (sex, age, medical risk factors). For the following categories 1-month and 1-year results were analysed: acute ischaemia (670 operations), critical limb ischaemia (853 operations), intermittent claudication (570 operations) and abdominal aortic aneurysm (282 operations).

Table 4 shows 30-day mortality after surgery for abdominal aortic aneurysm. The elective seem to be treated in an adequate way. Although there were no significant differences at rupture, the experience of surgeons in hospital seems to be of some importance. Having survived the first month it is known that patients operated on for aortic aneurysm have a near normal long-term survival.[36] Table 5 shows a similar analysis for acute ischaemia. District hospitals and inexperienced surgeons (<20 vascular cases per year) show suboptimal results, especially when dealing with

Table 4. 30-day mortality after surgery for abdominal aortic aneurysm related to hospital level and surgeon's case load

	Elective		*Rupture*	
Surgeon's case load (op./year)	*No. of Op.*	*Mortality %*	*No. of op.*	*Mortality %*
<20	25	4	22	50
20–50	78	4	43	21
>50	58	3	35	34
Hospital level				
University	98	4	43	21
County	52	4	40	35
District	11	0	17	53

Table 5. 30-day patency and clinical status after surgery for acute lower limb ischaemia related to hospital level and surgeon's case load

Surgeon's case load (op./year)	*Embolism Reconstruction patent No. of op.*	*Embolism Reconstruction patent Patient better %*	*Thrombosis Reconstruction patent No. of op.*	*Thrombosis Reconstruction patent Patient better %*
<20	263	46	99	32
20–50	121	65	84	61
>50	47	60	56	63
Hospital level				
University	173	67	104	53
County	175	48	109	55
District	83	36	26	8

thrombotic occlusion (acute on chronic ischaemia). Patients with critical limb ischaemia have an immediate threat of amputation. Figure 3 shows the frequency of amputation despite reconstruction to be significantly lower when reconstruction has been made to above the groin area (10 vs 19%). The 1-year mortality is high in this group of patients (19% as a total) and with no difference dependent on the site of distal anastomosis. It can be seen that 68% of the patients were living in their homes, 5% in service centres, 7% in geriatric wards and 1% in emergency wards. Outcome was not influenced by hospital level or surgical experience. There was no sex difference. In patients with intermittent claudication, where there is a certain infirmity but usually no limb threat, the decision to perform a reconstructive surgery must focus more directly on operative risks. Figure 4 shows, not surprisingly, that

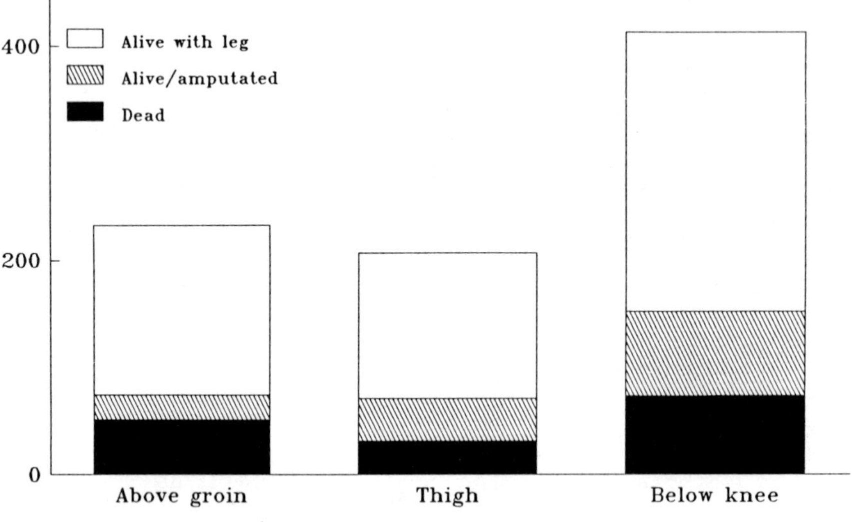

Fig. 3. Outcome 1 year after reconstruction in patients operated on because of critical low limb ischaemia in relation to the site for the distal anastomosis.

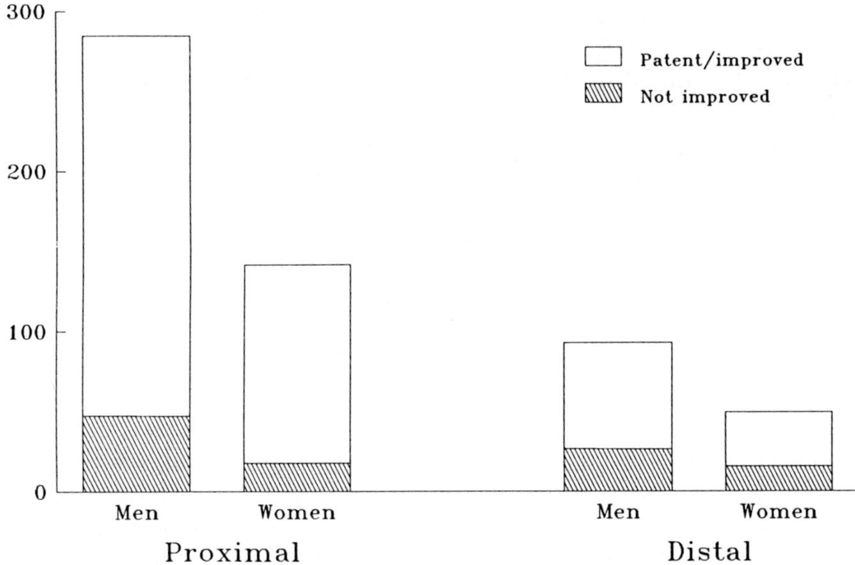

Fig. 4. Outcome 1 year after reconstruction for intermittent claudication in relation to the site for the distal anastomosis. Proximal means to the groin area distal to the popliteal artery above knee or further distally.

results are significantly better at 1-year follow-up in reconstructions with distal anastomosis in the groin area, 15% being unimproved vs 30% in claudicants operated on with a femorocrural bypass ($p < 0.001$). One interesting difference in indications is that only 10% of reconstructions for intermittent claudication were distal at university hospitals against 32% at county and district hospitals ($p < 0.000$). Surgical experience did not influence outcome, whereas the hospital level had some importance. In proximal reconstructions 1-year patency became significantly better when moving from district to university hospitals. There was no sex difference in outcome.

DISCUSSION

How to serve the whole population by a vascular registry is a very complex question, and analysis is not possible from any vascular registry published so far. A registry with such an aim must take the background population into account with exact epidemiological information and knowledge of the prevalence of the various diseases. We are far from that situation today. However, data are accumulating at least on some conditions, e.g. abdominal aortic aneurysm.[37] The selection process of patients offered surgery is also insufficiently known. One way of using the registry data for an analytical approach towards the utility of certain types of surgery in patients with a vascular problem is to use the methodology of decision analysis and in this way to calculate which outcome is a minimum to motivate surgical treatment.[38] We have used VRISS data together with data from various publications to analyse the role and value of reconstructive surgery in patients with critical limb ischaemia and intermittent claudication.[39,40]

When it is not feasible or practical to register the total population with peripheral vascular diseases, it would be a reasonable aim to register patients undergoing angiography and amputation (other than traumatic and for tumours). We have found even that too complicated and left it as an aim for the future.

The variables included in the data form may be discussed. Basically it was constructed as a modification of the record form used by Karmody *et al.*[24] and was found to work in the pilot study.[28] As already stated it is a compromise to optimize compliance and to guarantee registration both from highly specialized institutions and small district hospitals with rather few vascular cases a year. Although simple in structure the registry provides useful information and also a basis for a scientific approach to problems. Simplicity as a key factor to success with an overall registry has been stressed by Gruer *et al.*[21] and Plecha *et al.*[27] Rutherford[41] has rightly pleaded for uniform reporting routines and we have adopted criteria suggested by the Ad Hoc Committee for Reporting Standards.[31] However, in some instances there are controversial views and that can hardly fit into a vascular registry, which must be simple.

The validity and reproducibility have increased during the few years the registry has been in function. It seems important with continuous meetings and discussions to keep the compliance high and missing data low. One indication that the registry shows a fairly good function is the increasing number of hospitals joining the group after having had time to analyse it from outside. A similar registry is now starting in Finland (Lepäntalo, personal communication). It has also been used by Swedish health authorities as a functioning example of quality control within the health care system.[42] The optimal size of a registry is difficult to know. Perhaps that is reached now, covering half the Swedish population. However, when establishing other vascular registries in Sweden it would not be optimal to use different basic data than those having been shown to work in VRISS.

The use of record forms filled in by the surgeons and sent to the central registry will certainly be replaced by a personal computer system in the future. However, during the starting phase it has been valuable to have the possibility to check the individual protocols to find out where the difficulties and the missing data are. Whatever changes are made in reporting routines, it is vital that the basic data registered do not change without very strong indication. Otherwise potential alterations over time will be difficult to interpret.

Although only a little more than three years old the registry together with questionnaire data illustrates the increase of the vascular surgical volume in southern Sweden and also the spread of vascular surgical technology in peripheral direction within the health care system. Volume is the fairly easy part to register, and important to allow planning of resources in the form of number of surgeons, nurses, beds and so on. This is, however, not enough, especially not in an economy of restrained resources. As already indicated in the introductory remarks registration of volume must be linked to registration of outcome.[43] Quality assurance has become an important subject, in some countries even established legally (The Netherlands, Spain). At the same time registration of quality is very imprecise and there are huge methodological problems.[17] It is important that vascular surgeons take the responsibility in research activities dealing with quality control and assurance, and this is a major challenge for the future. If we as vascular surgeons do not go into this research activity others will force their solutions upon us.

The vascular audit or registry has a definite place in this process. In this chapter it has been illustrated by fairly simple outcome measures in the most common vascular surgical procedures. In analysing outcome and thereby defining suboptimal results it will hopefully be possible to make a more adequate choice for the surgeon in the future. One basic aim with a registry or audit is to decide on actions to correct deficiencies and then by continuing the registration show whether or not the outcome does change for the better.[19] Bad results are at least to some extent to be blamed on poor selection criteria and it is important to know when surgery is not the best treatment option, i.e., to be able to assess the appropriateness of operations.[13] How well and how often carotid endarterectomy is performed is not related to how strong an indication there is to perform it.[44] One way to improve appropriateness could be to use a registry system where the indications are well defined.

To analyse complications and thereby learn to avoid them is as important as to analyse the good results. A method of using adverse events as indicators for suboptimal performance has been suggested by the Joint Commission.[45] Some events like mortality and frequency of re-operations are signs of unsuccessful surgery, but as they reflect complex and multifactorial conditions we have found them less suitable for a straightforward quality control. More easily evaluated indicators in peripheral vascular surgery could be *re-operation* for occlusion within 1 month after a femoropopliteal bypass indicating a technical error or error in pre-or intraoperative judgement, graft infection within a month after elective vascular reconstruction, major amputation within a month of surgery for claudication and ipsilateral stroke within a month of surgery for transient ischaemic attack. Examining VRISS data for these events during 1987–1989 there were 111 cases in 5333 procedures.

This corresponds to 2.1% of all vascular procedures and results were stable during the three years, occurring in university hospitals in 1.6%, in county hospitals in 2.2% and in district hospitals in 1.8% of the procedures. Table 6 shows the indicators at the various hospital levels, no significant differences being seen. Further analyses will show whether or not these frequencies are acceptable for routine vascular surgery within a total population. For the individual patient these low-frequency events are, however, not acceptable. Moreover, they are often highly costly. It is therefore important to develop systems to identify errors of omission and commission and thereby possibilities to minimize their impact.[46,47]

For the future it is possible to expand the registry. One obvious need is to include data to make a more relevant quality analysis with social function of the patients after surgery, health indices and possibilities to make cost benefit approaches to the problems.[48] However, analysing the quality of life is still associated with difficult methodological problems.[49]

Now that the registry works it is another obvious aim to perform prospective studies on well-defined problems, e.g. types of surgery, adjuvant pharmacological treatment (to increase patency or decrease infections), comparison of grafts, comparison of surgical procedures and nonsurgical intraluminal interventions and so on. The number of patients in the registry is large and we believe it to be an ethical responsibility to use such registry for prospective research. In those cases the record form has to be modified into a study protocol for that specific project and used within a well-defined time limit, the basic variables being a common denominator in all protocols. The most informative surgical registry probably is the

Table 6. Indicators in peripheral vascular surgery 1987–89

	University hospital			*County hospital*			*District hospital*		
	No. of operations	*No. of indicators*	*%*	*No. of operations*	*No. of indicators*	*%*	*No. of operations*	*No. of indicators*	*%*
Reop. for occlusion	252	19	7.5	544	52	9.6	110	8	7.3
Graft infection	1257	6	0.5	1967	15	0.8	342	2	0.6
Major amputation	256	3	1.2	571	2	0.4	152	1	0.7
Ipsilateral stroke	61	2	3.3	63	1	1.6	0	0	—

prospective clinical trial but this must be limited in time. Routine outcome registration outside randomized prospective trials, on the other hand, will constantly be subject to changes and modifications on the basis of result analysis and feedback systems.

REFERENCES

1. Ernst CB, Rutkow IM, Cleveland RJ *et al*: Vascular surgery in the United States. Report of the Joint Society for Vascular Surgery–International Society for Cardiovascular Surgery Committee on Vascular Surgical Manpower. J Vasc Surg 6:611–612, 1987
2. Saether O, Myhre HO, Geiran O: Karkirurgi i Norge 1986. Tidskr Nor Lægeforen 109:23–26, 1989
3. Bergqvist D: Enkätsvar 1987: Ökning av artärkirurgi men stora regionala skillnader. Läkartidn 87:369–371, 1990
4. Luft HS, Bunker JP, Enthoven AC: Should operations be regionalized? The empirical relation between surgical volume and mortality. N Engl J Med 301:1364–1369, 1979
5. Squires JW, Johnson RE: Does the surgeon's annual case load make a difference in the quality of peripheral vascular surgery? A report of the mortality, morbidity, and long-term results of 101 procedures performed over 93 months. Arch Surg 120:781–785, 1985
6. Maeriki SC, Luft HS, Hunt SS: Selecting categories of patients for regionalization. Implications of the relationship between volume and outcome. Medical Care 24:148–158, 1986
7. Roos L, Cageorge S, Roos N, Danzinger R: Centralization, certification, and monitoring. Readmissions and complications after surgery. Medical Care 24:1044–1066, 1986
8. Hannan EL, O'Donnell JF, Kilburn H, Bernard HR, Yazici A: Investigation of the relationship between volume and mortality for surgical procedures performed in New York state hospitals. J Am Med Assoc 262:503–510, 1989
9. Hertzer NR, Avellone JC, Farrell CJ *et al*: The risk of vascular surgery in a metropolitan community. With observations on surgeon experience and hospital size. J Vasc Surg 1:13–21, 1984
10. Flood AB, Scott WR, Ewy W: Does practice make perfect? Part I: The relation between hospital volume and outcomes for selected diagnostic categories. Medical Care 22:98–114, 1984
11. Flood AB, Scott WR, Ewy W: Does practice make perfect? Part II: The relation between volume and outcomes and other hospital characteristics. Medical Care 22:115–125, 1984
12. Callow AD, Caplan LR, Correll JW *et al*: Carotid endarterectomy: what is its current status? Am J Med 85:835–838, 1988
13. Winslow CM, Solomon DH, Chassin MR *et al*: The appropriateness of carotid endarterectomy. N Engl J Med 318:721–727, 1988
14. Leape LL, Park RE, Solomon DH *et al*: Relation between surgeons' practice volumes and geographic variation in the rate of carotid endarterectomy. N Engl J Med 321:653–657, 1989
15. VRISS (Vascular Registry in Southern Sweden): Samband mellan volym och resultat-finns det inom svensk kärlkirurgi? Läkartidn 87:2564–2566, 1990

16. Amundsen S, Skjærven R, Trippestad A, Søreide O: Abdominal aortic aneurysms. Is there a relationship between surgical volume, surgical experience, hospital type and operative mortality? Acta Chir Scand 156:323–328, 1990
17. Wilkin A, McColl I: Surgical audit: the clinician's view. Theor Surg 1:195–206, 1987
18. Zook CJ, Moore FD: High-cost users of medical care. N Engl J Med 302:996–1002, 1980
19. Ashbaugh D, McKean R: Continuing medical education. The philosophy and use of audit. J Am Med Assoc 236:1485–1488, 1976
20. Campbell WB, Souter RG, Collin J, Wood RFM, Kidson IG, Morris PJ: Auditing the vascular surgical audit. Br J Surg 74:98–100, 1987
21. Gruer R, Gordon DS, Gunn AA, Ruckley CV: Audit of surgical audit. Lancet i:23–26, 1986
22. Clason AE, Stonebridge PA, Duncan AJ *et al*: Acute ischaemia of the lower limb: the effect of centralizing vascular surgical services on morbidity and mortality. Br J Surg 76:592–593, 1989
23. Sladen J: Morbidity audit, 1984, Canadian Society for Vascular Surgery. Can J Surg 30:3–4, 1987
24. Karmody AM, Fitzgerald K, Branagh M, Leather RP: Development of a computerized vascular registry for large-scale use. J Vasc Surg 1:594–600, 1984
25. Avellone JC, Beven EG, Hertzer NR *et al*: A regional specialty society as a model to monitor surgical care. J Am Med Assoc 240:2177–2180, 1978
26. Plecha FR, Avellone JC, Beven EG, DePalma RG, Hertzer NR: A computerized vascular registry: experience of the Cleveland Vascular Society. Surgery 86:826–835, 1979
27. Plecha FR, Bertin VJ, Plecha EJ *et al*: The early results of vascular surgery in patients 75 years of age and older: An analysis of 3259 cases. J Vasc Surg 2:769–774, 1985
28. VRISS (Vascular Registry in Southern Sweden): The vascular registry–a responsibility for all vascular surgeons? Eur J Vasc Surg 1:219–226, 1987
29. VRISS (Vascular Registry in Southern Sweden): Vascular Surgery in Southern Sweden–the first year experience of a vascular registry. Eur J Vasc Surg 3:563–569, 1989
30. Williams JG, Kingham MJ, Morgan JM, Davies AB: Retrospective review of hospital patient records. Br Med J 300:991–993, 1990
31. Ad Hoc Committee on Reporting Standards: Suggested standards for reports dealing with lower extremity ischemia. J Vasc Surg 4:80–94, 1986
32. Eriksson I, Hallén A, Simonsson N, Åberg T: Surgical classification of abdominal aortic aneurysms. Acta Chir Scand 145:455–458, 1979
33. Bergqvist D: Kartlaggning av arteriell kirurgi i Sverige. Stora regionala skillnader finns. Läkartidn 79:1891–1892, 1982
34. Bergqvist D: Enkät om svensk kärlkirurgi 1983: Antalet operationer har ökat markant men ännu är behovet troligen inte täckt. Läkartidn 82:3490–3491, 1985
35. Darke S: The provision of vascular surgery. Eur J Vasc Surg 1:217–218, 1987
36. Søreide O, Lillestøl J, Christensen O *et al*: Abdominal aortic aneurysms: survival analysis of four hundred and thirty-four patients. Surgery 91:188–193, 1982
37. Bengtsson H, Bergqvist D, Sternby NH: Increasing prevalence of abdominal aortic aneurysms—an autopsy-based study. (In prep.)
38. Doubilet P, McNeil BJ: Clinical decisionmaking. Medical Care 23:648–662, 1985
39. Troëng T, Bergqvist D, Janzon L, Jendteg S, Lindgren B: Reconstructive surgery or primary amputation in critical limb ischaemia—a decision analysis. J Vasc Surg 1991 (in press)
40. Troëng T, Bergqvist D, Janzon L, Jendteg S, Lindgren B: Surgery or conservative treatment in intermittent claudication—toss-up? (in prep.)
41. Rutherford RB: Computerized data management for the vascular surgeon: Introductory remarks. A plea for uniform reporting practices. J Vasc Surg 1:582–584, 1984
42. Spri: Kvalitetssäkring i kirurgi och anestesiologi. Sprirapport 289, Stockholm 1990
43. Ellwood P: Shattyck lecture—outcomes management. A technology of patient experience. N Engl J Med 318:1549–1556, 1988
44. Brook RH, Park RE, Chassin MR *et al*: Predicting the appropriate use of carotid endarterectomy, upper gastrointestinal endoscopy, and coronary angiography. N Engl J Med 323:1173–1177, 1990
45. O'Leary D: The joint commission looks to the future. J Am Med Assoc 258:951–952, 1987

46. Couch NP, Tilney NL, Rayner AA, Moore FD: The high cost of low-frequency events. The anatomy and economics of surgical mishaps. N Engl J Med 304:634–637, 1981
47. Troëng T, Janzon L: Assessing and monitoring of errors and complications in surgery. A review of rationales, obstacles and methods. Theor Surg 3:152–161, 1988
48. Bergqvist D, Jendteg S, Lindgren B: Standards for the cost-benefit approach to vascular surgery. Acta Chir Scand (Suppl) 555:105–110, 1990
49. Eypasch E, Troidl H, Wood-Dauphinée S *et al*: Quality of life and gastrointestinal surgery—a clinimetric approach to developing an instrument for its measurement. Theor Surg 5:3–10, 1990

How Can Thrombolytic Agents Influence Long-term Results of Arterial Bypass Grafts?

B. R. Hopkinson

Thrombolytic agents such as streptokinase, urokinase and more recently tissue plasminogen activators have all been used to dissolve clots in arteries, veins and occluded arterial bypass grafts. The first effective agent was produced by Tillott and Garner[1] in 1933 who found that proteases produced by streptococci had a fibrinolytic effect. Intravenous streptokinase was used in the 1960s for systemic thrombolysis to treat patients with acute ischaemia from arterial and venous causes, but fell into disrepute because many patients became allergic to the drug and others had serious bleeding problems.

Dotter *et al.*[2] described the low dose method of thrombolysis by injecting streptokinase directly into a clot via a radiologically placed arterial catheter. The dose required could be reduced to a twentieth. This technique proved to be much more effective and reliable than intravenous systemic therapy, presumably because the thrombolytic agent was directed to precisely where it was needed; there was a much lower allergic and haemorrhagic problem because of the lower dose released systemically. The difficulty was, of course, that skilled angiographic techniques were required to place the catheter accurately in the first place and in the 1970s these skills were not universally available. Slowly over the years since that time the techniques and skills required for the Dotter technique have become much more widely available and currently most radiological departments that regularly undertake angiography should be capable of using this method.

Advances in X-ray imaging such as digital subtraction angiography have enabled diagnostic films to be obtained using smaller intra-arterial catheters, and cause less local haemorrhagic complications than the larger catheters used before. On many occasions good quality angiograms can be obtained using intravenous digital subtraction techniques with minimal risk of haemorrhage from the venous puncture site. In the future the refinements of duplex ultrasound and magnetic resonance imaging may well make the puncture of arteries and veins unnecessary for the examination of peripheral arteries. Isotope imaging techniques are also being developed to enable recently formed clots to be identified using radioactively labelled platelets.[3] There is a hope here that the more recent the clot and the greater the turnover of platelets in it, the more it will enhance and help to identify not only where the clot is, but also which parts of the clot are more likely to be lysed.

Another advance which has enabled bleeding to be less troublesome is the routine use of the contralateral femoral artery to introduce the catheter for lysis. Advances in catheter manufacture have enabled the 'up and over' method to place a catheter via the contralateral femoral, 'up and over' the aorta and down into the thrombosed segment itself. Using this method the thrombolytic agent is much more dilute by the time it gets to the contralateral arterial puncture and there is less risk of any back perfusion of more concentrated lysing agent upto the femoral on an ipsilateral puncture site. The use of an introducer sheath through which the manoeuvres to advance or change the catheter can be performed have been advocated by Dawson *et al.*[4] to minimize trauma to the vessel as well as bleeding.

Advances in thrombolytic agents have also occurred since the first rather crude preparations of streptokinase were available. Acetylated Plasminogen-Streptokinase Activator Complex (Beecham Pharm.) (APSAC) is claimed by its manufacturers to be more 'clot specific' than streptokinase, but clinical work on peripheral arterial thrombosis has not yet substantiated their claim.[5] Urokinase[6] has been advocated in the USA as being better and safer than streptokinase but it has been generally too expensive to be used widely in the UK. More recently tissue plasminogen activator[7,8] and the genetically engineered recombinant tissue plasminogen activators (t-PA) have been introduced with claims of less bleeding, less reactions and more effective lysis of a clot. So far the agent is not widely available in the USA, although the centres that have used it have been enthusiastic about it. To date, although good individual results have been claimed for recombinant t-PA from different centres in England, no proper controlled trials have been performed to compare it with urokinase or streptokinase. Our own work in Nottingham suggests that it is better than APSAC when given intravenously and better than streptokinase when given intravenously or intra-arterially, but the evidence is not conclusive. To get proper controlled trials would be a very difficult task because of the relatively small number of cases presenting to any one centre and the extreme difficulty of matching cases within one centre, let alone with other centres in a multicentre trial. This trial, however, must be done some day because t-PA is much more expensive currently than the other available agents and its expense must be justified by proven clinical advantages. It may be that the centres that get better results with recombinant t-PA are now more skilled and experienced with the use of thrombolysis than when they started with streptokinase. The most useful attribute of recombinant t-PA is that it can be used repeatedly on the same patient with minimal risk of reaction, whereas streptokinase can commonly only be used once and can produce quite nasty reactions when patients are re-exposed to it. Perhaps the cheaper streptokinase should be used for the first course of thrombolysis and the more expensive t-PA held in reserve for any repeated treatment that may be required.

TIME FACTOR AND URGENCY OF THE SITUATION

The big disadvantage of thrombolysis, either intravenously or with the low dose intra-arterial method, is that it takes a long time to dissolve the offending clot and is certainly much slower than most surgical procedures: the time for lysis may vary from 12 to 72 hours. In our own practice, patients who have severe ischaemia with neurosensory and motor deficits are not thought to be appropriate for lysis and are sent off for immediate arteriogram with a view to urgent surgery. Our experience of urgent surgery for acute severe ischaemia with neurological deficit would suggest that surgery is very good for bypassing large vessels, such as those down to the level of the common femoral but the results for bypasses below the inguinal ligament to popliteal and distal vessels are not so good.

The big advantage of thrombolysis over surgery is that it enables the clot to be etched away more elegantly and delicately. The local damage created by the insertion of a fine intra-arterial thrombolysis catheter is very small compared with any surgical approach and it may be that, after all the clot has been removed by lysis, the offending stenosis which has caused the thrombosis can be identified and dealt with by a balloon dilatation before the lysing catheter is removed. Surgery is, of course, very good at clearing large vessels with the thrombectomy catheter but is really unreliable in its ability to remove clot from tibial and smaller vessels, whereas thrombolytic agents can often reach those parts quite easily and obtain an effective clearance of the run-off. Surgery can safely follow after thrombolysis because the biochemical effects of thrombolysis can be reversed but to undertake thrombolysis within a week of surgery is potentially hazardous because the most recent clot, that which is in the healing wound itself, is the most likely to be dissolved by the thrombolytic agent and thus cause local problems. If a situation is revealed by lysis that is clearly not going to respond to a simple balloon dilatation, surgery may be needed and can be quite safely performed at a convenient time. If thrombolysis is limited to patients with viable limbs and no neurological deficit, subsequent surgery or intervention by balloon dilatation can be performed as secondary procedures on planned angiographic or operating lists.

ESSENTIALS FOR GOOD THROMBOLYSIS

1. *A first class radiologist* who can reliably produce angiograms showing which vessels are patent from the aorta to the foot, and who can insert the lysing catheter well down into the offending clot, preferably by a remote entry point such as the contralateral femoral or brachial artery.

2. *Good nursing staff* are required to look after the patient, either on the ward or in the intensive treatment unit. They have to supervise the catheter and make sure that it stays in.

3. *An electrically driven syringe pump* is needed as a reliable way to regularly deliver the appropriate dose of thrombolytic agent.

4. *Facility for repeated angiograms* at 4 h, 6 h and then every 12 h until either lysis is complete or ceases to advance. In Nottingham we use a portable X-ray machine and a hand held injection of contrast medium to achieve this injecting directly down the thrombolytic catheter.

5. *Resident medical staff* are required to supervise the advancement or withdrawal of the catheter as lysis is seen to be taking place on the repeated angiograms.

6. *A skilful radiologist* is sometimes required to advance the catheter and to perform balloon dilatation on any residual stenoses revealed by the lysis before the catheter is removed.

7. *Enthusiastic surgeons* are required to deal with stenoses and occlusions that cannot be dissolved or dealt with by the radiologists. Patch angioplasties and inflow or outflow bypass procedures are often needed to augment flow past a recently thrombosed segment.

CAN THROMBOLYTIC AGENTS DECLOT VASCULAR GRAFTS?

It has been repeatedly shown that the most likely time for a graft to clot is within its first 24 h, and this is most often due to a technical error and repeat surgery is required to correct it. There is no place for thrombolytic agents in declotting vascular grafts during the first week after surgery; the cause is almost certainly a surgically correctable one or an error of selection in the first place and thrombolytic agents will simply dissolve the clot in the wound and create haemorrhagic problems. For grafts that clot after a week, and certainly ones that clot after they have been going for 4 weeks, there is a definite place for thrombolytic agents to be considered. Thrombosed grafts have been cleared quite successfully up to several weeks after the onset of the occlusion.

PLACE OF INTRAVENOUS SYSTEMIC THROMBOLYSIS

The simplest application of thrombolytic agents is to use them intravenously. This, of course, has a great appeal for centres where the necessary radiological skills to place intra-arterial catheters are not readily available. Although this technique may help to unblock a few grafts, the results are unreliable and the technique is not widely practised. If the graft is a woven or knitted Dacron there is always a great worry that the clot in the graft wall will dissolve, and there have been reports of quite serious bleeding straight through the graft. If the graft is within the abdomen, dangerous retroperitoneal bleeding may not be immediately recognized. There are a few reports of bleeding taking place straight through PTFE grafts but these are not so common. There is a certain logic in applying thrombolysis to clotted vein grafts, but published results for declotting vein grafts by intravenous thrombolytic agents are very poor indeed. The best report is by Earnshaw *et al.*[9] who in a retrospective survey of 19 carefully selected patients reported that 47% of thrombosed grafts were able to be lysed, but this did not mean that the grafts all continued to be patent. One patient died 3 days after treatment from unrelieved distal ischaemia despite apparently successful restoration of flow in an occluded aortobifemoral graft. Our own experience with intravenous lysis for occluded grafts in Nottingham show that none of the seven attempted had any evidence of initial lysis despite giving adequate doses for between 32 and 88 h. In this small series there were one major bleed, one minor bleed, two deaths and three patients came to Gritti–Stokes amputations, leaving only two patients' limbs still viable after 30 days.

THE USE OF INTRA-ARTERIAL LOW DOSE THROMBOLYSIS FOR THROMBOSED GRAFTS

The literature on this subject is rather confusing because generally the graft occlusions are a small number of cases reported within a larger series of acute arterial thromboses. Almost all authors agree that if you do not get the catheter directly into the clot within the graft there is a very remote chance of getting any lysis of clot in that graft.[10] They also agree that if the catheter can be introduced well into

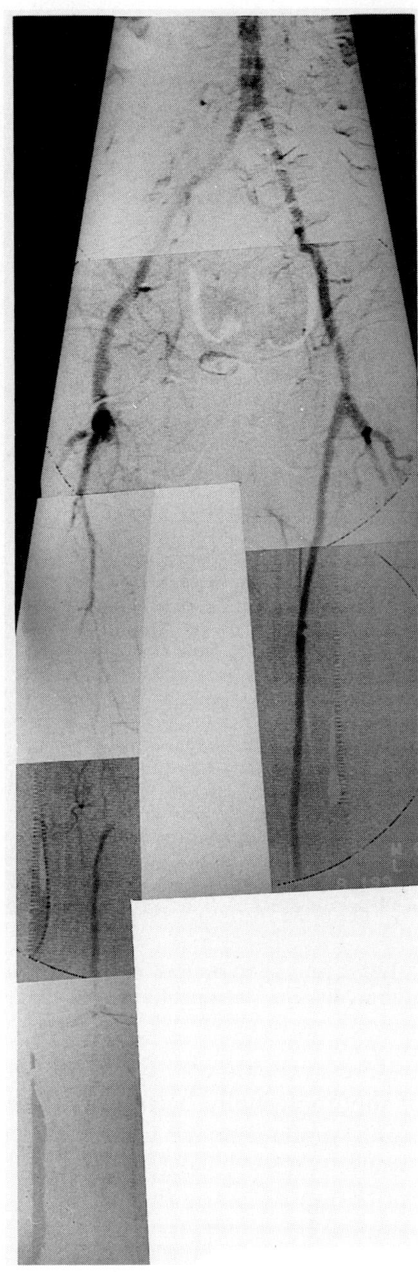

Fig. 1a. A composite picture from several DSA films showing a patent left femoropopliteal vein graft and an occluded right femoropopliteal vein graft refilling at the popliteal above the knee joint.

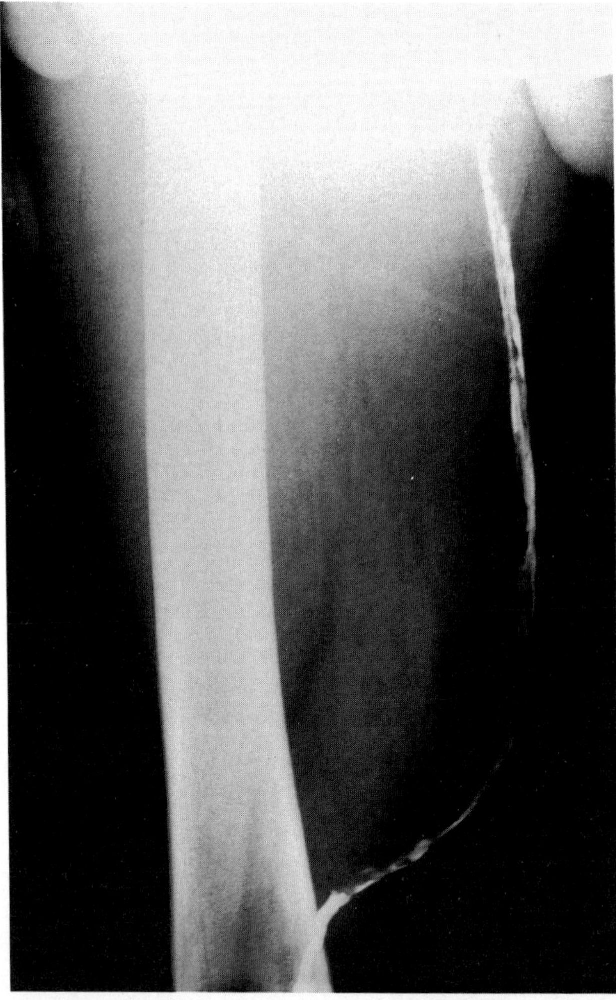

Fig. 1b. Thrombolysing catheter has been introduced from the top to the bottom of the occluded graft. Thrombolysis with streptokinase is beginning to take place.

the clot in the graft this is quite a reliable way of producing lysis of that clot in that graft. The results are probably marginally better for thrombolysis associated with polytetrafluoroethylene (PTFE) grafts than for vein grafts, and the improved results claimed for clotted PTFE grafts probably relate to the smooth and uniform nature of the wall and diameter of that graft in the first instance, whereas vein grafts are of variable diameter and seem to be subject to more specifically graft stenoses than are PTFE grafts. The experience described in the literature for thrombolysis of woven and knitted Dacron grafts is relatively small. Van Breda *et al.*[11] in 1984 reported 22 occluded grafts of which 14 were below the inguinal ligament, but only four were aortofemoral grafts. He concluded that there was more prospect of success in grafts distal to the inguinal ligament. Durham[12] reported good lysis of 17 Dacron

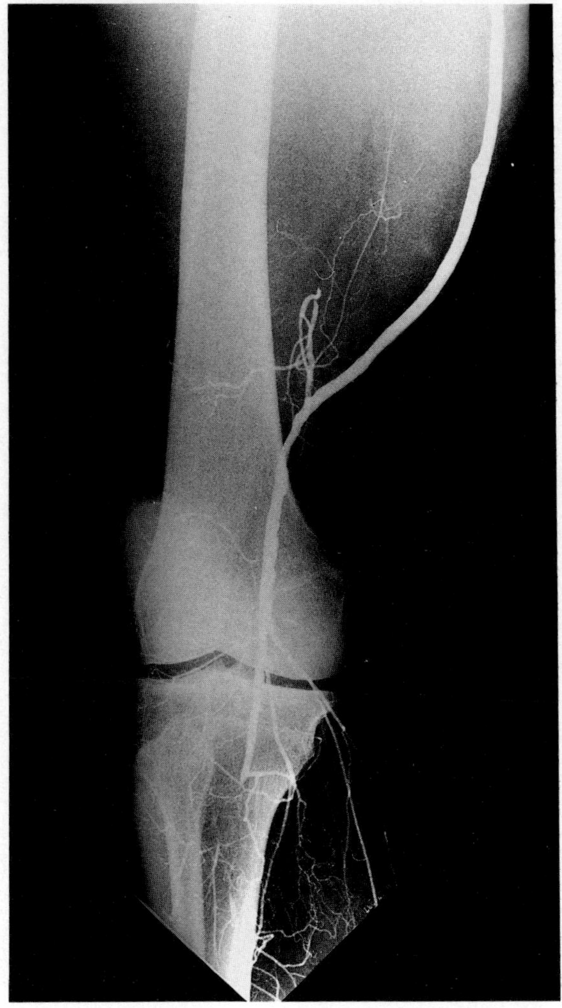

Fig. 1c. Complete thrombolysis of the graft has occurred but the thrombosis in the lower popliteal trifurcation persists.

grafts but felt that surgery was better for supra-inguinal grafts. Graor *et al.*[7] in 1986 reported 16 bypass grafts treated by t-PA, wherein two were Dacron grafts, seven were vein grafts and seven were PTFE. In 1984 Graor *et al.*[13] described a previous series using streptokinase to lyse 35 grafts, of which 12 were vein, 12 were PTFE and 11 were Dacron; he reported that six artificial grafts had significant extravasation of blood straight through the graft wall. In the British literature Walker and Giddings[14] in 1988 reported on seven vein grafts in which they achieved lysis in all and two aortobifemoral grafts wherein they achieved lysis in one. Despite 100% lysis of the seven vein grafts, all of them came to subsequent amputation; even the two patients with thrombosed aortofemoral grafts came to amputation despite the fact one of them had effective lysis and the other one suffered from significant

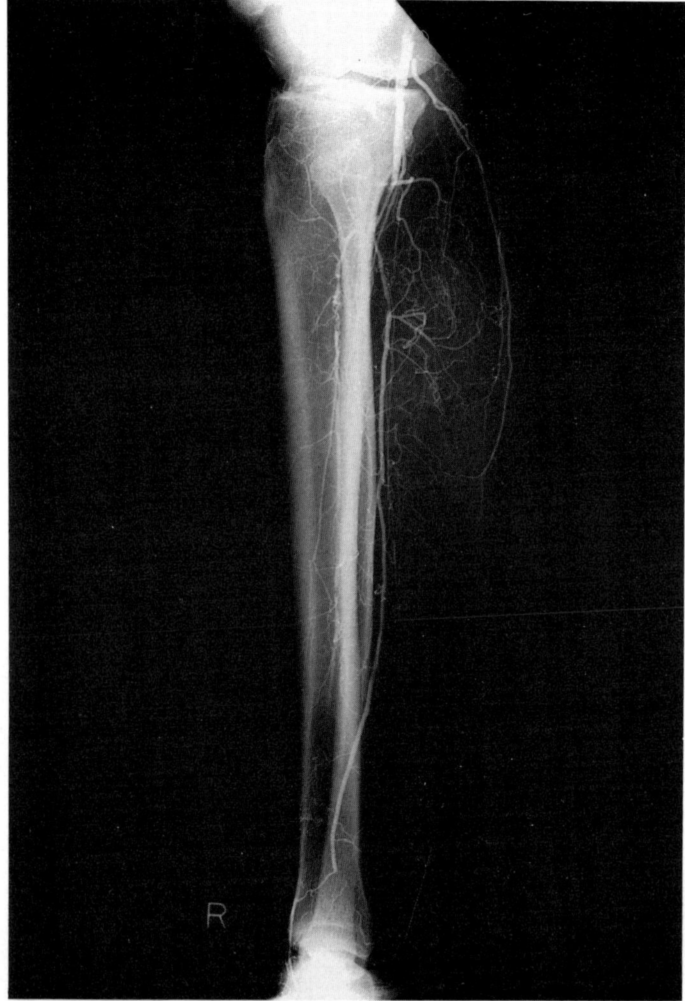

Fig. 1d. Despite continuing thrombolytic therapy the popliteal trifurcation remains occluded and is probably the reason why the graft clotted in the first place. An extension graft was performed to bypass the block from the lower end of the graft to the peroneal artery.

haemorrhage. In our own Nottingham series we have only attempted intra-arterial lysis on one Dacron graft; no lysis was achieved and the patient suffered a major haemorrhage. Al-Kutoubi describes (personal communication) one successful Dacron graft lysis and Plant (personal communication) one bleeding Dacron graft after 24 hours of lysis.

I think we can conclude that the use of thrombolytic agents for woven and knitted Dacron grafts is not very popular. The risks of haemorrhage straight through the graft are significant and it is probably wise to avoid thrombolytic agents for the treatment of thrombosed Dacron grafts, although a small number of successes have been reported.

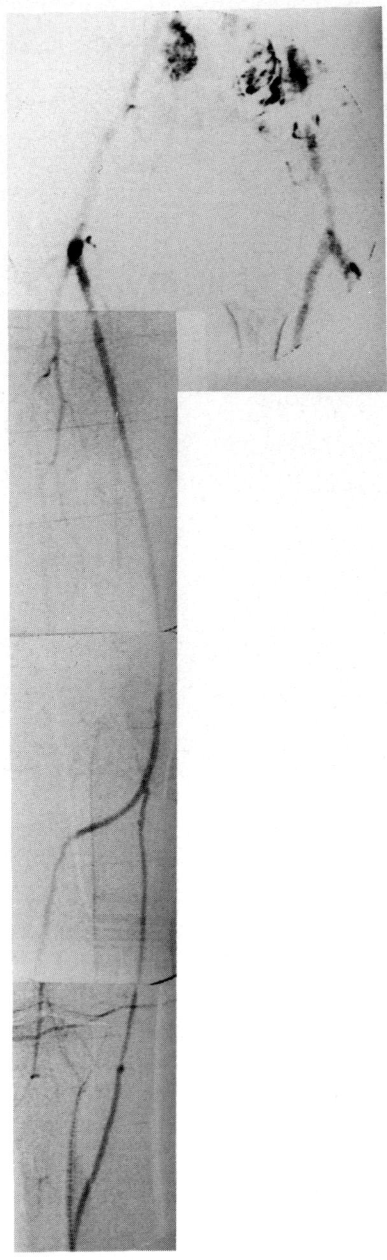

Fig. 1e. A composite DSA picture showing a patent extension graft from the lower end of the thrombolysed femoropopliteal graft going down to the peroneal. The saphenous vein from the lower leg was used for this graft. It continues to function well 9 months later.

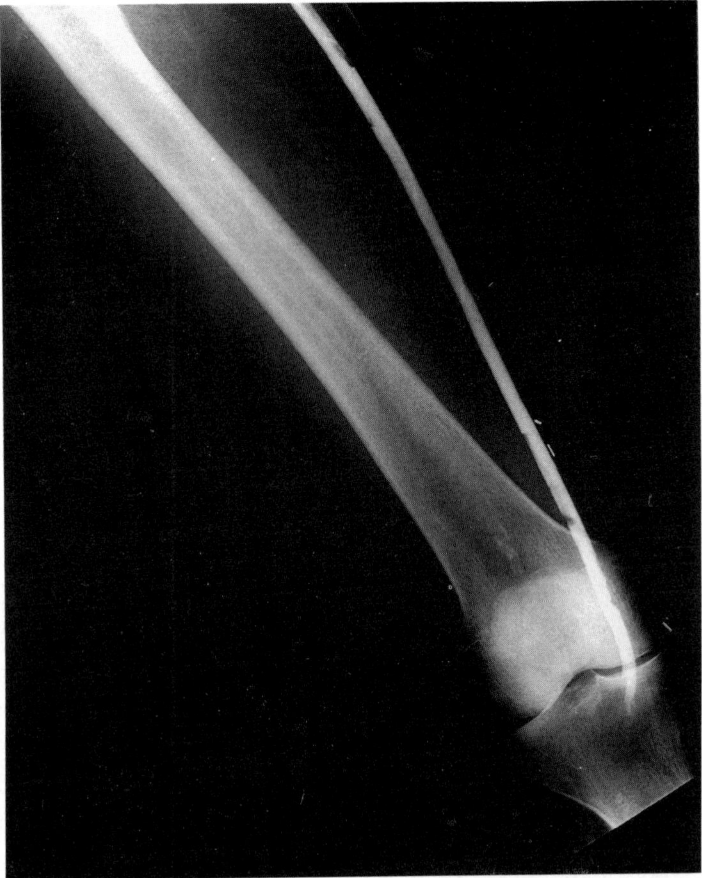

Fig. 2a. A Goretex graft that is being lysed with streptokinase. There is no apparent run-off yet and there is still some clot within the graft.

THROMBOLYSIS FOR INFRA-INGUINAL LIGAMENT GRAFTS

There is much more enthusiasm in the literature from thrombolysis of these more distal grafts than for aortic grafts. Hess[15] is clearly in favour but Perler *et al.*[16] are doubtful. Perler reported the use of low dose thrombolytic agents for two vein grafts and two PTFE grafts in the femoropopliteal position, and for four vein grafts and one PTFE graft in the femorotibial position, and concluded that low dose intra-arterial thrombolytic therapy is poorly efficacious and felt that surgery was much more appropriate for dealing with this problem. Le Bolt *et al.*[17] reported success in lysing 10 out of 14 vein grafts but only six out of 16 prosthetic grafts. Graor *et al.*[7] stated that if the catheter could not be placed in the graft no clinical or angiographic improvement occurred and described patients in whom graft lysis was complete but because there was no significant run-off the graft promptly re-occluded again. Al-Kutoubi (personal communication) also reported initial success in clearing clotted grafts below the inguinal ligament in seven of eight synthetic grafts and one of four vein grafts.

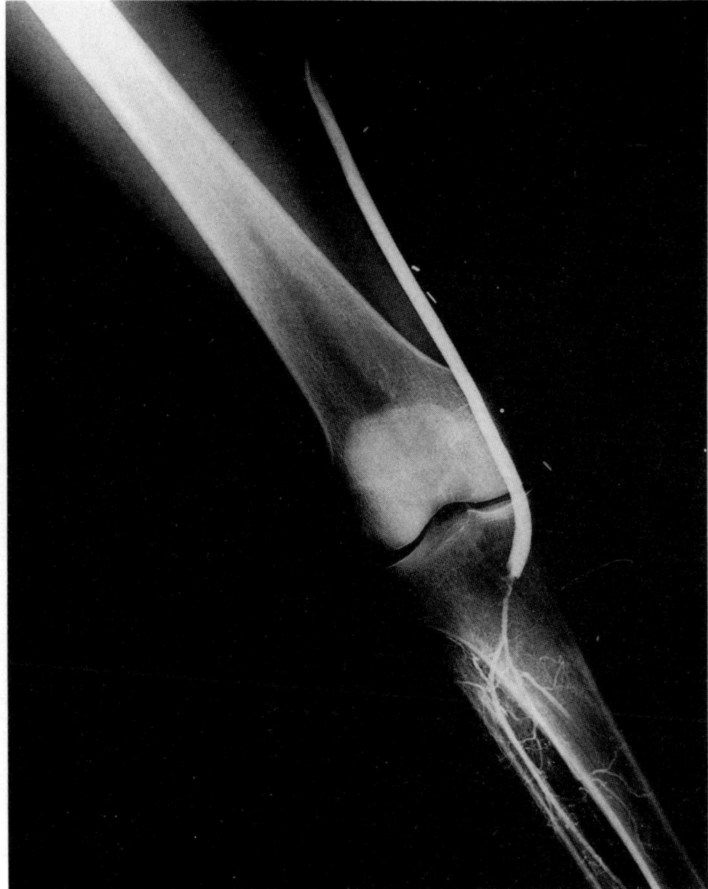

Fig. 2b. The graft is completely clear of clot and the run-off has now been revealed but there is a stenosis at the distal end of the graft. This was not dealt with by an angioplasty. The graft clotted within a week and the patient did not lose the leg.

In 1988 Graor *et al.*[18] reported the use of recombinant t-PA in 33 patients and compared it with a matched group of 38 patients undergoing surgical thrombectomy. They found that at 30 days 86% of the recombinant t-PA treated grafts were still patent, compared with only 42% of the surgically treated grafts. These good results were only achieved by submitting 91% of the recombinant t-PA treated patients to a second surgical procedure; 89% of the surgically treated patients also required a similar secondary surgical procedure.

In other words maintaining patency of declotted grafts, however they are declotted, requires much secondary surgical activity to correct the underlying cause of the graft failure. In the British literature a report from Blanshard and Hacking[19] documented extensive clearing of the graft thrombus in nine occluded PTFE grafts, and in six patients clinical improvement was achieved. Three patients required proxima anastomotic transluminal angioplasty, and one a distal anastomotic angioplasty but in two others the revealed stenosis was left alone. At the time of

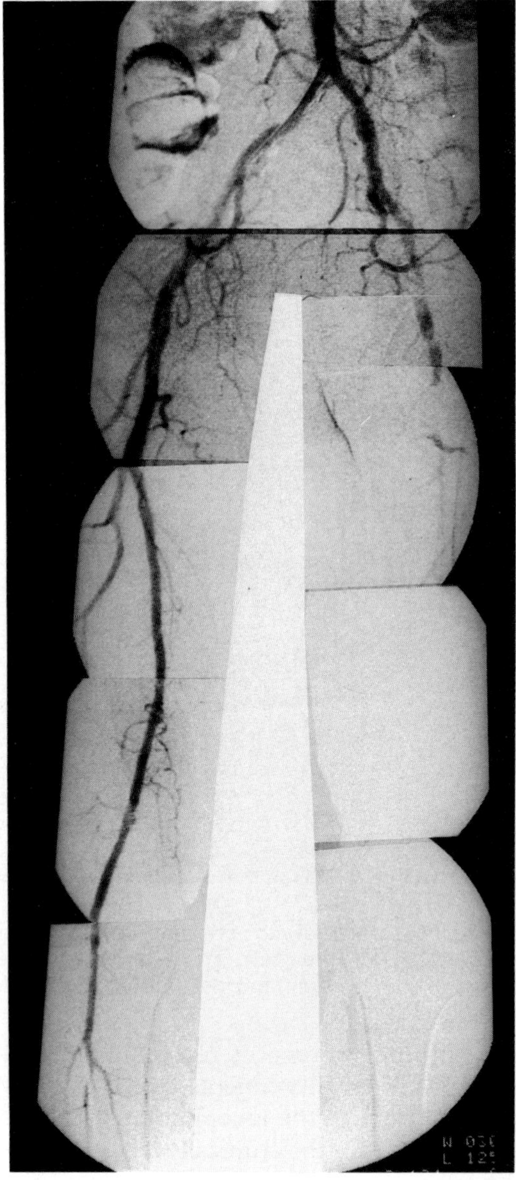

Fig. 3a. A composite DSA showing complete occlusion of an umbilical vein graft from the femoral to the tibial vessels.

discharge home from hospital, six of the nine patients had patent grafts and associated clinical improvement, but only two of these grafts were still patent at the time of reporting 7 to 8 months later. In our own series from Nottingham we have attempted intra-arterial clot lysis in 11 cases, eight vein grafts, one aortofemoral Dacron graft, one Goretex graft and one umbilical vein graft. We achieved lysis in all of the cases below the inguinal ligament but in only one case have we achieved any significant

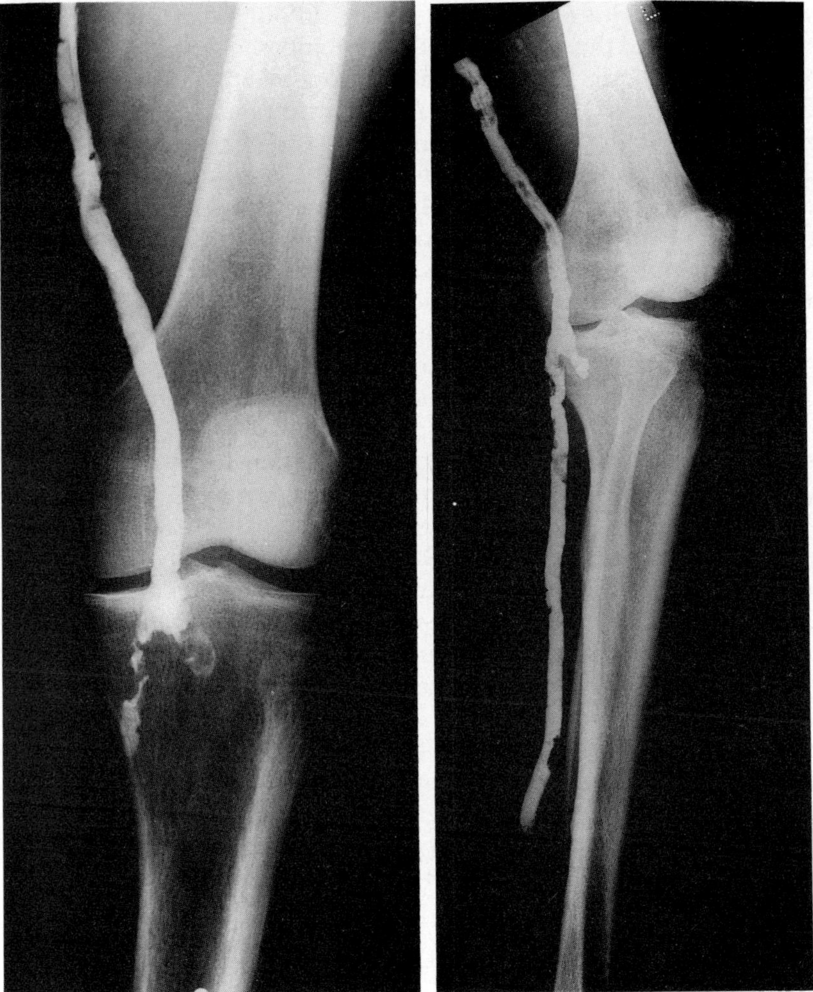

Fig. 3b. (Left) Thrombolysis catheter has been introduced down to just below the level of the knee joint and reveals that the original graft was a femoropopliteal bypass with further extension down to the posterior tibial vessels. **Fig. 3c.** (Right) Lysis is complete to the lower tibial anastomosis but no run-off from the graft can be detected at all. Graft promptly rethrombosed and the patient required an amputation above the knee.

long-term patency, and that was in a vein graft from the femoral to the popliteal (illustrated in Figs 1a–1e). An extension vein graft from the lower end of the thrombolysed vein graft was necessary to bypass a significant area of blockage in the lower popliteal and upper calf vessels. In all other cases the graft has rethrombosed. In five cases we had complications of minor bleeding and in two there were complications of major bleeding requiring blood transfusion. Two patients died within 30 days of treatment, one after an above knee amputation but no other patients came to amputation in this series. Case 2 is illustrated (Figs 2a,b) and shows a patient with a femoropopliteal PTFE graft that had been occluded for 14 days and after 32 h of intra-arterial streptokinase, was fully patent although minor bleeding occurred; the run-off was poor and the graft promptly rethrombosed within a week. The patient did not lose the leg. Case 3 demonstrates a patient with an umbilical vein graft occluded for 70 cm (Figs 3a,b,c). It was treated by intra-arterial t-PA for 50 h. There was complete lysis of the clot within the graft but there was no run-off and it rethrombosed within a day. It was complicated by major haemorrhage and the patient died within 30 days of thrombolysis following an above knee amputation.

A recent report for the use of thrombolytic agents in occluded vein grafts below the inguinal ligament is that from Belkin *et al.*[20] who claimed to have achieved good long-term patency of 22 vein grafts following successful thrombolysis. The good results of successful lysis were only achieved by additional procedures including percutaneous angioplasty, vein patch angioplasty and interposition vein grafts in 19 cases and suggests that in order to achieve good long-term results much additional surgery is required.

A most interesting experience is reported by Allen (personal communication) currently a Senior Registrar in Bath, from his time in Adelaide, Australia where their policy seems to have been to use intragraft thrombolysis on all possible occasions. Between 1981 and 1988 they treated 111 clotted grafts by thrombolysis, 91 PTFE grafts and 20 vein grafts. They inserted the catheter via the femoral artery in 23 cases, but put it directly into the graft itself in 88 cases. Of the 111, 82 achieved a certain degree of thrombolysis and went on to further surgery, eight of these being fully patent; 14 of the 20 vein grafts were cleared satisfactorily and of the six that were not clear, five went to amputation and one died. The evolving policy in Adelaide seems to be to insert a catheter directly into the thrombus in the graft in order to lyse the distal clot from the graft and clear as much run-off as possible before proceeding to a surgical clearance of the rest of the graft and the run-in. This is certainly a most interesting concept and deserves further study. It is interesting that they place their PTFE grafts subcutaneously in order to facilitate any subsequent thrombolysis that may be required.

CONCLUSION

Thrombolytic agents can clear clot from clotted grafts. The low dose intra-arterial technique of Dotter is more reliable and safer than systemic intravenous treatment, but 90% of successfully lysed grafts will require an additional manoeuvre, such as a transluminal angioplasty or a surgical procedure, to correct run-in and run-off problems. Definite caution should be exercised when attempting to clear Dacron grafts and to a lesser extent PTFE grafts because serious bleeding has been reported straight through the graft wall.

Streptokinase is a perfectly good lytic agent and is much cheaper than the newer and more expensive urokinase and t-PA. However, the more expensive drugs are safer and possibly more effective in their ability to clear clotted grafts.

ACKNOWLEDGEMENTS

I would like to thank my colleagues Mr G. S. Makin, Mr P. W. Wenham, Dr R. H. S. Gregson, Mr J. J. Earnshaw, Mr D. C. Berridge and Mr R. J. Lonsdale, without whose co-operation as a team effort none of this work would have been possible.

REFERENCES

1. Tillott WS, Garner RL: Fibrinolytic activity of haemolytic streptococci. J Exp Med 58:485–502, 1933
2. Dotter CT, Rosh J, Seman AJ: Elective clot lysis with low dose streptokinase. Radiology 111:31, 1974
3. Berridge DC: MD Thesis. University of Nottingham, 1989
4. Dawson K, Dex E, Platts A, Hamilton G: Groin haemorrhage complicating intra-arterial thrombolytic therapy: Choice of technique and agent. Paper read at the Vascular Surgical Society of Great Britain and Ireland: November, 1990
5. Earnshaw JJ, Westby JC, Makin GS, Hopkinson BR: The systemic fibrinolytic effect of BRL26921 during the treatment of acute peripheral arterial occlusion. Thromb Haem 55:259–266, 1986
6. Gardiner GA, Koltun W, Kandarpa K *et al*: Thrombolysis of occluded femoropopliteal grafts. Am J Roent 147:621–626, 1986
7. Graor RA, Risius B, Lucas FV *et al*: Thrombolysis with recombinant human tissue-type plasminogen activator in patients with peripheral artery and bypass graft occlusions. Circulation 74 (Suppl 1):1–15, 1986
8. Lonsdale RJ, Harrison JD, Berridge DC *et al*: Recombinant tissue plasminogen activator (rt-PA) is superior to streptokinase in peripheral arterial thrombolysis. Paper read at the Association of Surgeons of Great Britain and Ireland: 1991
9. Earnshaw JJ, Cosgrove C, Wilkins DC, Bliss BP: Acute limb ischaemia: The place of intravenous streptokinase. Br J Surg 77:1136–1139, 1990
10. Risius B, Graor RA, Geisinger MA *et al*: Recombinant human tissue-type plasminogen activator for thrombolysis in peripheral arteries and bypass grafts. Radiology 160:183–188, 1986
11. van Breda A, Robison JC, Feldman L *et al*: Local thrombolysis in the treatment of arterial graft occlusions. J Vasc Surg 1:103–112, 1984
12. Durham JD, Geller SC, Abbott MW *et al*: Regional infusion of urokinase into occluded lower extremity bypass graft: Long term clinical results. Radiology 172:83–87, 1989
13. Graor RA, Risius B, Young JR *et al*: Low dose streptokinase for selective thrombolysis: Systemic effects and complications. Radiology 152:35–39, 1984
14. Walker J, Giddings EB: A protocol for the safe treatment of acute lower limb ischaemia with intra-arterial streptokinase and surgery. Br J Surg 75:1189–1192, 1988
15. Hess H: Thrombolytic therapy in peripheral vascular disease. Br J Surg 77:1083–1084, 1990
16. Perler BA, White RI, Ernst CB, Williams GM: Low-dose thrombolytic therapy for infrainguinal graft occlusion: An idea whose time has passed? J Vasc Surg 2:799–805, 1985
17. LeBolt SA, Tisnado J, Cho S-R: Treatment of peripheral arterial obstruction with streptokinase: Results in arterial vs graft occlusions. Am J Roent 151:589–592, 1988
18. Graor RA, Risius B, Young JR *et al*: Thrombolysis of peripheral arterial bypass grafts: Surgical thrombectomy compared with thrombolysis. J Vasc Surg 7:347–355, 1988
19. Blanshard KS, Hacking PM: Fibrinolytic therapy for infra-inguinal synthetic graft occlusions. Clin Radiol 42:269–273, 1990
20. Belkin M, Donaldson MC, Whittemore AD *et al*: Observations on the use of thrombolytic agents for thrombotic occlusion of infrainguinal vein grafts. J Vasc Surg 11:289–296, 1990

Index